The Clinical Neurology of Old Age

Edited by

Raymond Tallis

Professor of Geriatric Medicine
Hope Hospital Department of Geriatric Medicine,
University of Manchester, UK

A Wiley Medical Publication

JOHN WILEY & SONS

Chichester · New York · Brisbane · Toronto · Singapore

Distributed in the United States of
America, Canada and Japan by
Alan R. Liss Inc., 41 East 11th Street,
New York, NY 10003, USA.

Library of Congress Cataloging-in-Publication Data:

The Clinical neurology of old age.

   1. Geriatric neurology.   I. Tallis, Raymond.
[DNLM: 1. Nervous System Diseases—in old age.
WL 100 C643]
RC346.C5425   1989   618.97'68   87–37130
ISBN 0 471 91108 9

British Library Cataloguing in Publication Data

The Clinical neurology of old age.
   1. Geriatric neurology
   I. Tallis, Raymond
   618.97'68   RC346
ISBN 0 471 91108 9

Printed in Great Britain
at the Alden Press, Osney Mead, Oxford

This book is dedicated with my love to my wife, Terry

Contents

Preface

The forebodings that attend the idea of old age are inspired less by the death that lies on the far side of it than by the misadventures with which it is cluttered. Among these, neurological diseases—the major cause of disability in the over 65s and by far the commonest reason for their dependency on others—are paramount. Their peculiarly invasive nature is typified by stroke, which may take away independence of movement, continence, the ability to make organized sense of even the simplest things, and the gift of expressing one's thoughts, feelings or even basic needs, and so deprive the sufferer of dignity and freedom and of much of what makes life seem worth living. The neurologically disabled elderly person may feel that he or she is being forced to live out a parody of old age.

The public response to the vast problem of the neurologically disabled elderly has been, to put it mildly, inadequate. If there has been greater awareness of the needs of this doubly disadvantaged group over the last few decades, this has mainly been stimulated by, and revolves around, concern over the economic implications. The failure to anticipate and meet the needs of the elderly neurologically disabled patient could be illustrated by the typical course of a stroke patient. Her illness will be diagnosed and initially managed in a hospital attuned to acute illness and geared to improving performance indicators that have little to do with quality of care. The junior staff who are responsible for day-to-day medical care will have little understanding of, or interest in, what is, after all, an incurable disease. Following acute management, or mismanagement, there may be transfer to a rehabilitation ward where the patient's status as 'a bed-blocker' will be less acute but where shortage of staff will mean very limited individual therapy and little opportunity to explore and respond to the individual patient's needs and those of her family. After this, she will have to survive in an outside world, where every amenity—housing, transport, shopping facilities, entertainment—is designed for the young and unimpaired, with the help of ramshackle, unreliable, complex, inadequate services. Alternatively, she may face institutional care where kindness, privacy, respect for her dignity and freedom may not be very much in evidence.

Confronted with these problems, it is not entirely surprising that those physicians who have been most concerned for the neurologically disabled elderly have concentrated their attention and energies on ensuring adequate clinical care and on improving access to services. Much has been learned over the last thirty years about providing services for this group of people who, along with their families, have difficulty 'penetrating the system'. What is now needed is the political will to implement this knowledge and the recognition that this cannot be cheap (though good care is often cheaper than mismanagement). The profession itself must move forward; and, although geriatricians must never lose their sense of responsibility for providing good services, nor their impulse to innovate in this sphere it is important that geriatric neurology should not remain for ever an infant specialty, borrowing its corpus of knowledge from those whose main concern is with younger patients. The time has come for a harder, longer, look at the phenomenology of neurological disease in old age. *The Clinical Neurology of Old Age* is an attempt to summarize what is known so far.

The first thing that may strike the reader looking at the contents page of this book is that it is not dominated, to the extent that might have been expected, by stroke, dementia and Parkinson's disease. In fact, the appearance of a relative under-representation of these conditions is misleading. Stroke, for example, has its own substantial chapter; but, in addition, the contents of the Section on Neurological Rehabilitation have a particular application to stroke, and cerebrovascular disease is a major consideration in the chapter on Neuroepidemiology of Old Age. Nevertheless, while it would be difficult to over-estimate the importance of stroke, Parkinson's disease and dementia, the scope of geriatric neurology extends beyond them. And this is reflected in the present text which aims to deal with the presentation and management of other common neurological diseases in the biologically aged patient, and also of rarer conditions. Moreover, it has to be recognized that many patients with neurological diseases usually associated with younger life—for example multiple sclerosis—now live on into old age. And there are other conditions, common in the elderly, of which it is true to say that most of what we think we know about them has been extrapolated from middle age or even youth. A typical instance here is epilepsy. Finally, there has been a conscious effort to bring to prominence conditions that tend to be relatively under-represented in the geriatric literature, though they are important in clinical practice, e.g. spinal cord disease.

This approach creates the opposite danger of replicating the curriculum of the classic textbooks of adult neurology and then merely suffixing every statement with 'in the elderly'. I have avoided this by allocating a substantial section to the influence of age on the pattern, presentation and management of neurological disease; by ensuring that the discussion of diseases that are common to earlier and later adult life is very much anchored in the conditions as they present in the elderly; and by ample recognition of problems that, because they may be multifactorial in origin, or because they represent final common pathways through which illness is expressed in the ageing nervous system, do not fit neatly into the classification schemes of the mediatric neurologist.

The importance of multiple pathology, of the cumulative effects of multiple sub-threshold impairments, of functional impact as well as neurological deficit, and of conditions such as recurrent acute confusional states, has been emphasized so that the terrain described here will be recognizable to the physician dealing with the elderly as that of his daily practice.

The situation of geriatric neurology is a 'noisy' one, in the communication engineer's sense. If we think of a disease, with its pathognomonic signs pointing to the diagnosis, as the 'signal', then the signal/noise ratio falls with advancing years. This is in part due to the influence of ageing on the presentation of disease; in part to the problem of separating age changes from neurological diseases; and in part to the way in which the co-occurrence of other diseases may increase the difficulty of obtaining a clear history and of eliciting clear-cut signs. Alas, this declining signal/noise ratio is often used to justify sloppy practices in the diagnosis and management of the elderly. Nevertheless, it does make life more difficult and justifies the problem-based approach adopted in some of the chapters of this book.

The caricature of the neurologist as a passive observer of human woe does not fit with the geriatrician's desire to intervene at all levels on behalf of his patients. There is therefore a major emphasis on practical aspects of management. As may be expected, there are many areas where there is uncertainty about the correct management. This has been clearly indicated. In some places, where the same question has been touched upon by two contributors, there has been conflict. For example, the reader will encounter different views as to the role of skull X-ray and isotope brain scanning in the investigation of the patient with a suspected space-occupying lesion. There are other places where there is a difference of emphasis; for example, in the discussions of the role of decompressive laminectomy in the management of spinal secondaries and of the relative merits of the treatments for post-herpetic neuralgia. I have allowed these differences to stand, seeing it as no part of an editor's task to create the impression of consensus where, in the absence of full knowledge, there must be room for disagreement.

In summary, I have attempted to keep to a middle

course between confining myself to the major neurological diseases of old age on the one hand and, on the other, a comprehensive textbook that runs the risk of replicating Brain and Walton in old age; and between on the one hand confining myself to conditions that have been well described in the biologically aged and on the other hand indicating the white spaces on the map. It is to be hoped that the vast number of references supporting the text will adequately sign-post the reader to deeper study. I also hope that a textbook of this size and scope will not only re-affirm the importance of geriatric neurology and promote good practice but also stimulate research. For if this book is a map of the current state of knowledge, it is also a map of our ignorance and of the areas most ripe for investigation. If this book succeeds in its aim, when the time comes to prepare a second edition, geriatric neurology will no longer be an infant science.

The Clinical Neurology of Old Age would not have been possible without Andrea Stewart and Beryl Drabble whose help throughout the editorial process has earned my lasting gratitude. I am grateful to Verity Waite of John Wiley and Sons Ltd who provided not only enormous editorial support during the long gestation but also psychotherapy. I should like to express my thanks to Professor Michael Hall for asking me to do this book. Finally, this seems to me to be a most appropriate place to acknowledge my great intellectual debt to Dr Lee Illis and Dr Michael Sedgwick of the Wessex Neurological Centre, whose stimulus and personal kindness consolidated my interest in matters neurological. In particular, their ambition to develop methods of neurological rehabilitation firmly grounded in neuroscience was a revelation to me in the three unforgettable years during which I had the privilege of working with them.

RAYMOND TALLIS
August 1988

Contributors

Rachel Angus   Senior Registrar, Department of Geriatric Medicine, Watford Road, Harrow, Middlesex HA1 3UJ

Keith Andrews   Director, Medical and Research Services, Royal Hospital and Home, West Hill, Putney, London SW15 3SW

Martin Binks   Lecturer in Psychology, University of Liverpool, Liverpool

G. A. Broe   Professor of Geriatric Medicine, Concord Repatriation Hospital, Sydney, NSW, Australia

Donald Calne   Professor and Head of Division of Neurology, Health Sciences Centre Hospital, 2211 Westbrook Mall, Vancouver, British Columbia, Canada V6T 1W5

Ted Cantrell   Senior Lecturer in Rehabilitation, Aids and Equipment Centre, Rehabilitation Unit, Southampton General Hospital, Tremona Road, Southampton SO9 4XY

Austin Carty   Consultant Radiologist, Royal Liverpool Hospital, Prescot Street, Liverpool 7

Peter Chin   Consultant Physician, Department of Geriatric Medicine, Cumberland Infirmary, Carlisle, Cumbria CA2 7HY

Iain Chisholm   Consultant Ophthalmic Surgeon, Southampton Eye Hospital, Wilton Avenue, Southampton SO9 4XW

Helen Creasey   Senior Lecturer in Geriatric Medicine, Concord Repatriation Hospital, Sydney, NSW, Australia

Ruth Eley   Principal Social Worker and Head of Department, Social Work Department, Royal Liverpool Hospital, Prescot Street, Liverpool 7

Susan Farr   Senior Occupational Therapist, Aids and Equipment Centre, Rehabilitation Unit, Southampton General Hospital, Tremona Road, Southampton SO9 4XY

James George   Consultant Geriatrician, Cumberland Infirmary, Carlisle, Cumbria CA2 7HY

Anne Gibson   Methodist Minister and Tutor, Wesley College, Henbury Road, Westbury-on-Trym, Bristol BS10 7QD

James Howe Consultant Physician in Medicine for the Elderly, Airedale General Hospital, Skipton Road, Steeton, Keighley, West Yorks BD20 6TD

B. M. Hubbard Research Fellow, Department of Pathology, Ninewells Hospital Medical School, Dundee

Peter Hudgson Consultant and Senior Lecturer in Neurology, Regional Neurological Centre, Newcastle General Hospital, West Gate Road, Newcastle-upon-Tyne NE4 6BE

Peter Humphrey Consultant Neurologist, Mersey Regional Department of Medical and Surgical Neurology, Walton Hospital, Liverpool L9 1AE

L. S. Illis Consultant Neurologist, Wessex Neurological Centre, Southampton General Hospital, Southampton; Clinical Senior Lecturer in Neurology, University of Southampton Medical School

Brian Livesley The University of London's Professor of the Care of the Elderly (Geriatrics), Charing Cross Hospital and Westminster Medical School, London

Michael Lye Professor of Geriatric Medicine, University Department of Geriatric Medicine, Royal Liverpool Hospital, Prescot Street, Liverpool L69 3BX

Ian Mackenzie Consultant Neuro-otologist, Neurosciences Department, Walton Hospital, Liverpool L9 1AE

Lindsay McLellan Professor in Rehabilitation, Consultant Neurologist, Rehabilitation Unit, Level C, West Wing, Southampton General Hospital, Tremona Road, Southampton SO9 4XY

Pauline Monro Consultant Neurologist, Atkinson Morley's Hospital, Copse Hill, Wimbledon, London SW20 0NE

P. G. Newrick Senior Medical Registrar, Department of Medicine, Bristol Royal Infirmary, Bristol BS2 8HW

R. K. Olney Assistant Professor, Department of Neurology, University of California, San Francisco, USA

P. O'Neill Consultant Neurosurgeon, The National Neurosurgery Centre, Beaumont Hospital, Dublin, Eire

Robin Philpott Consultant Psychogeriatrician, Royal Liverpool Hospital, Prescot Street, Liverpool 7

Jeremy Playfer Consultant Geriatrician, Royal Liverpool Hospital, Prescot Street, Liverpool 7

John Puxty Associate Professor, Geriatric Assessment Unit, Ottawa General Hospital, 501 Smyth, Ottawa, Ontario, Canada K1H 8L6

Michael Sharr Regional Neurosurgical Unit, Brook General Hospital, Shooters Hill Road, Woolwich, London SE18 4LW

Jollyon Smith   Consultant Clinical Neurophysiologist, University Hospital, Queen's Medical Centre, Nottingham NG7 2UH

Marian Squier   Consultant Neuropathologist, Neuropathology Department, The Radcliffe Infirmary, Oxford

Cameron Swift   Professor of Health Care of the Elderly, King's College School of Medicine and Dentistry, Denmark Hill, London SE5 9RS

Raymond Tallis   Professor of Geriatric Medicine, University of Manchester, Department of Geriatric Medicine, Clinical Sciences Building, Hope Hospital, Eccles Old Road, Salford M6 8HD

H. Teravainen   Division of Neurology, University of British Columbia, Vancouver, Canada

Gerald Tobin   Consultant Physician in Geriatric Medicine, Manor Park Hospital, Manor Park, Bristol BS16 2EW

J. Tsui   Division of Neurology, University of British Columbia, Vancouver, Canada

David Uttley   Consultant Neurosurgeon, Atkinson Morley's Hospital, Copse Hill, Wimbledon, London SW20 0NE

Hilmar M. Warenius   Professor of Radiation Oncology, Department of Radiation Oncology, Clatterbridge Hospital, Bebington, Wirral, Merseyside L63 4JY

John P. Wattis   Senior Lecturer and Consultant in the Psychiatry of Old Age, St James' University Hospital, Beckett Street, Leeds LS9

Christopher Wells   Consultant Anaesthetist and Director, Pain Relief Clinic, Walton Hospital, Rice Lane, Liverpool L9 1AE

SECTION ONE

The Influence of Age on the Pattern, Presentation and Management of Neurological Disease

Chapter 1

The Physical Ageing of the Neuromuscular System

Bethan M. Hubbard

Research Fellow, Department of Pathology, Ninewells Hospital Medical School, Dundee, UK

Marian Squier

Consultant Neuropathologist, The Radcliffe Infirmary, Oxford, UK

I The Central Nervous System
B. M. Hubbard

INTRODUCTION

The mechanisms of ageing and age-related disease in the human brain have attracted renewed interest in recent years. The reasons are twofold. Firstly, to aid the management of an increased number of elderly patients, more knowledge of the normal ageing process in all systems including the brain is required. Secondly, the advent of new technology, such as computerized axial tomography (now more commonly referred to as computed tomography, CT), automated image analysis and immunochemistry, has enabled the re-examination of known age-related tissue changes as well as the investigation of others which were previously unapproachable. The first section of the chapter will be concerned with recent observations on age-related changes in the human central nervous system. For more general reviews, the reader is referred to Tomlinson (1979),

and Tomlinson and Corsellis (1985). The considerable literature on ageing in animal systems is outwith the scope of this article.

CEREBRAL ATROPHY

Cerebral atrophy is a true age-related change since it occurs in all persons with advancing age. A mean average loss of some 100 grams in the total brain weight of both males and females between 25 and 70 years of age has been claimed in many reports (see Blinkov and Glezer, 1968; Korenschevsky, 1961). Not all investigators, however, agree about the absolute amount of weight lost (Tomlinson *et al.*, 1968) and one study failed to find a significant relationship between brain weight and age (Messert *et al.*, 1972). It is possible that the loss of brain mass in normal ageing is less than stated in early reports. Furthermore, comparison of the brain volume of

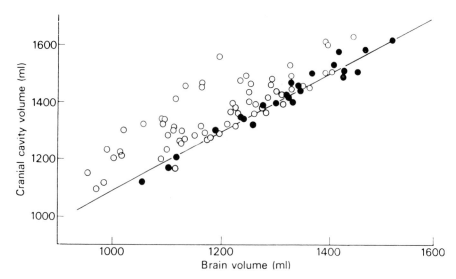

Figure 1.1. Cranial cavity volume plotted against brain volume; ●<55 years, ○>55 years. Males and females. (Davis and Wright, 1977.)

individuals with the cranial cavity volume indicates that the loss of brain mass may not be linear but instead an acceleration of brain atrophy occurs in advanced old age (Davis and Wright, 1977). In this study the ratio between brain volume and cranial cavity volume was found to be constant at $92.2 + 1.6\%$ (SEM) in adults of 20–55 years of age, whereas persons aged above 55 years showed a considerable deviation from this relationship, falling consistently to one side of the regression line (Figure 1.1).

A gradual increase in the average weight of the human brain during the last century has been observed (Miller and Corsellis, 1977). This secular effect is estimated at 0.5% per decade for males and 0.2% per decade for females. The percentage deficit per decade in the atrophy index as calculated from Davis and Wright's data and shown in Table 1.1 demonstrates clearly that, in spite of the secular effect, the human brain does show significant and apparently accelerated atrophy after 60 years of age.

In advanced old age (above 70 years), there is a change in the relative volume of both cortex and white matter but the loss of white matter is more pronounced. Figure 1.2 shows that the white matter volume falls by some 11% between 70 and 90 years of age compared to a 2–3% deficit of cortex (Anderson

TABLE 1.1   CEREBRAL ATROPHY WITH ADVANCING AGE (DATA OF DAVIS AND WRIGHT, 1977)

Age group	Atrophy index Brain volume/ cranial capacity	% Deficit per decade
40–49	91.81	—
50–59	91.74	0.076
60–69	89.60	2.33
70–79	87.05	2.85
80–89	84.19	3.28

et al., 1983), although there is evidence to suggest that between 20 and 50 years of age more cortex is lost than white matter (Miller *et al.*, 1980). A summary of age-related changes in the volume of the macroscopic components of the cerebral hemispheres is given in Table 1.2 (Hubbard and Anderson, 1983). Whether such deficits are global or localized to certain regions of the brain is not yet documented. A CT study has indicated reduced attenuation of white matter with age, suggesting a change in its composition (Zatz *et al.*, 1982). It is not unreasonable to suppose that further investigations of this type will eventually give more detailed information on regional losses of cortex and white matter.

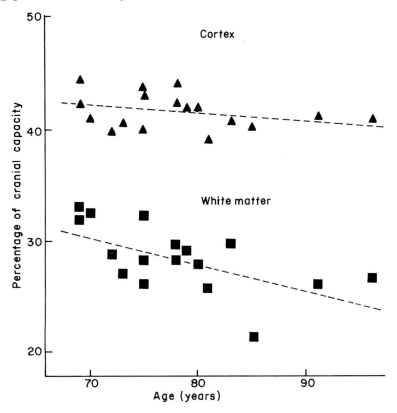

Figure 1.2. Volumes of cerebral cortex and white matter expressed as proportions of cranial capacity indicating less reduction of cortex ($r=0.38$) than white matter ($r=0.58$, $p<0.01$) in advanced old age. (*Reproduced by permission of Elsevier Science Publishers, Amsterdam from Anderson et al., 1983.*)

Recent evidence suggests that there may be differences in the rate of loss of brain mass in men and women. Early necropsy data are conflicting on this point. Some reports suggest that brain atrophy begins earlier in women than men (Bischoff, 1880; Ordy *et al.*, 1975) whereas others record no difference (Chernyshev, 1911; Pakkenberg and Voight, 1964). Computer tomography (CT) has provided the means of re-examining this problem: in a study of some 300 tomographic brain scans of hospital in-patients Hatazawa *et al.* (1982) found significant cerebral atrophy by the fifth decade in women but not until the sixth decade in men. These findings have been supported by a careful study of brain weights at necropsy (Hubbard and Anderson, 1983). In this investigation women showed the first significant deficit in brain weight in the sixth decade,

although the rate of loss slowed in the seventh decade. In contrast, males did not show a significant reduction in brain weight until the seventh decade. Thereafter, the decline was steady in both sexes. The reduction in brain weight between 40 and 90 years was estimated to be 2.92 g per year for women and 2.85 for men, but is should be noted that these figures were derived assuming a linear deficit with age which may not be correct as has been discussed above. Allowing for the secular effect of 0.44 g per year for women and 0.66 g for men, the authors suggest that sex differences in age-related brain atrophy may be absolute as well as relative. It is interesting that since similar trends are detectable in data presented by Bischoff in 1880 it is unlikely that such apparent sex differences in brain atrophy can be attributed so socio-economic conditions alone and

TABLE 1.2 THE VOLUME OF VARIOUS MACROSCOPICAL COMPONENTS OF THE CEREBRAL HEMISPHERES IN OLD AGE[a]

	Percentage of cranial capacity (mean±SD)			Age change: Deficit (%) 70–85 years	p[b]
	69–74 years	75–79 years	>80 years		
No. of cases	5	6	6		
Mean age (years)	70.6	76.7	85.8		
Cortex	41.7±1.8	42.5±1.5	40.7±1.0	2.6	NS
White matter	30.5±2.7	28.9±2.0	26.5±2.8	11.4	<0.01
Basal ganglia	5.54±0.49	5.10±0.71	4.77±0.54	8.1	<0.05
Total cerebrum	79.5±4.8	78.2±3.5	74.1±3.5	5.6	<0.01

[a] Reproduced by permission of Elsevier Science Publishers, Amsterdam, from Anderson *et al.* (1983).
[b] Spearman's rank correlation test.
NS, not significant.

must therefore reflect a real difference between the sexes.

In opposition to these reports, an independent CT study found the rate of brain atrophy to accelerate constantly with age in both sexes, but in the fourth and fifth decades the rate of decline in men was more than twice that for women (Takeda and Matsuzawa, 1984). This conflict could be due to different methods of measurement or to racial differences in the populations studied. Also, the assumption that brains of 20–30 year old persons are a representative standard for the comparison of older age groups has been criticized (Mintz and Jarvik, 1983). These are individuals who have either died prematurely or who have been given a CT scan for investigative purposes and are obviously not an entirely 'normal' sample. Some young males dying within this age range, for example, would most probably have had alcoholic brain atrophy. This would result in an urealistically low 'standard' value for young males and possibly even mask the timing of the onset of atrophy.

The advent of computed tomography has also renewed the question of age-related change in the ventricular volume of the brain. One such study (Barron *et al.*, 1976) has shown an exponential increase in ventricular size consistent with the findings of Davis and Wright (1977) on brain

atrophy. This report has been supported subsequently by a stereological necropsy study (Hubbard and Anderson, 1981). On the other hand, an investigation aimed at establishing normal standards for CT scans in the elderly found only a non-significant trend to larger ventricles with age, but this may have been due to a restriction of the study to persons over 62 years of age (Jacoby *et al.*, 1980). The extent of cerebral atrophy as assessed from ventricular appearances in CT scans would seem to be unreliable, since a reduction in brain volume is not always reflected by an increase in ventricular volume (Hubbard and Anderson, 1981). Hopefully, technical refinement will permit an accurate radiological measurement of the pericerebral space, a measurement which has already proved to be an accurate marker for cerebral atrophy in pathological studies (Davis and Wright, 1977).

NERVE CELL LOSS

The availability of computer assisted image analysis has renewed interest in the question of age-related nerve cell loss from the cerebral cortex. Automated image analysis, in addition to being objective and quicker than the traditional method of enumeration, also means that cell populations can be measured in terms of the area occupied by their cell bodies. This method avoids some of the problems of enumeration, in particular the 'split cell error' (Anderson *et al.*, 1983). Despite these technical advances recent image analysis studies have served mainly to confirm the findings achieved previously by traditional methods that nerve cell loss is universal in old age (Brody, 1955, 1970) and is therefore a true age-related change.

Cerebral Cortex

Three automated image analysis studies have been concerned with cell loss from the cerebral cortex as a result of increasing age (Henderson *et al.*, 1980; Anderson *et al.*, 1983; Miller *et al.*, 1984). Although the same image analyser was used in all three studies, the approaches to the problem have been quite different. Henderson *et al.* counted cell bodies in eleven areas of the neocortex over a wide age range. Anderson *et al.* made area proportion measurements of nerve cell bodies in two neocortical areas and two areas of the allocortex in advanced old age; whereas Miller *et al.* counted nucleolated neurones in the subiculum of the hippocampus in subjects between 15 and 96 years. There is general agreement that in the neocortex both large and small neurones decline in number with age. Considerable regional variation occurs, but the loss of large neurones seems to be consistently greater. Neocortical nerve cell loss estimated from cell counts has been calculated to be 36–60% between 18 and 95 years (Henderson *et al.*, 1980). This seems reasonably consistent with the loss of approximately 21.0% of the total neocortical neurone mass between 70 and 85 years of age as found by Anderson *et al.* (1983); 5% of this loss was considered to be due to shrinkage of nerve cell bodies and therefore actual cell loss after 70 years of age may be only 15–16%, i.e. an annual loss of about 1%. Expressing the data on nerve cell counts (Henderson *et al.*, 1980) in the same manner a loss of 1.1% per annum is evident above 70 years of age.

Data on the subiculum of the hippocampus are less easy to reconcile. The subiculum shows both pronounced atrophy and significant nerve cell loss with advancing age. This differs from other areas of the allocortex such as the cingulate gyrus where cellular shrinkage and not cell loss appears to be the major effect of age (Anderson *et al.*, 1983). Between 70 and 85 years of age the hippocampal subiculum is reported to shrink by some 24% (Anderson *et al.*, 1983) but there is some dispute regarding the actual amount of nerve cell loss. Enumeration of nucleolated neurones between 15 and 96 years has shown a fall of 3.6% per decade (Miller *et al.*, 1984). In contrast measurement of neurone area in advanced old age (70–85 years) showed a much larger deficit of 10% per decade (Anderson *et al.*, 1983). Such a discrepancy may in part be due to acceleration in the rate of neurone loss in advanced old age; sampling may also have contributed since considerable individual variation occurs.

Other Regions

Examination of various other discrete regions of the brain has shown that nerve cell loss is not a consistent feature of ageing. No evidence has been found for age-related nerve cell loss from the mammillary bodies (Wilkinson and Davies, 1978), the abducens nucleus (Vijayshankar and Brody, 1971), the inferior olive (Mongale and Brody, 1974), the ventral cochlear nucleus (Konigsmark and Murphy, 1970, 1972) or the trochlear nerve nucleus (Vijayashankar and Brody, 1973, 1977). By contrast above 60 years of age there is a significant cell loss in a number of other regions. The locus coeruleus loses 40–45% of its large melanin-filled neurones during adult life (Tomlinson *et al.*, 1981; Vijayashankar and Brody, 1979); this loss seems to take place in two phases, a rapid 27% loss between 65 and 71 years and a further but less dramatic reduction of about 13% between 75 and 87 years of age. In the cerebellum there is a mean reduction in Purkinje cells of 2.5% per decade during adult life, but mostly occurring after 60 years of age (Hall *et al.*, 1975). In the spinal cord loss of motor neurones from the lumbar sacral region seems to be negligible up to the age of 60 years; above this age there is a variable but significant loss of cells ranging from 5 to 50% but with a mean value of about 25% (Tomlinson and Irving, 1977). Age-related cell loss from the amygdaloid nucleus (Herzog and Kemper, 1980) and the substantia nigra (McGeer *et al.*, 1977) has also been reported.

THE DENDRITIC TREE

It is now evident that regression of the dendritic tree, which normally represents 95% of the receptor surface of cortical neurones, is another probable cause of cortical impairment with advancing age. Extensive qualitative changes including the loss of dendritic spines and basilar dendrites have been described in pyramidal cells of the temporal and frontal cortex (Scheibel *et al.*, 1977) and also in neurones of some areas of the limbic system (Scheibel, 1979). These events are probably a prelude to cell death. Conversely, there is some evidence to suggest that, in the face of nerve cell loss, the remaining viable cells show compensatory dendritic proliferation (Buell and Coleman, 1979, 1981). In the parahippocampal gyrus of mentally normal aged individuals neurones exhibit dendrites which are longer and more branched than those of adult persons and this elaboration of dendritic processes seems to continue into the tenth decade of life. Therefore, the ageing cortex would seem to contain both regressing dying neurones and surviving growing neurones (Buell and Colemen, 1979, 1981).

Dendritic growth of surviving neurones may account for the relative absence of neocortical atrophy in old age (Table 1.2). It is reasonable to suppose that the proliferating dendritic branches, which are chiefly located in the cortex, prevent cortical collapse from cell loss. By contrast, the extent of nerve cell fall out is more closely related to the degree of white matter loss, implying that there is no compensatory branching of axonal processes (Anderson *et al.*, 1983).

SENILE PLAQUES AND NEUROFIBRILLARY TANGLES

Senile plaques and neurofibrillary tangles, although frequently seen in the ageing brain, are not present in all elderly people nor are they exclusive to the ageing process. It is therefore debatable whether they are a normal age change. On the other hand senile plaques are a constant feature of senile dementia of Alzheimer type (SDAT) and Down's syndrome. Vast numbers of neurofibrillary tangles are found in SDAT, Down's syndrome and dementia pugilistica and smaller numbers in postencephalitic parkinson-ism, Parkinson-dementia complex of Guam and some other neuronal degenerative diseases (Tomlinson and Corsellis, 1984). Morphologically these lesions appear to be the same in all conditions cited.

Senile Plaques

The formation of senile plaques is a remarkable although inconsistent feature of the ageing human brain. Sometimes called argyrophilic plaques because of their affinity for silver stains they gradually accumulate after about 60 years of age and are exclusive to the grey matter, mostly occurring in the cerebral cortex but also in some deep grey matter structures such as the amygdaloid nucleus, the corpus striatum or in the brain stem, although rarely in the cerebellum (Tomlinson and Corsellis, 1984). Plaques are generally spherical and vary in size from 15 to 200 μm. Classically they comprise a central core and a surrounding halo when examined with silver or fluorescent methods (Figure 1.3).

Although first identified in 1892 (Blocq and Marinesco, 1892), it is only in recent years that the origin and in particular the composition of plaques has become better understood. Histochemistry and electron microscopy have both made important contributions. The central core of plaques has been shown to behave histochemically like amyloid. In particular, it has a great affinity for the dyes Congo Red and thioflavine T. The ultrastructure of plaques revealed by electron microscopy confirms a central core of amyloid fibrils surrounded by a large number of modified dendrites. Glial cell processes and occasional microglia are also seen. There is a five- to tenfold increase in the size of dendrites within plaques, mostly due to the accumulation of many small dense bodies derived from degenerating mitochondria. Intermingled with these enlarged dendrites are groups of helical filaments similar to those found in nerve cells showing neurofibrillary degeneration (Tomlinson and Corsellis, 1984).

Three types of plaques are described in the literature which are considered to represent three different stages in development (Terry and Wisniewski, 1972). The primitive plaque thought to be the earliest developmental stage consists of a few enlarged dendrites mostly presynaptic or axonal in

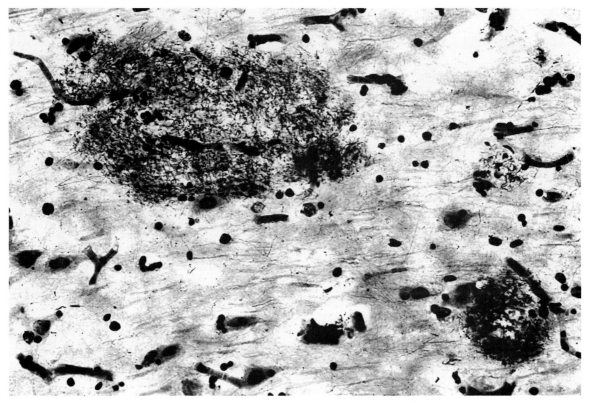

Figure 1.3. Senile plaque formation in the subiculum of the hippocampus of an 85 year old woman, illustrating different stages of development. King's silver impregnation, ×400.

origin. Associated amyloid fibrils are either few or completely absent, but there may be some glial cell involvement. By contrast the mature plaque shows a well-defined amyloid core surrounded by numerous dendrites, astrocytic processes and some glial cells. The final stage or 'burn out' plaque as it is sometimes called merely comprises the amyloid core. In addition, primitive and mature plaques show marked acetylcholinesterase (AChE) activity whereas this enzyme is present at low levels only in 'burnt out' plaques. Such observations have led to the suggestion that senile plaques form in association with the terminal dendrites of acetylcholine-secreting neurones, the cell bodies of which lie within the nucleus basalis of Meynert. This nucleus lies in the basal forebrain inferior to the globus pallidus and is the major source of neocortical cholinergic innervation (Gorry, 1963). It is postulated that dendrites

rich in AChE are early components of the plaque and that loss of these neurites results in the formation of 'burnt out' plaques with a corresponding reduction in cholinergic activity in the cortex (Price *et al.*, 1982).

Foci of positive staining for serum proteins observed in senile plaques led to the suggestion that plaque production may have an immunological basis (Ishii and Haga, 1976). However, a more recent investigation attributes such immunohistochemical staining to leakage of serum proteins from damaged vessels and post-mortem diffusion of these same molecules from vessels into the surrounding tissue (Mann *et al.*, 1982) and concludes that a positive staining reaction of this type does not necessarily mean that the formation of plaque amyloid involves an immunological mechanism. Alternatively, the discovery in plaque cores of

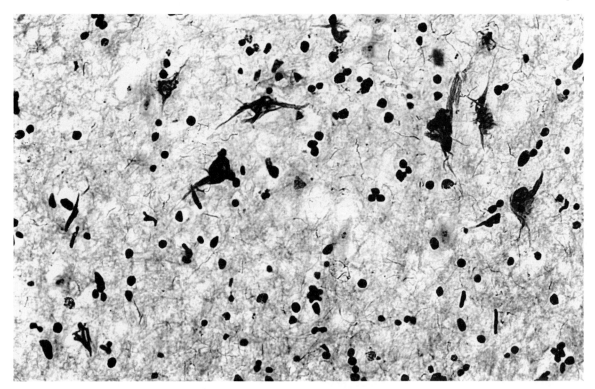

Figure 1.4. Neurofibrillary tangle formation in the subiculum of the hippocampus of a 91 year old woman. King's silver impregnation, ×400.

aluminium and silicon in the form of aluminosilicates has led to a new proposal that the initial stages of plaque production may involve inorganic components (Candy *et al.*, 1986).

Neurofibrillary Tangles

The formation of tangles within nerve cell bodies was first described by Alzheimer (1907a, 1907b). Eighty years later, the molecular basis of this apparent gradual cytoskeletal reorganization of some neurones is still not understood and little is known about the molecular origin and composition of these abnormal fibrous polymers (Rasool *et al.*, 1984).

Tangle formation as a feature of ageing tends initially to be confined to the hippocampus and parahippocampal gyrus (Figure 1.4). The numbers appearing in the hippocampus increase over 5 years of age and extensive clusters of tangles in this region are not uncommon in intellectually normal old persons (Morimatsu *et al.*, 1976). Even between 55 and 64 years of age the incidence has been shown to be as high as 43% (Ulrich, 1985) and by 90 years of age as many as 90% of persons have been reported to show tangle formation (Tomlinson, 1979), although an earlier study found a much smaller incidence (Ball, 1976). In later life the distribution is more widespread, affected neurones occurring regularly in the uncal area, the corticomedial part of the amygdaloid nucleus, the olfactory bulb and the nucleus basalis of Meynert (Tomlinson and Corsellis, 1984; Ulrich, 1985). The significance of neurofibrillary tangle formation affecting a large proportion of the apparently normal elderly population is not known; it is possible that some of these persons are showing early stages of SDAT, but in general there are clear quantitative differences between the normal elderly and patients with SDAT (Anderson and Hubbard, 1985).

Aluminium has been associated with the for-

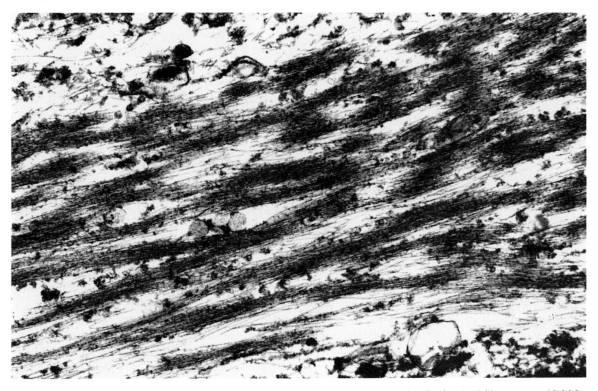

Figure 1.5. Electron micrograph of part of a neurofibrillary tangle showing detail of paired filaments. ×40 000.

mation of tangles. Most analyses have been carried out on brain samples from patients with SDAT but the findings seem to be the same for tangle-bearing brains from mentally normal old persons. Elevated aluminium levels have been reported in areas of the brain which contain large numbers of tangles (Crapper *et al.*, 1973). Furthermore, aluminium levels are said to be raised in all regions of the brain which in elderly persons are susceptible to tangle formation (McDermott *et al.*, 1977). This suggests that aluminium accumulation is an age-associated phenomenon and is consistent with an observed gradual increase in aluminium levels between infancy and 85 years of age (Markesbery *et al.*, 1981). X-ray micro-analysis of individual nerve cells has detected foci of aluminium within the nuclear region of a high percentage of neurones containing tangles while adjacent non-tangle-bearing neurones remain virtually aluminium free, suggesting that aluminium concentrations are tangle-specific (Perl and Brody, 1980). Another microprobe study has shown alumi-

nium to be present in other structures such as lipofuscin granules and in senile plaques as well as within tangles (Duckett and Galle, 1980). Whether or not aluminium plays a specific role in the pathogenesis of tangles remains therefore a controversial topic.

Much of the information acquired recently about the structure, origin and composition of neurofibrillary tangles has been achieved using brain tissue from SDAT patients but there is no evidence that these tangles differ in any way from those formed during normal ageing other than they are more numerous. Ultrastructurally, neurofibrillary tangles consist largely of bundles of paired helical filaments (Figure 1.5) (Terry, 1963; Kidd, 1964; Wisniewski *et al.*, 1976), although twisted and narrowed or straight tubules may also be present (Gibson *et al.*, 1976; Shibayama and Kitoh, 1978; Yagashita *et al.*, 1981). Paired helical filaments also occur in the neurites of senile plaques and are entirely a human phenomenon.

Immunological studies have provided some clues to the origins of tangles. Specific labelling of tangles with antisera raised against normal human neurotubules originally indicated that tangles may be derived from these components (Grundke-Iqbal *et al.*, 1979). Subsequent studies suggest instead that they are derived from neurofilaments but the relationship is not simple. Monoclonal antibody reactions indicate that neurofibrillary tangles share at least two antigenic determinants with normal neurofilaments (Anderton *et al.*, 1982). An antiserum highly specific for paired helical filaments has also been raised. This antiserum strongly labels tangles but shows no reaction with normal neurofilaments or any other brain protein currently tested (Ihara *et al.*, 1983). A hypothesis consistent with the available evidence states that tangles are heterogeneous regarding their filamentous content. They contain antigens which cross-react with neurofilaments and also antigens which appear to be unique to paired helical filaments and are not shared with normal neurofilaments (Rasool *et al.*, 1984).

NEUROCHEMISTRY

Age-related changes in the biochemistry of the human brain are various, e.g. alteration in the levels of nucleic acids, protein and lipids and a change in energy metabolism to mention but a few (Hahn, 1981; Shelanski and Selkoe, 1981; Horrocks *et al.*, 1981; Smith and Sokoloff, 1981). Recent years, however, have seen a considerable increase in our understanding of age-related changes in neurotransmitters; these imply functional impairment in the elderly and possibly point the way to replacement therapy.

Neurotransmitters are assessed either by direct measurement of the transmitters themselves or indirectly by the activities of neurotransmitter synthetic or degradative enzymes. Enzyme measurements are usually preferred since they require smaller tissue samples and in particular are more stable in post-mortem material (McGeer and McGeer, 1976). Synthetic enzymes are the more important since they are specific neuronal markers and reflect nerve cell integrity, whereas degradative enzymes are more widely distributed occurring in

glial cells as well as neurones or more than one neurotransmitter type (McGeer and McGeer, 1976). Measurement of binding or receptor sites for neurotransmitters in the brain is an alternative approach, also having the advantage that such binding sites show good post-mortem stability. However, binding sites which are independent of sodium ions are postsynaptic and therefore the information obtained does not relate directly to the function and integrity of specific nerve cell types.

Acetylcholine (ACh)

The cholinergic system has received considerable attention recently since it now seems that some aspects of human age-related cognitive and memory decline may be due to a reduction or malfunction of its activity (Drachman 1977; Bartus *et al.*, 1982). This is thought to relate to a loss of neurones from the nucleus basalis of Meynert, the main source of cholinergic innervation for the neocortex and hippocampus (Lewis and Shute, 1978), but detailed information on age-related changes in the numbers of these neurones is not yet available. Acetylcholine degrades rapidly post-mortem; therefore the ability of cholinergic neurones to produce acetylcholine is usually assessed by measuring the level of the synthesizing enzyme choline acetyltransferase (CAT) or the degradative enzyme acetylcholinesterase (AChE).

Evidence for normal age-related changes in the presynaptic cholinergic marker for CAT is inconclusive. Some investigators report a significant age-related decline in CAT levels of the cerebral cortex (Davies, 1979; Perry *et al.*, 1977; Perry and Perry, 1980) whereas others have failed to show any change at all (Spokes, 1979; Bowen *et al.*, 1979). Cortical biopsies of the temporal lobe have also proved negative in this respect (Bowen *et al.*, 1979). A recent more extensive post-mortem study of several areas of the cortex has shown small changes in CAT levels in some areas of frontal lobe only (Rossor, 1982). Age-related changes in CAT levels in the corpus striatum are also a controversial issue (Bartus *et al.*, 1982). Muscarinic cholinergic receptor binding in the cerebral cortex has been reported to decrease with increasing age (White *et al.*, 1977; Perry and Perry, 1980) although one investigation found no such change (Davies and Verth, 1978).

Monoamines

The effect of age on the dopaminergic and noradrenergic systems of the human brain has been extensively studied, especially the dopaminergic nigrostriatal system. It has been suggested that observed reductions in dopamine synthetic enzymes probably reflect impaired dopaminergic transmission which in turn may be responsible for the motor deficits characteristic of old age (McGeer *et al.*, 1977). Although one investigation found dopamine concentrations to be reduced with age (Carlson and Winblad, 1976), more recent comprehensive studies which examined both the substantia nigra and the corpus striatum failed to confirm this report (Spokes, 1979; Mackay *et al.*, 1982). In addition, the total number of dopamine binding sites, at least in the nucleus accumbens, shows a decrease with age when assessed with newly produced radioactively labelled ligands (Mackay *et al.*, 1982). These findings are unexpected since, if there really is a selective loss of the presynaptic nigrostriatal pathway with age, not only should dopamine levels be reduced but a loss of presynaptic input should result in an increase in postsynaptic receptors. It has been suggested that either receptor regulation is impaired or there is an additional loss of postsynaptic striatal neurones (Bugiani *et al.*, 1978). Alternatively, the brain may have some compensatory mechanism which serves to maintain neurotransmitter levels in the event of nerve cell loss (Rossor, 1985).

Regarding other monoamine neurotransmitters, noradrenaline concentrations in the hind brain have been reported by some to be reduced (Robinson *et al.*, 1972) with age but another study showed no significant change (Spokes, 1979). The latter report is at odds with the known age-related loss of cells from the locus coeruleus (Vijayashanker and Brody, 1979; Tomlinson *et al.*, 1981), the major source of noradrenergic projection to the forebrain, and may again indicate the brain's capacity for biochemical compensation in the face of nerve cell loss.

No change has been found with age in serotonin and its metabolite 5-hydroxy-indoleacetic acid (Robinson *et al.*, 1972). Data about the effect of age on adrenaline are presently unavailable.

Gamma-aminobutyric Acid (GABA)

The activity of gamma-aminobutyric acid and its biosynthetic enzyme, glutamic acid decarboxylase (GAD), are both reduced with age in a number of areas of the cortex (Spokes, 1979; Spokes *et al.*, 1980; Rossor *et al.*, 1982). In contrast GABA receptor binding sites are either increased or unchanged (Bowen *et al.*, 1979; Maggi *et al.*, 1979) Changes in the basal ganglia are less obviously age-related (Spokes *et al.*, 1980; Rossor, 1982). Since GABA is such a widespread neurotransmitter, being used by as much as one-third of all synapses, its decline may be responsible for many of the impaired functions of old age.

Other Neurotransmitters

Peptides are relatively newly discovered neurotransmitters and comparatively little is known about their function. Data on age-related changes are minimal. Substance P is claimed to be reduced in the hippocampus with advancing age (Crystal and Davies, 1982) whereas somatostatin and cholecystokinin appear to be unchanged (Davies *et al.*, 1980; Perry *et al.*, 1981). It is too early to comment on the functional implications of these observations.

In summary, there is little agreement about basic age-related changes in neurotransmitter systems and the implications in functional terms are even less clear apart perhaps from the cholinergic system and memory deficit, and catecholamines and hypokinesia. Clearly, this remains an area requiring further study.

II Peripheral Nerve and Muscle
M. V. Squier

Before discussing the structural changes in ageing peripheral nerve and muscle it is perhaps pertinent to review briefly the normal anatomy of the structures under consideration.

The functional unit is defined as the motor unit and consists of a motor nerve, its axon and the group of muscle fibres it supplies (Figure 1.6). The motor nerve cell bodies are found in the anterior horns of the central grey matter of the spinal cord. The axons from the motor nerve cells leave the spinal cord in the anterior root and run in the peripheral nerve to the muscles they supply. The axon branches and terminal twigs supply a number of fibres randomly dispersed throughout the muscle. The number of fibres supplied by a single nerve cell, and thus the size of the motor unit, varies between different muscles. In the major limb muscles there may be from 500 to 2000 muscle fibres in a single motor unit, while in the small muscles of the hand the number is only about 100 (Sissons, 1974).

Within the peripheral nerves the axons have a myelin sheath. Schwann cells, responsible for generating this covering, are seen at regular intervals along the length of the nerve. The tiny gaps between the segments of myelin produced by individual Schwann cells are known as nodes of Ranvier. The internode length of a myelin segment is regular and bears a consistent relationship to the diameter of the axon. After entering the muscle, the terminal branches of the nerves lose their myelin sheaths shortly before terminating in the neuromuscular junction. This consists of the terminal expansion of the axon and the specialized area of muscle membrane underlying it. The muscle membrane is folded in this region and a layer of amorphous basement-membrane-like material is seen between axon and muscle membrane and extends in continuity with the basement membrane covering each structure.

Muscle is made up of large numbers of long fibres of polygonal cross-section bound together by connective tissue. Each fibre has a mean diameter of between 10 and 100 μm, depending on age and the muscle of origin, and may be up to 10 cm in length

(Price, 1974). A muscle fibre is a syncytium of fused cells. The nuclei are found at the periphery and the major part of the cytoplasm is occupied by bundles of filaments of the contractile proteins, actin and myosin, in orderly array. The regular alignment of the myofilaments give rise to the cross-striation seen in skeletal muscle with the light microscope.

Between the filaments are other cellular organelles, the sarcoplasmic reticulum, and the T-system, mitochondria, Golgi apparatus, lipid droplets and glycogen.

The surface membrane of the fibre is known as the sarcolemma and outside this is a basement membrane. Between these two membranes are found satellite cells. These cells are relatively frequently seen in children, where their incidence relative to the intrinsic muscle nuclei is 10%; in adults the proportion drops to 2%. Satellite cells are thought to be stem cells capable of the repair of damaged muscle fibres (Landon, 1982).

Muscle fibres can be classified into several types on the basis of their metabolic properties. Type 1 fibres are 'slow' fibres depending on mitochondrial oxidative mechanisms for energy production. These fibres are used in slow movements, for example the maintenance of tone and posture. Type 2 'fast' fibres contain large amounts of glycogen and depend on glycolysis for energy production. The fibres are used in short bursts of vigorous activity and are readily fatigued. The fibres can be further subdivided into Types 2A, 2B and 2C.

Classification is usually made on the basis of adenosine triphosphatase (ATPase) activity. This enzyme is present in the muscle mitochondria, on the myosin filaments and free in the cytoplasm. Differential inhibition of these enzymes in tissue sections is possible by incubation of the sections in buffers of specific pH prior to staining. In this way the different fibre types are readily identified (Dubowitz and Brooke, 1973). A cross-section of normal muscle shows the Type 1 and Type 2 fibres to have a random mosaic distribution (Figure 1.7a). The metabolic type of a fibre is determined by its innervation

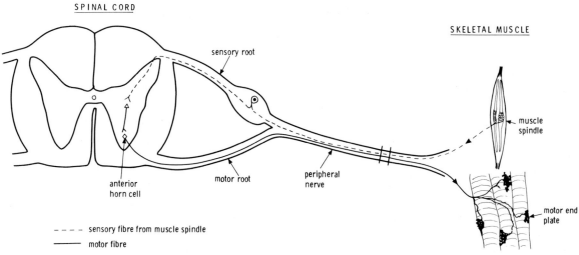

SPINAL CORD

SKELETAL MUSCLE

sensory root

muscle spindle

anterior horn cell

motor root

peripheral nerve

motor end plate

– – – – sensory fibre from muscle spindle

———— motor fibre

Figure 1.6. Diagram of components of the peripheral nerve and muscle.

(Buller *et al.*, 1960); thus all the fibres in a motor unit are of the same type.

AGE CHANGES IN PERIPHERAL NERVE AND NEUROMUSCULAR JUNCTION

Electrophysiological studies have shown a progressive fall in the number of functioning motor units after the age of 60 years in several different muscles (Campbell *et al.*, 1973; Sica *et al.*, 1974). Campbell *et al.* (1973) also showed that most of the surviving motor neurones innervate slow (or Type 1) muscle fibres. Progressive enlargement of remaining motor units suggests that they are 'taking over' and reinnervating muscle fibres which have lost their own nerve supply (Campbell *et al.*, 1973; Grimby and Saltin, 1983). This is consistent with the frequent observation of histological changes of denervation in aged muscle, as described below. Motor and sensory nerve conduction velocity slows after 60 years particularly in the distal parts of the axons (Dorfman and Bosley, 1979; Taylor, 1984).

Gutmann (1974) has defined other changes in the senile motor unit including an extreme decline in synthesis and release of transmitter and neurotrophic agents. This is related to slowed axoplasmic transport and results in a slowly progressing disturbance of neuromuscular connections. Most of Gutmann's

work is with laboratory animals and the relevance of these findings to man is uncertain.

Morphological studies of ageing human peripheral nerve are very few. After 60 years of age the relationship between internodal length and fibre diameter shows increasing variability. Evidence of demyelination and remyelination as well as axonal degeneration are seen more frequently. The densities of myelinated and unmyelinated fibres also decrease after 60 years (Lascelles and Thomas, 1966; Ochoa and Mair, 1969; Arnold and Harriman, 1970; Jacobs and Love, 1985). Reduplication of vascular basement membrane of the vasa nervorum and thickening of basement membrane of the perineurium is prominent in older subjects (Jacobs and Love, 1985).

In the distal parts of the axon spherical swellings are seen. These swellings contain filaments and granular material (Figure 1.8a–c). The subterminal axons undergo increased branching with enlargement and elaboration of motor end plates (Harriman *et al.*, 1970). Recently Oda (1984) has used some very elegant autoradiographical and histochemical methods to confirm these findings. He examined intercostal muscle from twelve autopsy cases from 32 to 76 years of age. With acetylcholinesterase methods the end plates of older subjects were seen to become fragmented and enlarged. Preterminal axons showed increased branching in older cases.

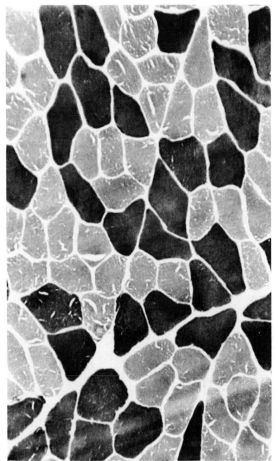

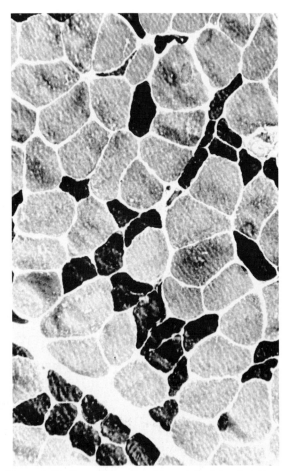

Figure 1.7a. Normal muscle showing a mosaic pattern of Type 1 fibres (pale) and Type 2 fibres (dark). ATPase pH 9.4, ×160.

Figure 1.7b. Type 2 atrophy. Almost all of the dark Type 2 fibres are smaller than the Type 1 fibres. ATPase pH 9.4, ×160.

Autoradiography with ^{125}I labelled alpha-bungarotoxin was used to demonstrate acetylcholine receptor sites. These were discrete, high density regions in the younger subjects but in older people the end plate contained a greater number of smaller conglomerates of receptors. In addition perijunctional acetylcholine receptor sites were seen in older subjects (Figure 1.9).

AGE CHANGES IN SKELETAL MUSCLE

It is a common observation that muscle strength and mass decline in old age. This may be primary and due to the process of ageing within the muscles themselves. However, muscle will also reflect changes in other parts of the motor unit (neuromuscular junction, peripheral nerve or anterior horn cell) and these structures may in turn be influenced by degeneration in higher centres of the nervous system.

Several groups of workers have measured the decline in muscle strength in elderly people (Larsson, 1978, 1982; Danneskiold-Samsoe *et al.*, 1984) which may be as much as 40% in the leg muscles and 30% in the arm (Grimby and Saltin, 1983). The decline is slightly greater for men than for women, but the ratio of strength to cross-sectional area of the quadriceps muscle remains constant in older men

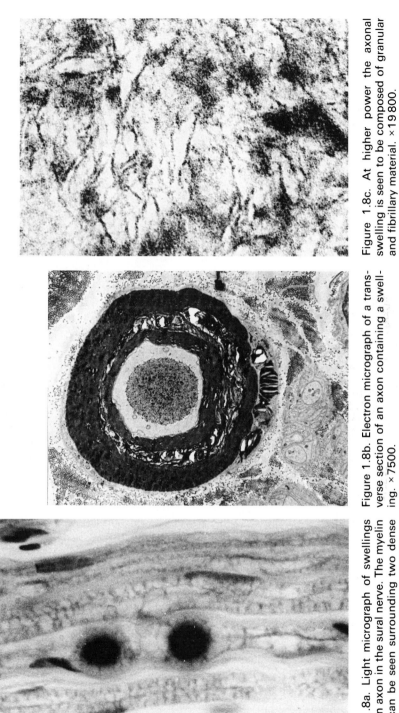

Figure 1.8a. Light micrograph of swellings within an axon in the sural nerve. The myelin sheath can be seen surrounding two dense bodies. Haematoxylin van Gieson, ×700.

Figure 1.8b. Electron micrograph of a transverse section of an axon containing a swelling. ×7500.

Figure 1.8c. At higher power the axonal swelling is seen to be composed of granular and fibrillary material. ×19 800.

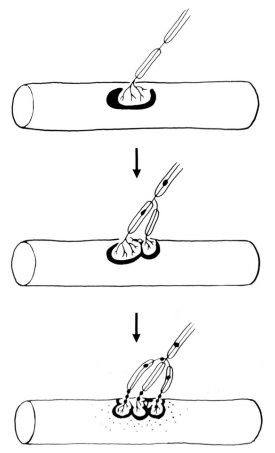

Figure 1.9. Schematic representation of age changes in human skeletal muscle end plates. Swellings appear on distal axons. Discrete dots on the muscle fibre surface represent extrajunctional acetylcholine receptors. The dense black rings indicate conglomerates of these receptors. (*Reproduced with modification by permission of Elsevier Science Publishers, Amsterdam from Oda, 1984.*)

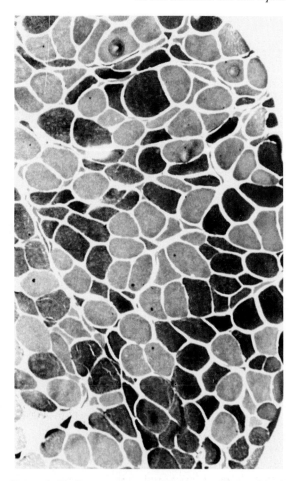

Figure 1.10. Denervation. Small angular fibres of both types are seen. The normal mosaic pattern of fibres is lost and there are small groups of fibres of similar metabolic type. ATPase pH 9.4, ×120.

and women (Young *et al.*, 1985). Speed of muscle movement also declines with age (McDonagh *et al.*, 1983).

Several methods have been used to quantify the loss of muscle mass. Indirectly methods include measurement of total excretion of creatinine and measurement of whole body potassium which reflects body cell mass. With these methods a decline of one-third is seen over 50 years; this is even greater by 80 years (Grimby and Saltin, 1983; Danneskiold-Samsoe *et al.*, 1984).

Direct measurements of individual muscle groups by ultrasound scanning (Young *et al.*, 1985), computed tomography (Imamura *et al.*, 1983) or at autopsy (Lexell *et al.*, 1983) have shown a similar loss.

Histological studies show that there is only a small decrease in the size of individual muscle fibres with ageing, of the order of 5–10% (Grimby and Saltin, 1983; Tomonaga, 1977), much less than the loss of total muscle bulk.

Lexell *et al.* (1983) studied cross-sections of vastus lateralis from six young (mean age 30 years) and six old (mean age 72 years) male subjects at autopsy.

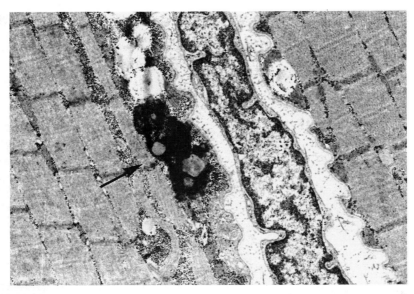

Figure 1.11. Electron micrograph of part of two muscle fibres. A granule of lipofuscin is seen beneath the surface membrane of one fibre (arrow). ×14 400.

They found the muscle to be 18% smaller in the older cases, while fibre numbers were reduced by 25%. They measured fibre size indirectly by counting the number of fibres per unit area and found no significant reduction in the older muscles. This method does not take into account the increase in interstitial connective tissue which occurs with age (Rubinstein, 1960), and may give a falsely high estimate of fibre size. They suggest that reduction in fibre numbers is the primary cause of ageing atrophy.

Biopsy studies have demonstrated a specific decrease in cross-sectional area of Type 2 fibres compared with Type 1 (Larsson, 1978, 1983; Larsson *et al.*, 1978; Tomonaga, 1977) (Figure 1.7b). This age-dependent atrophy is reversible. A group of elderly men regained muscle fibre diameters comparable with young controls after 15 weeks of weight training. Although physical strength improved it was not fully restored (Larsson, 1982). Type 2 atrophy was seen in 22% of diagnostic muscle biopsies from patients over 65 years (Squier, 1986).

Larsson has also shown a reduction in the proportion of Type 2 fibres with age which corresponds with the demonstration of Campbell *et al.* (1973) of preferential loss of 'fast' motor units. The change in fibre type proportion has not been consistently described (Grimby and Saltin, 1983).

This highlights the problem of studying human muscle, where biopsy samples are small and probably unrepresentative. Appearances vary between different muscle groups (Grimby *et al.*, 1982; Jennekens *et al.*, 1971) and within individual muscles (Mahon *et al.*, 1984; Lexell *et al.*, 1983). Further, inactivity produces considerable muscle atrophy (Imamura *et al.*, 1983; Young *et al.*, 1982) and preferential atrophy of Type 2 fibres (Engel, 1970; Dubowitz and Brooke, 1973).

The features of denervation have been described in a number of studies of ageing muscle (Grimby and Saltin, 1983; Jennekens, 1982b; Rubinstein, 1960; Tomlinson *et al.*, 1969; Tomonaga, 1977). The extent of the changes differs between different muscle groups, being more frequent in leg than arm muscles. Tomonaga (1977) found neuropathic changes to be the most common finding in the distal muscles of the lower extremity. However, by the ninth decade neurogenic change becomes apparent even in the proximal lower limb muscles (Jennekens, 1982b).

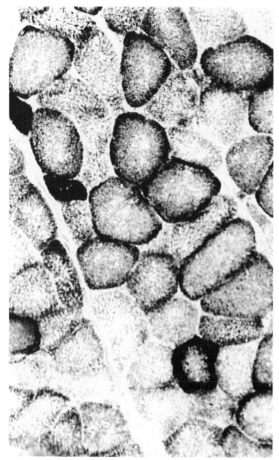

Figure 1.12. Light micrograph of a frozen section of muscle showing mitochondrial oxidative enzyme activity. Some small fibres are intensely stained throughout; in others there is a dense peripheral rim of stain—these correspond to 'ragged red fibres'. Succinate dehydrogenase, ×200.

Denervation is characterized by a number of histological and histochemical features. There is atrophy of both Type 1 and Type 2 fibres, being small and angular in outline and wedged between the larger normal hexagonal fibres. Others are reduced to a very small size and represented by clusters of basophilic, pyknotic nuclei with very little remaining sarcoplasm.

Denervation also causes an alteration in the normal checkerboard distribution of the fibre types (Figure 1.10). As a motor nerve degenerates, a neighbouring nerve may sprout and take over the supply of some of the muscle fibres which have been denervated. In this way the second neurone controls a larger 'motor unit'. The newly acquired fibres will assume the same metabolic functions as the parent motor unit and may undergo a switch in fibre type to do so. In this way the fibres of similar metabolic type become clustered and the mosaic pattern of the muscle fibre types is disturbed. The definition of a fibre type group depends on finding at least one fibre completely enclosed by fibres of its own type. In most cases this requires a group of ten to twelve fibres of the same metabolic type. If the process of denervation progresses then the larger motor units will also lose their supply and become atrophic resulting in atrophy of large groups of fibres.

Structural changes are also seen in denervated fibres. The small, angular, atrophic fibres frequently stain very deeply for oxidative enzymes. Larger fibres may show absence of enzyme activity in a central zone which is occasionally bordered by a rim of intensified enzyme activity. These fibres are called targetoid or target fibres and are seen frequently, but not specifically, in denervation (Jennekens, 1982a).

Lipofuscin, 'wear and tear' pigment, is a characteristic feature of older muscle fibres. Significant accumulation occurs after 60 years of age in the limb muscles but as early as 30 years in external ocular muscles (Rubinstein, 1960). This golden-yellow granular pigment collects just beneath the muscle membrane, usually close to nuclei. It contains lipid and stains brightly with fat stains (Figure 1.11). The chemical nature and origin of lipofuscin remains obscure but it is thought to be derived from lysosomal residual bodies (Shafiq *et al.*, 1978).

Interstitial connective tissue and fat increases with age (Rubinstein, 1960). Occasional necrotic fibres undergoing phagocytosis by histiocytes are seen (Shafiq *et al.*, 1978; Tomonaga, 1977; Jennekens *et al.*, 1971). There may be cellular infiltration of the muscles (Tomonaga, 1977). The proportion of muscle fibres with central nuclei is increased (Tomonaga, 1977; Jennekens *et al.*, 1971). This finding is usually understood to indicate that regeneration of the fibre has occurred following earlier necrosis (Cullen and Mastaglia, 1982). Nuclei may be deformed and small (Tomonaga, 1977).

Another finding is the presence of 'ragged red

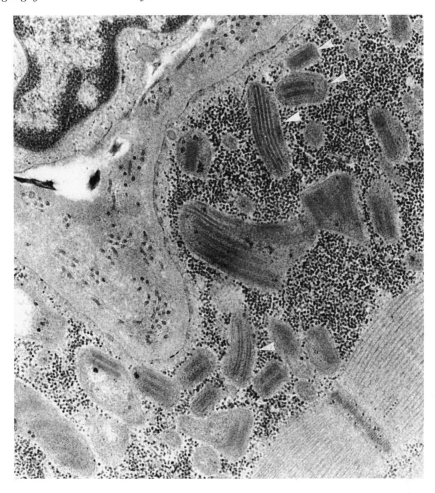

Figure 1.13. Electron micrograph of a group of abnormal mitochondria beneath the surface membrane of a muscle fibre. Most mitochondria contain paracrystalline inclusions (arrows). ×43 200.

fibres'. These are identified most easily with the trichrome stain as they have irregular, predominantly subsarcolemmal patches of red staining which correspond to areas of intense oxidative enzyme activity (Figure 1.12). With the electron microscope collections of mitochondria, some structurally abnormal, may be seen within these zones (Figure 1.13). Ragged red fibres are described in ageing muscle by Tomonaga (1977) and Jennekens *et al.* (1971) and possibly correspond to some of the changes in ageing external ocular muscles described by Rubinstein (1960). Ragged red fibres are also found in a number of myopathic conditions and are often associated with specific mitochondrial enzyme abnormalities (Carpenter and Karpati, 1984).

Ring fibres were also described (Jennekens *et al.*, 1971; Shafiq *et al.*, 1978; Tomonaga, 1977). In these fibres one or more myofibrils run obliquely or transversely around the longitudinal axis of a muscle fibre, usually at the periphery just beneath the surface membrane.

Ultrastructural changes noted in ageing muscle

include focal myofibrillar degeneration and streaming of Z lines, the formation of nemaline rods and cytoplasmic bodies, dilation of the sarcotubular system and thickening of capillary basement membrane (Shafiq *et al.*, 1978; Tomonaga, 1977).

CONCLUSIONS

There is relatively little information on normal ageing in human peripheral nerve and muscle due to the difficulty of examining normal tissue. The histology of muscle is altered by many factors which occur with increasing frequency in the elderly population; for instance disuse, vascular disease, cachexia, malignant disease, pressure palsies of peripheral nerves in bedridden people, and nerve damage from degenerative disease of the spine.

REFERENCES

I The Central Nervous System

Alzheimer, A. (1907a). Ueber eine eigenartige Erkrankung der Hirnrinde. *Allg. Z. Psychiat.*, **64**, 146–8.

Alzheimer, A. (1907b). Ueber eine eigenartige Erkrankung der Hirnrinde. *Zbl. Ges. Neurol. Psychiat.*, **18**, 177–9.

Anderson, J.M., and Hubbard, B.M. (1985). Age-related variations in the neuron content of the cerebral cortex in senile dementia of Alzheimer type. *Neuropathol. Appl. Neurobiol.*, **11**, 369–82.

Anderson, J.M., Hubbard, B.M., Coghill, G.R., and Slidders, W. (1983). The effect of advanced old age on the neurone content of the cerebral cortex. *J. Neurol. Sci.*, **58**, 233–44.

Anderton, B.H., Breinburg, D., Downes, M.J., Green, P.J., Tomlinson, B.E., Ulrich, J., Wood, J.N., and Kahn, J. (1982). Monoclonal antibodies show that neurofibrillary tangles and neurofilaments share antigenic determinants. *Nature*, **298**, 84–6.

Ball, M.J. (1976). Neurofibrillary tangles and the pathogenesis of dementia: a quantitative study. *Neuropathol. Appl. Neurobiol.*, **2**, 395–410.

Barron, S.A., Jacobs, L., and Kinkel, W.R. (1976). Changes in size of normal lateral ventricles during ageing determined by computerized tomography. *Neurology*, **26**, 1011–13.

Bartus, R.T., Dean, R.L., Beer, B., and Lippa, A. (1982). The cholinergic hypothesis of geriatric memory dysfunction. *Science*, **217**, 408–17.

Bischoff (1880). Cited by Blinkov, S.M., and Glezer, I.I. (1968). *The Human Brain in Figures and Tables*, Plenum Press, New York, p. 366.

Blinkov, S.M., and Glezer, I.I. (1968). *The Human Brain in Figures and Tables*, Plenum Press, New York, pp. 123–36.

Blocq, P., and Marinesco, G. (1892). Sur les lésions et la pathogènie de l'elipsie dite essentielle. *Sem. Med. (Paris)*, **12**, 445–6.

Bowen, D.M., Spillane, J.A., Curzon, G., Meier-Ruge, W., White, P., Goodhardt, M.J. *et al.* (1979). Accelerated ageing or selective neuronal loss as an important cause of dementia. *Lancet*, **i**, 11–14.

Brody, H. (1955). Organisation of the cerebral cortex, Part 3 (A study of ageing in the human cerebral cortex). *J. Comp. Neurol.*, **102**, 511–56.

Brody, H. (1970). Structural changes in the ageing nervous system. *Interdisc. Top. Geront.*, **7**, 9–21.

Buell, S.J., and Coleman, P.D. (1979). Dendritic growth in the aged human brain and failure of growth in senile dementia. *Science*, **206**, 854–6.

Buell, S.J., and Coleman, P.D. (1981). Quantitative evidence for selective dendritic growth in normal human ageing but not in senile dementia. *Brain Res.*, **214**, 23–41.

Bugiani, O., Salvarani, S., Perdelli, F., Mancardi, G.L., and Leonardi, A. (1978). Nerve cell loss with ageing in the putamen. *Eur. Neurol.*, **17**, 286–91.

Candy, J.M., Klinowski, J., Perry, E.K., Fairbairn, A., Oakley, A.E., Carpenter, T.A., Atack, J.R., Blessed, B., and Edwardson, J.A. (1986). Aluminosilicates and senile plaque formation in Alzheimer's Disease. *Lancet*, **i**, 354–6.

Carlsson, A., and Winblad, B. (1976). Influence of age and time interval between death and autopsy on dopamine and 3 methoxytyramine levels in human basal ganglia. *J. Neurol. Trans.*, **38**, 271–6.

Chernyshev, S.P. (1911). Cited by Blinkov, S.M., and Glezer, I.I. (1968). *The Human Brain in Figures and Tables*, Plenum Press, New York, p. 337.

Crapper, D.R., Krishnan, S.S., and Dalton, A.J. (1973). Brain aluminium distribution in Alzheimer's disease and experimental neurofibrillary degeneration. *Science*, **180**, 511–13.

Crystal, H.A., and Davies, P. (1982). Neurotransmitter-related enzymes in senile dementia of the Alzheimer type. *Brain Res.*, **171**, 319–27.

Davies, P. (1979). Neurotransmitter-related enzymes in senile dementia of the Alzheimer type. *Brain Res.*, **171**, 319–27.

Davies, P., Katzman, R., and Terry, R.D. (1980). Reduced somatostatin-like immunoreactivity in cerebral cortex from cases of Alzheimer's disease and Alzheimer senile dementia. *Nature*, **288**, 279–80.

Davies, P., and Verth, A.H. (1978). Regional distribution of muscarinic acetylcholine receptor in normal and Alzheimer-type dementia brains. *Brain Res.*, **138**, 385–92.

Davis, P.J.M., and Wright, E.A. (1977). A new method for measuring cranial cavity volume and its application to the assessment of cerebral atrophy at autopsy. *Neuropathol. Appl. Neurobiol.*, **3**, 341–58.

Dayan, A.D., and Lewis, P.D. (1985). The central nervous system—neuropathology of ageing. In: Brocklehurst, J.C. (ed.) *Textbook of Geriatric Medicine and Gerontology*, Churchill Livingstone, Edinburgh, pp. 268–93.

Drachman, D.A. (1977). Memory and cognitive function in man: does the cholinergic system have a specific role? *Neurology*, **27**, 783–90.

Duckett, S., and Galle, P. (1980). Electron-microprobe studies of aluminium in the brains of cases of Alzheimer's disease. *J. Neuropathol. Exp. Neurol.*, **39**, 350.

Gibson, P.H., Stones, M., and Tomlinson, B.E. (1976). Senile changes in the human neocortex and hippocampus compared by the use of the electron and light microscopes. *J. Neurol. Sci.*, **27**, 389–405.

Gorry, J.R. (1963). Studies on the comparative anatomy of the ganglion basale of Meynert. *Acta Anat.*, **55**, 51–104.

Grundke-Iqbal, L., Wisniewski, H.M., Johnson, A.B., and Terry, R.D. (1979). Evidence that Alzheimer neurofibrillary tangles originate from neurotubules. *Lancet*, **i**, 578–80.

Hahn, von H.P. (1981). Nucleic acids in the ageing brain and the concept of ageing. In: Davison, A.N., and Thompson, R.H.S. (eds) *The Molecular Basis of Neuropathology*, Edward Arnold, London, pp. 579–90.

Hall, T.C, Miller, A.K.H., and Corsellis, J.A.N. (1975). Variations in the human Purkinje cell population according to age and sex. *Neuropathol. Appl. Neurobiol.*, **1**, 267–92.

Hatazawa, J., Ito, M., Yamaura, H., and Matsuzawa, T. (1982). Sex differences in brain atrophy during ageing: A quantitative study with computed tomography. *J. Am. Geriat. Soc.*, **30**, 253–39.

Henderson, G., Tomlinson, B.E., and Gibson, P.H. (1980). Cell counts in human cerebral cortex in normal adults throughout life using an image analysing computer. *J. Neurol. Sci.*, **46**, 113–36.

Herzog, A.G., and Kemper, T.L. (1980). Amygdaloid changes in ageing and dementia. *Arch. Neurol. (Chic.)*, **37**, 625–9.

Horrocks, L.A., Van Rollins, M., and Yates, A.J. (1981). Lipid changes in the ageing brain. In: Davison, A.N., and Thompson, R.H.S. (eds.) *The Molecular Basis of Neuropathology*, Edward Arnold, London, pp. 601–30.

Hubbard, B.M., and Anderson, J.M. (1981). Age, senile dementia and ventricular enlargement. *J. Neurol. Neurosurg. Psychiatry*, **44**, 631–5.

Hubbard, B.M., and Anderson, J.M. (1983). Sex differences in age-related brain atrophy. *Lancet*, **i**, 1447–8.

Ihara, Y., Abraham, C., and Selkoe, D.J. (1983). Antibodies to paired helical filaments in Alzheimer's disease do not recognize normal brain proteins. *Nature*, **304**, 727–30.

Ishii, T., and Haga, S. (1976). Immunoelectronmicroscopic localization of immunoglobulins in amyloid fibrils of senile plaques. *Acta Neuropathol. (Berl.)*, **36**, 243–9.

Jacoby, R.J., Levy, R., and Dawson, J.M. (1980). Computed tomography in the elderly. 1. The normal population. *Br. J. Psychiatry*, **136**, 249–55.

Kidd, M. (1964). Alzheimer's disease. An electron microscopical study. *Brain*, **87**, 307–20.

Konigsmark, B.W., and Murphy, E.A. (1970). Neuronal populations in the human brain. *Nature*, **197**, 192–3.

Konigsmark, B.W., and Murphy, E.A. (1972). Volume of the ventral cochlear nucleus in man: Its relationship to neuronal population and ageing. *J. Neuropathol. Exp. Neurol.*, **31**, 304–16.

Korenschevsky, V. (1961). In: Bourne, G.H. (ed.) *Physiological and Pathological Ageing*, Karger, Basel and New York.

Lewis, P.R., and Shute, C.D. (1978). Cholinergic pathways in the CNS. In: Iversen, L.L., Iversen, S.D., and Snyder, S.H. (eds.) *Handbook of Psychopharmacology*, Vol. IX, Plenum Press, New York, pp. 315–56.

McDermott, J.R., Smith, A.L., Iqbal, K., and Wisniewski, H.M. (1977). Aluminium and Alzheimer's disease. *Lancet*, **ii**, 710–11.

McGeer, P.L., and McGeer, E.G. (1976). Enzymes associated with the metabolism of catecholamines, acetylcholine and GABA in human controls and patients with Parkinson's disease and Huntingdon's Chorea. *J. Neurochem.*, **26**, 65–76.

McGeer, P.L., McGeer, E.G., and Suzuki, J.S. (1977). Ageing and extrapyramidal function. *Arch. Neurol. (Chic.)*, **34**, 33–5.

Mackay, A.V.P., Iversen, L.L., Rossor, M., Spokes, E.G.S., Bird, E., Arregui, A. *et al.* (1982). Increased brain dopamine and dopamine receptors in schizophrenia. *Arch. Gen. Psychiatry*, **39**, 991–7.

Maggi, A., Schmidt, M.J., Ghetti, B., and Enna, S.J. (1979). Effect of ageing on neurotransmitter receptor binding in rat and human brain. *Life Sci.*, **24**, 367–74.

Mann, D.M.A., Davies, J.S., Hawkes, J., and Yates, P.O. (1982). Immunohistochemical staining of senile plaques. *Neuropathol. Appl. Neurobiol.*, **8**, 55–61.

Markesbery, W.R., Ehmann, D.W., Hossain, T.I.M., Alauddin, M., and Goodwin, D.T. (1981). Instrumental neutron activation analysis of brain aluminium in Alzheimer disease and ageing. *Ann. Neurol.*, **10**, 511–16.

Messert, B., Wannamaker, B.B., and Dudley, A.W. (1972). Revaluation of the size of the lateral ventricles of the brain. *Neurology (Minneap.)*, **22**, 941–51.

Miller, A.K.H., Alston, R.L., and Corsellis, J.A.N. (1980). Variations with age of the volume of grey and white matter in the cerebral hemispheres of man—Measurements with an image analyser. *Neuropathol. Appl. Neurobiol.*, **6**, 119–32.

Miller, A.K.H., and Corsellis, J.A.N. (1977). Evidence for a secular increase in human brain weight during the past century. *Ann. Hum. Biol.*, **4**, 253–7.

Miller, A.K.H., Alston, R.L., Mountjoy, C.Q., and Corsellis, J.A.N. (1984). Automated differential cell counting on a sector of the normal human hippocampus: the influence of age. *Neuropathol. Appl. Neurobiol.*, **10**, 123–41.

Mintz, J., and Jarvik, L.F. (1983). Sex differences in brain atrophy during ageing. *J. Am. Geriatr. Soc.*, **31**, 187–9.

Monagle, R.D., and Brody, H. (1974). The effects of age upon the main nucleus of the inferior olive in the human. *J. Comp. Neurol.*, **155**, 61–6.

Morimatsu, M., Hirai, S., Muramatsu, A., and Yoshikawa, M. (1975). Senile degenerative brain lesions and dementia. *J. Am. Geriatr. Soc.*, **23**, 390–406.

Ordy, J.M., Kaack, B., and Brizzee, K.R. (1975). Lifespan neurochemical changes in the human and nonhuman primate brain. In: Brody, H., Harman, D., and Ordy, J.M. (eds.) *Clinical, Morphologic and Neurochemical Aspects of the Ageing Central Nervous System*, Plenum Press, New York, pp. 133–89.

Pakkenberg, H., and Voight, J. (1964). Brain weight of the Danes. *Acta Anat. (Basel)*, **56**, 297–307.

Perl, D. P., and Brody, A.R. (1980). Alzheimer's disease: x-ray spectrometric evidence of aluminium accumulation in neurofibrillary tangle-bearing neurones. *Science*, **208**, 297–9.

Perry, E.K., and Perry, R.H. (1980). The cholinergic system in Alzheimer's disease. In: Roberts, P.J. (ed.) *Biochemistry of Dementia*, John Wiley & Sons, Chichester, pp. 135–83.

Perry, E.K., Gibson, P.H., Blessed, G., Perry, R.H., and Tomlinson, B.E. (1977). Neurotransmitter enzyme abnormalities in senile dementia. *J. Neurol. Sci.*, **34**, 247–65.

Perry, E.K., Blessed, G., Tomlinson, B.E., Perry, R.H., Crow, T.J., Cross, A.J. *et al.* (1981). Neurochemical activities in human temporal lobe related to ageing and Alzheimer-type changes. *Neurobiol. Ageing*, **2**, 251–6.

Price, D.L., Whitehouse, P.J., Struble, R.G., Coyle, M.R., Clark, A.W., Delong, M.R., Cork, L.C., and Hendreen, J.C. (1982). Alzheimer's disease and Down's Syndrome. *Ann. N.Y. Acad. Sci.*, **396**, 145–64.

Rasool, C.G., Abraham, C., Anderton, B.H., Haugh, M., Kahn, J., and Selkoe, D.J. (1984). Alzheimer's Disease: Immunoreactivity of neurofibrillary tangles with antineurofilament and anti-paired helical filament antibodies. *Brain Res.*, **310**, 249–60.

Robinson, D.S., Nies, A., Davis, J.N., Bunney, W.E., Davis, J.M., Colburn, R.W. *et al.* (1972). Ageing, monoamines, and monoamine-oxidase levels. *Lancet*, **i**, 290–1.

Rossor, M.N. (1982). Neurotransmitters and CNS disease: dementia. *Lancet*, **i**, 290–1.

Rossor, M.N. (1985). The central nervous system—neurochemistry of the ageing brain and dementia. In: Brockelhurst, J.C. (ed.) *Textbook of Geriatric Medicine and Gerontology*, Churchill Livingstone, Edinburgh, pp. 294–308.

Rossor, M.N., Garrett, N.J., Johnson, A.L., Mountjoy, C.Q., Roth, M., and Iversen, L.L. (1982). A postmortem study of the cholinergic and GABA systems in senile dementia. *Brain*, **105**, 313–30.

Scheibel, A.B. (1979). The hippocampus: organisational patterns in health and senescence. *Mech. Age. Dev.*, **9**, 89–102.

Scheibel, M.E., Tomiyasu, U., and Scheibel, A.B. (1977). The ageing human Betz cell. *Expt. Neurol.*, **56**, 598–609.

Shelanski, M.L., and Selkoe, D.J. (1981). Protein changes in the ageing brain. In: Davison, A.N., and Thompson, R.H.S. (eds.) *The Molecular Basis of Neuropathology*, Edward Arnold, London, pp. 591–600.

Shibayama, H., and Kitoh, J. (1978). Electron microscopic structure of the Alzheimer neurofibrillary changes in a case of atypical senile dementia. *Acta Neuropathol. (Berl.)*, **41**, 229–34.

Smith, C.B., and Sokoloff, L. (1981). The energy metabolism of the brain. In: Davison, A.N., and Thompson, R.H.S. (eds.) *The Molecular Basis of Neuropathology*, Edward Arnold, London, pp. 104–131.

Spokes, E.G.S. (1979). An analysis of factors influencing measurements of dopamine, noradrenaline, glutamate decarboxylase and choline acetylase in human post mortem brain tissue. *Brain*, **102**, 333–46.

Spokes, E.G.S., Garrett, N.J., Rossor, M.N., and Iversen, L.L. (1980). Distribution of GABA in post-mortem brain tissue from control, psychotic and Huntingdon's Chorea subjects. *J. Neurol. Sci.*, **48**, 303–13.

Takeda, S., and Matsuzawa, T. (1984). Brain atrophy during ageing: A quantitative study using computed tomography. *J. Am. Geriatr. Soc.*, **32**, 520–7.

Terry, R.D. (1963). The fine structure of neurofibrillary tangles in Alzheimer's disease. *J. Neuropathol. Exp. Neurol.*, **22**, 629–42.

Terry, R.D., and Wisniewski, H.M. (1972). Ultrastructure of senile dementia and of experimental analogs. In: Gaitz, C.M. (ed.) *Advances in Behavioral Biology*, Plenum Press, New York, pp. 89–116.

Tomlinson, B.E. (1979). The ageing brain. In: Thomas Smith, W., and Cavanagh, J.B. (eds.) *Recent Advances in Neuropathology*, Churchill Livingstone, Edinburgh, pp. 129–59.

Tomlinson, B.E., Blessed, G., and Roth, M. (1968). Observations on the brains of non-demented old people. *J. Neurol. Sci.*, **7**, 331–56.

Tomlinson, B.E., and Corsellis, J.A.N. (1984). Ageing and

the dementias. In: Hume Adams, J., Corsellis, J.A.N., and Duchen, L.W. (eds.) *Greenfield's Neuropathology*, Edward Arnold, London, pp. 951–1025.

Tomlinson, B.E., and Irving, D. (1977). The numbers of limb motor neurones in the human lumbosacral cord throughout life. *J. Neurol. Sci.*, **34**, 213–19.

Tomlinson, B.E., Irving, D., and Blessed, G. (1981). Cell loss in the locus coeruleus in senile dementia of Alzheimer type. *J. Neurol. Sci.*, **49**, 419–28.

II Peripheral Nerve and Muscle

Arnold, N., and Harriman, D.G.F. (1970). The incidence of abnormality in control human nerves studied by single axon dissection. *J. Neurol. Neurosurg. Psychiatry*, **33**, 55–61.

Buller, A.J., Eccles, J.C., and Eccles, R.M. (1960). Interactions between motorneurones and muscles in respect of the characteristic speeds of their responses. *J. Physiol.*, **150**, 417–39.

Campbell, M.J., McComas, A.J., and Petito, F. (1973). Physiological changes in ageing muscles. *J. Neurol. Neurosurg. Psychiatry*, **36**, 179–82.

Carpenter, S., and Karpati, G. (1984). *Pathology of Skeletal Muscle*, Churchill Livingstone, New York.

Cullen, M.J., and Mastaglia, F.L. (1982). Pathological reactions of skeletal muscle. In: Mastaglia, F.L., and Walton, J. (eds.) *Skeletal Muscle Pathology*, Churchill Livingstone, Edinburgh, pp. 88–139.

Danneskiold-Samsoe, B., Kofod, V., Munter, J., Grimby, G., Schnohr, P., and Jensen, G. (1984). Muscle strength and functional capacity in 78–81 year old men and women. *Eur. J. Appl. Physiol.*, **52**, 310–14.

Dorfman, L.J., and Bosley, T.M. (1979). Age-related changes in peripheral and central nerve conduction in man. *Neurology*, **29**, 38–44.

Dubowitz, V., and Brooke, M.H. (1973). *Muscle Biopsy: A Modern Approach*, Saunders, London.

Engel, W.K. (1970). Selective and non-selective susceptibility of muscle fibre types. *Arch. Neurol.*, **22**, 97–117.

Grimby, G., Danneskiold-Samsoe, B., Huid, K., and Salton, B. (1982). Morphology and enzymatic capacity in arm and leg muscles in 78–81 year old men and women. *Acta Physiol. Scand.*, **115**, 125–34.

Grimby, G., and Saltin, B. (1983). The ageing muscle (mini review). *Clin. Physiol.*, **3**, 209–18.

Gutmann, E. (1974). Age changes in the neuromuscular system and aspects of rehabilitation medicine. In: Buerger, A.A., and Tobis, J.S. (eds.) *Neurophysiologic Aspects of Rehabilitation Medicine*, Charles C. Thomas, Springfield, Ill., pp. 42–61.

Harriman, D.G.F., Taverner, D., and Wolf, A.L. (1970). Ekbom's syndrome and burning paraesthesiae. *Brain*, **93**, 393–406.

Imamura, K., Ashida, H., Ishikawa, T., and Fujii, M. (1983). Human major psoas muscle and Sacrospinalis

muscle in relation to age: A study by computed tomography. *J. Gerontol.*, **38**, 678–81.

Jacobs, J.M., and Love, S. (1985). Qualitative and quantitative morphology of human sural nerve at different ages. *Brain*, **108**, 897–924.

Jennekens, F.G.I. (1982a). Neurogenic disorders of muscle. In: Walton, J., and Mastaglia, F.L. (eds.) *Skeletal Muscle Pathology*, Churchill Livingstone, Edinburgh, pp. 204–34.

Jennekens, F.G.I. (1982b). Disuse, cachexia and ageing. In: Walton, J., and Mastaglia, F.L. (eds.) *Skeletal Muscle Pathology*, Churchill Livingstone, Edinburgh, pp. 605–20.

Jennekens, F.G.I., Tomlinson, B.E., and Walton, J.N. (1971). Histochemical aspects of five limb muscles in old age: an autopsy study. *J. Neurol. Sci.*, **14**, 259–76.

Landon, D.N. (1982). Skeletal muscle—normal morphology, development and innervation. In: Mastaglia, F.L., and Walton, J. (eds.) *Skeletal Muscle Pathology*, **1**, 1–87.

Larsson, L. (1978). Morphological and functional characteristics of the ageing skeletal muscle in man: a cross sectional study. *Acta Physiol. Scand. (Suppl.)*, **458**, 1–36.

Larsson, L. (1982). Physical training effects of muscle morphology in sedentary males at different ages. *Medicine and Science in Sports and Exercise*, **14 (3)**, 203–6.

Larsson, L. (1983). Histochemical characteristics of human skeletal muscle during ageing. *Acta Physiol. Scand.*, **117**, 469–71.

Larsson, L., Sjodin, B., and Karlsson, J. (1978). Histochemical and biochemical changes in human skeletal muscle with age in sedentary males, age 27–65 years. *Acta Physiol. Scand.*, **103**, 31–9.

Lascelles, R.G., and Thomas, P.K. (1966). Changes due to age in internodal length in the sural nerve in man. *J. Neurol. Neurosurg. Psychiatry*, **29**, 40–4.

Lexell, J., Henriksson-Larsen, K., Winblad, B., and Sjostrom, M. (1983). Distribution of different fibre types in human skeletal muscles: effects of ageing studied in whole muscle cross section. *Muscle and Nerve*, **6**, 588–95.

McDonagh, M.J.N., White, M.J., and Davies, C.T.M. (1984). Different effects of ageing on the mechanical properties of human arm and leg muscles. *Gerontology*, **30**, 49–54.

Mahon, M., Toman, A., Willan, P.L.T., and Bagnall, K.M. (1984). Variability of histochemical and morphometric data from needle biopsy specimens of human quadriceps femoris muscle. *J. Neurol. Sci.*, **63**, 85–100.

Ochoa, J., and Mair, W.G.P. (1969). The normal sural nerve in man. *Acta Neuropathol. (Berl.)*, **13**, 217–39.

Oda, K. (1984). Age changes in motor innervation and Ach receptor distribution on human skeletal muscle fibres. *J. Neurol. Sci.*, **66**, 327–38.

Price, H.M. (1974). Ultrastructure of the skeletal muscle fibre. In: Walton, J.N. (ed.) *Disorders of Voluntary Muscle*, Churchill Livingstone, Edinburgh, pp. 31–67.

Rubinstein, L.J. (1960). Ageing changes in muscle. In:

Bourne, G.H. (ed.) *The Structure and Function of Muscles*, Vol. III, Academic Press, London, pp. 209–26.

Shafiq, S., Lewis, S.G., Dimino, L.C., and Schutta, H.S. (1978). Electron microscopic study of skeletal muscle in elderly subjects. In: Kaldor, G., and DiBattista, W.J. (eds.) *Ageing in Muscle*, Raven Press, New York, pp. 65–85.

Sica, R.G.P., McComas, A.J., Upton, A.R.M., and Longmire, D. (1974). Motor unit estimations in small muscles of the hand. *J. Neurol. Neurosurg. Psychiatry*, **37**, 55–67.

Sissons, H.A. (1974). Anatomy of the motor unit. In Walton, J.N. (ed.) *Disorders of Voluntary Muscle*, Churchill Livingstone, Edinburgh, pp. 1–19.

Squier, M.V. (1986). The pathology of neuromuscular disease in the elderly. In: Griffiths, R.A., and McCarthy, S.T. (eds.) *Degenerative Neurological Disease in the Elderly*, Wright, Bristol, pp. 119–29.

Taylor, P.K. (1984). Non linear effects of age on nerve conduction in adults. *J. Neurol. Sci.*, **66**, 223–34.

Tomlinson, B.E., and Corsellis, J.A.N. (1984). Ageing and the dementias. In: Hume Adams, J., Corsellis, J.A.N., and Duchen, L.W. (eds) *Greenfield's Neuropathology*, Edward Arnold, London, pp. 951–1025.

Tomlinson, B.E., and Irving, D. (1977). The numbers of limb motor neurones in the human lumbosacral cord throughout life. *J. Neurol. Sci.*, **34**, 213–19.

Tomlinson, B.G., Walton, J.N., and Rebeiz, J.J. (1969). The effects of ageing and of cachexia upon skeletal muscles: a histopathological study. *J. Neurol. Sci.*, **9**, 321–46.

Tomlinson, B.E., Irving, D., and Blessed, G. (1981). Cell loss in the locus coeruleus in senile dementia of Alzheimer type. *J. Neurol. Sci.*, **49**, 419–28.

Tomonaga, M. (1977). Histochemical and ultrastructural changes in human skeletal muscle. *J. Am. Geriat. Soc.*, **25**, 125–31.

Ulrich, J. (1985). Alzheimer changes in nondemented patients younger than sixty-five: possible early stages of Alzheimer's disease and senile dementia of Alzheimer type. *Ann. Neurol.*, **17**, 273–7.

Vijayshankar, N., and Brody, H. (1971). Neuronal population in human abducens nucleus. *Anat. Rec.*, **169,** 447.

Vijayshankar, N., and Brody, H. (1973). The neuronal population of the nuclei of the trochlear nerve and the locus coeruleus in the human. *Anat. Rec.*, **172**, 421–2.

Vijayashankar, N., and Brody, H. (1977). Aging in the human brain stem: a study of the nucleus of the trochlear nerve. *Acta Anat.*, **99**, 169–72.

Vijayshankar, N., and Brody, H. (1979). A quantitative study of the pigmented neurones in the nuclei locus coeruleus and subcoeruleus in man as related to aging. *J. Neuropath. Exp. Neurol.*, **38**, 490–7.

White, P., Hiley, C.R., Goodhardt, M.J., Carrasco, L.H., Keet, J.P., Williams, I.E.I., and Bowen, D.M. (1977). Neocortical cholinergic neurones in elderly people. *Lancet*, **ii**, 668–70.

Wilkinson, A., and Davies, I. (1978). The influence of age and dementia on the neurone population of the mamillary bodies. *Age and Ageing*, **7**, 151–60.

Wisniewski, H.M., Narang, H.K., and Terry, R.D. (1976). Neurofibrillary tangles of paired helical filaments. *J. Neurol. Sci.*, **27**, 173–81.

Yagashita, S., Itah, T., Wang, N., and Amano, N. (1981). Reappraisal of the fine structure of Alzheimer's neurofibrillary tangles. *Acta Neuropath. (Berl.)*, **54**, 239–46.

Young, A., Hughes, I., Round, J.M., and Edwards, R.H.T. (1982). The effect of knee injury on the number of muscle fibres in the human quadriceps femoris. *Clin. Sci.*, **62**, 227–34.

Young, A., Stokes, M., and Crowe, M. (1985). The size and strength of the quadriceps muscles of old and young men. *Clin. Physiol.*, **5**, 145–54.

Zatz, L.M., Jernigan, T.L., and Ahumuda, A.J. (1982). White matter changes in cerebral computed tomography related to aging. *J. Comput. Assist. Tomogr.*, **6**, 19–23.

The Clinical Neurology of Old Age
Edited by R. Tallis
© 1989 John Wiley & Sons Ltd

Chapter 2

Changes in Mental Functioning associated with Normal Ageing

Martin Binks

Lecturer in Psychology, University of Liverpool, Liverpool, UK

INTRODUCTION

This review, though not exhaustive, discusses the effects of normal ageing on cognition, personality and emotion. All have recently been treated more extensively (Birren and Schaie, 1985). The effects of normal ageing on mental functioning are relevant to assessment and rehabilitation, and provide a baseline from which pathological states emerge (Woods and Britton, 1985).

Most studies use cross-sectional experimental designs. These cannot separate age differences from characteristics that vary between the generations studied. Generations differ in the duration and type of education they have had, in upbringing, and in the chance and choice of work. When these variations between generations are relevant to psychological variables, cross-sectional conclusions generalize to adjacent generations but no further. Variations between generations in nutrition, exposure to disease and access to effective medical care may also limit generalization from cross-sectional studies of medical variables. Longitudinal designs are flawed in different ways. Sequential designs (Palmore, 1978) can sometimes separate age effects from generation and time-of-measurement effects but their use has largely been restricted to studies of personality and intelligence. A further characteristic of many of the studies referred to in this chapter is that volunteer subjects are typically above average in intelligence and socioeconomic status. When the range of subjects is extended it rarely reaches those who are below average.

Descriptive studies of mental functioning and age have evolved in the last two decades into explanatory studies using the cognitive paradigm based on objective behavioural data such as speed of performance or the probability and type of error (Cohen, 1983). The aim is to identify how knowledge about the world and events that occur around the subject are represented mentally and how cognitive processes establish, revise, retain and use those representations. A small set of representations and processes combine in different ways to explain cognition and how ageing affects it (Kausler, 1982; Salthouse, 1982).

Although cognitive psychology includes analyses of intelligence and problem solving, these are not prominent issues in the medical care of the elderly; they have been reviewed by Labouvie-Vief (1985) and Rabbitt (1977) respectively. Language and memory have greater relevance for the assessment and management of the elderly. In such studies subjects are typically over 65 years of age.

LANGUAGE

Language skills such as naming and defining remain stable until 70 and the modest but significant declines thereafter in group mean performance arise from a minority who show large declines (Obler and Albert, 1985).

Most studies of communicating with old people focus on their competence in perception of thematic structure, comprehension and memory. Studies typically present spoken material at moderate rates (around 120 words per minute) and match age groups on their performance on auditory aspects of intelligence such as digit span or spoken vocabulary to control audibility. Petros *et al.* (1983) asked subjects to allocate idea units within Japanese folk tales to four levels of importance to the theme. There were no effects of age or years of education. Old subjects were not handicapped in perceiving the thematic structure of this text despite its origin in another culture. However, old subjects may make less use of such organization in comprehension and learning.

Cohen (1979) separated comprehension of spoken text from remembering it by controlling the conditions of learning and retention and then comparing recall of facts with recall of inferences drawn from these facts. Subjects of average education made significantly more errors in recalling inferences than facts and this difference increased significantly with age. Cohen's subjects were attending a geriatric day hospital but were selected for the absence of confusion. Old, highly educated subjects made significantly more errors in recalling inferences than similar young subjects. Since there were no age differences for highly educated subjects in the recall of factual information, they were unlikely to have forgotten the inferences more rapidly than the young, but either drew fewer inferences or were less able to consolidate them for long-term use. There is support for both of these explanations. Light *et al.* (1982) supported the first explanation since old, highly educated subjects drew significantly fewer correct inferences from sets of three related sentences even when all sentences were recalled correctly and with high confidence. The second explanation (the poor consolidation of inferences) was supported by testing comprehension after minimum delay, and by testing memory after a delay filled with mental activity to prevent rehearsal. After hearing a passage, highly educated subjects were asked to recog-

nize changes in a printed version (Cohen and Faulkner, 1981). For semantic changes there were no significant age differences at 10 seconds (an approximation to comprehension) but there was a significant age decline after 25 seconds. Although exact wording was rapidly forgotten by both age groups, meaning was appreciated but forgotten more rapidly by old subjects than by the young. This suggests that even the highly educated people used in this study have difficulty consolidating a detailed, non-redundant topic before coping with a subsequent topic.

Clinical Implications of Age Differences in Language

Age differences in retaining the meaning and implications of speech arise more from forgetting than from understanding. These difficulties can be reduced if the speaker paces the presentation using the old person's verbal and gestural signs of understanding and provides a written reminder of the material that the old person has understood but may forget. The reduced recall of inferences by the old suggests that all important parts of communication should be explicit. These implications apply more strongly to subjects of average education since they have the additional handicap of forgetting facts. This may reduce the context that facilitates the retention of inferences.

MEMORY

Normal old people often complain of a reduction in the speed and consistency of recall. Intermittent but complete failure to learn and to recall are prominent early symptoms of dementia. Consequently it is important to establish which memory tasks are age sensitive and which are age resistant before seeking explanations in terms of particular memory processes.

Memory Complaints

Old people have been asked to make systematic reports of their memory problems. Zelinski *et al.* (1980) assessed the types of problems and ways of coping with them in a wide range of memory situations. There were two ways whereby individuals differed in their self-evaluation of memory. The first indicated rare memory failures, while the second indicated rare use of memory aids and good ability for remembering recent and remote past events. These characteristics were significantly more common in subjects below 40 than those above 60. Hulicka (1982) aggregated a similar range of assessments and found a significant age trend in self-assessed memory but with 38% of the decline occurring by 44, followed by stability until 70 when a further major decline occurred. Cavanaugh *et al.* (1983) compared diary reports from groups with mean ages of 28 and 59 and found significant differences in that the old reported 30% more failures, were more upset by them, forgot more names, regular routines, objects and locations. The young forgot when stressed, the old when their routine was disrupted. A significant doubling of the frequency of difficulties of remembering proper names was found between ages 47 and 70 by Cohen and Faulkner (1986) in a questionnaire study. The problematic names were available in memory but were temporarily inaccessible since many were recalled hours later by all ages. However, the old were significantly less likely to find retrieval failure accompanied by hunches about or attributes of the target names, so they were unable to start to reconstruct the missing names.

Although most studies confirm an increase in overall memory problems with old age, two exceptions occur when reports were limited to the frequency of memory failures assessed by estimates of absolute frequency (varying from 'not at all in the past three months' to 'more than once a day') (Sunderland *et al.*, 1984). In two studies old subjects reported significantly fewer memory failures than the young. It is unlikely that old subjects forget how often their memory fails or are reluctant to report their frequency (Rabbitt, 1982). The second exception occurred when no significant overall effects of age were found for the total scores on the Every-day Memory Questionnaire and Cognitive Failures Questionnaire (Martin, 1986). However, old subjects reported significantly more problems than the young with simple rote learning and the recall of names. This contrasts with significantly fewer problems in organizing their lives, including remembering appointments. This was confirmed by independent records of missed appointments with the experimenter.

The opportunity to use well-established routines may explain the divergence between self-report and observational studies of memory failures (Harris, 1984). In a laboratory study of pattern comparison, subjects had to remember to indicate how long their comparisons took before stating their conclusion; thus time stress was likely and compensatory strategies prevented. The number of presses omitted was nine times greater for the old. In a small field study of telephoning at appointed times, old subjects forgot less often and were less often late than the young. When the old were persuaded to reduce compensatory strategies such as diaries, they performed at the same level as the young.

Clinical implications of age differences in memory complaints

Interviews should cover the types of memory failure and compensating adjustment adopted as well as the frequency of memory failures. The extent of memory failures in old age could be modified by the avoidance of risk situations and by minimizing failure with compensatory strategies such as a diary or setting up a visible reminder (Harris, 1984). These offer better prospects for improving memory in the elderly than mnemonic strategies (Robertson-Tchabo, 1980). Since direct observation of forgetfulness is very time consuming, Sunderland *et al.* (1984) in their study of head-injured patients recommended substituting either a questionnaire completed by a younger person who spends a large part of the day in social contact with the subject, or a daily checklist completed by the subject. Similar procedures may contribute to the assessment of some subjects who are forgetful in old age. The questionnaire has greater validity but a well-briefed informant will not usually be available. The checklist will be more widely usable but reduces rather than avoids the underestimation of memory problems because of forgetting them.

Memory for Past Events

The stereotype that old people remember the events of remote decades more accurately than the recent past misrepresents normal old people. Since events from different decades may vary in memorability, Butters and Albert (1982) used famous people and events matched for the probability of recall by 50 year olds and found that 70 year olds recalled less. No age group was more accurate for remote decades with unaided recall. When recall failed, Moscovitch (1982) provided semantic and phonemic cues and found that the old had more memories available but they were more inaccessible for the remote than for the recent decades. Based on the topics introduced in conversation, Hulicka (1982) found that three old people with intact memory chose to recall events from all decades of their lives, but selected the past far more often than young and middle-aged subjects.

Subject-performed tasks (break the piece of chalk, look in the mirror) provide a new way of studying memory for recent events. When subjects heard such an instruction, were given the object and performed the action themselves, their immediate and delayed recall showed trivial differences between 23 and 70 year olds. In contrast both types of recall showed a significant deterioration with age when the action was not permitted despite the presence of the object (Bäckman, 1985). Thus it is the performance of actions or the subjects' monitoring of them that suppresses an age difference in memory for familiar past events. However, when the past events used were a series of previously performed unfamiliar cognitive tasks each lasting several minutes (Kausler and Hakami, 1983), old subjects recalled significantly fewer tasks than young subjects. The only exception was the absence of age differences in recall of problem-solving tasks which may have been more demanding or more distinctive than the other perceptual-motor and memory tasks. A subsequent study found that old subjects' recognition hit rate but not their false alarm rate was slightly but significantly worse than that of young subjects (Kausler *et al.*, 1985a). Thus the age difference cannot be fully explained by a retrieval deficit.

Despite finding age differences in remembering which activities had occurred, Kausler *et al.* (1985a) found that old subjects monitored the frequency of planning and executing activities with the same accuracy as young subjects but were significantly more variable. In an experiment with a task series

taking about an hour, Kausler *et al.* (1985b) showed that both old and young subjects could exceed chance performance in recalling the quarter of the series to which a task had been assigned. However, old subjects were slightly but significantly less accurate in remembering when activities occurred. Applying these assessments to Bäckman's task may identify further aspects of memory for past events that are insensitive to ageing yet assess orientation in time.

Clinical implications of age differences in memory for past events

When normal old people emphasize the past, this may reflect preference rather than competence. Asking old people for important personal events in each decade of their lives would indicate how much was readily accessible in recall but cueing by relatives or by mementoes may well show that much more was available with help. Studies of memory for subject-performed tasks and for assessment procedures suggest ways of collecting data on memory functioning within existing medical assessment and treatment settings if patients experience a sequence of tests or participate in a series of activities such as those used in behavioural assessments of the activities of daily living. Cooper (1982) provided a protocol for assessing memory using the subtests and test contents of the Wechsler Intelligence subscales. Memory assessment in other settings would be analogous.

Memory Processes

Age differences in memory vary greatly in magnitude and are absent for some tasks and materials. This diversity is clarified by two ways of classifying memory. In the first, a memory of the occurrence of an event is established by encoding, becomes weaker or modified during storage, and is accessible if the retrieval task distinguishes it from other memories. In the second, the number of different events which occur in the retention interval between encoding and retrieval is either less than four to eight (primary memory and working memory) or greater than eight (secondary memory) (Craik and Rabinowitz, 1984).

In primary memory situations, encoding and retrieval receive undivided attention since remembering is the entire task. Age differences in accuracy are slight for subjects of high verbal ability (Craik, 1971), while significant age differences in encoding, but not in storage or retrieval, occur for subjects of average ability (Binks and Sutcliffe, 1972). However, significant slowing has occurred by age 70 (Waugh *et al.*, 1978). In working memory situations attention is divided or switched between firstly, encoding and retrieving and secondly, using the memories as components of a larger task. The significant age differences which occur in backward digit span (Bromley, 1958), running digit span (Parkinson *et al.*, 1980) and mental addition (Wright, 1981) indicate a reduction in working memory.

In secondary memory situations, more than eight items or events must be remembered for more than 30 seconds and age differences are often large and significant. They can sometimes be reduced if the conditions of encoding and retrieval elicit the mental activity that young subjects engage in spontaneously but which old subjects neglect, or do inefficiently (Craik and Rabinowitz, 1984). When learning which words have been paired for a laboratory task, old subjects show a production deficiency or inefficiency in that they generate a linking word or image to aid learning significantly less often than the young do, yet improve significantly after training in the use of such mediators (Kausler, 1982, p. 383). When learning a list of words old subjects encode the general aspects such as category membership as effectively as do the young, but make significantly less use of aspects specific to each word such as the context sentence in which it occurs or the association that they were required to generate to it (Rabinowitz *et al.*, 1982). Additional time for encoding helped the young significantly more than the old when no guidance was given for encoding, but helped both age groups equally when there was a semantic encoding question such as 'Taller than a man?' for each list of concrete nouns (Craik and Rabinowitz, 1985). Thus slow encoding was a less effective explanation than the failure of old subjects to use an available encoding strategy. This was insufficient to remove the age deficit although the addition of assistance with retrieval by the use of a recognition test was of greater benefit to the old group at the shortest encoding time.

Unfortunately, the common situation of a conversation among a group of people is likely to combine the effects of age declines in attention, comprehension and memory. Rabbitt (1981) found that the recall of four statements, each spoken by a different person, produced no age differences but when old subjects also had to recall the speaker or both the speaker and the recipient, they had little success. This failure was reduced if the recipient was named or if a statement was a direct reply to the previous statement and contained a phrase from it. Replying to one of three statements produced a larger age decline in the recall of other people's statements than did listening to someone else's reply to that statement. However, old people remembered the replies that they had made themselves.

Clinical implications of age differences in memory processes

Craik and Rabinowitz (1984) suggest that semantic processing at encoding is important for establishing distinctive memories. Old subjects are less likely to do this when the material or the task is unfamiliar or when they must generate a new procedure for coping. Coping with novelty is constrained by processes which are less efficient, less flexible and more demanding in old age. Familiar situations, habitual expectations and responses limit the impact of such changes and guidance with encoding or retrieval compensates for them if there is also time to implement the guidance. A one-to-one conversation helps old people to remember if it uses partial recapitulations and explicit connections between issues. Leading questions which ensure that the old people themselves repeat or summarize important points should turn to good advantage their preference for remembering their own contributions.

Although most aspects of cognition change with age in difficult or novel situations, remedial measures are possible for some aspects; simpler or familiar situations can defer the onset of changes.

PERSONALITY AND EMOTION

The sparse literature on mood and emotion in normal old age prevents clear conclusions, but shows the need to be alert in detecting unsupported stereotypes about ageing.

Emotion, mood and personality can be distinguished in three ways (Schultz, 1982). Strong emotions such as fear involve high arousal for some minutes and produce behaviour intended to change the environment. Moods or moderate emotions such as grief involve moderate arousal for hours or days in normal individuals but longer in the psychiatrically ill, with the main effects being a change in the perception of the self and the environment. Personality differs from mood in that it lasts for years.

THE STABILITY OF PERSONALITY

There are three ways of describing an individual's personality: the trait approach, the psychoanalytical approach and the interactional approach which qualifies the effects of traits or psychoanalytical coping styles by identifying environments or situations which modify their effects. There are three aspects of the stability of personality: what is typical of the group, how an individual is ranked within the group and the relationship between aspects of personality. Most studies of ageing and personality have taken a life-span approach with the minority of data drawn from those over 65. Consequently the mean age of the oldest group of subjects must be specified in each study. These studies describe personality on the threshold of old age and offer a tentative basis for extrapolation up to 70.

The Trait Approach to Personality

The major studies have used the trait approach and show more stability than change in mean levels over 8 to 10 years. Two of these studies have used the Cattell 16PF questionnaire in a cross-sectional design and found few significant main or interaction effects of time and cohort. The Duke study (Seigler *et al.*, 1979) sampled men and women, aged 46–70 from an American health insurance plan. The Boston study of male armed forces veterans included a wider range of socio-economic status than the Duke study, except in those aged 50—the oldest group (Costa and McCrae, 1978). In both studies the short-term retest reliability of the individual traits

was around 0.50. This was low enough for true change with age to be hard to detect against a background of unreliability. In the Baltimore study male volunteers in scientific, professional or managerial jobs completed the Guilford-Zimmerman Temperament Survey (GZTS). In up to 10 years of follow-up with cross- and time-sequential designs, Douglas and Arenberg (1978) found that even the significant age effects were small. The level of somatic complaints elicited by the Cornell Medical Index showed significant stability when retested 8 to 17 years later (correlation 0.72) and was strongly related to neuroticism (GZTS Emotional Stability scale with reversed scoring) but was not related to age up to 70 (Costa and McCrae, 1985). Thus hypochondriasis did not increase in old males and a comparison of current with past levels of somatic concerns may help in distinguishing consistent elevated levels of somatic concerns in chronic neurosis from a recent rise in acute depression in old age.

The rank order of individuals relative to their peers is little changed by their idiosyncratic histories of life events or by ageing since the retest correlation often declines little from a few weeks to 10 years. In the 16PF most traits had stabilities of about 0.50 in the Boston study (Costa and McCrae, 1978). For the GZTS all stabilities exceeded 0.59.

The final aspect of the stability of traits concerns the grouping of specific traits into broader clusters or factors. In the Boston study, Costa and McCrae (1976) found three clusters in the Cattell 16PF: Neuroticism, Extroversion and Openness to Experience. The Neuroticism and Extroversion clusters were stable in a cross-sectional study of groups of men with mean ages of 32, 44 and 60. They were also replicated in a 9 year longitudinal study (Costa and McCrae, 1977–8) which also showed that Openness to Experience was stable for all age groups. In the Baltimore study, Costa *et al.* (1980) showed that Neuroticism and Extroversion were consistent factors in the GZTS across times of measurement, longitudinal retesting and age groups with mean ages of 37, 52 and 68.

Although personality traits are almost as stable across decades as they are in short-term retest reliability, in part this is due to selecting the traits and items which are most stable. More importantly the trait approach ignores the effects of assessing equivalent rather than identical situations and behaviours. In young subjects a retest reliability of 0.8 may fall to a cross-situational consistency of 0.3 (Mischel and Peake, 1982). Further reductions in cross-situational consistency may arise from variations with age in the situations and purposes which elicit behaviour and in the presence or probability of rewards and punishments which maintain or suppress behaviour. Since these have not been studied, the above literature may well overestimate the stability of personality. The emphasis on traits and their clusters hides the potential changes in validity of individual items that may occur with age. Items that ask about depressed mood may be using concepts rarely used by old people and which have socially undesirable connotations for that age group. In contrast, young people may use the same concepts over-inclusively to include boredom and with little sense of social undesirability.

The Psychoanalytical Approach to Personality

Psychoanalysis has drawn attention to defence mechanisms or styles of coping with life events. These aspects of personality suggest types of adjustment to ageing which correlate with life satisfaction and level of activity in social roles for subjects aged 53 to 83 drawn from a wide range of socio-economic status (Neugarten *et al.*, 1980). Small sample sizes in this cross-sectional study meant that most types were represented by fewer than ten individuals. Similar methods were used by Maas and Kuypers (1974) in a longitudinal study of the life styles at 30 and 70 years of age for 142 subjects of high socio-economic status. The men showed little change in the types of life styles in old age. Similar stability was found for two of the life styles of women (visiting, husband-centred). In contrast, change was common in the other four life styles of women (work-centred, group-centred, uncentred, disabled-disengaged). This sex difference was associated with more pressure and opportunity for change produced by the social and geographical environments of women which had greater effects on their lives than on the lives of men. Most subjects were satisfied with their life styles and

coped well with difficulties with little sign of an age decline. When personality or life style caused problems in old age, these were usually the continuation of young adult problems which were not overcome when they first occurred. Although both studies have relied heavily on case-study and projective test methods to support inferences about unconscious processes, with the consequent risk of low reliability and difficult replication, there is agreement about the stability of coping styles as men age.

The conscious experience and behavioural expression of coping were assessed by self-report questionnaire in a cross-sectional study of the Baltimore sample (McCrae, 1982). There were significant age differences in the nature of stressful life events during the previous year, with fewer challenges and more threats of present or future danger for those over 65, but no age differences in the frequency of the need to adjust to the consequences of past events. Subjects were asked about ways that they had used to cope with their own most stressful event from the last year. Those over 65 made significantly less use of immature styles of coping such as escapist fantasy and of hostile reactions than those below 50. The evidence was less consistent for significant declines in mature styles of coping such as positive thinking, self-adaptation and humour. Thus healthy old people of high socio-economic status did not show widespread regression from the mature coping strategies of middle age.

The Interaction Approach to Personality

Although this is a central issue in theories of personality (Mischel and Peake, 1982; Houts *et al.*, 1986), it has rarely been applied to ageing and then only to high-level business executives (Heckhausen, 1983). Environmental opportunities and contingencies may modify the expression of personality in old age.

Clinical Implications of the Apparent Stability of Personality

Although each approach provides evidence for the stability of personality in old age, the evidence is not sufficiently strong to justify an expectation of stability as the starting point for the assessment and management of old people with medical problems. However, all approaches suggest that it is worth asking old people and those who know them well about the old person's personality and coping styles in middle age. This is valuable either as the starting point from which changes in coping during old age must start, or as the stability that persists throughout old age for the majority of old people who do not develop psychopathology. Both uses of reports of personality in middle age provide realistic expectations of the constraints on management so that a modest improvement for each emerging problem, rather than an enduring cure, is sufficient success (Costa and McCrae, 1986).

MOOD AND EMOTION

Self-reports of happy, sad and neutral moods were not noticeably different when those over 65 were compared with younger subjects (Cameron, 1975). However, it may be important to distinguish between types of events. Familiar events may make less impact on the old due to adaptation to repetition. Their impact may be briefer if there is a well-practised course of corrective action or compensatory adjustment. New events such as retirement may be pleasant but need not be. Bereavement and illness become more likely so there is greater risk of unpleasant emotion and reduced control of the outcome of new events in old age (Schultz, 1982). Moreover, many studies do not distinguish between actual and expected events yet the strength of emotion may depend upon the extent of this discrepancy as much as the frequency of events (Thomae, 1970).

Emotional responses and their expression in behaviour were studied by Malatesta and Kalnok (1984) using ratings made by subjects aged 17 to 88 drawn from middle or high socio-economic status groups living in the community. Those over 65 did not report changes in the type of affect or in the frequency or intensity of emotion compared with their experiences in earlier decades. The life events that elicited emotion had largely similar consequences for all age groups with two exceptions. The only age differences in emotions which were both

significant and large concerned sadness, which was caused less often by personal losses but more often by physical problems for old subjects, and anger, which was caused more often by personal losses but less often by meeting responsibilities for old subjects. Old subjects were significantly more likely than young subjects to say that they ought to conceal emotion but there were no corresponding age differences in the inhibition of the expression of emotion. Apparent age differences in the expression of emotion may arise from the behaviour expected of the old rather than their experience of emotion.

PATHOLOGICAL MENTAL FUNCTIONING

The previous sections outline some features of cognition and mood in the elderly to provide a baseline of normal ageing from which emerge pathologies of cognition and mood. Age changes in this baseline represent either a gradual 'continuous decline' or an abrupt 'terminal drop' preceding fatal illness (Rabbitt, 1986). The baseline guides the selection of pathology resistant measures to estimate premorbid function. Comparing this with measures sensitive to particular pathologies should aid the early detection and assessment of the severity of psychopathology (Binks and Davies, 1984).

Clarifying Uncertain Complaints

Occasionally, performance on a cognitive task may underestimate ability due to the subject's poor motivation or exaggerated complaints. If assessment starts with patently legible material which shrinks to normal large print the exaggerated complaint may be abandoned (Binks and Davies, 1985). In more resistant cases the suspicions raised by inconsistencies of deficits may be explored using two-alternative forced-choice responses to a random series of events that the subject denies being able to understand or remember (Pankrantz, 1983). The simulation of random responding is so difficult that exaggeration ceases or produces a statistically unlikely pattern of responding. Hannay and James (1981) suggested that recognition tasks might identify exaggeration by a rate of false alarms that is rarely found in verified disability. Schacter (1986) found that psychiatrists and psychologists could not distinguish genuine from simulated forgetting, but found that simulators showed significantly reduced confidence in the likelihood of improving when assisted by recognition or cued recall test formats. Extending this behavioural approach to the elderly may help to remotivate the subject who exaggerates complaints and to justify determined rehabilitation of them.

The following sections deal with the two commonest psychopathologies of old age: dementia and depression. The discussion is restricted to behavioural data since clinical structured interviews and mental status questionnaires are dealt with elsewhere (Copeland *et al.*, 1986; Roth *et al.*, 1986; Teseri *et al.*, 1984). Although there is a considerable literature on the cognitive changes associated with dementia and depression in comparison with normal ageing (Grant and Adams, 1986; Woods and Britton, 1985), the validity of differential diagnosis using cognitive changes is rarely demonstrated. Either clear-cut severe cases are used (Kendrick *et al.*, 1979) or data are presented (Kopelman, 1986) but await an explicit analysis of differential diagnosis (Binks, 1987). Few studies meet the methodological requirements identified by Jorm (1986).

Cognition in Dementia

Since a major feature of dementia is an acquired global intellectual deterioration, intelligence test verbal-performance discrepancy scores and characteristic profiles of subtests have been sought as signs of dementia. Fuld (1983) reported a Wechsler Adult Intelligence Scale (WAIS) profile that discriminated dementia of the Alzheimer's type from normal ageing and multi-infarct dementia. However, even the use of the revision (WAIS-R) and the clarity of confirmatory factor analysis fail to identify the cognitive processes underlying the subtests (O'Grady, 1983). The use of intelligence tests validated against cognitive processes (Hunt, 1983) and selected for their relevance to dementia would provide a more rational assessment of the global intellectual deterioration in dementia.

There has been greater success in clarifying the nature of the memory impairment in dementia. Although primary memory is impaired in dementia

(Kopelman, 1985), Morris (1984) showed that dementia did not impair the contribution of verbal rehearsal to immediate memory span (the inner voice or articulatory loop). However, dementia greatly increased the vulnerability of working memory to distraction by simple tasks such as finger tapping or suppression of articulatory rehearsal, both of which had little effect on the retention of normal old people (Morris, 1986). Thus in tests of immediate memory span the backward version is a more sensitive measure than the forward version which minimizes working memory. Spilich (1983) performed a propositional analysis of text recall from secondary memory and found that working memory was used for randomly selected propositions by memory impaired old people, while normal old people selected by importance.

In several secondary memory situations, dementia produced significantly reduced learning, but when items were exposed for longer to remove this difference in encoding, the rate of forgetting was no greater (Kopelman, 1985). When the multi-trial learning task is modified so that reminding is selective and restricted to those items not recalled on the latest attempt, it is possible to separate primary and secondary memory retrieval, secondary memory storage and consistent retrieval. Although demented subjects were significantly worse than controls on all measures of selective reminding, primary memory retrieval was the least impaired, particularly for the mildly demented who neglected secondary memory while concentrating on primary memory (Ober *et al.*, 1985). The moderately demented showed a significantly greater increase with trials in secondary memory storage but failed to retrieve these items consistently, so their total recall did not benefit from their equal emphasis on primary and secondary memory.

Remote memory has been investigated in dementia using the famous people test (Albert *et al.*, 1979). Wilson *et al.* (1981) found that the recall deficit was similar for all decades. Moscovitch (1982) provided semantic and then phonemic cues if free recall failed and found that the earliest decades were the best recalled and matched the performance of normal old people. The effect of dementia was greatest on the most recent decades. The failure to benefit from such cues might discriminate dementia from normal ageing.

Although subject-performed tasks are age resistant, they are dementia sensitive when tested by free recall (Winblad *et al.*, 1985). The mild, but not the moderately, demented improved more for subject-performed tasks than for sentences when tested by cued recall. Thus cueing may maximize the accessibility of recent personal events in mild dementia.

The effects of dementia on language have been described but less often explained (Obler and Albert, 1985). Fluency, as in naming members of a category such as 'animals', is impaired in mild dementia (Martin and Fedio, 1983) and arises from less systematic and less exhaustive searching rather than the loss of conceptual distinctions that define a category (Diesfeldt, 1985; Ober *et al.*, 1986). In moderate dementia semantic errors are detected and corrected less often than syntactic or phonological errors (Bayles, 1982).

Cognition in Depression

Establishing the nature of the cognitive impairment in pure depression might identify features which would reduce the frequency of confusion with dementia. Studies rarely follow-up to exclude either cases in which the underlying dementia progresses to reduce self-awareness of cognitive impairment and thereby the depressive reaction to dementia, or cases in which successful treatment of depression reveals an underlying dementia. Consequently, such cases cloud the comparison of cognitive impairment in depression and dementia. In addition, most studies of cognition in depression include a wide range of ages; very few are restricted to cases over 65.

Cognitive impairment in depression could be either a secondary side-effect of somatic and affective symptoms (pseudodementia), or an intrinsic central symptom itself (Jorm, 1986). An intrinsic impairment would only subside when depression was successfully treated, while a secondary impairment could be modified before the treatment of depression. The results of Weingartner *et al.* (1981a) suggest that passive encoding of word lists in secondary episodic memory is a secondary effect of depression since obvious organization of the list greatly reduced the

memory deficit for depressed subjects with mean age 38. Caution may be a secondary effect of depression in unpaced secondary memory recognition tasks where, by comparison with normal old people, false alarm rates reduced more than hit rates in depression (Miller and Lewis, 1977; Larner, 1977), but not when the affective tone of the material was varied (Dunbar and Lishman, 1984) or in a paced primary memory task (Hilbert *et al.*, 1976). The status of other cognitive deficits in depression is even less clear. Hilbert *et al.* (1976) found that depressed patients were significantly slower to start searching sub-span digit lists but were no slower than controls once started. Cronholm and Ottosson (1961) compared immediate and 3 hour delayed recall and found that the proportional and absolute amounts forgotten were only slightly greater for depressed patients with mean age 50 than for controls. The discrimination of real from fictitious names of people who had been famous in the past but were no longer so was worse for depressed patients mean age 49 than controls (Frith *et al.*, 1983), but was significantly improved after treatment. However, this study adopted the assumptions of signal detection theory without supporting evidence (Richardson, 1979).

Clinical Implications of Cognition in Depression and Dementia

Assistance with the differential diagnosis of depression and dementia in old age must be very tentative at present since few studies include normal, depressed and demented old subjects. Those that do often find that demented subjects perform no better than chance (Hilbert *et al.*, 1976; Miller and Lewis, 1977). Thus, early preclinical cases of dementia are needed and must be compared with older depressed subjects than those used in the indicative studies of Weingartner (1981a, 1981b).

ACKNOWLEDGEMENTS

I am grateful to Professor D. B. Bromley and Mr J. J. Downes for constructive comments on an earlier draft.

REFERENCES

Albert, M.S., Butters, N., and Levin, J. (1979). Temporal gradients in the retrograde amnesia of patients with alcoholic Korsakoff's disease. *Arch. Neurol.*, **36**, 211–16.

Bäckman, L. (1985). Further evidence for the lack of adult age differences on free recall of subject-performed tasks: the importance of motor action. *Hum. Learn.*, **4**, 79–87.

Bayles, K.A. (1982). Language function in senile dementia. *Brain Lang.*, **16**, 265–80.

Binks, M.G. (1987). Clinical tests of memory as sensitive and specific signs of dementia. *Br. J. Psychiat.*, **150**, 719–20.

Binks, M.G., and Davies, A.D.M. (1984). The early detection of dementia. A baseline from healthy community dwelling old people. In: Bromley, D.B. (ed.) *Gerontology: Social and Behavioural Perspectives*, Croom Helm, London, pp. 7–13.

Binks, M.G., and Davies, A.D.M. (1985). The contribution of the National Adult Reading Test to the detection of dementia amongst community dwelling old people. In: Butler, A. (ed.) *Ageing: Recent Advances and Creative Responses*, Croom Helm, London, pp. 241–9.

Binks, M.G., and Sutcliffe, J. (1972). The effects of age and verbal ability on short-term recognition memory. *Bull. Br. Psychol. Soc.*, **25**, 146.

Birren, J.E., and Schaie, K.W. (Eds.) (1985). *Handbook of the Psychology of Aging*, second edition, Van Nostrand Reinhold, New York.

Bromley, D.B. (1958). Some effects of age on short-term learning and remembering. *J. Gerontol.*, **13**, 398–406.

Butters, N., and Albert, M.S. (1982). Processes underlying failures to recall remote events. In: Cermak, L.S. (ed.) *Human Memory and Amnesia*, Erlbaum, Hillsdale, New Jersey, pp. 257–74.

Cameron, P. (1975). Mood as an indicant of happiness: age, sex, social class and situational differences. *J. Gerontol.*, **30**, 216–24.

Cavanaugh, J.C., Grady, J.G., and Perlmutter, M. (1983). Forgetting and the use of memory aids in 20 to 70 year olds' everyday life. *Int. J. Aging Hum. Devel.*, **17**, 113–22.

Cohen, G. (1979). Language comprehension in old age. *Cognit. Psychol.*, **11**, 412–29.

Cohen, G. (1983). *The Psychology of Cognition*, second edition, Academic Press, London.

Cohen, G., and Faulkner, D. (1981). Memory for discourse in old age. *Discourse Processes*, **4**, 253–65.

Cohen, G., and Faulkner, D. (1986). Memory for proper names: age differences in retrieval. *Br. J. Devel. Psychol.*, **4**, 187–97.

Cooper, S. (1982). The post-Wechsler memory scale. *J. Clin. Psychol.*, **38**, 380–7.

Copeland, J.R.M., Dewey, M.E., and Griffith-Jones, H.M. (1986). A computerised psychiatric diagnostic system and case nomenclature for elderly subjects: GMS and AGECAT. *Psychol. Med.*, **16**, 89–99.

Costa, P.T., Jr, and McCrae, R.R. (1976). Age differences in personality structure: a cluster analytical approach. *J. Gerontol.*, **31**, 564–70.

Costa, P.T., Jr, and McCrae, R.R. (1977–8). Age differences in personality structure revisited: Studies in validity, stability and change. *Int. J. Aging Hum. Devel.*, **8**, 261–75.

Costa, P.T., Jr, and McCrae, R.R. (1978). Objective personality assessment. In: Storandt, M., Siegler, I.C., and Elias, M.F. (eds.) *The Clinical Psychology of Aging*, Plenum Press, New York, pp. 119–43.

Costa, P.T., Jr, and McCrae, R.R. (1985). Hypochondriasis, neuroticism, and aging. *Am. Psychol.*, **40**, 19–28.

Costa, P.T., Jr, and McCrae, R.R. (1986). Personality stability and its implications for clinical psychology. *Clin. Psychol. Rev.*, **6**, 407–24.

Costa, P.T., Jr, McCrae, R.R., and Arenberg, D. (1980). Enduring dispositions in adult males. *J. Personality Soc. Psychol.*, **38**, 793–800.

Craik, F.I.M. (1971). Age differences in recognition memory. *Q. J. Exp. Psychol.*, **23**, 316–23.

Craik, F.I.M., and Rabinowitz, J.C. (1984). Age differences in the acquisition and use of verbal information: a tutorial review. In: Bouma, H., and Bouwhuis, D.G. (eds.) *Attention and Performance X: Control of Language Processes*, Erlbaum, London, pp. 471–99.

Craik, F.I.M., and Rabinowitz, J.C. (1985). The effects of presentation rate and encoding task on age-related memory deficits. *J. Gerontol.*, **40**, 309–15.

Cronholm, B., and Ottosson, J. (1961). Memory functions in endogenous depression. *Arch. Gen. Psychiatry*, **5**, 193–7.

Diesfeldt, H.F.A. (1985). Verbal fluency in senile dementia: an analysis of search and knowledge. *Arch. Gerontol. Geriat.*, **4**, 231–9.

Douglas, K., and Arenberg, D. (1978). Age changes, cohort differences, and cultural change on the Guilford-Zimmerman Temperament Survey. *J. Gerontol.*, **33**, 737–47.

Dunbar, G.C., and Lishman, W.A. (1984). Depression, recognition memory and hedonic tone: a signal detection analysis. *Br. J. Psychiatry*, **144**, 376–82.

Frith, C.D., Stevens, M., and Johnstone, E.C. (1983). Effects of ECT and depression on various aspects of memory. *Br. J. Psychiatry*, **142**, 610–17.

Fuld, P.A. (1983). Psychometric differentiation of the dementias. In: Reisberg, B. (eds.) *Alzheimer's Disease*, The Free Press, New York, pp. 201–10.

Grant, I., and Adams, K.M. (1986). *Neuropsychological Assessment of Neuropsychiatric Disorders*, Oxford University Press, New York.

Hannay, H.J., and James, C.M. (1981). Simulation of a memory deficit on the continuous recognition memory test. *Percept. Motor Skills*, **53**, 51–8.

Harris, J.E. (1984). Remembering to do things: a forgotten

topic. In: Harris, J.E., and Morris, P.E. (eds.) *Everyday Memory Actions and Absent-mindedness*, Academic Press, London, pp. 71–92.

Heckhausen, H. (1983). Concern with one's competence: developmental shifts in person-environment interaction. In: Magnusson, D., and Allen, V.L. (eds.) *Human Development: an Interactional Perspective*, Academic Press, New York, pp. 167–85.

Hilbert, N.M., Niederehe, G., and Kahn, R.L. (1976). Accuracy and speed of memory in depressed and organic aged. *Educ. Gerontol.*, **1**, 131–46.

Houts, A.C., Cook, T.D., and Shadish, W.R. (1986). The person-situation debate: a critical multiplist perspective. *J. Personality*, **54**, 52–105.

Hulicka, I.M. (1982). Memory functioning in late adulthood. In: Craik, F.I.M., and Trehub, S. (eds.) *Aging and Cognitive Processes*, Plenum Press, New York, pp. 331–51.

Hunt, E. (1983). On the nature of intelligence. *Science*, **219**, 141–6.

Jorm, A.F. (1986). Cognitive deficit in the depressed elderly: a review of some basic unresolved issues. *Aust. N. Z. J. Psychiatry*, **20**, 11–22.

Kausler, D.H. (1982). *Experimental Psychology and Human Aging*, Wiley, New York.

Kausler, D.H., and Hakami, M.K. (1983). Memory for activities: adult age differences and intentionality. *Devel. Psychol.*, **19**, 889–94.

Kausler, D.H., Lichty, W., and Davis, R.T. (1985a). Temporal memory for performed activities: intentionality and adult age differences. *Devel. Psychol.*, **21**, 1132–8.

Kausler, D.H., Lichty, W., and Freund, J.S. (1985b). Adult age differences in recognition memory and frequency judgments for planned versus performed activities. *Devel. Psychol.*, **21**, 647–54.

Kendrick, D.C., Gibson, A.J., and Moyes, I.C.A. (1979). The revised Kendrick Battery: clinical studies. *Br. J. Soc. Clin. Psychol.*, **18**, 329–40.

Kopelman, M.D. (1985). Multiple memory deficits in Alzheimer-type dementia: implications for pharmacotherapy. *Psychol. Med.*, **15**, 527–41.

Kopelman, M.D. (1986). Clinical tests of memory. *Br. J. Psychiatry*, **148**, 517–25.

Labouvie-Vief, G. (1985). Intelligence and cognition. In: Birren, J.E., and Schaie, K.W. (eds.) *Handbook of the Psychology of Aging*, second edition, Van Nostrand Reinhold, New York, pp. 500–30.

Larner, S. (1977). Encoding in senile dementia and elderly depressives: a preliminary study. *Br. J. Soc. Clin. Psychol.*, **16**, 379–90.

Light, L.L., Zelinski, E.M., and Moore, M. (1982). Adult age differences in reasoning from new information. *J. Exp. Psychol. Learning, Memory and Cognition*, **8**, 435–47.

Maas, H.S., and Kuypers, J.A. (1974). *From Thirty to Seventy*, Jossey-Bass, San Francisco.

McCrae, R.R. (1982). Age differences in the use of coping mechanisms. *J. Gerontol.*, **37**, 454–60.

Malatesta, C.Z., and Kalnok, M. (1984). Emotional experience in younger and older adults. *J. Gerontol.*, **39**, 301–8.

Martin, A., and Fedio, P. (1983). Word production and comprehension in Alzheimer's disease: the breakdown of semantic knowledge. *Brain Lang.*, **19**, 124–41.

Martin, M. (1986). Ageing and patterns of change in everyday memory and cognition. *Hum. Learn.*, **5**, 63–74.

Miller, E., and Lewis, P. (1977). Recognition memory in elderly patients with depression and dementia: a signal detection analysis. *J. Abnorm. Psychol.*, **86**, 84–6.

Mischel, W., and Peake, P.K. (1982). Beyond déjà vu in the search for cross-situational consistency. *Psychol. Rev.*, **89**, 730–55.

Morris, R.G. (1984). Dementia and the functioning of the articulatory loop system. *Cognit. Neuropsychol.*, **1**, 143–57.

Morris, R.G. (1986). Short-term forgetting in senile dementia of the Alzheimer's type. *Cognit. Neuropsychol.*, **3**, 77–97.

Moscovitch, M. (1982). A neuropsychological approach to perception and memory in normal and pathological aging. In: Craik, F.I.M., and Trehub, S. (eds.) *Aging and Cognitive Processes*, Plenum Press, New York, pp. 55–78.

Neugarten, B.L., Crotty, W.J., and Tobin, S.S. (1980). Personality types in an aged population. In: Neugarten, B.L. *et al.* (eds.) *Personality in Middle and Late Life*, Arno Press, New York, reprint of 1964 edition, pp. 158–87.

Ober, B.A., Koss, E., and Friedland, R.P. (1985). Processes of verbal memory failure in Alzheimer-type dementia. *Brain Cognit.*, **4**, 90–103.

Ober, B.A., Dronkers, N.F., Koss, E., Delis, D.C., and Friedland, R.P. (1986). Retrieval from semantic memory in Alzheimer-type dementia. *J. Clin. Exp. Neuropsychol.*, **8**, 75–92.

Obler, L.K., and Albert, M.L. (1985). Language skills across adulthood. In: Birren, J.E., and Schaie, K.W. (eds.) *Handbook of the Psychology of Aging*, second edition, Van Nostrand Reinhold, New York, pp. 463–73.

O'Grady, K.E. (1983). A confirmatory factor analysis of the WAIS-R. *J. Consult. Clin. Psychol.*, **51**, 826–31.

Palmore, E. (1978). When can age, period and cohort be separated? *Social Forces*, **57**, 282–95.

Pankratz, L. (1983). A new technique for the assessment and modification of feigned memory deficit. *Percept. Motor Skills*, **57**, 367–72.

Parkinson, S.R., Lindholm, J.M., and Urell, T. (1980). Aging, dichotic memory, and digit span. *J. Gerontol.*, **35**, 87–95.

Petros, T., Tabor, L., Cooney, T., and Chabot, R.J. (1983). Adult age differences in sensitivity to semantic structure of prose. *Devel. Psychol.*, **19**, 907–14.

Rabbitt, P.M.A. (1977). Changes in problem solving ability in old age. In: Birren, J.E., and Schaie, K.W. (eds.) *Handbook of the Psychology of Aging*, first edition, Van Nostrand Reinhold, New York, pp. 606–25.

Rabbitt, P.M.A. (1981). Talking to the old. *New Society*, **55**, 140–1.

Rabbitt, P.M.A. (1982). Development of methods to measure changes in activities of daily living in the elderly. In: Corkin, S., Davis, K.L., Growdon, J.H., Usdin, E., and Wurtman, R.J. (eds.) *Alzheimer's Disease: A Report of Progress*, Raven Press, New York, pp. 127–31.

Rabbitt, P.M.A. (1986). Memory impairment in the elderly. In: Bebbington, P.E., and Jacoby, R. (eds.) *Psychiatric Disorders in the Elderly*, The Mental Health Foundation, London, pp. 101–19.

Rabinowitz, J.C., Craik, F.I.M., and Ackerman, B.P. (1982). A processing resource account of age differences in recall. *Can. J. Psychol.*, **36**, 325–44.

Richardson, J.T.E. (1979). Signal detection theory and the effects of severe head injury upon recognition memory. *Cortex*, **15**, 145–8.

Robertson-Tchabo, E.A. (1980). Cognitive-skill training for the elderly: why should 'old dogs' acquire new tricks? In: Poon, L.W., Fozard, J.L., Cermak, L.S., Arenberg, D., and Thompson, L.W. (eds.) *New Directions in Memory and Aging*, Erlbaum, Hillsdale, New Jersey, pp. 511–17.

Roth, M., Tyme, E., Mountjoy, C.Q., Huppert, F.A., Hendrie, H., Verma, S., and Goddard, R. (1986). CAMDEX a standardised instrument for the diagnosis of mental disorder in the elderly with special reference to the early detection of dementia. *Br. J. Psychiatry*, **149**, 698–709.

Salthouse, T.A. (1982). *Adult Cognition*, Springer, New York.

Schacter, D.L. (1986). Feeling-of-knowing ratings distinguish between genuine and simulated forgetting. *J. Exp. Psychol.: Learning, Memory, and Cognition*, **12**, 30–41.

Schultz, R. (1982). Emotionality and ageing: a theoretical and empirical analysis. *J. Gerontol.*, **37**, 42–51.

Seigler, I.C., George, L.K., and Okun, M.A. (1979). Cross-sequential analysis of adult personality. *Devel. Psychol.*, **15**, 350–1.

Spilich, G.J. (1983). Life-span components of text processing: structural and procedural differences. *J. Verb. Learn. Verb. Behav.*, **22**, 231–44.

Sunderland, A., Harris, J.E., and Gleave, J. (1984). Memory failures in everyday life following severe head injury. *J. Clin. Neuropsychol.*, **6**, 127–42.

Teseri, J.A., Golden, R.R., and Gurland, B.J. (1984). Concurrent and predictive validity of indicator scales developed for the Comprehensive Assessment and Referral Evaluation Interview Schedule. *J. Gerontol.*, **39**, 158–65.

Thomae, H. (1970). Theory of ageing and cognitive theory of personality. *Hum. Devel.* **13**, 1–10.

Waugh, N.C., Thomas, J.C., and Fozard, J.L. (1978). Retrieval time from different memory stores. *J. Gerontol.*, **33**, 718–24.

Weingartner, H., Cohen, R.M., Murphy, D.L., Martello, J., and Gerdt, C. (1981a). Cognitive processes in depression. *Arch. Gen. Psychiatry*, **38**, 42–7.

Weingartner, H., Kaye, W., Smallberg, S.A., Ebert, M.H., Gillin, J.C., and Sitaram, N. (1981b). Memory failures in progressive idiopathic dementia. *J. Abnorm. Psychol.*, **80**, 187–96.

Wilson, R.S., Kaszniak, A.W., and Fox, J.H. (1981). Remote memory in senile dementia. *Cortex*, **17**, 41–8.

Winblad, B., Hardy, J., Bäckman, L., and Nilsson, L.-G. (1985). Memory function and brain biochemistry in normal aging and in senile dementia. *Ann. N.Y. Acad. Sci.*, **444**, 255–68.

Woods, R.T., and Britton, P.G. (1985). *Clinical Psychology with the Elderly*, Croom Helm, London.

Wright, R.E. (1981). Aging, divided attention and processing capacity. *J. Gerontol.*, **36**, 605–14.

Zelinski, E.M., Gilewski, M.J., and Thompson, L.W. (1980). Do laboratory tests relate to self-assessment of memory ability in the young and old? In: Poon, L.W., Fozard, J.L., Cermak, L.S., Arenberg, D., and Thompson, L.W. (eds.) *New Directions in Memory and Aging*, Erlbaum, Hillsdale, New Jersey, pp. 519–44.

The Clinical Neurology of Old Age
Edited by R. Tallis
© 1989 John Wiley & Sons Ltd

Chapter 3

The Influence of Age on Neurological Recovery

L.S. Illis

Consultant Neurologist, Wessex Neurological Centre, Southampton General Hospital, and Clinical Senior Lecturer in Neurology, University of Southampton Medical School, Southampton, UK

Recovery of function following a lesion in the central nervous system (CNS) has always been an intriguing and puzzling phenomenon for the neurologist, neuroscientist and those in the field of rehabilitation. In the last 20 years or so, following a long period of relative lack of interest and even cynicism, the phenomenon has attracted increasing attention. Clearly, if the mechanisms of recovery were known, not only would the organization of the CNS be more fully understood, but also methods for aiding recovery in man would become more rational and systematic.

Until relatively recently it was a common belief (still perpetuated in many textbooks) that nervous system connections are laid down during development and subsequent changes are due only to loss of nerve cells. This imposed a serious, if not insurmountable, restriction on understanding recovery of function after injury. In the last two decades, however, there has been increasing evidence of the great structural and functional adaptability of even the adult nervous system in response to partial lesions and to alterations in the environment. This response is manifested in changed connectivity due to the formation of new synapses or unmasking of pre-existing but relatively little used synapses. How the process of recovery works, why it does not work more efficiently, and similar questions remain unanswered.

Even more uncertain is the influence of age on neurological recovery. In this review, an attempt will be made to outline determinants of recovery in the central nervous system and to give some idea of the way in which age might influence these determinants. The fact that problems of recovery and the problems of ageing are under intensive investigation mean that much of what will be said in this review will, thankfully, be outdated over the next few years.

The ageing process is a complex, widespread and non-uniform change involving mental, sensory, motor, autonomic, metabolic and endocrine functions. Species, individual and organ differences support the belief that, to a large extent, ageing is genetically determined, though the rate of ageing may be environmentally influenced. The diversity of the functions affected by the ageing process makes it virtually certain that the nervous system is involved in the regulation of this process. The anatomical or histological changes which occur in the normal ageing process are still ill-defined and this makes them difficult to distinguish from changes which are secondary to age-related disease, such as cerebrovascular disease.

Since ageing within individuals is displayed in a non-uniform way, it follows that not all parts of the central nervous system will age at the same time—a fact well known in clinical neurology. If one area is changing (ageing) more rapidly than another, this may have effects, not only within the ageing area but also on other areas of the central nervous system in neuronal contact with the affected part. We know that lesions in the central nervous system produce progressive alterations in the intact nervous system. This is not entirely of theoretical interest. At the present time it is not possible to halt or slow down the ageing process, but if the ageing process is having a deleterious effect on relatively intact or relatively normal parts of the central nervous system then this may, at least theoretically, be amenable to treatment.

SOME EFFECTS OF AGEING

Cellular changes

Reports of global brain cell loss with age reminds one of advertisements for dandruff treatment. They are not based on fact. Some experimental studies show no loss of nerve cells with age (Brizzee *et al.*, 1968; Diamond *et al.*, 1977) but most studies suggest that the CNS neurone population does decline with age, but in a non-uniform way. For example the striatum, substantia nigra, locus coeruleus and dorsal nucleus of the vagus show most degenerative change, whereas other brain stem nuclei show relatively little alteration (Bugiani *et al.*, 1978; Corsellis, 1976; Peng and Lee, 1979). There is a marked loss of cells in the monoaminergic neuronal systems (Teravainen and Calne, 1983). The overall decline of neurone population with age, neglecting the heterogeneous pattern, is roughly of the order of 60–70% at the age of 80–90 years, compared to age 20 years (Brody, 1955; Henderson *et al.*, 1980).

Dendrites

Loss of terminal dendrites and dendritic spines has been demonstrated in pyramidal neurones of rat cortex (Feldman and Dowd, 1974; Feldman, 1976) and also the human pre-frontal and temporal cortex (Scheibel, 1978). Changes in the dendritic trees include a decrease in arborization and often irregularities and blunting of processes. Diamond and Connor (1984), however, point out that although the alteration in dendritic morphology may be an

effect of ageing these changes may also be influenced by the environment.

Myelin

With increasing age there is a decrease in the total brain myelin by some 30% (Berlet and Volk, 1980). The major change is in lipid synthesis. Considerably more work has been done on myelin in the peripheral nervous system (Jacobs and Love, 1985). With age there appears to be an alteration in the ratio of axon diameter to fibre diameter (g ratio), the ratio normally increasing with increasing fibre size. Over the age of about 60 years degeneration and demyelination of myelinated fibres becomes increasingly common: with age there is an increase in the number of axons with thick myelin sheaths and therefore an abnormally low g ratio. The cause of the changes in peripheral nerve in the elderly is not known. They may be related to loss of anterior horn cells with age or the prevalence of degenerative disease with age. It has some significance with regard to central nervous system functioning. Presumably if the axon/myelin diameter ratio alters then the speed of conduction along these nerves will alter. This means that the pattern of impulses impinging on the central nervous system will alter both temporally and spatially. This will have an effect on the pattern of stimulation of central nervous system cells at successively higher levels. In this way, even an apparently small change with age in the peripheral nervous system may have an effect in the central nervous system.

Synapse Density

Synapse density is much easier to measure in animals than in humans for obvious reasons of difficulties with fixation. As far as is known, the density of synapses on the cell surface is much the same in all animals. In the cat, the density of synaptic terminals is similar on both cell body and dendrite and there is no correlation between the size of bouton and its position on the cell or dendrite surface (Illis, 1964a; 1964b). The density of synaptic endings is about 20 per 100 μm^2 (Wyckoff and Young, 1956). It has been estimated that a large central nervous system may have 30 000 or more synaptic terminals or, put

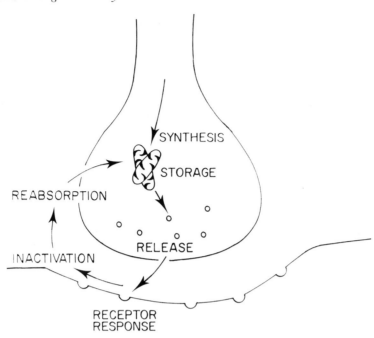

Figure 3.1. Possible stages where synaptic transmission may fail or be reduced with age.

another way, there are units in the central nervous system which have 30 000 or more inputs from diverse sources and one output ending in many places. This synaptic zone is the truly unique aspect of the central nervous system in that it is an area of discontinuity and one where all integration must take place. Unfortunately not much is known about age-related changes in this area. Houttenlocher (1979) has indicated that the synaptic density in human frontal cortex drops about 13% with age—comparing patients over the age of 74 with those below the age of 74.

Neurotransmitters

Neurotransmitters have been studied by Ordy and Brizzee (1975) and Ordy (1982) amongst others. There appears to be a reduction in choline acetyltransferase and in acetylcholinesterase. Cholinergic receptors are reduced (Freund, 1980) as are dopamine receptors (Makman *et al.*, 1979; Govoni *et al.*, 1977). Noradrenaline falls by about half by the ninth decade. There is a 25% fall in muscarinic receptors (Nordberg *et al.*, 1982) and an even bigger fall in nicotinic receptors (about 40%) between the ages of 60 years and 90 years.

One of the effects of these alterations in neurotransmitters, together with alteration in conduction is that there is a considerable alteration in the central processing of signals (see Table 3.1 and Figure 3.1).

In summary, there are age-related changes in the peripheral nervous system which may produce a deleterious effect on CNS function, and there are alterations in nerve cells, dendrites, myelin and neurotransmission in the CNS. One would expect all of these changes to be reflected in altered function. It is not surprising, therefore, that with age there is slowing in the performance of various motor tasks and an increased latency of any kind of sensory evoked response. Does this mean that there must be an inexorable decline of function with age and little, if any, chance of recovery after a lesion; or is limited recovery still a possibility?

THE NATURE OF RECOVERY OF FUNCTION

Some aspects of the early recovery of function after a lesion in the central nervous system can be readily understood and explained by the transient and reversible changes which occur at or near the edge of

TABLE 3.1   FACTORS ALTERING CENTRAL PROCESSING

Decrease in conduction velocity in peripheral nerves	Dorfman and Bosley (1979) Norris *et al.* (1953)
Increased latencies in multi-synaptic pathways	Dorfman and Bosley (1979) Chambers *et al.* (1966)
Impaired synaptic potentiation	Lanfield *et al.* (1978)
Decreased conduction at neuromuscular junction	Smith (1979)
Loss of receptors	Freund (1980)—cholinergic Makman *et al.* (1979)—dopamine Greenberg and Weiss (1978)—adrenergic
Abnormal synaptic calcium transport	Sun and Seaman (1977)

the lesion and reflect reversible damage to nerve cells and reversible metabolic and circulatory changes. The long-term recovery of function cannot be explained in these ways.

Although this may represent something of a simplification, it is possible to identify two opposing views as to the nature of recovery of function. One view comes from von Monakow's concept of 'diaschisis' (von Monakow, 1914). This has become a rather fashionable concept. It was originally suggested as the explanation for spontaneous recovery after a lesion in the CNS. If a part of the CNS is destroyed, a distant (and intact) part with which it was in neuronal contact stops functioning. After a period of time the 'depressed' area recovers its ability to function.

Although von Monakow was unable to explain the mechanism of recovery, it was clear that it would be due to removal of 'depression' rather than to structural reorganization of the CNS. Even so, this is less an explanation than a re-description, although some recent work suggests physiological or pharmacological mechanisms.

The second view invokes the concept of the plasticity of the CNS. It is assumed that recovery of function is consequent upon a reorganization of the nervous system directed towards a re-establishment of the structural and physiological basis of the function originally lost. This is analogous to Le Chatelier's principle: if a system is in equilibrium and one of the conditions of the system is altered, the system will adjust itself in such a way as partially to neutralize the change of condition. This principle, well known in physical and chemical science, was first applied to biological systems (specifically recovery) in 1967 (Illis, 1967b). The anatomical and physiological basis for this view lies in observations on axonal sprouting and unmasking of new synapses. Recovery of function may be due to opening up of paths not normally or previously used by the organism, or to reorganization of the intact nervous system after a lesion has occurred, or to both mechanisms.

Neurotransmitters and the Effects of Lesions

Studies of the effect of a lesion in the CNS indicate that the clinical effects are not due solely to destruction of certain pathways present in the normal or intact CNS but also to a gradual alteration of the entire CNS which may take place over a period of time following a lesion (see Illis, 1982).

In the same way it might be expected that the effects of ageing will be in part due to depletion of certain pathways and in part to gradual alteration of the remainder of the CNS as it reacts to this process. The application of von Monakow's concept of diaschisis here may be perhaps best understood by looking at the pharmacology of the central nervous system and the pharmacological changes which may be produced by injury.

There are at least three types of communication between nerve cells: point-to-point or fast transmission; neuromodulation, involving the indirect alteration of postsynaptic conductance by altering neurotransmitter release or by altering postsynaptic responsiveness (this is seen with encephalins, opiates, benzodiazepines); and neurohormonal communication where there is no synaptic contact but long-lasting changes of target cells following stimulation of specific peptidergic neurones. In contrast to fast point-to-point transmitters such as gamma-aminobutyric acid (GABA), glycine, L-glutamate and L-aspartate, monoamine release is associated with diffuse neural pathways and with nerve cells localized mostly in the brain stem and with diffuse ramifications to wide terminal fields so that very large numbers of cells may be affected. It is generally accepted that these pathways, which use catecholamines (adrenaline, noradrenaline and dopamine), are modulatory (Iversen, 1982). The noradrenergic system, originating mostly from brain stem nuclei (locus coeruleus), innervates the cerebral cortex, cerebellum, hippocampus, hypothalamus and spinal cord, and, indeed, ramifies to virtually the entire CNS.

Endogenous opiates may interact with other physiological systems, particularly in the autonomic nervous system. Opioids are co-stored with catecholamines in sympathetic ganglia and adrenal medulla and may be released with catecholamines and under the same controls as them. The opioid antagonist, naloxone, has been used as a blocking agent to investigate endogenous opiate function and in the treatment of a variety of neurological disorders. In the spinal injured cat, naloxone has been reported to decrease neurological impairment and increase spinal cord blood flow (Faden *et al.*, 1981; Young *et al.*, 1981). Improvement has been reported in stroke (Baskin and Hosobuchi, 1981), experimental hemiplegia (Baskin *et al.*, 1982) and subacute necrotizing encephalopathy (Brandt *et al.*, 1980). It would seem that pharmacological reversal of neurological deficit is not only a possibility but that at least part of the clinical picture is produced by pharmacological changes acting via a neuromodulatory system.

The amenability of damage involving the catecholamine system to treatment raises questions as to the true nature of such a deficit. It suggests an explanation of the previously purely descriptive concept of diaschisis. Unilateral cortical ablation in rat and cat produces a specific deficit which can be altered pharmacologically (Feeney *et al.*, 1982) by a single injection of amphetamine providing that the animal is kept mobile. The reversal of neurological deficit does not occur if the animal is confined—from which it may be inferred that sensory feedback is essential for recovery. This can be retarded or reversed by catecholamine antagonists such as phenoxybenzamine (Feeney *et al.*, 1983) and can be blocked by haloperidol when given early after the injury. The reversal of deficit and the time scale is such that it cannot be due to a direct pharmacological effect on the original, primary, damage but must be an effect on disturbed function remote from the lesion. This would be compatible with the suggestion already made that original insult to the CNS produces its effects not only by direct damage but also indirectly by causing functional abnormality of other areas of CNS. The noradrenaline system, with its widespread ramifications to a broad target area and its modulatory effect, is an obvious candidate for the pharmacological basis for diaschisis—alone or in conjunction with the neuropeptide system.

Recent biochemical and histological work supports the hypothesis of remote effects of cortical injury. Following unilateral ligation of the middle cerebral artery in rats bilateral reduction in noradrenaline has been found in the cortex and in the locus coeruleus (Robinson *et al.*, 1977; 1979; 1980). Similarly, abnormal cerebrospinal fluid (CSF) monoamine activity has been found in man after stroke (Meyer *et al.*, 1974). Following unilateral cortical injury, a change in oxidative metabolism in uninjured cortical areas can be demonstrated and these changes may be modified by lesions of the locus coeruleus (Dail *et al.*, 1981). Since the cells of the locus coeruleus are in the brain stem and injury is restricted to cortical tissue, these changes indicate that a remote reaction to brain injury may occur, perhaps through damage to a terminal projection site of the locus coeruleus in the cortex.

The implication of this work, in relation to rehabilitation in man, is that damage to a particular area of the CNS produces not only irreparable damage but also 'functional' damage. It is possible that appropriate drug therapy administered during the rehabilitation programme may accelerate recovery by alleviation of the 'functional' damage although clearly it is unlikely to have any effect on the primary damage. Since there is a reduction in neurotransmitters with age, any drug treatment used in rehabilitation must cope with the additional fact that an ageing brain has a relative deficit in neurotransmitters quite apart from the direct effects of injury.

Formation of Synaptic Contacts and Sprouting of Intact Fibres

The mature nervous system contains far fewer nerve cells than are present during embryonic life and it is not known what stimulus or reaction is responsible for the survival of some developing neurones and the death of others. It appears that developing neurones must make synaptic contact with appropriate target cells in order to survive (Purves and Nja, 1978). The organization at synaptic level as the nervous system develops and matures probably involves the elimination of synapses via a mechanism known as contact inhibition. When appropriate cells are contacted, nerve growth ceases so that neurones carry a finite number of terminals. If some of these degenerate due to axonal injury then uninjured axons sprout to fill the local sites available and consequently expand the synaptic field of the injured axons. Sprouting continues into adult life. It is not known whether sprouting is triggered only by degeneration metabolites, or whether all terminals have a constant tendency to sprout, though sprouting is normally limited by adjacent boutons as suggested by the concept of contact inhibition. Removal of contact inhibition will result in continuous remodelling of the intact nervous system or reorganization and regeneration of the damaged nervous system. The sprouting of uninjured axons to fill local sites available and the expansion of synaptic fields of uninjured axons means that function will alter as the relative contribution of afferent axons to larger cells changes. Collateral sprouting is recognized as a widespread phenomenon and has been demonstrated in peripheral, central and autonomic systems

(Edds, 1953; Murray and Thompson, 1957; Liu and Chambers, 1958; Illis, 1967b, 1973a, 1973b; Raisman, 1969; Lynch *et al.*, 1973).

Although the fact of sprouting is fairly well established, its significance is uncertain. It is not known whether it is really a form of regeneration and an attempt to restore normal function, or a random response resulting in haphazard and inappropriate activity. And, as mentioned above, it is still not known whether sprouting is initiated by the lesion or is a natural continuing process in the normal CNS.

Sprouting alone cannot explain early changes occurring in the nervous system following injury. Moreover the alteration of relative contributions of terminals to a target site will produce an abnormal connectivity which, though contributing to the altered clinical state, is not necessarily contributing to recovery.

Unmasking of Existing Synapses

In the last 8 years a new and important aspect of plasticity has been uncovered by the work of Wall and his colleague (Merrill and Wall, 1978). One of the very important features of this work is that many of the experiments were carried out in *adult* animals. The experiments demonstrate that when nerve cells are de-afferented and therefore lose their normal input, they begin to respond to new inputs, i.e. inputs which in the intact animal elicit no response. Unmasking is seen not only following degeneration but also when there is a change of afferent bombardment producing a central alteration of receptive fields (Devor and Wall, 1976).

This work has definite implications for rehabilitation in neurological deficit in man. For example, in both sprouting and unmasking, previously unused or little used pathways now take on a more significant role. Goldberger and Murray (1974) have demonstrated the occurrence of reflex activity unmasked by chronic de-afferentation. Faganel and Dimitrijevic (1982) studied ankle jerks after conditioning with noxious electrical stimuli applied to thoracic, lumbar and sacral dermatomes in patients with clinically complete spinal cord injury. Painful cutaneous stimulation applied to the skin produces a reflex contraction withdrawal. In patients with a complete transverse lesion the induced excitation spreads to adjacent and more distant cranial and caudal segments both ipsilaterally and contralaterally (Sherrington, 1910). This spread of reflexes, not seen in the normal or intact spinal cord, reflects altered anatomy and physiology.

The alteration in anatomy can be explained in terms of sprouting and/or unmasking since the existence of crossed monosynaptic afferents and the spread over adjacent and distant segments has been demonstrated anatomically (Illis, 1967a; 1973a). The alteration in physiology is on the basis of such anatomy. That is, in the intact spinal cord, the anatomical substrate is present but is 'masked' by a dominant system of connections. One effect of a lesion is to alter this dominance (Illis, 1967b). The new responses of the partially denervated CNS following a lesion or the altered responses of an ageing nervous system in which different parts of the CNS age at different rates, could be due to disinhibition or unmasking of different afferents either by alteration of inhibition (disinhibition of synaptic inhibition) or by denervation hypersensitivity. There appears to be an immediate development of new receptive fields followed by a later development of new inputs.

Recovery

We have already discussed several theories of recovery. A further theory is based on the rather ill-defined concept of 'substitution'. A different part of the nervous system takes over the task of controlling a particular function lost as the result of a lesion. This theory is perhaps one of the most popular in textbooks of neurology and has a certain amount of appeal because of its simplicity. It is, however, empty unless the precise pathways involved, and the mechanisms by which substitution takes place, can be demonstrated.

As indicated above, it would appear that recovery in the nervous system can be at least partially explained in pharmacological, anatomical and physiological terms. Indeed, determinants of recovery may be listed, however tentatively (see Goldberger and Murray, 1978; Devor, 1982; Illis, 1982). It is only by basing rehabilitation or therapeutic stategies

upon such pharmacology, physiology and anatomy that any progress is likely to be made. As an example of such therapeutic rehabilitation strategies one may look at the effect of external stimulation.

Repetitive electrical stimulation has been used in the treatment of various neurological diseases, especially multiple sclerosis and spinal cord injury, and has been shown to produce improvement in spasticity, bladder control and pain (see Illis *et al.*, 1983; Sherwood, 1985). The influence of stimulation on recovery following CNS lesions is now widely accepted in Europe but less generally accepted in the USA. The use of environmental stimulation in promoting recovery from brain damage has also been the subject of considerable research. Goldman and Lewis (1978), for example, have shown that the effect of environmental stimulation in accelerating recovery is due not simply to a training effect; that recovery does not occur if there is extensive damage or involvement of critical areas; that the earlier environmental stimulation is provided the better the chances of recovery; and that recovery is inversely related to age. If identical lesions are suffered by infants and adults, and the same postoperative environmental stimulation is provided, the recovery of function is seen only in those animals operated on as infants.

CONCLUSION

This short review has indicated some of the mechanisms of recovery and their relevance to ageing populations. Many of the barriers to recovery are the same irrespective of age but clearly age itself produces changes in the central nervous system which will have an adverse affect on any process of recovery. It will therefore affect the application of therapeutic procedures. Nevertheless, such approaches to rehabilitation are really in their infancy and the fact that the patient is old should not rule out the use of soundly based therapeutic procedures. Rather, an ageing population should be an encouragement and a stimulus to further study.

REFERENCES

Baskin, D.S., and Hosobuchi, Y. (1981). Naloxone reversal of ischaemic neurological deficits in man. *Lancet*, **ii**, 272.

Baskin, D.S., Kiech, C.F., and Hosobuchi, Y. (1982). Naloxone reversal of ischaemic deficits in baboons is not mediated by systemic effects. *Life Sci.*, **31**, 2201.

Berlet, H.H., and Volk, B. (1980). Age related micro-heterogeneity of myelin basic protein isolated from human brain. In: Amaducci, I. (ed.) *Ageing of the Brain and Dementia*, Raven Press, New York, p. 81.

Brandt, N.J., Terenius, L., Jacobsen, B.B., Klinken, L., Nordus, A., Brandt, S., Blegvad, K., and Yssing, M. (1980). Hyper-endorphin syndrome in a child with necrotising encephalopathy. *N. Engl. J. Med.*, **303**, 914.

Brizzee, K.R., Sherwood, N., and Timiras, P.S. (1968). A comparison of various depth levels in cerebral cortex of young adults and aged Long-Evans rats. *J. Gerontol.*, **23**, 289–97.

Brody, H. (1955). Organisation of the Cerebral Cortex. III. A study of ageing in the human cerebral cortex. *J. Comp. Neurol.*, **102**, 511.

Bugiani, O., Salvarani, S., Perdelli, F., Mancardi, G.L., and Leonardi, A. (1978). Nerve cell loss in the putamen. *Eur. Neurol.*, **17**, 286.

Chambers, W.P., Dunihue, P.N., Smith, C.J., Blanchard, R.R., Taylor, C.H., and Hill, D.B. (1986). Effect of vasopressin and adrenal steroids on cortical responses evoked at mid-brain level in aged rats. *Gerontologia*, **12**, 65.

Corsellis, J.A.N. (1976). Ageing and dementias. In: Blackwood, W. and Corsellis, J.A.N. (eds.) *Greenfield's Neuropathology*, Edward Arnold, London.

Dail, W.G., Feeney, D.M., Murray, H.M., Linn, R.T., and Boyson, M.G. (1981). Responses to cortical injury: II widespread depression of the activity of an enzyme in cortex remote from a focal injury. *Brain Res.*, **211**, 79.

Devor, M. (1982). Plasticity in the adult nervous system. In: Illis, L.S., Sedgwick, E.M., and Glanville, H.J. (eds.) *Rehabilitation of the Neurological Patient*. Blackwell Scientific, Oxford, pp. 44–84.

Devor, M., and Wall, P.B. (1976). Dorsal horn cells with proximal cutaneous receptive fields. *Brain Res.*, **118**, 325.

Diamond, M.C., and Connor, J.R. (1984). Morphological measurements in the ageing rat cerebral cortex. In: Scheff, S.W. (ed.) *Ageing and Recovery of Function in the CNS*, Plenum Press, New York.

Diamond, M.C., Johnson, R.E. and Gold, M.W. (1977). Changes in neuron and glia number in the young, adult and ageing rat occipital cortex. *Behav. Biol.*, **20**, 409–18.

Dorfman, L.J., and Bosley, T.M. (1979). Age related changes in peripheral and central nerve conduction in man. *Neurology (Minneap.)*, **29**, 38.

Edds, M.V. (1953). Collateral nerve regeneration. *Quart. Rev. Biol*, **28**, 260–276.

Faden, L., Jacobs, T.P., Mougey, E., and Holaday, J.W. (1981). Endorphins in experimental spinal injury: therapeutic effect of naloxone. *Ann. Neurol.*, **10**, 325.

Faganel, J., and Dimitrijevic, M.R. (1982). Study of propiospinal interneurone system in man: cutaneous exteroceptive conditioning of stretch reflexes. *J. Neurol. Sci.*, **56**, 155.

Feeney, D.M., Gonzalez, A., and Law, W.A. (1982). Amphetamine, haloperidol and experience interact to affect rate of recovery after motor cortex lesion. *Science*, **217**, 855.

Feeney, D.M., Houda, D.A., and Salo, A.A. (1983). Phenoxybenzamine reinstates all motor and sensory deficits in cats fully recovered from sensorimotor cortex ablations. *Fed. Am. Soc. Exp. Biol.*, **42**, 1157.

Feldman, M.L. (1976). Ageing in the morphology of cortical dendrites. In: Ordsy, J.M., and Brizzee, K.R. (eds.) *Neurobiology of Ageing*, Raven Press, New York, p. 211.

Feldman, M.L., and Dowd, C. (1974). Ageing in rat visual cortex: light microscopic observations on layer V pyramidal apical dendrites. *Anat. Rec.*, **178**, 355.

Freund, G. (1980). Cholinergic receptor loss in brain of ageing mouse. *Life Sci.*, **26**, 371.

Goldberger, M.E., and Murray, M. (1974). Restitution of function and collateral sprouting in the cat spinal cord: The deafferented animal. *J. Comp. Neurol.*, **158**, 37–54.

Goldberger, M.E., and Murray, M. (1978). Recovery of movement and axonal sprouting may obey some of the same laws. In: Cotman, C.W. (ed.) *Neuronal Plasticity*, Raven Press, New York, pp. 73–96.

Goldman, P.S., and Lewis, M.E. (1978). Developmental biology of brain damage and experience. In: Cotman, C.W. (ed.) *Neuronal Plasticity*, Raven Press, New York, pp. 291–310.

Govoni, S., Loddo, P., Spano, P.F., and Trabucci, M. (1977). Dopamine receptor sensitivity in brain and retina of rats during ageing. *Brain Res.*, **138**, 565.

Greenberg, L.H., and Weiss, B. (1978). α-Adrenergic receptors in aged rat brain. *Science*, **201**, 61.

Henderson, G., Tomlinson, B.E., and Gibson, P.H. (1980). Cell counts in human cerebral cortex in normal adults throughout life using an image analysing computer. *J. Neurol. Sci.*, **46**, 113.

Houttenlocher, P.R. (1979). Synaptic density in human frontal cortex—developmental changes in effects of ageing. *Brain Res.*, **163**, 195.

Illis, L.S. (1964a). Spinal cord synapses in the cat: normal appearances. *Brain*, **87**, 543.

Illis, L.S. (1964b). Spinal cord synapses in the cat: reaction at motorneurone surface. *Brain*, **87**, 555.

Illis, L.S. (1967a). The relative densities of monosynaptic pathways to cells and dendrites in the ventral horn. *J. Neurol. Sci.*, **4**, 259.

Illis, L.S. (1967b). The mononeurone surface and spinal shock. In: Williams, D. (ed.) *Modern Trends in Neurology*, Series 4, Butterworths, London, pp. 53–68.

Illis, L.S. (1973a). An experimental model of regeneration in the CNS: I synaptic changes. *Brain*, **96**, 47.

Illis, L.S. (1973b). An experimental model of regeneration in the CNS: II glial changes. *Brain*, **96**, 61.

Illis, L.S. (1982). Determinants of recovery. *Int. Rehab. Med.*, **4,** 166.

Illis, L.S., Read, D.J., Sedgwick, E.M., and Tallis, R.C. (1983). Spinal cord stimulation in the United Kingdom. *J. Neurol. Neurosurg. Psychiatry*, **46,** 299.

Iversen, L.I. (1982). Neurotransmitters and CNS disease. *Lancet*, **ii,** 914.

Jacobs, J.M., and Love, S. (1985). Qualitative and quantitative morphology of human sural nerve at different ages. *Brain*, **108,** 897–924.

Lanfield, P.W., McGaugh, J.L., and Lynch, G. (1978). Impaired synaptic potentiation in the hippocampus of aged, memory-deficient rats. *Brain Res.*, **150,** 85.

Liu, G.N., and Chambers, W.W. (1958). Intraspinal sprouting of dorsal root axons. *Arch. Neurol. Psychiatry*, **79,** 44–61.

Lynch, G., Deadwyler, S., and Cotman, C. (1973). Postlesion axonal growth produces permanent functional connections. *Science*, **180,** 1364–6.

Makman, M.H., Ahn, H.S., Thal, L.J., Sharpless, N.S., Dvorkin, B., Horowitz, S.G., and Rosenfeld, M. (1979). Ageing and monoamine receptors in brain. *Fed. Proc.*, **38,** 1922.

Merrill, E.G., and Wall, P.B. (1978). Plasticity of connections in the adult nervous system. In: Cotman, C.W. (ed.) *Neuronal Plasticity*, Raven Press, New York, pp. 97–111.

Meyer, J.S., Welch, K.M., Okamoto, S., and Shimazu, K. (1974). Disorder neurotransmitter function. Demonstration by measurement of norepinephine and 5HT in CSF of patients with recent cerebral infarction. *Brain*, **97,** 655–64.

Monakow, C., von (1914). *Dass Grosshirn und die Abbaufunktion Durch Kortikale*, Bergman, Herde Wiesbaden.

Murray, J.G., and Thompson, J.W. (1957). The occurrence and function of collateral sprouting in the sympathetic nervous system of the cat. *J. Physiol.*, **135,** 133.

Nordberg, A., Adolfson, R., and Marcusson, J. (1982). Cholinergic receptors in the hippocampus in normal ageing and dementia of Alzheimer type. In: Giacobini, E., Filogama, G., and Giocabini, G. (eds.) *The Ageing Brain: Cellular and Molecular Mechanisms of Ageing in the Nervous System. Ageing*, Vol. 20. Raven Press, New York, p. 231.

Norris, A.H., Shock, N.W., and Wagman, I.H. (1953). Age changes in the maximum conduction velocity of motor fibres of human ulnar nerves. *J. Appl. Physiol.*, **5,** 589.

Ordy, J.M. (1982). Geriatric psychopharmacology: drug modification of memory and emotionality in relation to ageing human and non-human primate brain. In: Hoffmeister, F., and Muller, C. (eds.) *Brain Function in Old Age*, Springer-Verlag, Berlin, p. 435.

Ordy, J.M., and Brizzee, K. (1975). *Neurology of Ageing*, Plenum Press, New York.

Peng, M.T., and Lee, L.R. (1979). Regional differences of neuron loss of rat brain in old age. *Gerontology*, **25,** 205.

Purves, D., and Nja, A. (1978). Trophic maintenance of synaptic connections in autonomic ganglia. In: Cotman, C.W. (ed.) *Neuronal Plasticity*, Raven Press, New York, pp. 27–47.

Raisman, G. (1969). Neuronal plasticity in the septal nuclei of the adult rat. *Brain Res.*, **14,** 25.

Robinson, R.G., Bloom, F.E., and Battenberg, E.L. (1977). A fluorescent histochemical study of changes in noradrenergic neurons following experimental cerebral infarction in the rat. *Brain Res.*, **132,** 259.

Robinson, R.G., and Coyle, J.T. (1979). Lateralisation of catecholaminergic and behavioural response to cerebral infarction in the rat. *Life Sci.*, **24,** 943.

Robinson, R.G., and Coyle, J.T. (1980). The differential effect of right versus left hemispheric cerebral infarction on catecholamines and behaviour in the rat. *Brain Res.*, **188,** 63.

Scheibel, A.B. (1978). Structural aspects of the ageing brain. Spine systems and dendrite arbor. In: Katzman, R., Terry, R.D., and Bick, K.L. (eds.) *Alzheimer's Disease. Senile Dementia and Related Disorders*, Raven Press, New York, p. 11.

Sherrington, C.S. (1910). *The Integrative Action of the Nervous System*, Constable, London.

Sherwood, A.M. (1985). Electrical stimulation of the spinal cord in movement disorders. In: Myklebust, J.B., Cusick, J.F., Sances, J., and Larson, S.T. (eds.) *Neural Stimulation*, Vol. I, CRC Press, Florida, pp. 111–46.

Smith, D.O. (1979). Reduced capabilities of synaptic transmission in aged rats. *Exp. Neurol.*, **150,** 650.

Sun, A.Y., and Seaman, R.N. (1977). The effect of ageing on synaptosomal Ca2 transport in the brain. *Exp. Ageing Res.*, **3,** 1.

Teravainen, H., and Calne, D.B. (1983). Motor system in normal ageing and Parkinson's disease. In: Katzman, R., and Terry, R. (eds.) *The Neurology of Ageing*, F.A. Davis Company, Philadelphia.

Wyckoff, R.W.G., and Young, J.Z. (1956). The motor-neurone surface. *Proc. Roy. Soc.*, **B139,** 18.

Young, W., Flamm, E.S., Demopoulos, H.G., Tomasula, J.H., and Decrescito, V. (1981). Effects of naloxone on post traumatic ischaemia in experimental spinal contusion. *J. Neurosurg.*, **55,** 209.

Chapter 4

The Neuroepidemiology of Old Age

G. A. Broe

Professor of Geriatric Medicine, Concord Repatriation Hospital, Sydney, Australia

Helen Creasey

Senior Lecturer in Geriatric Medicine, Concorde Repatriation Hospital, Sydney, Australia

There are several different approaches to the problem of determining the frequency of neurological disorders with age. One approach is to study differences in cognitive, behavioural and sensorimotor performances with age, both cross-sectionally and longitudinally in normal subjects. Generally, such studies have not been performed on a random sample but rather on individuals selected on the basis of absence of specific clinical diseases. Thus, by definition, such subjects are known not to have classical neurological diseases.

A second approach has been to study a random sample of the elderly to determine the presence or absence of a series of symptoms, signs, syndromes or diseases and estimate disability and dependence. This approach allows some measure of the relative importance of neurological disease in the elderly in terms of the burden to the health care system and the needs for services. The only epidemiological survey attempting to measure the prevalence of neurological disease in the elderly by resultant disability and dependence is that of Akhtar *et al.* (1973), who looked at a random community sample of 808 people aged 65 years and over. Twenty-eight per cent (227) of the individuals studied showed significant disability in that they required assistance to live in their own homes. This disability rose dramatically with

advancing age from 12% in the group aged 65 to 69 years, to more than 80% in those aged 85 years and over. By contrast, dependency (defined as disability for self-care) was rare under the age of 85 years, but was present in approximately 25% over that age. The major cause of disability in all the individuals was neurological, accounting for just under half of the total (48%), and the cause of 93% of the dependence (see Table 4.1). There were numerous

TABLE 4.1 CAUSES OF DISABILITY AND DEPEN-DENCY IN THE ELDERLY: RANDOMLY SELECTED SAMPLE OF PEOPLE 65 YEARS AND OVER (GLAS-GOW-KILSYTH STUDY) (AKHTAR *ET AL.*, 1973)

	Disability $n=227$ (%)	Dependence $n=227$ (%)
Neurological	48	93
Cardiorespiratory	38	18
Joint	24	30
Functional psychiatric	22	11
Obesity	16	11
Visual	11	15
Other	8	18

TABLE 4.2 PREVALENCE (%) OF NEUROLOGICAL DISORDERS IN COMMUNITY ELDERLY (BASED ON RANDOM SAMPLE, GLASGOW-KILSYTH STUDY)

Disorder	Age group		
	65–74 (n=488)	75+ (n=320)	65+ (=808)
Dementia	4.3	14.1	8.2
Senile	2.5	10.9	5.8
Vascular	1.4	2.5	1.9
Other[a]	0.4	0.6	0.5
Stroke	7.0	7.8	7.3
Parkinsonism	1.6	1.6	1.6
Essential tremor	0.8	3.1	3.7
Other diagnoses[b]	4.1	6.3	4.0
Non-diagnostic motor signs			
Unilateral	1.6	2.5	2.0
Bilateral	0.6	2.5	1.4
	(n=227)	(n=81)	(n=308)
Gait disorder	4.4	32.1	11.7
Transient ischaemic attack (TIA)	8.4	9.9	8.7

[a] Alcohol related; traumatic.
[b] Peripheral nerve lesions (8); traumatic lesions (5); cervical myelopathy (4); epilepsy (3); congenital lesions (3); neuralgias (3); motor neurone disease, multiple sclerosis, pituitary tumour, chorea, uraemic encephalopathy; neurofibromatosis (1 each).

types of neurological disease, but only four were common. Their contributions towards total disability were: dementia (21%) consisting of 6% associated with and 11% without cerebrovascular disease; stroke without dementia (11%); parkinsonism (3%); and a disorder of balance and gait (13%). Seventy-seven per cent of the dependent group were demented, while 97% showed some organic brain disease.

A third approach to the neuroepidemiology of ageing has taken the classic method of measuring the incidence and/or prevalence of specific disorders in the population in relation to age. Only one study has looked at the prevalence of all neurological disorders in a random sample of the elderly living in the community (Broe *et al.*, 1976) (see Table 4.2). Other studies have focused on those disorders which clinically appear important and common in old age. The definitions of the diseases are, however, usually those developed on a younger population and then applied to elderly individuals. This creates some problems in case finding as will be shown later. The major diseases studied using this approach are stroke, the dementias and parkinsonism (see Table 4.3).

These individual disorders will be considered in greater detail below. First, however, some of the results of the studies using the healthy elderly and the disabled elderly will be reviewed.

THE HEALTHY ELDERLY AND NEUROLOGICAL OLD AGE

The pathological changes that occur in the nervous system with ageing are dealt with in Chapter 1, the psychological changes in Chapter 2 and the findings on neurological examination in Chapter 5. Nevertheless, it will be useful to review some aspects of the neurological manifestations of ageing here. These need to be distinguished from specific neurological diseases; otherwise diagnostic errors are likely,

TABLE 4.3 NEUROLOGICAL DISEASES IN THE ELDERLY: LITERATURE REVIEWS

	Prevalence/100 000	Reviewer
Severe dementia	600–27 800	Cooper and Bickel (1984)
Mild dementia	5 400–52 700	Henderson (1986)
Stroke	2 930–7 000	Kannel and Wolf (1983)
Parkinsonism	80–1 400	Kessler (1978)
Primary CNS tumour	20–90	Schoenberg (1978)
Motor neurone disease	9–19	Li, T-m. *et al.*, 1985
Epilepsy	200–500	Grimley-Evans and Caird (1982)

making any estimate of the incidence or prevalence of a particular neurological disorder in the elderly inaccurate.

Pathological changes in the nervous system have been extensively studied worldwide and show general reductions in brain weight and volume with age in individuals considered not to have neurological disease in life. This atrophy is more apparent in certain regions of the brain, especially the limbic and insular gyri of the temporal lobes and the parasagittal frontal and parietal gyri (Tomlinson *et al.*, 1968). Complementary microscopic studies have revealed accumulations of new structures and substances with age (e.g. plaques, tangles, lipofuscin) while more limited studies have shown areas of neuronal loss, which appear to be both anatomically and biochemically specific. There are two important features in all these studies: first, there is overlap between young and old individuals with regard to cell counts, brain weights and volumes; and secondly, there appear to be both phases of accelerated change (such as decrease in brain weight after age 70) and phases of regression (such as a decline in plaques and tangles in the over 90 year age group) (see review, Creasey and Rapoport, 1985). There is some evidence that part of these ageing changes, such as the numbers of non-diseased subjects with plaques, may show variations around the world. The Japanese and Dayan found incidence figures around 30% in non-demented elderly while Tomlinson, Wildi and Gellerstadt report nearly 80% involvement (Matsuyama and Nakamura, 1978). MacDonald Critchley (1931a) commented that plaques had not been found in Turks. Certain of these age-related changes (such as

plaques and tangles) are known to occur in greater degree in disease states (Blessed *et al.*, 1968) whereas others have no known functional significance (such as lipofuscin accumulation). These changes may be important both in misclassification of 'normal' ageing changes as disease and vice versa. Our understanding of the interaction between normal senescence and disease requires further study.

Prominent clinical characteristics associated with ageing are changes in mobility and mentation. However, scientific study of these changes in relation to the known morphological ageing changes of the nervous system has been scanty. Definitions of health differ in degree: for some studies, it is the absence of a major disorder (such as dementia) while in others it may require absence of a large number of disease states both symptomatic and those detectable in a battery of screening tests. By far the most sophisticated of these have been the cross-sectional and longitudinal studies of cognition performed by psychologists. These are far too complex and varied to be reviewed here. However, a brief example is the Wechsler Adult Intelligence Scale (WAIS) which was standardized on a random sample of the population of the USA and shows marked declines in some areas of testing with age. This cross-sectional view differs from those of longitudinal samplings which show some functions hold or even continue to improve with age, such as vocabulary, while others decline almost universally, such as reaction time, both simple and choice, and the ability to store new information (see review, Birren and Schaie, 1985).

The neurological examination has been used to measure the changes to the nervous system in old age. One of the earliest studies using this approach was that of Howell (1949) who studied 200 Chelsea Pensioners without known neurological disease and found a variety of deficits. He used the list of clinical impressions of disordered neurological functioning unique to the elderly and postulated to be due to old age by MacDonald Critchley (1931b). Howell found major changes including loss of reflexes, especially ankle jerks; reduced vibration sense in the lower limbs; impairment of pupillary reactions; abnormal dysmetria and reductions in other sensory modalities. He noted these changes could not be easily attributed to one or several of the known pathological changes.

Skre (1972) also used neurological examination to study changes in a series of signs with age on a random sample of five equally sized 10 year age groups ($n = 373$). He found with age significant increases in minor pareses, deformities, loss of proprioception in hands and feet, and ataxia. He noted that there were few individuals over age 65 years who did not have some abnormality, and that those of poor sociovocational status showed more abnormalities.

Potvin *et al.* (1980) attempted to quantitate the sensorimotor changes detectable on neurological examination, in a functional sense. He found in 61 non-neurologically diseased men, chosen to represent each year from age 20 to 80 years, that there were large declines in hand-force steadiness, speed of hand–arm movements, one-legged balance with eyes closed and vibration sense with age. When assessed in terms of loss of daily living skills, deficits were less in amount but still significant.

Jacobs and Grossman (1980) showed that the frequency of elicitation of primitive reflexes increased with advancing age in normal adults, the palmomental reflex appearing in the third decade and being present in over 50% of subjects in the eighth decade. The snout and corneomandibular reflexes appeared later and showed less frequent occurrence.

More sophisticated approaches to assessment of neurological function in life have included use of neurophysiological measures. Electroencephalographic changes have been found in both cross-sectional as well as longitudinal studies. Less extensive work has been done with nerve conduction studies, cerebral blood flow, and cerebral metabolic studies. Because of the technical and time requirements, such studies can rarely address whole populations, so their usefulness in epidemiological work is limited (Creasey and Rapoport, 1985).

Changes in peripheral nerve input and primary sensory input (both somatosensory and the special senses—vision, hearing, smell and taste) are often viewed as causes of an observed reduction in function. However, measured changes cannot always fully explain the disorders of integrated function of the individual. They may conceivably contribute to poorer brain functioning by creating a state of relative sensory deprivation or by providing misinformation. However, dysfunction of the special senses (visual and auditory) in old age has been shown to relate more closely with functional psychiatric than organic neurological disease (Eastwood *et al.*, 1985).

The importance of these studies of the neuroepidemiology of old age lies in the definition of changes which can occur in old people in the absence of defined neurological disease. This may determine whether or not an abnormal finding is listed or attributed to 'normal' ageing. As none of these studies has any pathological correlations, it is not possible to decide the normality of any of these changes at present.

NEUROLOGY OF OLD AGE: DISABILITY AND DEPENDENCE

As mentioned previously, the only study addressing this question is that of Akhtar *et al.* (1973). Here we shall consider some aspects of this study in more detail. In the group aged 75 years and over, two neurological disorders were of major importance in causing disability: dementia and senile gait disorder, these showing a dramatic rise in prevalence in those over 75 years of age. Two other disorders (stroke and parkinsonism) also were significant as causes of disability. Three of these disorders (stroke, dementia and parkinsonism) have been the subject of individual incidence and prevalence studies, which will be discussed later. The fourth disorder, that of gait impairment, remains a poorly defined entity both clinically and pathologically. In this study it affected 31% of the elderly 75 years and over living at home. While impairment of gait in the elderly is well known clinically and has been studied extensively with regard to specific complications such as falls and fractured neck and femur, the assessment of the neurological and neuropathological deficits which are associated with this disorder has yet to be reported. The disorder occurs in the absence of any definable disease of the nervous system, in particular in the absence of stroke, dementia or parkinsonism. Clinically, it is associated with other features of neurological ageing including flexed posture and limited upgaze, poor convergence and loss of ankle jerks. There also appears to be an associated mild mental decline as noted by Adams (1977).

A preliminary case-control study of this disorder (Broe, 1986) has shown that it is the gait disordered elderly who show the neurological and psychometric changes attributed at times to normal ageing in cross-sectional studies of the type mentioned in the last section. This study distinguished a group of gait disordered but otherwise normal healthy individuals living in the community and compared them to an age and sex matched group of non-gait disordered, community living individuals. Testing showed that the gait disordered subjects were not only impaired on heel–toe walking but also had a slower and more ataxic spontaneous gait pattern. Neurological examination in these two groups showed significant differences, the gait disordered being more flexed in posture, slower in individual limb movements, having more action tremor and more often absent ankle jerks and impaired vibration sense (see Table 4.4). This same group showed significantly greater impairment of upward gaze and convergence. Psychometric assessment revealed impairment in memory retrieval and adaptive abilities. Whether this group has the clinical manifestations of the known pathological changes associated with ageing, or whether the gait disorder at least in some cases represents the earlier manifestation of one of the classical neurological diseases of the aged (dementia being the only one of comparable prevalence) is unknown. However, the differences found in this subgrouping of the not classically diseased elderly suggest that some of the differences found in the

TABLE 4.4 NEUROLOGICAL SIGNS AND AGEING

	Normal gait*		Senile gait†	
	(%)	n‡	(%)	n‡
Defective upgaze	15	(39)	44	(16)
Positive glabella tap	18	(39)	31	(16)
Benign memory loss	23	(39)	44	(16)
Reduced vibration sense	19	(41)	52	(24)
Action tremor	19	(41)	52	(24)
Absent ankle jerks	14	(80)	44	(40)

Based on Kilsyth and Lidcombe studies, Broe *et al.* (1976) and Broe (1986).
* Able to heel–toe walk ten paces.
† Not able to heel–toe walk ten paces.
‡ Number tested.

'healthy elderly' studies may be attributed to group heterogeneity. In support of the gait disordered elderly constituting a separate clinical group is the finding of a recent study of a random population sample in Finland, where postural sway, which had been previously shown by Brocklehurst to be associated with impaired vibration sense, increased with age along with increased vibratory threshold of the ankles (Eva and Heikkinen, 1985).

Thus the two disorders (dementia and gait disorder) most commonly found in the earlier disability study may be considered to involve processes seen to a lesser degree in normal ageing. In terms of health care requirement, this study suggests that the major burden of disability does not arise until after age 75 and that most of it is due to dementia of degenerative type and to disorders of gait and balance. There is the additional problem, associated with the latter, of falls. Studies of the increasing incidence of falls with age show that many, particularly those associated with hip fractures or mortality, have an intrinsic reason and that the commonest intrinsic reason is a neurologically abnormal gait (Nickens, 1985).

Although the elderly with senile gait disorder constitute a separate clinical group this is a syndrome of multiple aetiology rather than a specific clinical diagnosis. The neurology of senile gait disorder includes an extrapyramidal component with slowing of movement and reduced step length; a cerebellar component with a mildly widened gait base and increased sway; a peripheral nerve component with

TABLE 4.5 STROKE INCIDENCE AND PREVALENCE BY AGE, SINGLE STUDIES

Reference	Age group			Country
	55–64	65–74	75+	
Incidence (per 100 000 per year)				
Matsumoto *et al.* (1973)	375	1115	2240	USA
Kuller (1978)	670	800	1365	USA
Eckstrom *et al.* (1969)	325	600	2300	USA
Eisenberg *et al.* (1964)	405	955	2215	USA
Sivenius *et al.* (1985)	525	1187	2332	Finland
	50–59	60–69	70+	
Johnson *et al.* (1967)	475	1105	3785	Japan
Ashok *et al.* (1986)	248	304	371	Libya
Li, S-c. *et al.* (1985a)	400	1000	1700	China
Prevalence (per 100 000)				
	55–64	65–74	75+	
Matsumoto *et al.* (1973)	1550	3510	7245	USA
Schoenberg *et al.* (1986)	2505	4206	5906	USA
Kannel and Wolf (1983)	810	3560	5970	USA
	50–59	60–69	70+	
Heyman *et al.* (1971)	2415	3115	7800	USA
Epstein *et al.* (1965)	1500	2500	7500	USA
Li, S-c. *et al.* (1985a)	2000	3000	4000	China

reduced ankle jerks and distal vibration sense; and, in a broad sense, a cognitive component with mild slowing of information processing and impairment of adaptive abilities.

Senile gait disorder probably represents the summation or convergence of a number of presumably pathological processes affecting the nervous system without any one of these being sufficiently advanced for the diagnosis of a specific neurological disease to be sustained. The concept of summation of different subclinical pathologies to produce a clinical disorder is an important one in geriatric medicine and underlies other common neurological syndromes of ageing, for example, acute confusional states and incontinence. Further study of senile gait disorder is clearly required to elucidate its neurological components and to determine the risk factors underlying them.

SPECIFIC NEUROLOGICAL DISORDERS OF INCREASING PREVALENCE IN OLD AGE

Stroke

In the age group between 45 and 74 years, the incidence of stroke is so much higher than for other neurological diseases that misclassification of neurological diseases as stroke is a minimal problem. A consensus of studies of incidence and prevalence suggests an incidence of 2/1000/year and a prevalence of 7–12/1000 of stroke for all ages (Kannel and Wolf, 1983) (Table 4.5). In those under 65 years of age, stroke is often considered by clinical type (TIA, RIND*, completed stroke), pathological type (ischaemic, thrombotic, embolic, haemorrhagic) and underlying disease process (atheroma, arteritis,

* Reversible ischaemic neurological deficit

hypertension, valvular heart disease). Most epidemiological studies in the elderly do not define the type of stroke. While this may be justified by the knowledge that almost all strokes in the elderly are due to age-associated vascular disease with ischaemic infarction as the major pathological process, some problems do arise from the fact that other neurological diseases of ageing may be misclassified as stroke, leading to overreporting of stroke rates. This is particularly seen in the recording of dementia due to vascular disease which has been grossly overreported in the past. However, it may in part be balanced by an underreporting of stroke seen in patients of nursing homes, the majority of whom are old.

While some causes of stroke in the younger patient are rare in the elderly or have not been found to be associated with stroke in the elderly (such as mitral valve prolapse), there are other causes of stroke which appear to be unique to or at least largely confined to the elderly. In this regard, only a few will be mentioned:

1   retrograde carotid arteritis seen in herpes zoster ophthalmicus, which can result in carotid occlusion and major stroke;
2   giant cell arteritis, which may involve the intracranial vessels;
3   amyloid angiopathy, which is a cause of non-hypertensive intracerebral haemorrhage in the elderly;
4   lastly mitral annulus calcification, which can cause emboli in the elderly.

While all authors agree that stroke prevalence and incidence rise with age, there is some dispute as to whether this is linear or exponential. This may be related to local overall differences in rates—rather than to a difference in age-related rates—as are seen in the Japanese (Tanaka *et al.*, 1985) versus European figures (e.g. Sivenius *et al.*, 1985), or the differences in blacks versus whites in the USA (e.g. Schoenberg *et al.*, 1986). Few studies extend into the very old (over 75 years, or over 85 years), so that secular effects on the incidence and prevalence now known to be occurring in the 45 to 65 year age group are not known for this group.

Considering the majority of studies, the stroke prevalence rate over all ages can be set at 7–12/1000 in males, rising from age 55 years to reach 100/1000

in the over 75 year age group. Incidence rates also rise with age becoming more apparent in the over 65 age group (from 2/1000/year for all ages to 35/1000/year for the over 75 age group). While one study suggested increased incidence after age 75 years as compared with 65 years (4–16/1000/year versus 10–35/1000/year) (see Table 4.5) another showed no change in prevalence after age 65, with a rate around 80/1000 (Broe *et al.*, 1976).

The sex ratio is not as marked as for coronary artery disease, and incidence is related to rates of hypertension and diabetes. The age-specific mortality rate rises with age, as does the severity, morbidity, case fatality rate of stroke and the period of hospitalization required to treat the acute stroke and the likelihood of hospitalization with any stroke (Wade *et al.*, 1984; 1985). It has been suggested that it is the increased severity which causes the increased morbidity and mortality, as one study showed equivalent rates of recovery over a 6 month period following stroke given equal deficits at outset, independent of age. Hemiplegia rather than monoplegia, perceptual disorder and incontinence are more frequent clinical findings in the elderly with stroke.

The factors found to be associated with an increased risk of stroke in younger subjects, such as obesity, smoking, social class, occupation, serum lipids and control of hypertension, have not been well studied in the elderly. Evidence from the Framingham study would suggest that past history of hypertension and its duration, as well as past obesity may be associated with increased risk of stroke at all ages (Wolf *et al.*, 1977). Associated vascular disease is a common accompaniment of stroke in the elderly, particularly congestive cardiac failure with arrhythmia of any type and peripheral vascular disease. ECG findings of arrhythmias are also frequent. The implication of these associations is not clear: what their role is in the cause or outcome of stroke has not been defined. The Framingham study showed that isolated syncope, which has increasing prevalence with age, is not associated with an increased risk of either stroke or myocardial infarction (prevalence rising from 13.9/100 000 in the 45 to 54 year age group to 55.9/100 000 in the 75 and over age group) (Savage *et al.*, 1985). With regard to other vascular disease, subarachnoid haemorrhage has been shown as declining in incidence in males with age while increasing in incidence in females with age, the reason for this being unclear (males falling from 19.7/100 000 in the 54–74 age group to 4.7/100 000 in the 75 plus age group while females rise from 28.1 to 41.2/100 000 over the same age groups) (Bonita and Thomson, 1985).

Dementia

Dementia is the most important cause of disability and dependency. Moreover, regardless of age over 65 years, poor mental function is the best predictor of mortality, especially when combined with poor functional capacity and urinary incontinence, two markers of the severity of the dementing process (Campbell *et al.*, 1985a, 1985b). Further, it is the most important determinant of chronic institutionalization of the elderly, which is the major economic health cost to Western governments. According to Cooper and Bickel (1984) 'Field-surveys have consistently revealed a high prevalence in elderly populations, most estimates for severe and moderately severe forms of dementia lying between 5 and 8% of those aged over 65 years. The life-time cumulative risk of becoming severely demented by the age of 80 has been estimated from population-based longitudinal data at between 15 and 20%.' Behind these kinds of figures and predictions lies a complicated body of information beset by many problems.

The common causes of dementia in the elderly are two: Alzheimer's disease (AD) and vascular dementia, usually called multi-infarct dementia (MID). The relative incidence and prevalence of these two types of dementia is based solely on autopsy data. Figures quoted vary little: British data show a frequency of dementia of 4.4% in the 65 and over age group (Tomlinson, 1970) with 57% AD, 21% MID and 21% a mixture of AD and MID, while a Swiss series (Todorov *et al.*, 1975) yielded figures of 36% dementias due to AD, 22% due to MID and 43% due to a mixture of AD and MID. The claim that such series do reflect the relative rates of these disorders in the living population, despite all the limitations and biases inherent in autopsy studies, is supported by the similarities of the incidence of dementia in a general autopsy population and that in a population survey. In a series of 2804 general autopsies, levels of plaques and tangles known to be associated with dementia in life were found in 477 individuals, or 16.4% (Matsuyama and Nakamura, 1978). This group had an average age at onset of 73.5 years and average age at death of 78.5 years which is in keeping with the ages at which dementia becomes clinically frequent.

However, the situation is made more complicated by the fact that the pathological features of the two major causes of dementia are not unique to the demented (Blessed *et al.*, 1968). Both the hallmarks of AD (plaques and tangles) and of MID (stroke) are found at autopsy in non-demented individuals. For example, a Japanese study of 617 consecutive non-demented brains (Matsuyama and Nakamura, 1978) showed all individuals over 80 contained tangles and only a handful did not have plaques. The number of tangles and the incidence of plaques declined after age 90. The type of plaque also appeared to change in that younger subjects had more 'primitive' plaques while the older ones had more 'mature' plaques. This study also showed that there was an increase in the numbers of tangles found in the later years of the study (autopsies performed from 1968 to 1972) than in the earlier years (autopsies performed from 1957 to 1964). Similarly Tomlinson *et al.* (1968) found tangles, plaques and lacunae in many of his non-demented brains. Thus the use of autopsy data alone cannot yield a true picture of the incidence of clinical disease in life.

Yet there is no clinically accurate method of reliably distinguishing either of these diseases in life. The diagnosis of dementia in the field is hampered by lack of a simple sensitive and specific test. For example, Rocca *et al.* (1986) report that Alzheimer's disease in life can be diagnosed with only about 70–75% sensitivity and specificity (Molsa *et al.*, 1985). Further, attempts to separate AD from MID in life have also shown that the differentiation of pure AD or pure MID from a mixture of both diseases is very difficult. As dementia is not a direct cause of death, use of death certificates to define frequency will underestimate the rate of this disease. Clinical studies have also shown that a significant minority of the elderly who have been labelled demented may be found on more extensive study or review and further investigation to be suffering from a treatable or

TABLE 4.6   DEMENTIA INCIDENCE AND PREVALENCE BY AGE GROUP, SINGLE STUDIES

Country	Age group			Reference
	65–74	75–84	85+	
Incidence (per 100 000 per year)				
Finland	56	374	1 144	Rocca *et al.* (1986)
	60–69	70–79	80–89	
Sweden	37	210	270	Rocca *et al.* (1986)
Sweden	29	186	458	Rocca *et al.* (1986)
USA	288	1 307	3 248	Rocca *et al.* (1986)
Prevalence (per 100 000)				
	65–74	75–84	85+	
USA	1 100	4 300	16 800	Weissman *et al.* (1985)
Finland	359	1 910	6 295	Rocca *et al.* (1986)
Finland	1 700	6 300	14 800	Rocca *et al.* (1986)
Japan	400	3 275	10 575	Rocca *et al.* (1986)
	60–69	70–79	80+	
Britain	2 300	3 900	2 200	Kay (1972)
Denmark	0	190	13 200	Kay (1972)
Japan	2 300	5 900	19 800	Kay (1972)
Sweden	0	980	3 890	Rocca *et al.* (1986)

reversible condition (Cooper and Bickel, 1984). Autopsy series of presumed MID and AD have also included several cases in which no pathological brain disease could be found. All these factors make any estimate of clinical incidence or prevalence difficult and different findings may be attributed to the methods used to cope with the above problems. However, real differences may also be obscured by methodological differences.

Unlike vascular disease, dementia (especially AD) is rare under age 60 years, though prevalence and incidence figures for all adult ages do not exist. However, over 65 years of age, the incidence and prevalence of dementia has been the subject of a series of studies (Table 4.6). Unfortunately, comparisons are difficult because of differences in the definition of dementia, method of classification of impairment (some use only one category of impairment, others several) and the method of case ascertainment, each with its own source of biases. Despite these major technical problems, surprisingly similar trends emerge, with the prevalence of dementing illnesses for the total age group 65 years and over being estimated at around 5%. It rises dramatically with increasing age, especially in the over 75 and over 80 year age groups, reaching about 20% in the latter. Typical ranges given are 23–70/1000 for ages 65 to 75 years, 40–200/1000 for ages 75 to 84 years and 150–300/1000 for the over 85 age group (Nilsson and Persson, 1984; Weissman *et al.*, 1985; Sulkava *et al.*, 1985; Kay *et al.*, 1964). When classified by severity, figures of 44/1000 severe and 120/1000 mild to moderate dementia are reasonable estimates for the over 65 year age group. Prevalence studies show this marked increase occurs with age, whether measured in Britain, Scandinavia or the USA, though the latter two show smaller age- and sex-specific ratios than the first. Japanese figures appear lower than any of these and do not rise so dramatically in the very old (Henderson, 1983).

The prevalence of so-called 'mild-dementia' reported from field surveys has varied enormously from less than 5% (2.6% being the lowest quoted by Henderson and Huppert, 1984) to over 60% of those aged 65 years and over. The outcome of this group is unclear and as yet insufficient numbers have been followed to autopsy to define the pathological homogeneity of this group. Follow-up mortality data, however, suggest that these subjects have an increased mortality rate compared with their mentally intact peers.

Age-specific mortality rates in the USA show increases from 1.2/100 000 for the 60–65 year age group to 11.6/100 000 for those over 85 years (Chandra et al., 1986). The annual incidence rates from several studies show an increase from 10.5/100 000/year for the 60–65 year age group to 280–3248/100 000/year for those over 85 years (Nilsson, 1984; Chandra et al., 1986; Jonsson and Hallgrimsson, 1983). The reason for the wide range in incidence rates between different populations cannot be assessed at the present time for lack of accurate compatible data. Such information is scanty. Hagnell's unbiased community 25 year prospective study of the population of 'Lundby' (Hagnell et al., 1981) showed a fall in the cumulative risk of moderate to severe age psychosis between 1947–1957 and 1957–1972, from 0.57 to 0.46 for males and 0.64 to 0.44 for females. This study included both MID and AD. One might suggest the decline in incidence of dementia may be related to the documented decline in stroke over the same period. However, another follow-up study of 22 octagenarian twins showed a corrected rate for the development of dementia of 16% between the mean ages of 84 and 89, compatible with a late drop in the increasing incidence of dementia with very old age (Jarvik et al., 1982). Against these data, however, is the prevalence study performed on a population survey in Finland where the prevalence rate rose from 20% in the over 85 year age group to 30% in the over 90 year age group on both cross-sectional and 5 year longitudinal follow-up study, suggesting the incidence remained unchanged (Haavisto et al., 1985). Patterns for mortality from dementia in the USA also showed an increase in age-adjusted mortality rates for dementia between 1971 and 1978 (Chandra et al., 1986).

As case definition becomes more refined, and perhaps with the aid of yet to be developed tools, a more accurate picture of the incidence and prevalence of individual dementias may become available.

The other major theme in the epidemiological study of the dementias has been the search for putative risk factors using the case-control method. The early studies of Larsen and Akesson established the association between vascular dementia and hypertension and the presence of atherosclerotic disease (Hagnell et al., 1981). More recent attempts to find risk factors for AD have yielded some common and some conflicting associations. Heston's autopsy based study (Heston et al., 1981) found significant associations with a family history of dementia and Down's syndrome as well as a family history of lymphoproliferative disease. Heyman et al. (1984) found a family history of dementia and previous or intercurrent history of thyroid disease as well as past history of head injury to be significant. Mortimer et al. (1985) confirmed the head injury finding while Amaducci et al. (1986) did not. These studies face the same case definition problems cited above, with the exception of Heston's post-mortem based study. Nevertheless case-control studies hold out the promise of providing clues about the cause of this major neurological problem in the elderly.

Parkinsonism

Parkinsonism, like dementia, is essentially a disorder of ageing, with a negligible incidence below 50 years of age and a prevalence rising from 25/100 000 in the decade 50–59 to over 2000/100 000 (2%) in the population 70 years of age and over (Kurtzke and Kurland, 1983; Li, S-c. et al., 1985b; Li, T-m. et al., 1985; Broe et al., 1976). Incidence rates, reported by Kurtzke and Kurland (1983), show a rise from 10/100 000/year at age 50 to 140/100 000/year at age 70. Some difficulties in measuring incidence and prevalence in the very old arise because of the slow onset and somewhat different clinical presentation with less prominent tremor, greater symmetry and more prominent posture and balance deficits and greater autonomic involvement. Incidence rates depend heavily on definition and, as parkinsonism is not a primary cause of death, it is difficult to discover its frequency from death certificates. Prevalence figures are thus more reliable, but cases need to be distinguished from senile gait impairment mentioned previously and from essential tremor, both conditions which rise dramatically in prevalence in the very old (over 75 years). The former disorder rises from 40/1000 in the decade 65 to 75 years of age to 240/1000 in the over 75 year age group, while the latter rises from 10/1000 to 40/1000 in the same age periods, both prevalence rates exceeding those of Parkinson's disease (Broe *et al.*, 1976).

Several other rarer extrapyramidal disorders such as progressive supranuclear palsy also appear to be largely confined to the elderly.

Motor Neurone Disease

Motor neurone disease increases in prevalence and incidence with age, though less dramatically than the disorders previously discussed, rising from 1/100 000 under age 50 to 10/100 000 in the over 70 year age group (Juergens *et al.*, 1980; Li, T-m. *et al.*, 1985).

Other Neurological Disorders in Old Age

Several neurological disorders show either no major change in incidence or prevalence with age, or a decline. For many of these there are no satisfactory studies extending into the very old. For example, while community studies suggest a decline in the incidence of clinically significant cerebral tumours with age, autopsy series suggest that asymptomatic tumours, particularly meningiomas, rise in incidence (Annegers *et al.*, 1980). More of the clinically significant tumours in the elderly are malignant, and many are metastatic (Walker *et al.*, 1985).

There is no age-related rise in trauma to the nervous system, with the exception of chronic subdural haematomas. In one series, 50% of all chronic subdural haematomas occurred in the over 64 year age group and were associated with head injury in only half of the cases. This group accounted for most of the deaths and half of the poor outcomes in a series of 114 cases of adult chronic subdural haematomas (Cameron, 1978). Despite this, the majority of elderly individuals treated surgically do well (Patrick and Gates, 1984).

The incidence of peripheral neuropathies, especially Guillain–Barré syndrome, is unchanged with

age. Earlier studies showed no rise in the incidence of epilepsy in old age but more recent studies contradicted this. The epidemiology of epilepsy is discussed in Chapter 15.

Certain diseases show idiosyncratic features in the elderly. Encephalitis of unknown cause and meningitis from a variety of rarer pathogens (such as *Listeria*) are more common with age. This differential susceptibility is most likely related to changes in immune function with ageing, in that age-associated changes in overall incidence and prevalence of encephalitides and meningitides are not marked.

The marked age-associated increase in the incidence of herpes zoster may also represent a reactivation of a latent virus, and a reflection of changes in the immune function of the elderly. Giant cell arteritis may also be considered in this category: a systemic susceptibility to a disease process with ageing which may manifest in the nervous system.

Interestingly, several neurological disorders associated with immune abnormalities, such as myasthenia gravis and multiple sclerosis are thought to have an immunological basis. They are relatively rare in the elderly, though myasthenia gravis may not uncommonly present after 60 (see Chapter 25). One might postulate that the known age changes in immune function render the very old less susceptible to these diseases. Age-related immunological changes may be important in the clinical occurrence of the paraneoplastic myasthenic syndrome (see Chapter 21).

IMPLICATIONS FOR HEALTH CARE PLANNING AND FUTURE SERVICE NEEDS

Dementia is the principal cause of disability and dependence in old age. The implications of this have been spelled out by Cooper and Bickel (1984).

More than half the total of 1.2 million persons currently resident in homes for the aged and dependent in the USA show some degree of cognitive impairment and it would appear that over half of all such mentally infirm home residents require maximum or intermediate grade nursing care. The total costs of care are prodigious. There can thus be no question as to the desirability of methods of early detection, if these promise to lead to a reduction in chronic disability and dependence on institutional care.

Moreover, the potential for reducing the demand for community services for those at home would be even greater, given that the majority of demented persons live outside of institutions.

Health programme planners have taken this marked age increase in prevalence to imply major increases in needs with rising absolute numbers of cases in the next 20 years. This is supported by the observed increasing prevalence with time (a doubling of age-specific prevalence from 1949 to 1959) which has been attributed to increased duration of disease. This more than offsets any possible projections from the one study which suggests that the age-specific incidence may be falling.

Given that there is at present no specific therapy for dementia, medical care is chiefly aimed at supporting independent functioning in the community for as long as possible and at minimizing the distress to the care givers. The level of such services is best determined by field studies of prevalence of varying degrees of impairment in functional terms. Such short-term needs are acute and of crisis proportion at the present time. The longer-term aim of field studies must remain, however; namely to define the pattern of illness with the hope of finding clues to the causes of dementia in old age and thus to allow preventive and curative treatments to be developed.

Studies of morphological changes in the nervous system of individuals currently classified as *not* neurologically diseased suggests that the brain acquires damage during life which is age-related but not necessarily age-caused. It may be hypothesized that tangles, plaques and cell loss reduce the brain's capacity to function optimally, though this may not be clinically apparent. Studies of living subjects, classified as non-neurologically diseased, indeed show quantifiable changes in neurological functioning with age which usually fall short of clear-cut disease. There is little understanding of the link between the pathological and neurophysiological changes with age or between these two and any individual's health and needs. Knowledge of the causes of these changes may allow some of the 'normal' ageing of the nervous system seen currently in populations of old people to be reversed or

prevented. We do not know if these changes are biological or innate, or if they represent acquired deficits, which may have their origins in insults occurring at any stage of life after conception. Several studies have shown that the declines are negatively correlated with high socio-economic and occupational status, which may reflect either greater initial potential, less susceptibility to decline or less exposure to environmental hazards. This requires further study if the burden of ageing per se on health care and services is not to increase even more.

With regard to the classic neurological diseases, it is evident that the need for health care and the greatest demand for services arises from the dementias. However, it must not be forgotten that 35% of all brain tumours occur after age 60; and that two-thirds of all strokes occur in the over 60s. Given reduced reserves in the brains of such individuals one might predict greater resultant needs and demands on the health service system by such individuals. Hence the need to study the neurological functional disabilities of all elderly individuals.

REFERENCES

Adams, R. (1977). The neurology of aging, involution and senescence. In: Adams, R.D., and Victor, M. (eds.) *Principles of Neurology*, McGraw Hill, New York, pp. 376–410.

Akhtar, A.J., Broe, G.A., Crombie, A., McLean, W.M.R., Andrews, G.R., and Caird, F.L. (1973). Disability and dependence in the elderly at home. *Age Ageing*, **2**, 102–10.

Amaducci, L.A., Frariglioni, L., Rocca, W.A., Fieschi, C., Livrea, P., Pedone, D., Bracco, L., Lippi, N., Gandolfo, C., Bino, G., Prencipe, M., Bonatti, M.L., Givotti, F., Carella, F., Tavolato, B., Ferla, S., Lenzi, G.L., Carolei, A., Gambi, A., Grigoletto, F., and Schoenberg, B.S. (1986). Risk factors for clinically diagnosed Alzheimer's disease: a case-control study of an Italian population. *Neurology (Cleveland)*, **36**, 922–31.

Annegers, J.F., Schoenberg, B.S., Okazak, H., and Kurland, L.T. (1980). Primary intracranial neoplasms in Rochester, Minnesota (1935–1977). In: Rose R.C. (ed.) *Clinical Neuro-epidemiology*, Pitman Medical, Tunbridge Wells, pp. 366–71.

Ashok, P.P., Radhakrishnan, K., Sridharan, R., and El-Mangoush, Ma. (1986). Incidence and pattern of cerebrovascular diseases in Benghazi, Libya. *J. Neurol. Neurosurg. Psychiatry*, **49**, 519–23.

Birren, J.E., and Schaie, K.W. (1985). *Handbook of the*

Psychology of Aging, second edition, Van Nostrand Reinhold, New York.

Blessed, G., Tomlinson, B.E., and Roth, M. (1968). The association between quantitative measurements of dementia and of senile change in the cerebral gray matter of elderly subjects. *Br. J. Psychiatry*, **114**, 797–811.

Bonita, R., and Thomson, S. (1985). Subarachnoid haemorrhage: epidemiology, diagnosis, management and outcome. *Stroke*, **16**, 591–4.

Broe, G.A. (1986). Brain ageing and the dementia syndrome. In: Anderson, V., Ponsford, J., and Snow, P. (eds.) *Proceedings of 10th Annual Brain Impairment Conference*, The Australian Society for the Study of Brain Impairment, Richmond, Victoria, Australia, pp. 116–30.

Broe, G.A., Akhtar, A.J., Andrews, G.R., Caird, F.I., Gilmore, A.J.J., and McLennan, W.J. (1976). Neurological disorders in the elderly at home. *J. Neurol. Neurosurg. Psychiatry*, **39**, 362–6.

Cameron, M.M. (1978). Chronic subdural haematoma: a review of 114 cases. *J. Neurol. Neurosurg. Psychiatry*, **41**, 834–9.

Campbell, A.J., Diep, C., Reinken, J., and McCosh, L. (1985a). Factors predicting mortality in a total population sample of the elderly. *J. Epidemiol. Comm. Health*, **39**, 337–42.

Campbell, A.J., Reinken, J., and McCosh, L. (1985b). Incontinence in the elderly: prevalence and prognosis. *Age Ageing*, **14**, 65–70.

Chandra, V., Bharucha, N.E., and Schoenberg, B.S. (1986). Patterns of mortality from types of dementia, in the United States 1971 and 1973–1978. *Neurology (Cleveland)*, **36**, 204–8.

Cooper, B., and Bickel, H. (1984). Population screening and the early detection of dementing disorders in old age: a review. *Psychol. Med.*, **14**, 81–5.

Creasey, H., and Rapoport, S.I. (1985). The aging human brain. *Ann. Neurol.*, **17**, 2–10.

Eastwood, M.R., Corbin, S.L., Reed, M., Nobbs, H., and Kedward, H.B. (1985). Acquired hearing loss and psychiatric illness: an estimate of prevalence and comorbidity in a geriatric setting. *Br. J. Psychiatry*, **147**, 552–6.

Eckstrom, P.T., Brand, F.R., Edlavitch, S.A., and Parrish, H.M. (1969). *Public Health Rep.*, **84**, 878–82.

Eisenberg, H., Morrison, J.T., Sullivan, P., and Foote, F.M. (1964). Cerebrovascular accidents. Incidence and survival rates in a defined population, Middlesex County, Connecticut *J.A.M.A.*, **189**, 883–8.

Epstein, F.H., Francis, T., Jr, Hayner, N.S., Johnson, B.C., Kjelsberg, M.O., Napier, J.A., Ostrander, L.D., Jr Payner, M.W., and Dodge, H.J. (1965). Prevalence of chronic diseases and distribution of selected physiologic variables in a total community, Tecumseh, Michigan. *Am. J. Epidemiol.*, **81**, 307–22.

Eva, P., and Heikkinen, E. (1985). Postural sway during standing and unexpected disturbance of balance in random samples of men of different ages. *J. Gerontol.*, **40**, 287–95.

Grimley-Evans, J., and Caird, F.L. (1982). Epidemiology of neurological disorders in old age. In: Caird, F.I. (ed.) *Neurological Disorders in the Elderly*, Wright PSG, Bristol, pp. 1–16.

Haavisto, H.V., Heikinheimo, R.J., Mattila, K.J., and Rajala, S.A. (1985). Living conditions and health of a population aged 85 years or over: a five-year follow up study. *Age Ageing*, **14**, 202–8.

Hagnell, O., Lanke, J., Rossman, B., and Ojesjo, L. (1981). Does the incidence of age psychosis decrease? A prospective longitudinal study of a complete population investigated during the 25 year period, 1947–1972: the Lundby study. *Neuropsychobiology*, **7**, 201–11.

Henderson, A.S. (1983). The coming epidemic of dementia. *Aust. N.Z. J. Psychiatry*, **17**, 117–27.

Henderson, A.F. (1986). The epidemiology of Alzheimer's disease. *Br. Med. Bull.*, **42**, 3–10.

Henderson, A.S., and Huppert, F.A. (1984). The problem of mild dementia. *Psychol. Med.*, **14**, 5–11.

Heston, L.L., Mastri, A.R., Anderson, V.E., and White, J. (1981). Dementia of the Alzheimer type: clinical genetics, natural history and associated conditions. *Arch. Gen. Psychiatry*, **38**, 1085–90.

Heyman, A., Karp, H.R., Heyden, S., Bartel, A., Cassel, J.C., Tyroler, H.A., and Hames, C.G. (1971). Cerebrovascular disease in the biracial population of Evans County, Georgia. *Arch. Intern. Med.*, **128**, 949–55.

Heyman, A., Wilkinson, W.E., Stafford, J.A., Helms, M.J., Sigmon, A.H., and Weinberg, T. (1984). Alzheimer's disease—a study of epidemiological aspects. *Ann. Neurol.*, **15**, 335–41.

Howell, T.H. (1949). Senile deterioration of the central nervous system. *Br. J. Med.*, **i**, 56–8.

Jacobs, L., and Grossman, M.D. (1980). Three primitive reflexes in normal adults. *Neurology (N.Y.)*, **30**, 184–8.

Jarvik, L.F., Ruth, V., and Matsuyama, S.S. (1980). Organic brain syndrome and aging. A six-year follow-up of surviving twins. *Arch. Gen. Psychiatry*, **37**, 280–6.

Johnson, K.G., Yano, K., and Kato, H. (1967). Cerebral vascular disease in Hiroshima, Japan. *J. Chronic Dis.*, **20**, 545–59.

Jonsson, A., and Hallgrimsson, J. (1983). Comparative disease patterns in the elderly and the very old: a retrospective autopsy study. *Age Ageing*, **12**, 111–17.

Juergens, S.M., Kurland, L.T., Okazaki, H., and Mulder, D.W. (1980). ALS in Rochester, Minnesota, 1925–1977. *Neurology (N.Y.)*, **30**, 463–70.

Kannel, W.B., and Wolf, P.A. (1983). Epidemiology of cerebrovascular disease. In: Ross Russell, R.W. (ed.) *Vascular Disease of the Central Nervous System*, second edition, Churchill Livingstone, Edinburgh, pp. 2–3.

Kay, D.W.K. (1972). Epidemiological aspects of organic

brain disease in the aged. In Gaitz, C.M. (ed.) *Aging and the Brain*, Plenum Press, New York, pp. 13–27.

Kay, D.W.K., Beamish, P., and Roth, M. (1964). Old age mental disorders in Newcastle upon Tyne. Part 1: a study of prevalence. *Br. J. Psychiatry*, **110**, 146–58.

Kessler, I.I. (1978). Parkinson's disease in epidemiologic perspective. In: Schoenberg, B.S. (ed.) *Epidemiology of Neurologic Diseases. Advances in Neurology*, Vol. 19, Raven Press, New York, pp. 335–84.

Kuller, L.H. (1978). Epidemiology of stroke. In: Schoenberg, B.S. (ed.) *Epidemiology of Neurologic Diseases. Advances in Neurology*, Vol. 19, Raven Press, New York, pp. 281–312.

Kurtzke, J.F., and Kurland, L.T. (1983). The epidemiology of neurologic disease. In: Baker, A.B., and Baker, L.H. (eds.) *Clinical Neurology*, Vol. 4, Harper and Row, Philadelphia, pp. 55–60.

Li, S-c., Schoenberg, B.S., Wang, C-c., Cheng, X-m., Bolis, C.L., and Wang, K-j. (1985a). Cerebrovascular disease in the People's Republic of China: Epidemiological and clinical features. *Neurology (Cleveland)*, **35**, 1708–13.

Li, S-c., Schoenberg, B.S., Wang, C-c., Cheng, X-m., Rui, D.Y., Bolis, C.T., and Schoenberg, D.G. (1985b). A prevalence survey of Parkinson's disease and other movement disorders in the People's Republic of China. *Arch. Neurol.*, **42**, 655–7.

Li, T-m., Swach, M., and Alberman, E. (1985). Morbidity and mortality in motor neurone disease: comparison with multiple sclerosis and Parkinson's disease: age and sex specific rates and cohort analyses. *J. Neurol. Neurosurg. Psychiatry*, **48**, 320–7.

MacDonald Critchley (1931a). The neurology of old age. *Lancet*, **i**, 1119–27.

MacDonald Critchley (1931b). The neurology of old age. Clinical manifestations in old age. *Lancet*, **i**, 1221–30.

Matsumoto, N., Whisnant, J.P., Kurland, L.T., and Okazaki, H. (1973). Natural history of stroke in Rochester, Minnesota, 1955 through 1969: an extension of a previous study, 1945 through 1954. *Stroke*, **4**, 20–9.

Matsuyama, H., and Nakamura, S. (1978). Senile changes in the brain in the Japanese: incidence of Alzheimer's neurofibrillary change and senile plaques. In: Katzmann, R., Terry, R.D., and Bick, K.L. (eds.) *Alzheimer's Disease: Senile Dementia and Related Disorders, Aging*, Raven Press, New York, Vol. 7, pp. 289–97.

Molsa, P.K., Paljarvi, L., Rinne, J.O., Rinne, U.K., and Sako, E. (1985). Validity of clinical diagnosis in dementia: a prospective clinicopathological study. *J. Neurol. Neurosurg. Psychiatry*, **48**, 1085–90.

Mortimer, J.A., French, L.R., Hutton, J.T., and Schuman, L.M. (1985). Head injury as a risk factor for Alzheimer's disease. *Neurology (Cleveland)*, **35**, 264–7.

Nickens, H. (1985). Intrinsic factors in falling among the elderly. *Arch. Intern. Med.*, **145**, 1089–93.

Nilsson, L.V. (1984). Incidence of severe dementia in an urban sample followed from 70 to 79 years of age. *Acta Psychiatr. Scand.*, **70**, 478–86.

Nilsson, L.V., and Persson, G. (1984). Prevalence of mental disorders in an urban sample examined at 70, 75 and 79 years of age. *Acta Psychiatr. Scand.*, **69**, 519–27.

Patrick, D., and Gates, P.C. (1984). Chronic subdural haematoma in the elderly. *Age Ageing*, **13**, 367–9.

Potvin, A.R., Syndulko, K., Tourtellote, W.W., Lemmon, M.S., and Potvin, J.H. (1980). Human neurological function and the aging process. *J. Am. Geriatr. Soc.*, **28**, 1–9.

Rocca, W.A., Amaducci, L.A., and Schoenberg, B.S. (1986). Epidemiology of clinically diagnosed Alzheimer's disease. *Ann. Neurol.*, **19**, 415–24.

Savage, D.D., Corwin, L., McGee, D.L., Kannel, W.B., and Wolf, P.A. (1985). Epidemiologic features of isolated syncope: the Framingham study. *Stroke*, **16**, 626–9.

Schoenberg, B.S. (1978). Epidemiology of primary nervous system neoplasms. In: Schoenberg, B.S. (ed.) *Epidemiology of Neurologic Diseases, Advances in Neurology*, Vol. 19, Raven Press, New York, pp. 475–95.

Schoenberg, B.S., Anderson, D.W., and Haerer, A.F. (1986). Racial differentials in the prevalence of stroke. *Arch. Neurol.*, **43**, 565–8.

Sivenius, J., Heironen, O.P., Pyroala, K., Salonen, J., and Riekkinen, P. (1985). The incidence of stroke in the Kuopio area of east Finland. *Stroke*, **16**, 188–92.

Skre, H. (1972). Neurological signs in a normal population. *Acta Neurol. Scand.*, **48**, 575–606.

Sulkava, R., Wikstrom, J., Aroman, A., Raitasalo, R., Lehtinen, V., Lahtela, K., and Palo, J. (1985). Prevalence of severe dementia in Finland. *Neurology (Cleveland)*, **35**, 1025–9.

Tanaka, H., Hayashi, M., Date, C., Imai, K., Asada, M., Shoji, H., Okazaki, K., Yamamoto, H., Yoshikawa, K., Shimada, T., and Lee, S.I. (1985). Epidemiologic studies of stroke in Shibota, a Japanese provincial city: preliminary report on risk factors for cerebral infarction. *Stroke*, **16**, 773–80.

Todorov, A.B., Go, R.C.P., Constantinidis, J., and Elston, R.L. (1975). Specificity of the clinical diagnosis of dementia. *J. Neurol. Sci.*, **26**, 81–98.

Tomlinson, B.E., Blessed, G., and Roth, M. (1968). Observations on the brains of nondemented old people. *J. Neurol. Sci.*, **11**, 205–42.

Tomlinson, B.E., Blessed, G., and Roth, M. (1970). Observations on the brains of demented old people. *J. Neurol. Sci.*, **11**, 205–42.

Wade, D.T., Langton-Hewer, R., and Wood, V.A. (1984). Stroke: the influence of age upon outcome. *Age Ageing*, **13**, 357–62.

Wade, D.T., Wood, V.A., and Hewer, R.L. (1985). Recovery after stroke: the first 3 months. *J. Neurol. Neurosurg. Psychiatry*, **48**, 7–14.

Walker, A.E., Robins, M., and Weinfeld, E.D. (1985).

Epidemiology of brain tumors: the national survey of intracranial neoplasms. *Neurology*, **35**, 219–26.

Weissman, M.M., Myers, J.K., Tischler, G.L., Holzer, III C.E., Leaf, P.J., Orraschel, H., and Brody, J.A. (1985). Psychiatric disorders (DSM = III) and cognitive impairment among the elderly in a US urban community. *Acta Psychiatr. Scand.*, **71**, 366–79.

Wolf, P.A., Dawber, T.R., Thomas, H.E., Colton, T., and Kannel, W.B. (1977). Epidemiology of stroke. In: Thompson, R.A., and Green, J.R. (eds.) *Advances in Neurology*, Vol. 16, Raven Press, New York, pp. 8–14.

Chapter 5

The Neurological Examination
of the Elderly Patient

James George

Consultant Geriatrician, Cumberland Infirmary, Carlisle, UK

Neurological examination in old age requires a modified approach. Allowance needs to be made for the possible presence of signs due to normal ageing, and also for disease affecting other systems which may mask or mimic neurological signs. Furthermore, examination should be extended to encompass functional aspects and provide a basis for rehabilitation. In common with younger patients, however, most diagnoses can be established from the history, and examination must always be preceded by a thorough history. In this chapter, history-taking is discussed, followed by consideration of the neurological signs attributed to ageing. Finally, important practical aspects of the neurological examination of the elderly are described.

HISTORY-TAKING

History-taking may be more difficult in the elderly, requiring patience and skill. There may be memory loss, which makes accurate timing of symptoms difficult, and older patients tend to have low expectations of health and are less forthcoming about their symptoms.

The symptoms of neurological disease are described elsewhere in this volume. All elderly patients should be asked about their mobility both inside and outside the home. It is useful to ask if they are able to do their own shopping and collect their own pension, as this gives a measure of walking ability. There may be particular difficulties inside the home, and patients should be routinely asked how they manage stairs; a patient may deny a problem at first but further questioning reveal that stairs are being climbed on all fours! Patients should also be asked about their self-care such as washing (including ability to get in and out of the bath), dressing and cooking and whether there has been any recent change in these activities. Drug history is also important, as adverse reactions to drugs, particularly those acting on the central nervous system, are a common reason for admission to hospital (Williamson and Chopin, 1980). Corroborative evidence from relatives and neighbours is often helpful. A phone call to someone who knows the patient well can save considerable time and unnecessary investigation. The telephone is a valuable neurological tool.

NEUROLOGICAL SIGNS ASSOCIATED WITH AGEING

Since the classic paper of Critchley (1931) there have been numerous studies describing abnormal neurological signs in apparently healthy elderly (Table 5.1).

TABLE 5.1   NEUROLOGICAL SIGNS ASSOCIATED WITH AGEING

	Critchley (1931)	Howell (1949)	Klawans et al. (1971)	Prakash and Stern (1973)	Kokmen et al. (1977)	Carter (1979)	Potvin et al. (1980)
Age	Not given	65–91 years	65–74 years	69–94 years	61–84 years	>70 years	20–80 years
No.	—*	200	927	100	51	100	61
Subjects	—	Chelsea Pensioners	Subjects receiving financial aid	Patients in geriatric wards	Community volunteers	Patients in medical wards	Community volunteers
Limitation upward gaze	Common	—	—	—	20%	Common	
Pupillary changes	Small sluggish pupils common	28% reacted poorly to light and accommodation	—	34% reacted poorly to light 12% reacted poorly to accommodation	—	8% reacted poorly to light and accommodation	—
Muscle wasting	Common in hands	—	—	77% wasting dorsal interossei	—	50% wasted hands	—
Resting tremor (not parkinsonian)	Common involving head and arms	—	—	7% head 43% arms	—	—	Nil
Tendon reflexes	Loss of ankle jerk common	70% loss ankle jerks 23% loss knee jerks	70% loss ankle jerks 11% loss knee jerks	38% loss ankle jerks 26% loss knee jerks	18% loss ankle jerks	31% loss ankle jerks 13% loss knee jerks	—
Plantar response	Usually flexor	5% extensor	0.2% extensor	3% equivocal			
Sensation	General reduction especially vibration	30% loss vibration ankles 24% loss pain touch and temperature	84% loss vibration	31% loss vibration ankles	100% loss vibration (legs>arms)	57% loss vibration ankles	Vibration sense lost. No loss touch or 2-point discrimination
Gait	Flexed posture small steps	—	—	8% ataxic 56% short steps	—	—	Normal

* No data quoted.

Neuro-ophthalmological Signs and Ageing

Visual acuity declines with age in about 12% of the elderly population but in some individuals may actually improve (Milne, 1979). Limitation of convergence and irregular pupils with diminished reactivity to light and accommodation have all been described in normal old age (Critchley, 1931; Skre, 1972; Prakash and Stern, 1973). Pupil diameter gradually decreases from the age of 15 onwards but the explanation for this is not known (Loewenfeld, 1979). Chamberlain (1971) found a progressive loss of upward gaze from fifteen onwards and speculates that this is due to 'disuse'. The corneal reflex is often lost in normal elderly people (Rai and Elias-Jones, 1979).

Motor Signs and Ageing

Atrophy of the intrinsic hand muscles, especially the dorsal interossei, has been found in as many as three-quarters of elderly inpatients without neurological disease (Prakash and Stern, 1973). A striking feature is that, despite muscle wasting, power is relatively preserved (Carter, 1979). There is, however, a decline in muscle power with age, affecting the legs more than the arms and this affects the dominant more than the non-dominant side (Potvin et al., 1980).

Critchley (1931) found that increased tone was common in old age, especially in the legs. However, in a study of hospital inpatients over the age of 50 without neurological symptoms, 75% were found to have radiological evidence of cervical spinal canal narrowing (Pallis et al., 1954). Thus isolated increased tone may be the sole manifestation of trivial cervical cord compression and not represent a genuine ageing process.

Paratonia or gegenhalten is an increase in tone in both extension and flexion which is increased even more if the patient is asked to relax or the limb is displaced quickly, but is paradoxically reduced if the limb is displaced slowly. It is occasionally found in the elderly but seems to be related to diffuse cerebral disease (Jenkyn et al., 1977), rather than uncomplicated ageing. Similarly, nuchal rigidity is sometimes found in cognitively impaired patients and in these

circumstances does not necessarily indicate meningitis (Puxty et al., 1983).

Essential tremor is common in the elderly, often involving the head (Prakash and Stern, 1973). There is a slight decline in coordination and dexterity with age (Potvin et al., 1980), but frank intention tremor on the finger–nose test is not a feature of old age (Howell, 1949). Generalized chorea is sometimes found in the elderly, and most cases are probably due to late onset Huntington's chorea (Critchley, 1956) or are a consequence of levodopa therapy. On the other hand, orofacial dyskinesia, not drug related or part of Huntington's chorea, is occasionally seen and its prevalence increases with age (Klawans and Barr, 1982), suggesting that this is a true ageing phenomenon.

The gait of elderly people has been observed to show change, with shortening of stride, flexed posture and diminished associated movements (Critchley, 1931). These changes suggest an extrapyramidal disturbance due to ageing, for which there is biochemical evidence (McGeer et al., 1977). Potvin et al. (1980) found that although their very fit elderly showed no deterioration in tandem gait (timed walking, heel to toe, along a straight line, without support) they did have difficulty balancing on one leg, especially with their eyes closed. This may explain the predisposition of the elderly to falls (Overstall et al., 1977).

An idiopathic gait disorder associated with old age has been described (Sabin, 1982). This consists of a very hesitant, shuffling gait with a marked tendency to fall backwards and difficulty turning. Often when the patient is examined in bed, the leg movements are normal. Suggested causes include a frontal lobe apraxia, normal pressure hydrocephalus, an extrapyramidal disturbance, multiple cerebral infarction, cervical myelopathy or a peripheral neuropathy (Sabin, 1982). Sudarsky and Ronthal (1983) investigated 50 elderly neurological patients with a previously unexplained gait disorder and found causes in 86%. Common causes, in their series, were multiple sensory deficits (peripheral neuropathy with proprioceptive loss and visual or vestibular impairment), cervical myelopathy, multiple cerebral infarction and previously undetected Parkinson's disease.

Reflex Changes and Ageing

Many authors (Critchley, 1931; Howell, 1949; Milne and Williamson, 1972; Prakash and Stern, 1973) have described loss of ankle reflexes to be common in the elderly with occasional loss of other tendon reflexes also. However, a more recent study (Impallomeni *et al.*, 1984) found loss of ankle jerks rare in the elderly, provided consideration was given to timing and method of testing. Absence of ankle jerks may be the first clue to a peripheral neuropathy in the elderly (Huang, 1981) as with the young.

Abdominal reflexes are often absent in normal elderly but extensor plantar responses are rare (Prakash and Stern, 1973). Loss of the jaw jerks also seems to be common (Prakash and Stern, 1973). The snout reflex consists of a pursing–pouting movement when the examiner presses firmly with the index finger over the philtrum of the upper lip. The grasp reflex consists of flexion of the fingers with adduction of the thumb in response to stroking the palm of the hand. These primitive reflexes have been found to be common in normal elderly (Jacobs and Gosman, 1980). The subjects, however were not screened with formal neuropsychometric testing and the snout and grasp reflex have been shown to correlate significantly with performance on cognitive tests (Tweedy *et al.*, 1982).

Sensory Signs and Ageing

Hearing is progressively impaired with age (Milne, 1977) and sense of smell may also be impaired (Prakash and Stern, 1973). Loss of vibration sense, particularly at the ankles, is universally recognized and has been quantified (Bloom *et al.*, 1984). Position sense is preserved in old age (Howell, 1949; Potvin *et al.*, 1980). Howell (1949) found impairment for light touch, pain and temperature but admitted that documentation was difficult. In contrast, Potvin *et al.* (1980) found no loss in touch sensation or two point discrimination with age. There is gradual slowing of nerve conduction velocities with age (Dorfman and Bosley, 1979). Tactile inattention on bilateral simultaneous stimulation is uncommon in normal old people (Kokmen *et al.*, 1977).

FUNCTIONAL CHANGES AND AGEING

Potvin *et al.* (1980) investigated changes in performance with age in simulated activities of daily living. Sixty-one right-handed volunteers, between the ages of 20 and 80 years, were examined. There was an average 30% decline in speed of performance in such tasks as putting on a shirt, undoing buttons, cutting with a knife and rising from a chair. However, accuracy in performance of these tasks is maintained in old age (Potvin *et al.*, 1973) and it seems that speed is sacrificed for accuracy (Welford, 1962).

Clinical Significance of Neurological Signs due to Ageing

The neurological signs described above have been found in apparently normal old people and have been attributed to the ageing process. However, these signs may also be caused by neurological diseases common in the elderly such as dementia, cervical myelopathy or peripheral neuropathy. The data are derived mainly from cross-sectional studies with non-random samples of subjects. Some of the signs observed may be due to lifelong differences between generations rather than ageing effects. Also, it is often difficult to exclude subclinical neurological disease. There is a need for more data from longitudinal studies. Meanwhile, many of the signs described are best regarded as 'soft signs'. They may be clinically significant but need to be interpreted in conjunction with the presence or absence of other related signs and symptoms. In dealing with the individual patient, the clinician should not attribute abnormal neurological signs to old age without considering other underlying causes.

IMPORTANT PRACTICAL ASPECTS OF THE NEUROLOGICAL EXAMINATION IN THE ELDERLY

Comprehensive descriptions of the neurological examination are given in standard neurological texts and only those aspects considered to be particularly relevant to the elderly are discussed here. A proposed scheme is given in Table 5.2. It is essential that the neurological examination is methodical and systematic although the precise order of examination is not important. A few general points need to be mentioned before considering the areas of special interest in the elderly.

General examination should include auscultation of the neck for bruits and measurement of blood pressure, both lying and standing, as postural hypotension is common in the elderly.

First impressions of posture, and facial features are very useful and can be diagnostic, as with Parkinson's disease.

Conscious level is assessed in the same way as with younger patients, using the Glasgow Coma Scale (Teasdale and Jennett, 1974). There is a tendency to assume that all unconscious elderly patients have suffered a stroke, whereas other causes of coma such as hypoglycaemia are also common and need to be considered. A good history (using the telephone if necessary) and a complete general examination are mandatory in any elderly unconscious patient.

Papilloedema is a less common manifestation of raised intracranial pressure in the elderly (Godfrey and Caird, 1984).

Fasciculation confined to the calves is not usually significant.

Essential tremor is common and it is important to distinguish it from parkinsonian tremor. It is not accompanied by rigidity, is more likely to involve the head, and is usually absent at rest.

Mental State

Dementia may go unrecognized unless specifically sought. A simple questionnaire test, such as the abbreviated mental test score (Table 5.3), tests memory and orientation and is quick, portable and reliable. However, questionnaire tests can be misleading if the patient is deaf, dysphasic, depressed or physically unwell. The Kew test (Hare, 1978) has more localizing value as it includes assessment of parietal and temporal lobe function and is also easy to administer at the bedside. A comprehensive review of mental status tests is given by Strub and Black (1985).

Speech

Aphasia may be defined as loss of ability to formulate, express or understand the meaning of spoken

TABLE 5.2   SCHEME FOR NEUROLOGICAL EXAMINATION IN THE ELDERLY

General
  Posture and facial features
  Involuntary movements
  Blood pressure lying and standing
  Auscultation for neck bruits

Mental status
  Conscious level
  Mental test score
  Special testing for aphasia and apraxia

Cranial nerves
Motor
  Wasting and fasciculation
  Power, tone and coordination
Reflexes
Sensation
Gait
Assessment of activities of daily living
Assessment of aids

TABLE 5.3   ABBREVIATED MENTAL TEST SCORE (HODKINSON, 1972)

1.   Age
2.   Time
3.   Address for recall at end of test
4.   Year
5.   Name of hospital
6.   Recognition of two persons
7.   Date of birth
8.   Year of First World War
9.   Name of present Monarch
10. Count backwards 20–1

words, due to a lesion of the language area of the dominant cerebral hemisphere. In common usage the terms aphasia and dysphasia have come to be interchangeable. Before testing for aphasia it is important to check that the patient's hearing and vision are satisfactory. By assessing spontaneous speech (fluent or non-fluent), comprehension, repetition of words and phrases and naming or word finding, the major types of aphasia can be recognized at the bedside (Table 5.4). Naming of objects can be tested by asking the patient to identify parts of a

TABLE 5.4 RECOGNITION OF THE COMMON TYPES OF APHASIA

Type of aphasia	Spontaneous speech	Compre-hension	Naming
Wernicke's	Fluent	Poor	Impaired
Broca's	Non-fluent	Good	Impaired
Global	Severe non-fluent	Very poor	Impaired

watch. Naming is impaired in all types of aphasia and is a useful screening test. Comprehension can be tested by asking the patient to point to objects about the room. The task can be made more complex by asking the patient to point out a series of objects in sequence.

In *fluent* aphasias (e.g. Wernicke's aphasia), the lesion is posteriorly situated in the dominant hemisphere. Word output is normal or increased with frequent incorrect words or sounds resulting in meaningless speech. This type of aphasia can be easily misdiagnosed as confusion or a psychosis.

In *non-fluent* aphasias (e.g. Broca's aphasia), word output is low consisting mainly of nouns. In Broca's aphasia the lesion is anteriorly situated in the dominant hemisphere and is usually accompanied by a hemiparesis.

In *global* aphasia there is virtually no word output and comprehension is severely impaired. Global aphasia is due to a lesion of the whole perisylvian region. The prognosis is poor but what little recovery there is tends to occur after 6 months (Sarno and Levita, 1981). Global aphasia and Wernicke's aphasia seem to be more common with increasing age (Eslinger and Damasio, 1981).

Dysarthria, which is a disorder of articulation of speech, must be distinguished from aphasia and in the elderly a common cause is poorly fitting dentures.

Apraxia

Apraxia is defined as the inability to carry out a purposive movement, the nature of which the patient understands, in the absence of severe motor paralysis, sensory loss or ataxia. It indicates a focal disturbance of the parietal lobes and can represent a barrier to recovery from stroke (Adams and Hurwitz, 1963). It is important to test for constructional and dressing apraxia in the elderly. Constructional apraxia can be tested for by asking the patient to copy a simple line drawing of a house. Picture drawing tests are a useful screening test for visuospatial perception problems as well as constructional apraxia and are of prognostic value in stroke patients (Andrews *et al.*, 1980). Dressing apraxia is assessed by observing the patient put on a jacket or coat. Dressing apraxia is due to a lesion of the non-dominant hemisphere whereas constructional apraxia may be due to a lesion in either hemisphere. For a comprehensive description of the various forms of apraxia and how to test for them, the reader is referred to Strub and Black (1985).

Vision and Hearing

Vision and hearing assessment is very important in the elderly, but is all too often neglected. Visual fields should be assessed and visual acuity formally measured. A Snellen 3 metre distance chart and a standard reading chart should be available on every ward. Simple assessment of vision will reveal many remediable problems (Fenton *et al.*, 1975). Deafness is also common and may be due to wax or be improved with the provision of a hearing aid (Crammond and Gabb, 1980).

Muscle Power

Testing of power in the elderly is performed in the same way as in younger patients. If weakness is present it is important to try and identify the type of weakness; whether due to a pyramidal tract lesion, a lower motor neurone lesion or a muscular lesion.

Reflexes

For eliciting the tendon reflexes and for examination of tone the patient should be relaxed. It may be necessary to delay testing until the patient has settled in hospital. Apart from deciding whether the reflexes are normal, increased or decreased, it is important to compare the reflexes from both sides of the body, in order to localize a neurological lesion. Tendon reflexes may be diminished in the elderly due to stiffness of the joints. Similarly deformities of the toes are very common in the elderly and may make elicitation of the plantar response difficult or impossible.

Sensation

Sensory testing requires the cooperation and interest of the patient; this is not always possible. Sensation is tested in the same way in the elderly as in young patients. It should be remembered that vibration sense is often lost distally but that position sense is maintained. The thumb-finding test is a useful test for position sense applicable to the elderly (Caird and Judge, 1979). The patient's arm is held up by the sleeve and the patient is asked to grasp his thumb with the opposite hand with eyes closed. Visuospatial perception should also be assessed by asking the patient to copy simple line drawings, as described previously.

Gait

Every elderly patient should be watched rising from a suitable chair, walking a few paces and turning round. It is not always possible to classify abnormal gaits in the elderly as 'spastic', 'ataxic', 'waddling', etc., as many abnormal gaits are due to non-neurological disease such as osteoarthritis and disorders of the feet. A practical approach is to classify gait as safe or unsafe (especially on turning) as this is of most concern to the patient. If the gait is unsafe then the cause needs to be ascertained and rehabilitation efforts directed towards achieving safer mobility, perhaps with the use of a walking aid.

Assessment of Aids

Elderly patients are often reliant on aids and a complete examination should always include assessment of mobility aids, dentures, spectacles and hearing aids to ensure that these items are appropriate and in good working order (Mulley, 1985).

Functional Assessment

Assessment of the patient's performance in activities of daily living is of tremendous practical importance

and is usually carried out with the help of an occupational therapist. There are numerous scales for the formal assessment of ability in washing, dressing, and cooking. An ideal scale should be easy to use, valid and repeatable, sensitive to minor change and applicable to a wide range of different diseases. The Katz scale (Katz *et al.*, 1963) and the Barthel scale (Mahoney and Barthel, 1965) meet these requirements most closely and have been used successfully in old people. It is better to use a well-established scale rather than create a new one. Most of the difficulties in activities of daily living should be predictable from the preceding neurological examination. Sometimes, however, patients perform less well than expected; in such cases apraxias, perception difficulties and depression should always be considered.

At the completion of the functional assessment, it should be possible to predict if the patient can manage at home, with or without support, or needs residential care. It is important, however, not to reach a final conclusion without involving the patient and relatives as well as all members of the rehabilitation team, thereby ensuring that all possible remediable conditions have been treated or excluded. Often a final assessment needs to be made in the patient's own home.

Assessment of the Patient in the Home

No account of examination of the elderly patient would be complete without emphasizing the extra information which can be gained by visiting the patient at home (Arcand and Williamson, 1981). A neglected house or garden suggests lack of energy or initiative. Incontinence may be evident from the odour. Heating, access to the toilet, bathing facilities, stairs and rails, medication containers and food and cooking facilities should all be noted. Home assessment is also a valuable opportunity for patients and carers to identify particular problems within the home.

Abbreviated Neurological Examination

It is useful to have an abbreviated scheme for neurological examination for elderly patients in whom no neurological disease is suspected.

Mental status should be assessed using the abbreviated mental test score. Cranial nerves are examined, omitting sense of smell, but not forgetting visual acuity. The arms are then outstretched and any falling away, when the eyes are closed, is noted. Fine finger movements and grip are then tested. Power is examined in the legs by testing straight leg raising and foot dorsiflexion. The tendon reflexes and the plantar response are then examined. Sensory testing can be limited to appreciation of fine touch, pinprick and position sense in the hands and feet. Finally the patient should be watched rising from a chair, walking a few yards and turning round. Using this simple scheme, most important neurological abnormalities will be detected.

CONCLUSION

Neurological examination in the elderly is an intriguing and often satisfying challenge which few doctors can avoid—intriguing because of the background of changes due to ageing and coexisting disease; satisfying, because if a practical functional approach is adopted, remediable problems will be discovered. The examination should be completed by communicating results to the patient and the rehabilitation team and maintaining a clear record in the case notes.

REFERENCES

Adams, G.F., and Hurwitz, L.J. (1963). Mental barriers to recovery from strokes. *Lancet*, **ii**, 533–7.

Andrews, K., Brocklehurst, J.C., Richards, B., and Laycock, P.J. (1980). The prognostic value of picture drawings by stroke patients. *Rheumatol. Rehabil.*, **19**, 180–8.

Arcand, M., and Williamson, J. (1981). An evaluation of home visiting of patients by physicians in geriatric medicine. *Br. Med. J.*, **283**, 718–20.

Bloom, S., Till, S., Sonksen, P., and Smith, S. (1984). Use of a biothesiometer to measure individual vibration thresholds and their variation in 519 non-diabetic subjects. *Br. Med. J.*, **288**, 1793–5.

Caird, F.I., and Judge, T.G. (1979). *Assessment of the Elderly Patient*, Pitman Medical, London, p. 86.

Carter, A.B. (1979). The neurological aspects of ageing. In: Rossman, I. (ed.) *Clinical Geriatrics*, J.B. Lippincott, Philadelphia, pp. 292–316.

Chamberlain, W. (1971). Restriction in upward gaze with advancing age. *Am. J. Ophthalmol.*, **71**, 341–6.

Crammond, G.W., and Gabb, P. (1980). Impaired hearing in the elderly. *Br. Med. J.*, **280**, 612.

Critchley, M. (1931). The neurology of old age. Clinical manifestations in old age. *Lancet*, **i**, 1221–30.

Critchley, M. (1956). Neurological changes in the aged. *J. Chronic Dis.*, **3**, 459–77.

Dorfman, L.J., and Bosley, T.M. (1979). Age related changes in peripheral and central nerve conduction in man. *Neurology*, **29**, 38–44.

Eslinger, P.J., and Damasio, A.R. (1981). Age and type of aphasia in patients with stroke. *J. Neurol. Neurosurg. Psychiatry*, **44**, 377–81.

Fenton, P.J., Arnold, R.C., and Wilkins, P.S.W. (1975). Evaluation of vision in slow stream wards. *Age Ageing*, **4**, 43–8.

Godfrey, J.B., and Caird, F.I. (1984). Intracranial tumour in the elderly: diagnosis and treatment. *Age Ageing*, **13**, 152–8.

Hare, M. (1978). Clinical checklist for diagnosis of dementia. *Br. Med. J.* **ii**, 266–7.

Hodkinson, H.N. (1972). Evaluation of a mental test score for assessment of mental impairment in the elderly. *Age Ageing*, **1**, 233–8.

Howell, T.H. (1949). Senile deterioration of the central nervous system. A clinical study. *Br. Med. J.*, **i**, 56–8.

Huang, C.Y. (1981) Peripheral neuropathy in the elderly: A clinical and electrophysiological study. *J. Am. Geriatr. Soc.*, **29**, 49–54.

Impallomeni, M., Kenny, R.A., Flynn, M.D., Kraenzlin, M., and Pallis, C.A. (1984). The elderly and their ankle jerks. *Lancet*, **i**, 670–3.

Jacobs, L., and Gosman, M.D. (1980). Three primitive reflexes in normal adults. *Neurology*, **30**, 184–88.

Jenkyn, L.R., Walsh, D.B., Culver, C.M., and Reeves, A.G. (1977). Clinical signs in diffuse cerebral dysfunction. *J. Neurol. Neurosurg. Psychiatry*, **40**, 956–66.

Katz, S., Ford, A.B., Moskowitz, R.W., Jackson, B.A., and Jaffe, M.W. (1963). Studies of illness in the aged. *J.A.M.A.*, **185**, 914–19.

Klawans, H.L., and Barr, A. (1982). Prevalence of spontaneous lingual-facial-buccal dyskinesias in the elderly. *Neurology (N.Y.)*, **32**, 558–9.

Klawans, H.L., Tufo, H.M., Ostfield, A.M., Shekelle, R.B., and Kilbridge, J.A. (1971). Neurologic examination in an elderly population. *Dis. Nerv. Syst.*, **32**, 274–9.

Kokmen, E., Bossemeyer, R.W., Barney, J., and Williams, W.J. (1977). Neurological manifestations of ageing. *J. Gerontol.*, **32**, 411–19.

Loewenfeld, I.E. (1979). Pupillary changes related to age. In: Thompson, H.S. (ed.) *Topics in Neuro-ophthalmology*, Williams and Wilkins, Baltimore, pp. 124–50.

McGeer, P.L., McGeer, E.G., and Suzuki, J.S. (1977). Ageing and extrapyramidal function. *Arch. Neurol.*, **34**, 33–5.

Mahoney, F.I., and Barthel, D.W. (1965). Functional

evaluation: the Barthel index. *Md. State Med. J.*, **14**, 61–5.

Milne, J.S. (1977). A longitudinal study of hearing loss in older people. *Br. J. Audiol.*, **11**, 7–14.

Milne, J.S. (1979). Longitudinal studies of vision in older people. *Age Ageing*, **8**, 160–6.

Milne, J.S., and Williamson, J. (1972). The ankle jerk in older people. *Geront. Clin.*, **14**, 86–8.

Mulley, G.P. (1985). *Practical Management of Stroke*, Croom Helm, London.

Overstall, P.W., Exton-Smith, A.N., Imms, F.J., and Johnson, A.L. (1977). Falls in the elderly related to postural imbalance. *Br. Med. J.*, **i**, 261–4.

Pallis, C., Jones, A.M., and Spillane, J.D. (1954). Cervical spondylosis. *Brain*, **77**, 274–89.

Potvin, A.R., Tourtellotte, W.W., Pew, R.W., Albers, J.W., Henderson, W.G., and Snyder, D.N. (1973). The importance of age effects on performance in the assessment of clinical trials. *J. Chronic Dis.*, **26**, 699–717.

Potvin, A.R., Syndulko, K., Tourtellotte, W.W., Lemmon, J.A., and Potvin, J.H. (1980). Human neurologic function and the ageing process. *J. Am. Geriatr. Soc.*, **28**, 1–9.

Prakash, C., and Stern, G. (1973). Neurological signs in the elderly. *Age Ageing*, **2**, 24–7.

Puxty, J.A.H., Fox, R.A., and Horan, M.A. (1983). The frequency of physical signs usually attributed to meningeal irritation in elderly patients. *J. Am. Geriatr. Soc.*, **31**, 590–2.

Rai, G.S., and Elias-Jones, A. (1979). The corneal reflex in elderly patients. *J. Am. Geriatr. Soc.*, **27**, 317–18.

Sabin, T.D. (1982). Biological aspects of falls and mobility limitations in the elderly. *J. Am. Geriatr. Soc.*, **30**, 51–8.

Sarno, M.T., and Levita, E. (1981). Some observations on the nature of recovery in global aphasia after stroke. *Brain Lang.*, **13**, 1–12.

Skre, H. (1972). Neurological signs in a normal population. *Acta Neurol. Scand.*, **48**, 575–606.

Strub, R.L., and Black, F.W. (1985). *The Mental Status Examination in Neurology*, F.A. Davis Company, Philadelphia.

Sudarsky, L., and Ronthal, M. (1983). Gait disorders among elderly patients. A survey study of 50 patients. *Arch. Neurol.*, **40**, 740–3.

Teasdale, G., and Jennett, B. (1974). Assessment of coma and impaired consciousness. A practical scale. *Lancet*, **ii**, 81–3.

Tweedy, J., Reding, M., Garcia, C., Schulman, P., Deutsch, G., and Antin, S. (1982). Significance of cortical disinhibition signs. *Neurology (N.Y.)*, **32**, 169–73.

Welford, A.T. (1962). On changes of performance with age. *Lancet*, **i**, 335–9.

Williamson, J., and Chopin, J.M. (1980). Adverse reactions to prescribed drugs in the elderly: a multicentre investigation. *Age Ageing*, **9**, 73–80.

Chapter 6

Neuroradiological Investigation of the Elderly

Austin Carty

Consultant Radiologist, Royal Liverpool Hospital, Liverpool, UK

INTRODUCTION

Modern discussion about the limited availability of medical resources may have distracted attention from another constraint perhaps narrower than any politically imposed financial cut. This is the capacity of patients to endure medical care and profit from it. Osler pointed out that one feature which distinguishes humans from the lower animals is their apparently limitless capacity to take medicine. But even he could not have foreseen the marathon of high technology to which our patients are expected to submit.

Sadly, even extreme old age may confer little if any immunity to the investigating zeal of physicians. This attitude is perhaps less culpable in laboratory investigation where the participation of the patient generally ceases with the furnishing of a specimen. However, the elderly patient who is subjected to a gamut of imaging investigations is expected to remain a willing and cooperative participant throughout. His consent may be no more than formal; it is seldom informed. He is turned over to strangers often, but by no means always, sympathetic to minimizing his discomfort. He is thrust into unfamiliar surroundings; his name is frequently forgotten and his genuine interest in the course of an examination and the significance of its findings may be summarily dismissed. In short, elderly patients often feel that they are messed about in X-ray departments and they are often right.

The purpose of this chapter is to summarize the imaging techniques available for neurological investigation, to state what they involve for the patient, to highlight their strengths and their weaknesses and, finally, to discuss their application to some clinical conditions commonly found in the aged. In this way it is hoped that those physicians who have been charged with the care of the aged will investigate with precision when they should and show restraint when investigations might be judged to satisfy clinical curiosity rather than further patient welfare. Happy is the physician whose skill justly prompts him to manage his patient on clinical grounds alone.

IMAGING TECHNIQUES

Chest X-ray

Even in the absence of clinical evidence of disease in the chest there can be no good reason for denying an elderly patient who has come to hospital a chest X-ray. A possible exception is the patient who has had a normal chest film within the previous 6 months. Chest films are cheap, easy on the patient and particularly useful in excluding serious disease— notably malignancy or tuberculosis. Even if it is difficult to move the patient to the X-ray department a good quality posteroanterior (PA) film can be obtained using a mobile apparatus with the patient sitting on the side of the bed. Enough bones are displayed on a good quality chest film to go a long way towards excluding disseminated bony malignancy. Lateral views should not be requested as a routine even in the knowledge that there is disease in one side of the chest: they will be done at the discretion of the radiologist.

Skull X-rays

It is tempting, even traditional, to ask for skull X-rays on all elderly patients with even the mildest loss of cerebral function. The skull film is virtually useless in the investigation of neurological disease. Tress (1983) reviewed 1000 patients who had computed tomography (CT) and skull films and found that in only five (0.5%) was the management changed because of an abnormality detected on a skull film and not at CT. He further observed that in only two (0.2%) cases was a plain film abnormality found that was not visible on the lateral view alone. For this reason, a skull examination should be done only if bone disease, including fracture, is suspected. The examination should be confined to a single lateral view with a horizontal X-ray beam and meticulous attention to accurate laterality. Further views should be done only at the direction of the radiologist except in trauma cases where an anteroposterior (AP) (Towne's) view is probably justified if facilities for CT scan are not to hand.

Bone changes, such as those due to Paget's disease (Figure 6.1), myeloma or metastases (Figure 6.2) will be obvious. Erosion of the dorsum sellae may point to the possibility of intracranial disease, but the absence of such changes *does not exclude serious and possibly remediable intracranial disease*. Changes in the sella can only be interpreted on accurate lateral views in which the orbital plates of the frontal bones and the anterior clinoid processes are superimposed. It is usually possible to distinguish the generalized thinning of bone at the sella commonly found in the elderly from the changes of raised intracranial pressure (RICP) because the lamina dura of the dorsum sellae is preserved in the involutional skull but lost in RICP. (The changes are subtle and do not reproduce well on a printed page.) Confusing shad-

ows may be cast in the region of the sella by calcification in the carotid siphon, but an awareness of the possibility usually makes the diagnosis easy (Figure 6.3). Thickening of the inner table of the skull, notably in the frontal region (hyperostosis frontalis interna, Figure 6.4), may prompt a search for possible meningioma. It is usually, though not always, bilateral and symmetrical, often spectacular and always innocent.

Use of the horizontal beam, either with the patient upright or brow-up, not only increases the chances of an accurate lateral view, but makes possible the detection of air fluid levels either in the sphenoid sinuses or within the calvarium in those cases where a communication between the cerebrospinal fluid (CSF) spaces and the air-containing sinuses has been opened by a skull fracture.

Classically, one is urged to seek displacement of the pineal in cases of suspected mass lesions. However, even in the elderly, the pineal is not always sufficiently calcified to be seen on plain films. Furthermore, even slight rotation on the AP film leads to error in interpretation and a normally situated pineal *does not exclude a mass lesion*.

It will be seen, therefore, that although clues to the presence of intracranial disease may be found on plain films and these will always warrant further investigation, serious disease frequently fails to show plain film changes. The plain X-ray of the skull is thus a poor discriminator and its time-hallowed place in neurological investigation is no longer justified.

Echo-encephalography

This technique employs ultrasound to detect displacement of the midline structures and ventricular system caused by tumours. It has been advocated for over 20 years as a screening test and has found continuing favour in a few isolated centres. It has, however, never attained wide popularity and should not now be included in the mainstream of neurological imaging techniques.

Isotope Brain Scan

There will be predictable brain uptake of certain radiopharmaceuticals following intravenous injec-

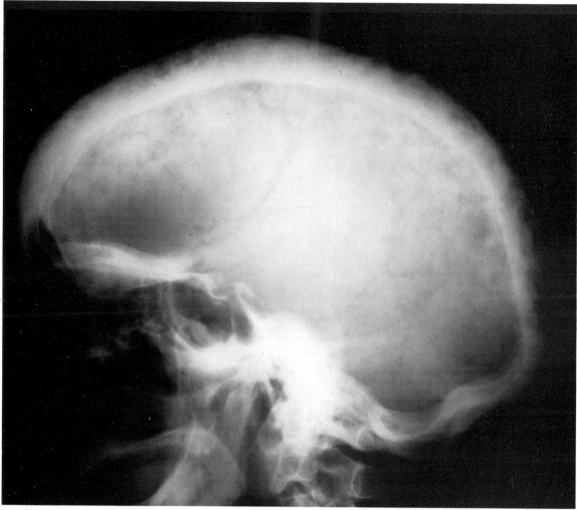

Figure 6.1. Paget's disease of the skull. Note thickening of skull vault and general basilar invagination.

tion and this may be altered in various disease states. Modern nuclear medicine departments favour the use of technetium 99m DTPA. Diseases which affect the blood–brain barrier will lead to increased uptake in the affected area. Thus, tumours, abscesses, infarcts and subdural haematomas may all lead to increased uptake. The changes are not particularly specific but the distribution of increased uptake will normally give a clue to the nature of the pathology. For example, increased uptake along the distribution of the territory of a known artery points to infarction as the cause.

The technique is simple. Isotope is injected and the patient is examined 30–45 minutes after injection. The gamma camera detector is placed to take counts at the front, back, both sides and the vertex of the skull. It is generally better to move the camera than alter the position of the patient. Each count takes 3 minutes and it is important that the patient remains still throughout. The scanning procedure takes about half an hour in all.

Isotope brain scanning has an overall sensitivity of 75–93% compared with 93–98% for CT. The specificity of CT in tumours is about 90% but that of

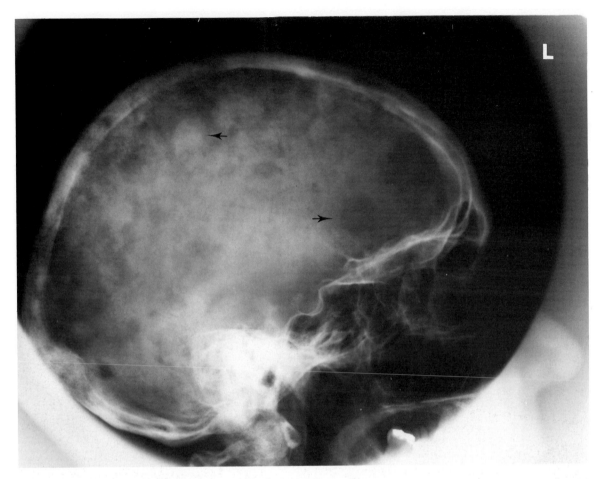

Figure 6.2. Metastases from breast carcinoma. Note mixture of lytic and sclerotic deposits of various sizes. No change in the thickness of the skull vault.

isotope scanning is considerably lower (Harbert, 1986). Isotope brain scanning is still very widely used in the UK largely because general physicians and geriatricians have restricted access to brain CT. Generally speaking, if there is a choice between isotope and CT scanning, CT is to be preferred. There is little difference in cost. It is to be hoped that the wider availability of CT machines will make isotope brain imaging obsolete. Patients often get referred on for brain CT after an isotope study. Few are referred for an isotope study after brain CT. Most neurosciences departments have abandoned isotope brain scanning.

CT Brain Scanning

Computed tomography (CT) (obsolete synonyms CAT scan; EMI scan) has revolutionized the investigation of brain disease. It has been available in prototype form since 1971 and has come into increasingly wide clinical use during the past decade.

The equipment consists of an X-ray source which is rotated through a full circle around the patient's head. The partially attenuated X-ray beam which emerges from the patient's head is intercepted by an array of detectors which give off a numerical signal related to the intensity of the X-ray beam. The

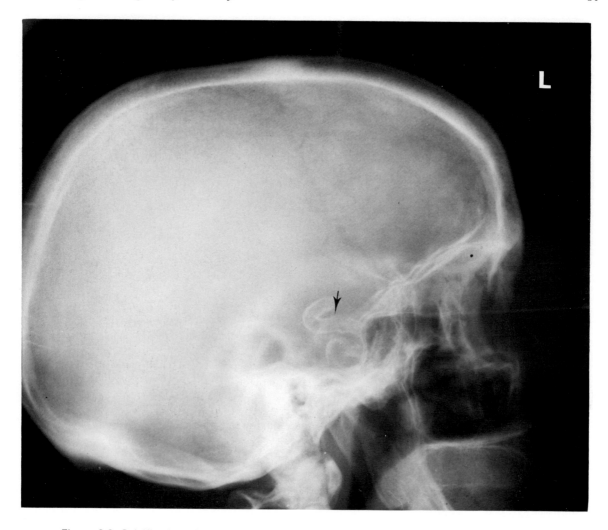

Figure 6.3. Calcification of the carotid siphon projected through and above the pituitary fossa.

numerical or digital signals are analysed by computer and an analogue image is reconstructed displaying the axial anatomy of the slice examined.

The resolution of the images is extremely high and devoid of artefact on modern machines. Furthermore, disease which alters the blood–brain barrier allows escape of conventional iodinated contrast medium into lesions thus enhancing the image in many diseased states. While some artefact is cast by bone, particularly in the posterior fossa, the scope for confirming, and more particularly excluding, intracranial disease by modern CT is very great. The

decision whether to enhance an examination with contrast medium rests with the supervising radiologist. A scan judged as acceptable unenhanced by a competent radiologist will be up to 99% accurate. That is to say if no lesion is seen on the unenhanced scan only one in 100 such cases rescanned with contrast will reveal disease not previously detected. The risk of missing an isodense subdural haematoma is remote with a modern machine.

Modern scanners are equipped with wide aperture gantries and there is no justification for a feeling of claustrophobia. A routine examination can be

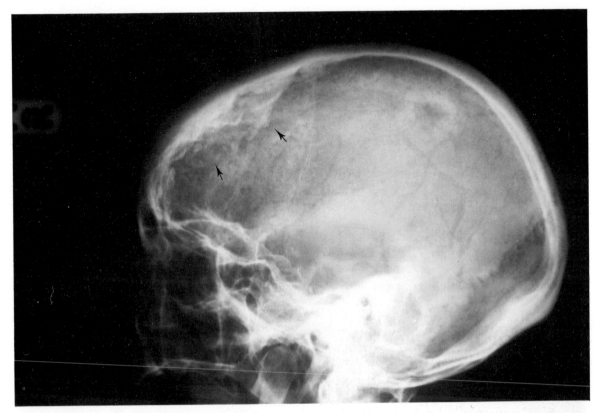

Figure 6.4. Hyperostosis frontalis interna. Note thickening of the inner table in the frontal region.

completed in 10 minutes. Patients can be scanned in a dynamic mode whereby up to a dozen slices can be completed within a minute. The use of general anaesthesia can now be confined to those patients who cannot be kept still by reassurance alone. Such patients should have their CT done in specialized neurosurgical units. Sedation for brain scanning may be very risky and is not advised for use in a general CT department.

The radiation dose in a modern CT brain scan is higher than it was with earlier models and is now about equivalent to 15–20 plain skull films. This is seldom an important consideration in the elderly.

With the advent of new machines and the replacement of earlier generation dedicated brain scanners has come a marked increase in the resolution of images. Improved resolution makes interpretation easier. In many circumstances, diagnostic accuracy can be improved by scanning heads after administra-

tion of contrast medium. Ideally, all brain scans should be done without contrast and repeated with contrast where necessary. This would, however, lead to a vastly increased workload and most CT departments who scan heads proceed to enhancing scans with the notable exception of patients suspected of having a haemorrhage, recent infarction or head injury. Any radiographic contrast medium suitable for intravascular use is acceptable and the usual dose is 15–20 g of iodine given as a bolus. The usual guidelines about the use of non-ionic agents apply, but will not be discussed here (Grainger, 1986). The basis of the use of contrast medium is that many brain lesions, notably tumours, presumably by causing permeability of the blood–brain barrier, take up contrast medium while the surrounding brain does not. Lesions are thus easier to detect and the enhancement pattern may give additional clues to the nature of the lesion. The reason for not enhancing cases of suspected haemorrhage is that the lesions are already radiodense and the accuracy of diagnosis might be diminished by contrast. There is some evidence (Kendall and Pullicino, 1980) that contrast medium may extend the zone of neurone injury or death in cases of recent infarction. Basic interpretation of brain CT should be within the scope of physicians with responsibility for the care of neurologically ill patients. Subtleties of interpretation may be left to radiologists and all practitioners should have access to the expert opinions of neuroradiologists where required. A knowledge of basic brain anatomy can be refreshed remarkably quickly from the recesses of undergraduate memory with the aid of axial images. For further information, the interested reader is referred to more detailed texts (Baddeley, 1984; Moseley, 1986; Valentine *et al.*, 1981).

Recent haemorrhage is more dense to X-rays than brain and looks white on the image (Figure 6.5).

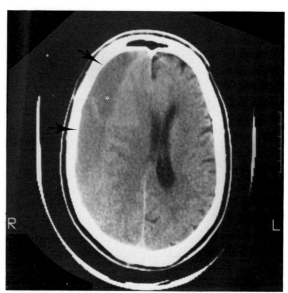

Figure 6.6. Old subdural haematoma. Note hypodense area between the inner table and the cerebral hemisphere. Displacement of midline structures.

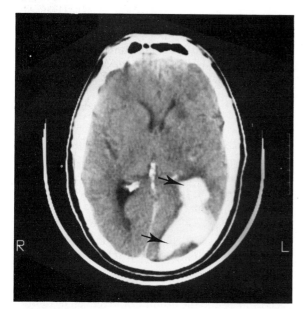

Figure 6.5. Recent haemorrhage on CT. Note triangular increased density immediately lateral to the posterior horn of lateral ventricle.

With the passage of time, haematoma becomes less dense, passing through a phase of being isodense to brain between 10 and 20 days and thereafter being hypodense, i.e. a darker shade of grey (Figure 6.6).

Haemorrhage and haematoma usually exercise a mass effect and this is recognized by the displacement of landmarks.

Infarcts may contain areas of haemorrhage when recent, but they are generally hypodense. They are often found in the territory of a known artery or vein and seldom cause a mass effect. Indeed, because they cause atrophy, they may displace landmarks towards them.

Tumours in the elderly are frequently metastatic. Metastases generally enhance and are surrounded by oedema which is hypodense (Figure 6.7). The extent of oedema may appear very great relative to the size of the enhancing tumour. Tumour and oedema cause mass effects. Metastases are usually multiple and if so, diagnosis is easy. Sometimes only a solitary metastasis is obvious. In such instances, a careful search should be made in the region of the frontal lobes or the posterior fossa, where a subtle distortion of the fourth ventricle may point to the second deposit and clinch the diagnosis. It is important also to reassess the chest film.

Abscess is always difficult. Classical rim enhancement, central hypodensity of gas formation cannot be relied on. Clinical suspicion is a great help. It is so

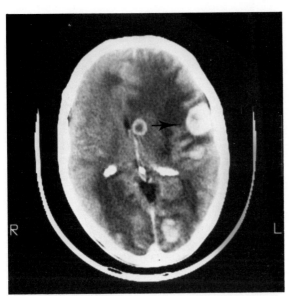

Figure 6.7. Hypodense metastases within the brain, on CT. Multiple lesions of varying sizes with mass effect.

much easier to find a needle in a haystack if you know that it is a needle you are looking for.

For all its excellence, brain CT is a resource which is limited by its cost and the overall dearth of scanners. Clinicians *must* exercise restraint in their requests. It is easy to fall in for a habit of asking for head CT in the Micawber-like hope that something will turn up. This is irresponsible (Leading Article, 1979). CT radiologists are at least as busy as clinicians, but both should be capable of finding time to discuss the possible value of a scan in an aged patient before 'pressing the button'.

Cerebral Angiography

The cerebral circulation can be opacified by the selective introduction of contrast medium into major vessels. This is usually done by selective arterial catheterization but there are some radiologists who favour direct puncture of the carotid artery in the neck. There is no place in modern radiology for attempts to puncture the vertebral artery percutaneously. The advent of digital subtraction angiography (DSA), a computer technique whereby the contrast of enhanced vessels is multiplied by computer techniques, makes it possible to examine the extracranial vascular system following an intravenous injection. Intravenous DSA techniques are fraught with the risk of artefact from swallowing movement but in spite of this many vascular surgeons are prepared to operate on the basis of the images obtained in up to 90% of intravenous DSA studies. The use of DSA coupled with selective arterial catheterization means that contrast medium can be reduced in both concentration and volume. This, coupled with the use of non-ionic agents, has eliminated toxic effect related to the high osmolality of conventional contrast agents used in classical angiography. The advance has also made possible the use of smaller bore catheters which are more manoeuvrable and less likely to damage the intima.

DSA machines are increasingly but not universally available in the UK.

Magnetic Resonance Imaging (MRI)

(Synonym (obsolete) nuclear magnetic resonance (NMR).) This is a new exciting imaging technique particularly applicable to the brain and spine. Tissue protons can be caused to behave as gyromagnets if the body is placed in a strong magnetic field and they precess. If they are excited by a radiofrequency energy their precession is deflected and then rebounds when the radiofrequency is removed. The rebound causes the emission of a radiosignal and this can be intercepted and analysed in a variety of sequences to produce images. Images so obtained can be presented axially, coronally and sagittally. The anatomical detail in the brain, particularly in the posterior fossa, is exquisitely fine because bony structures give no signal. The spine can be imaged sagittally along its full length. Having said this it must be emphasized that the interpretation of abnormalities displayed is still in a largely experimental stage and the promise of MRI will be fulfilled with painstaking research whereby MRI findings are correlated with CT, neurosurgical and autopsy observations. It should not be regarded as a tool yet available for routine clinical use. The patient for MRI is motored into a fairly long narrow tunnel. The resemblance between this position and that of the departing coffin at a crematorium is inescapable. For this reason, perhaps, a significant minority of patients (including the elderly) will not tolerate MRI because of a sense of claustrophobia. Furthermore, data acquisition for each set of images requires the patient to remain quite still for several minutes. Failure to remain still results in an unacceptable degradation of image quality.

Spinal Radiology

Plain films of the spine can be obtained with little fuss. Back pain and neck pain are common in the elderly and may be associated with motor or sensory changes either related to peripheral nerves or long tracts. It is unusual to see spinal films of a patient over 60 years without evidence of degenerative disease. It is a largely futile exercise to attempt to correlate the X-ray signs of disc degeneration, facet joint disease and osteophytosis with the clinical neurological signs. The real value of spinal films is to confirm or exclude the presence of disease other than degenerative disease, i.e. neoplasms (usually metastatic, Figure 6.8) or infections. Demineralization of bone is common in the aged and is usually due to osteoporosis. Osteoporosis in the spine shows as poorly mineralized vertebral bodies with the accentuation or etching of their cortical margins. Vertebral bodies may be biconcave as a result and compression fractures are common.

Osteomalacia (rickets) is less common but has a pathognomonic sign, the Looser zones. These are small 'bites' of unossified osteoid usually found on the inner aspects of the femoral necks, the obturator rings and the lateral borders of the scapulae (Figure 6.9).

Myelography

Myelograms in the aged should be confined to identifying the site and nature of spinal compression threatening the long tracts. If a patient develops an acute long tract or cauda equina neurological deficit, the implication is that there is a compressing lesion, neoplastic or infective. Plain films may be negative but if progressive symptoms and objective neurological signs are present, *urgent* myelography should be done in consultation with neurosurgeons.

Modern myelograms use non-ionic water-soluble iodinated contrast agents which are safe for use throughout the spine. The procedure is often arduous for the patient who may have to be tilted in a manner similar to the ritual for burial at sea. In the presence of severe degenerative changes lumbar puncture may require great skill for the radiologist and fortitude from his patient. The elderly should not be expected to submit to such procedure unless it represents the pathway to a major decision about management, usually neurosurgical or radiotherapeutic. Myelograms should not be requested in the aged without prior consultation with a neurologist, neurosurgeon or radiotherapist.

Spinal CT (see also Chapter 17)

Good resolution of intraspinal structures requires contiguous slices no thicker than 5 mm. Eight or 10 mm slices are often unacceptable. It follows that without accurate clinical and plain film localization of a lesion, a vast number of slices will be required. Localization of spinal lesions is notoriously difficult

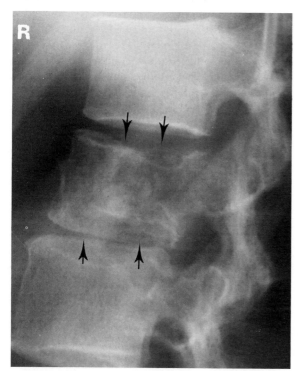

Figure 6.8. Metastases in a lumbar vertebral body.

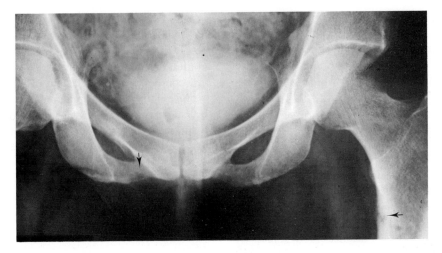

Figure 6.9. Osteomalacia. Note Looser zones of diminished density in the cortex (arrows).

and for these reasons, CT is disappointing in the initial investigation of spinal cord compression syndromes in the elderly despite the attractions of its relative non-invasiveness. It is superficially attractive to consider CT for investigation of the neurological complications of cervical spondylosis, but unless a neurosurgeon is involved and is seriously considering decompression or other procedure, such investigation confers little benefit to the patient.

SELECTED CLINICAL CONDITIONS

Stroke

Imaging investigations should not usually be required to confirm the diagnosis of stroke. Claims may be made that CT should be done to distinguish haemorrhage from infarction. Few, if any, stroke patients will have haemorrhage to the extent that surgical evacuation will be considered. Similarly, there will be relatively few cases in which anticoagulation will be considered, though the indications for antiplatelet therapy are widening. In such cases, however, a prior CT scan is mandatory.

Plain skull films have little to offer, but it is hard to resist the demands for them and easier to comply with a single lateral view which will at least confirm or exclude bony lesions. Chest films are important to exclude serious unsuspected chest disease, but it may be better to wait for 3 to 4 days when the patient is more stable and can sit up for a proper chest film.

Transient Ischaemic Attack (TIA)

Before these patients are subjected to invasive radiological investigation, it is necessary to decide whether or not they are to be considered for surgery (usually carotid endarterectomy) rather than managed conservatively. If surgery is being considered, investigation should await consultation with the surgeon. The implication then is that there is stenosis or, more likely, an ulcerated plaque (Figure 6.10) and the surgeon will want a route map before operation. It may be preferable to precede angiography by Doppler ultrasound studies to rule out occlusion of the carotid artery. In most cases where the facility exists, intravenous arch arteriography with digital subtraction (DSA) will show the origins of the great vessels, carotid bifurcations and carotid siphons in sufficient detail. Otherwise arteriography must be done either by catheter or direct carotid puncture according to local practice.

Head Injury

The difficulty about head injury in the elderly is that the patient may present in a confused or semiconscious state without evidence of having sustained a head injury. Having established that there has indeed been a head injury, a process of triage must be applied. Most accident and emergency departments have guidelines as to when to do a skull X-ray, when

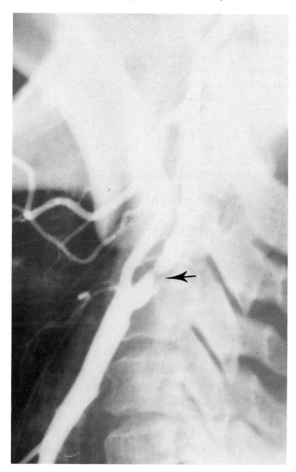

Figure 6.10. Internal carotid atheromatous plaque.

to admit for observation, when to do CT and when to refer urgently to the neurosurgeons. Ideally, CT is the cornerstone of management of the patient who is clinically unstable following head injury and it should be available on a 24 hour basis in all district general hospitals (Report of Working Party, 1986). In these circumstances, CT should be done without prior skull X-rays. In the less than ideal circumstances under which most of us practise, a single lateral and AP (Towne's) film should be done in all but the most trivially affected patient who has had a head injury. The presence of a fracture greatly increases the likelihood of intracranial bleeding. Furthermore, if an elderly patient who has previously been alert persists in confusion following

head injury for more than 12 hours, CT is strongly advised even if there is no evidence of skull fracture (Galbraith, 1987; see also Chapter 18).

Subdural Haematoma

If this diagnosis is being seriously considered, then the investigation of choice is a CT scan. Although a quick unenhanced scan is all that is needed, the provision of this facility is at best patchy, as has already been pointed out. An isotope brain scan is next best. A skull X-ray is rarely helpful.

Carotid angiography is obsolete in the primary investigation of suspected subdural haematoma. In the occasional case in which it is employed it will be done only after CT.

Suspected Spinal Compression

A level should be established clinically, if possible. If there are upper motor neurone signs the lesion is likely to be L1 or above. A chest X-ray may reveal a primary or destructive bony change in the ribs. Plain X-rays of the spine should concentrate on the suspected level. If bony destruction is contained by an intervertebral disc it is likely to be due to malignancy of which the vast majority in this age group are metastatic. If the process affects vertebrae on either side of a disc, infection is more likely and urgent neurosurgical advice should be obtained. A neurosurgeon may advise transfer for investigation at his unit or may ask for myelography or CT to be arranged. If so, this should be carried out as a matter of urgency.

General Impairment of Mental Function

This problem is dealt with elsewhere in more detail (see Chapter 27). From the point of view of imaging, the clinician must be alerted to the clinical pointers which raise the possibility of potentially remediable intracranial disease such as chronic subdural haematoma, normal pressure hydrocephalus and some brain tumours. If the clinical case is a good one, the patient, however elderly, deserves CT and should not be fobbed off with skull X-rays, isotope scans or other inferior imaging techniques. It is important to remember, however, that there are very many extracranial causes of acute and chronic confusion. Some of these may be identified by the simplest of all imaging tests—the chest film.

REFERENCES

Baddeley, H. (1984). *Radiological Investigation: A Guide to the Use of Medical Imaging in Clinical Practice*, John Wiley, Chichester.

Galbraith, S. (1987). Head injuries in the elderly. *Br. Med. J.*, **294,** 325.

Grainger, R.G. (1986). In: Grainger, R.G., and Allison, D.J. (eds.) *Diagnostic Radiology*, Vol. 1, Chapter 7, Churchill Livingstone, Edinburgh, pp. 99–109.

Harbert, J.C. (1986). In: Grainger, R.G., and Allison, D.J.

(eds.) *Diagnostic Radiology.*, Vol. 3, Churchill Livingstone, Edinburgh, p. 1862.

Kendall, B.E., and Pullicino, B. (1980). Intravascular contrast media in ischaemic lesions. II: Effect on prognosis. *Neuroradiology*, **19,** 241–3.

Leading Article (1979). Chronic subdural haematoma. *Br. Med. J.*, **i,** 433–4.

Moseley, I.F. (section ed.) (1986). Section 9: The Central Nervous System. In: Grainger, R.G., and Allison, D.J. (eds.) *Diagnostic Radiology: An Anglo-American Textbook of Imaging*, Vol. III, Churchill Livingstone, Edinburgh.

Report of the Working Party on Head Injuries. (1986) Royal College of Surgeons of England.

Tress, B.M. (1983). The need for skull radiographs in patients presenting for CT. *Radiology*, **146,** 87–9.

Valentine, A.R., Pullicino, P., and Bannan, E. (1981). *A Practical Introduction to Cranial Computed Tomography*, Heinemann, London.

The Clinical Neurology of Old Age
Edited by R. Tallis
© 1989 John Wiley & Sons Ltd

Chapter 7

Clinical Neurophysiology
in the Elderly

Jollyon Smith

Consultant Clinical Neurophysiologist, University Hospital, Queen's Medical Centre, Nottingham, UK

Neurophysiological tests, particularly the electro-encephalogram (EEG), are widely used but frequently misunderstood by clinicians (Matthews, 1964); indeed, almost every statement in this chapter could be prefaced by the remark 'Contrary to beliefs firmly held in some quarters . . . .' Although those who write neurophysiological reports have occasionally been criticized for alleged 'obliquity of thought and ambiguity of expression' (Matthews, 1972), an appropriately requested neurophysiological investigation usually produces an informative result (Critchley, 1978). Dissatisfaction with EEG reports most often arises from an inappropriate request, and such requests are still received in spite of several recent reviews of the neurophysiological tests in the elderly (McGeorge, 1981; Roberts and Caird, 1982; Evans, 1985). A further factor leading to a gulf between users and providers of the service is that results are frequently misinterpreted or ignored, even when expressed with neither circumlocution nor equivocation. This chapter is therefore written in the hope of providing clear guidance on the proper use and interpretation of neurophysiological investigations for those involved in the care of elderly patients.

The decision to request a test in a particular patient should depend upon satisfactory answers to two questions:

1   What abnormalities can the test demonstrate?
2   How would knowledge of such abnormalities affect the management of this patient?

It should not be necessary to emphasize that if none of the possible results would alter management, then the investigation should not be undertaken. In the elderly a further consideration is whether the patient is capable of benefiting from any change in management; for example, clear demonstration of a tumour may not be useful in a patient whose general condition precludes operation. These points are frequently forgotten by doctors who cheerfully submit frail patients to uncomfortable investigations, including the vagaries of the ambulance service, in a dogged and blinkered pursuit of a diagnosis. Clinicians should also beware of requesting investigations simply because a research report mentions abnormalities in a certain group of patients. Many such reports are studies of a condition which has been confidently diagnosed by other methods, and the abnormalities described, while being of great interest, do not contribute to the diagnosis. For example, EEG abnormalities have been reported in both psychopaths and dements, but presence or absence of EEG abnormalities does not alter the fact that a particular patient either is psychopathic (or demented), or he is not.

ELECTROENCEPHALOGRAPHY

An EEG involves the recording of the small differences in electrical potential (often less than 50 microvolts) between pairs of electrodes attached to the scalp in standardized positions. A modern routine record consists of either eight or sixteen channels recorded from various combinations of at least 21 electrodes. The duration of recording is about 30 minutes, and a similar time is taken by a skilful technician in applying and removing the electrodes; more time and the assistance of a second technician may be called for in an uncooperative patient. Activation by photic stimulation is used routinely at all ages. Hyperventilation produces little change in the elderly because of diminished responsiveness of the cerebral vessels to falling arterial $P\text{CO}_2$, and so this form of activation is not often used over the age of 60, and is never used in the presence of chest or heart disease, or if raised intracranial pressure is suspected. Sleep occasionally activates EEG abnormalities, and a longer record may be necessary to ensure a period of natural sleep. Stopping anticonvulsant drugs does not materially increase the probability of a diagnostic EEG abnormality, and carries a serious risk of precipitating a fit or even status epilepticus. Most EEG departments simultaneously record one lead of the ECG and this is of special importance in the elderly, where episodes of altered consciousness often have a cardiac origin. Further details of recording technique may be found in Scott (1976) and in Kiloh *et al.* (1981).

The EEG undergoes a process of maturation from birth, and specific changes are known to accompany ageing in normal adults. In particular, the alpha rhythm, a sinusoidal oscillation of potential, at a frequency of 8–13 Hz, over the occipital region while the patient is alert and relaxed with the eyes closed, shows a fall in frequency of about 1 Hz for each decade over 60, although a frequency below 8 Hz is abnormal at any age. Intermittent slow activity (theta, 4–8 Hz, and delta, below 4 Hz) may also appear in elderly subjects who are free of neurological symptoms. It is not entirely clear to what extent these changes merely reflect physiological ageing, or the increasing incidence of subclinical cortical atrophy and cerebrovascular disease with advancing age. This complex subject has been reviewed by Obrist (1976), Busse and Wang (1979) and by Torres *et al.* (1983). For practical purposes, the range of normality of the EEG becomes wider with increasing age; nevertheless the occasional octogenarian can be found whose EEG is indistinguishable from that of a 20 year old.

The EEG is simply a graph of voltage against time (Scott, 1976). It therefore gives an indication of cortical function for the duration of the recording, and any inferences about function at other times are entirely speculative, as are conclusions about underlying structural changes. The EEG of a normal subject is entirely different during sleep, mental activity or under the influence of many drugs. Similarly, patients suffering from encephalitis or severe metabolic encephalopathy have grossly abnormal records while radiological investigations fail to show any definite abnormality in such cases. EEG recording and radiology are thus complementary; each type of investigation has its own capabilities, and the indications for each are different.

The indications for EEG recording may be divided into those related to epilepsy or suspected epilepsy, and those concerned with continuous diffuse disturbances of cortical function (Table 7.1). Suspected epilepsy constitutes the commonest single indication, but is the field in which routine EEG recording is most disappointing. This is because the commonest question asked by the clinician ('Are the attacks epileptic?') cannot be answered with certainty unless the recording includes a typical attack. Attacks are rarely so frequent that one will occur during a standard routine 30 minute recording. The vast majority of EEGs are therefore recorded between attacks (inter-ictal), and can only give an indication of the probability that attacks are epileptic.

An inter-ictal EEG may be broadly classified into one of four categories according to the nature and degree of departure from normality:

1   Normal.
2   Mild, non-specific abnormalities.
3   Specific abnormalities (not paroxysmal), which may be related to the cause of epileptic attacks.
4   A paroxysmal or seizure discharge.

TABLE 7.1   SUMMARY OF INDICATIONS FOR EEG RECORDING IN THE ELDERLY

1. Epilepsy

   What type of epilepsy?

   Is there an underlying cause for fits (e.g. possible tumour) requiring further investigation?

   What is the risk of attacks in future? (especially after a single fit)

   Are the attacks epileptic? Only answered by a recording *during* an attack; rarely necessary if clinical assessment adequate

2. Undiagnosed coma, stupor or confusion

   Especially minor status, encephalopathy or encephalitis

3. Subacute intellectual impairment

   Especially Jakob–Creutzfeldt disease

A normal record does not in any way exclude the diagnosis of epilepsy; some patients subject to life-long attacks have a normal inter-ictal record. Non-specific abnormalities, such as poorly localized theta activity, have no significance with respect to the diagnosis of epilepsy. More than half the inter-ictal records in adults are either normal or show non-specific abnormalities. Specific abnormalities, such as localized delta waves or focal spikes, although relatively uncommon, are very helpful if the diagnosis of epilepsy is established, since they suggest a focal cortical disturbance as the cause of the fits, and carry the implication that radiological investigation should be considered. When a paroxysmal discharge occurs in an inter-ictal record, this increases the probability, but does not prove conclusively, that the patient's attacks are epileptic. In elderly patients with fits of recent onset such discharges are extremely rare, and the presence of bilateral discharges similar to those seen in children with primary generalized epilepsy, especially if photosensitivity is also demonstrated, raises the possibility of drug effects, alcohol withdrawal or other metabolic disturbance as the cause of the fits.

Thus, a routine EEG can only rarely indicate whether attacks are likely to be epileptic. However, if the diagnosis of epilepsy is established, the EEG may indicate the probable type of epilepsy, and give some guidance as to the need for further investigation. The EEG gives *no* information on the need for anti-convulsant treatment in newly diagnosed cases, the adequacy of treatment in those already receiving it,

or whether treatment may safely be stopped.

A particular problem is posed by the holder of a driving licence who has a single fit. Here the EEG can make a definite contribution, since the finding of any abnormality associated with an increased risk of further fits means that, under present regulations, the licensing authority must be informed that a prospective disability exists and the licence surrendered. Absence of such abnormalities after a single fit should lead to loss of the licence for only one year, provided other investigations are normal (Pond and Espir, 1976). There are *no* circumstances under which the result of an EEG would permit a patient to drive if he was disqualified for other reasons.

A routine EEG cannot determine with certainty whether intermittent symptoms are due to focal fits or transient ischaemic attacks. If the EEG shows a non-specific focal abnormality the safest course is to assume that the explanation is an area of infarction that is otherwise asymptomatic (Harrison and Marshall, 1977) rather than an epileptogenic focus. This is because the result of failing to prevent cerebral emboli, namely a devastating stroke, is very much more serious than leaving focal fits untreated.

Since the only conclusive evidence of the epileptic nature of attacks is provided by a recording of a typical attack, efforts have been made to prolong the recording so as to increase the probability that it will include an attack. This can be done in several ways (Binnie, 1983). A routine EEG may be extended to last for several hours, in some cases with cable or radio telemetry to permit the patient to move around, rather than being confined to a couch. Alternatively four or eight channels of EEG may be recorded on a portable cassette tape recorder, similar to that used for 24 hour ECG recording. Indeed, the value of the procedure is greatly enhanced if the EEG and ECG are recorded simultaneously, in view of the frequency with which cardiac arrhythmias cause transient symptoms in the elderly. In particularly difficult cases concurrent video recording may be necessary to elucidate the nature of attacks, and may give valuable additional information, such as surreptitious ingestion of drugs when the patient thinks that he is not being observed. Recordings made under less than ideal conditions may present difficulties of interpretation, particularly the distinction between artefacts and paroxysmal activity, but the problems are well recognized and not insurmountable (Docherty, 1981; Blumhardt and Oozeer, 1982). These methods are extremely time-consuming, and have yet to be fully evaluated or be made generally available.

An EEG is indicated in patients with acute confusion, delirium, stupor or coma, in whom the diagnosis remains obscure after clinical examination and simple investigations such as blood sugar estimation, chest X-ray, etc. (Obrecht *et al.*, 1979). The EEG may show evidence of metabolic encephalopathy, especially hepatic (triphasic waves), the specific features of herpes encephalitis, or evidence of drug intoxication, especially with barbiturates or benzodiazepines (fast activity), or lateralized abnormalities suggesting the presence of a subdural haematoma (Luxon and Harrison, 1979). If the history strongly suggests the possibility of subdural haematoma, then appropriate radiological investigation should be undertaken immediately, since an EEG cannot exclude the presence of haematoma. The finding of a prominent slow wave focus in a patient with an encephalitic illness raises the question of a cerebral abscess. The unusual condition of minor status may occasionally present as acute confusion in the elderly (see Chapter 15), and can be diagnosed only by means of the EEG (Schwartz and Scott, 1971); firm diagnosis of a prolonged post-ictal confusional state may be more difficult (Godfrey *et al.*, 1982).

The EEG has a limited place in the investigation of insidious impairment of cerebral function (dementia) in the elderly. In the two commonest causes of dementia, Alzheimer's disease and multiple infarcts, the EEG abnormality simply parallels the deterioration of intellect, and has no diagnostic significance, although the EEG may form part of research protocols to give independent confirmation of the degree of cerebral impairment in demented patients (Christie, 1979). The eminently treatable causes of dementia (communicating hydrocephalus, myxoedema), although affecting the EEG, cannot be diagnosed by means of the EEG (Smith and Kiloh, 1981). The EEG is sometimes used in an attempt to distinguish between depression and dementia, an abnormal EEG being taken as evidence of an organic cause for mental impairment. This is not entirely reliable, since the presence of an EEG abnormality does not rule out a good response to antidepressant treatment. The only firm indication for an EEG in a demented patient is dementia of rapid progression, together with other signs (myoclonus, cortical blindness, etc.) suggesting a diagnosis of Creutzfeldt–Jakob disease (Masters *et al.*, 1979). This condition is associated with a typical EEG pattern of repetitive periodic complexes. Unfortunately, the typical features may not appear until the terminal stages of the disease, so that negative EEGs do not exclude the diagnosis. If Creutzfeldt–Jakob disease is suspected this should be made clear in the EEG request, since special precautions will be necessary while applying electrodes. Although a typical EEG greatly increases the likelihood of the diagnosis in the presence of appropriate clinical features, the EEG alone is never diagnostic, since almost identical EEGs may be found in patients with other conditions, especially encephalitis and hepatic encephalopathy. An EEG is *not* indicated in patients with syncope, migraine or headache, since there are no EEG features that would contribute to the diagnosis or management in any of those conditions. After a stroke, a localized EEG abnormality is to be expected, and clearing of this abnormality after a few weeks confirms the absence of a tumour (Roseman *et al.*, 1952). However, the distinction between vascular lesions and tumours can be made much more reliably today by

means of non-invasive radiological examination, so
that an EEG is no longer indicated in stroke patients.
The EEG should not be used as a screening test to
exclude the presence of a cerebral tumour. Although
the EEG is usually abnormal in glioma of the brain,
it is frequently normal, or shows only a slight
disturbance, in patients with meningiomas. The
EEG is therefore not a reliable screening procedure.

Evoked Potentials

An evoked potential (or evoked response) is defined
as the sequence of potential changes in any part of
the brain following deliberate stimulation of a sense
organ, sensory nerve, etc. (Chang, 1959). Clinical
applications of such techniques rely upon signal
averaging to extract the low amplitude responses,
which occur at fixed intervals after each stimulus,
from the randomly occurring spontaneous activity
upon which they are superimposed. Digital averaging equipment is now available in most clinical
neurophysiology departments, and with the addition
of suitable stimulators the responses evoked by
visual, auditory and somatosensory stimuli can be
readily recorded in a single session if necessary
(Clarke, 1984). Full details of recording technique
and interpretation are given by Halliday (1982).

There are marked changes in evoked responses
due to ageing in normal subjects. In general the
latency of all responses increases with age, and
amplitudes tend to fall, even in the absence of lens
opacities, conductive hearing loss, etc. The precise
changes with age are different in each sensory
modality, and in the visual system depend upon the
characteristics of the pattern stimulus used (Halliday, 1982). There are also significant differences
between elderly males and females.

The commonest clinical application of evoked
response recording is in the detection of clinically
silent lesions in the diagnosis of multiple sclerosis
(Deltenre *et al.*, 1973; Khoshbin and Hallett, 1981).
In particular, visual and auditory responses may be
helpful in demonstrating extra lesions in patients
with progressive spastic paraplegia, many of whom
are eventually found to have multiple sclerosis.
Statistical differences have been reported in the

cervical somatosensory responses between cervical
spondylotic myelopathy and myelopathy due to
multiple sclerosis (Ganes, 1980), but the differences
are not sufficiently reliable to be clinically useful in
individual cases. Besides, previously undiagnosed
multiple sclerosis is unlikely to be encountered in the
elderly. Evoked responses are most useful in demonstrating integrity of sensory pathways, for example in
patients with sensory loss due to hysteria or mal-
ingering (Halliday, 1972), as part of the preoperative assessment of patients with dense cataracts, or in
the objective assessment of visual acuity (Howe *et al.*,
1981) and hearing (Gibson, 1978). Evoked responses
are also used to monitor the state of sensory pathways
during operations for pituitary adenoma, acoustic
neuroma, and for spinal tumour or unstable spinal
fracture (Grundy, 1983).

Recent research has suggested that demented
patients, and particularly those with Alzheimer's
disease, may show specific evoked response abnormalities. Delays have been reported in the P300, a
cognitive response depending upon recognition of
the stimulus (Brown *et al.*, 1982; Syndulko *et al.*,
1981). Similarly, the flash-evoked visual response is
said to be delayed in demented patients, even when
the response to pattern reversal is normal (Wright *et
al.*, 1984; Danesi *et al.*, 1985). The full significance of
these fascinating findings has yet to be determined.
Diagnostic applications are likely to be limited, and
must await full correlation with pathology.

ELECTROMYOGRAPHY AND NERVE
CONDUCTION STUDIES

Many aspects of the function of the peripheral
nervous system are amenable to electrophysiological
investigation. Nerve conduction velocities and
action potential amplitudes are easily measured,
neuromuscular transmission can be assessed, and the
features of motor units and their recruitment may be
recorded by muscle sampling with a needle electrode. Full details of all these techniques are readily
available in standard textbooks, for example Goodgold and Eberstein (1983) or Kimura (1983). Three
of the commonest measurements (maximum nerve
conduction velocity, sensory action potential ampli-

tude and motor unit duration) show changes with age suggesting a gradual loss of sensory and motor axons. Maximum velocities in both motor and sensory nerves fall by about 0.1 m/s per year after the age of 40, and sensory potential amplitudes fall by about 10% over the age of 60 (Behse and Buchthal, 1971; Dorfman and Bosley, 1979). The mean duration of motor units almost doubles between the ages of 3 and 75 years (Buchthal, 1957), indicating a fall in the number of units, with re-innervation by surviving nerve fibres. Since techniques vary, each clinical neurophysiology department will have its own normal values, and all studies in elderly patients should include comparison with age matched controls.

Nerve conduction studies can usually distinguish between axonal and demyelinating neuropathy, the former producing a reduction in amplitude of sensory potentials with only slight reduction in velocity, while the latter produces prominent slowing (velocities less than 60% of normal). This may be helpful in identifying the relatively rare cases of demyelinating neuropathy, some of which may respond to steroid treatment. Detailed study of a number of nerves may help in distinguishing between peripheral neuropathy and mononeuritis multiplex, a distinction which is occasionally of practical significance. Nerve conduction measurements are certainly not indicated automatically in all patients with suspected peripheral neuropathy; in the majority of cases the diagnosis can be made on clinical grounds, and the cause of the neuropathy (e.g. diabetes, vitamin B12 deficiency) cannot be determined by electrophysiological methods.

Isolated peripheral nerve lesions can be localized and their severity assessed by means of nerve conduction studies. This leads to the commonest single reason for such tests, namely suspected compression of the median nerve in the carpal tunnel. Sunderland (1978) describes nerve conduction studies as an 'unnecessary luxury' when a firm diagnosis can be made from the characteristic clinical features, and electrophysiological tests are indicated only when a clinician dealing regularly with the carpal tunnel syndrome is unsure of the diagnosis. The characteristic finding is reduction of median nerve velocities across the wrist, with reduction of sensory potential

amplitudes. Sensory conduction is affected before motor, and refined methods may be necessary to demonstrate the abnormality in early cases (Smaje, 1982; Mills, 1985).

Nerve conduction studies are particularly valuable in cases of ulnar nerve palsy, firstly to confirm the presence of an ulnar nerve lesion and exclude other causes of wasting or paraesthesiae in the hand, and secondly to determine the site of the lesion, usually elbow or wrist. In patients with a mild lesion which can be treated conservatively, and in those with a palsy following a single episode of trauma to the nerve, conduction studies in general make no contribution to the management. Electrophysiological methods are occasionally necessary in other nerve compression syndromes, particularly the peroneal nerve at the head of the fibula and the tarsal tunnel syndrome, and may also be used to distinguish a peripheral nerve lesion from a spinal root lesion. Here electromyography may supplement clinical examination by confirming the distribution of muscles affected.

In patients with myasthenia gravis and the Eaton–Lambert myasthenic syndrome repetitive nerve stimulation can usually demonstrate the disorder of neuromuscular junctions (Elmquist and Lambert, 1968; Ozdemir and Young, 1977). However, in myasthenia gravis the response to Tensilon (edrophonium) is usually diagnostic, making neurophysiological tests unnecessary. When all other tests fail to demonstrate the abnormality, single fibre electromyography with measurement of neuromuscular jitter may be necessary (Stålberg, 1980).

Sampling of muscle activity using a needle electrode (electromyography or EMG) permits detection of abnormal spontaneous activity, found in neuropathic conditions, polymyositis and myotonias, together with measurements of features of motor units and an estimate of their number from the recruitment pattern. In neuropathic conditions motor unit numbers fall, and in chronic cases partial reinnervation leads to an increase in duration and complexity of surviving units. Myopathic conditions show a decrease in the number of fibres per unit, and thus in the duration of each unit, but the total number of units remains constant until the late stages. There have been many exciting developments in electromyography recently; limitation of space precludes more than a mention of single fibre electromyography (Stålberg and Trontelj, 1979), interference pattern analysis (Forster *et al.*, 1984) and accurate motor unit counting (Ballantyne and Hansen, 1974). In spite of considerable research in electromyography, the technique is incapable of doing more than making the distinction between myopathic and neuropathic weakness and wasting, and may not even be capable of that in advanced cases (Barwick, 1981). The EMG is never diagnostic, except perhaps in polymyositis and the myotonias, and can never indicate the *cause* of a myopathy or neuropathy.

Motor neurone disease poses a special problem for the electromyographer. An EMG is requested almost automatically in patients in whom such a diagnosis is suspected. This is not always appropriate, since the firm diagnosis of motor neurone disease depends upon a combination of clinical and electrical features (Peacock *et al.*, 1979). The proper role of the EMG in the diagnosis of motor neurone disease is to exclude the presence of other conditions, particularly neuropathy or myopathy, and to confirm the presence of widespread denervation, often found in many muscles that do not appear to be affected clinically. In eleven elderly patients referred for EMG with suspected motor neurone disease, George and Twomey (1983) were able to confirm the diagnosis in only one, an alternative diagnosis was made in two and the EMG was equivocal or normal in eight. This suggests a need for more detailed clinical assessment before referral for EMG.

This section would be incomplete without a reminder that the presence of a cardiac pacemaker of 'demand' type constitutes an absolute contraindication to electrical stimulation of peripheral nerves, and severe angina or uncontrolled cardiac tachyarrhythmias are relative contraindications.

In conclusion, it should be emphasized that a request for any neurophysiological test really amounts to a referral for the specialist opinion of a clinical neurophysiologist. Full discussion of difficult cases will allow the neurophysiologist to indicate the most effective approach to investigation. Occasionally he will be able to point out that the proposed investigation will not provide useful information in a particular case, and this expert advice should be respected since it will save the patient from the discomfort of an unnecessary procedure.

REFERENCES

Ballantyne, J.P., and Hansen, S. (1974). A new method for the estimation of the number of motor units in a muscle. 1. Control subjects and patients with myasthenia gravis. *J. Neurol. Neurosurg. Psychiatry*, **37**, 907–15.

Barwick, D.D. (1981). Clinical electromyography. In: Walton, J. (ed.) *Disorders of Voluntary Muscle*, fourth edition, Churchill Livingstone, Edinburgh, pp. 952–75.

Behse, F., and Buchthal, F. (1971). Normal sensory conduction in the nerves of the leg in man. *J. Neurol. Neurosurg. Psychiatry*, **34**, 404–14.

Binnie, C.D. (1983). Telemetric EEG monitoring in epilepsy. In: Pedley, T.A., and Meldrum, B.S. (eds.) *Recent Advances in Epilepsy*, Churchill Livingstone, Edinburgh, pp. 155–78.

Blumhardt, L.D., and Oozeer, R. (1982). Problems encountered in the interpretation of ambulatory EEG recordings. In: Stefan, H., and Burr, W. (eds.) *Mobile Long Term EEG Monitoring: Proceedings of the MLE Symposium, Bonn, 1982*, G. Fischer, Stuttgart, pp. 37–54.

Brown, W., Marsh, J.T., and La Rue, A. (1982). Event related potentials in psychiatry: differentiating depression and dementia in the elderly. *Bull. Los Angeles Neurol. Soc.*, **47**, 91–107.

Buchthal, F. (1957). *An Introduction to Electromyography*, Scandinavian University Books, Copenhagen.

Busse, E.W., and Wand, H.S. (1979). The electroencephalographic changes in late life: a longitudinal study. *J. Clin. Exp. Gerontol.*, **1**, 145–58.

Chang, H-T. (1959). The evoked potentials. In: Field, J., and Magoun, H.W. (eds.) *Neurophysiology Vol. 1. Section 1 of Handbook of Physiology*, American Physiological Society. Washington DC, pp. 299–314.

Christie, J.E. (1979). Neurophysiology of dementia. In: Glen, A.I.M., and Whalley, L.J. (eds.) *Alzheimer's Disease*, Churchill Livingstone, Edinburgh, pp. 90–2.

Critchley, E.M.R. (1978). Electroencephalography today. *J. Roy. Soc. Med.*, **71**, 473–6.

Clarke, S.A. (1984). Pattern VEPs, BAEPs and SEPs recorded from healthy subjects in a single session. *J. Electrophysiol. Technol.*, **10**, 83–91.

Danesi, M.A., Huxley, P., and Murray, N.M.F. (1985). Flash and pattern VEPs in dementia. *Electroenceph. Clin. Neurophysiol.*, **61**, S196.

Deltenre, P., Vercruysse, A., Van Nechael, C., Ketelaer, P., Capon, A., Colin, F., and Manil, J. (1979). Early diagnosis of multiple sclerosis by combined multimodal evoked potentials: results and practical considerations. *J. Biomed. Eng.*, **1**, 17–21.

Docherty, T.B. (1981). Ambulatory electroencephalogram monitoring in routine clinical practice. *J. Electrophysiol. Technol.*, **7**, 141–65.

Dorfman, L.J., and Bosley, T.M. (1979). Age related changes in peripheral and central nerve conduction in man. *Neurology (N.Y.)*, **29**, 38–44.

Elmquist, D., and Lambert, E.H. (1968). Detailed analysis of neuromuscular transmission in a patient with the myasthenic syndrome associated with bronchogenic carcinoma. *Mayo Clin. Proc.*, **43**, 689–713.

Evans, B.M. (1985). Special investigations. (A) Electroencephalography. In: Hildick-Smith, M. (ed.) *Neurological Problems in the Elderly*, Baillière Tindall, London, pp. 39–43.

Forster, A., Mills, K.R., Morton, H.B., and Willison, R.G. (1984). On-line 'turns' analysis of the human electromyogram. *J. Physiol. (Lond.)*, **360**, 3P.

Ganes, T. (1980). Somatosensory conduction times and peripheral, cervical and cortical evoked potentials in patients with cervical spondylosis. *J. Neurol. Neurosurg. Psychiatry*, **43**, 683–9.

George, J., and Twomey, J.A. (1983). Electrophysiological investigation of peripheral neuromuscular disorders in the elderly. *Age Ageing*, **12**, 50–3.

Gibson, W.P.R. (1978). *Essentials of Clinical Electric Response Audiometry*, Churchill Livingstone, Edinburgh.

Godfrey, J.W., Roberts, M.A., and Caird, F.I. (1982). Epileptic seizures in the elderly: II, Diagnostic problems. *Age Ageing*, **11**, 29–34.

Goodgold, J., and Eberstein, A. (1983). *Electrodiagnosis of Neuromuscular Diseases*, third edition, Williams and Wilkins, Baltimore.

Grundy, B.L. (1983). Intraoperative monitoring of sensory evoked potentials. *Anesthesiology*, **58**, 72–87.

Halliday, A.M. (1972). Evoked responses in organic and functional sensory loss. In: Fessard, A., and Lelord, G. (eds.) *Activités Évoquées et leur Conditionnement Chez l'Homme Normal et en Pathologie Mentale*, Editions Inserm, Paris, pp. 189–212.

Halliday, A.M. (ed.) (1982). *Evoked Potentials in Clinical Testing*, Churchill Livingstone, Edinburgh.

Harrison, M.J.G., and Marshall, J. (1977). Evidence of silent cerebral embolism in patients with amaurosis fugax. *J. Neurol. Neurosurg. Psychiatry*, **40**, 651–4.

Howe, J.W., Mitchell, K.W., and Robson, C. (1981). Electrophysiological assessment of visual acuity. *Trans. Ophthalmol. Soc. UK.*, **101**, 105–8.

Khoshbin, S., and Hallet, M. (1981). Multimodality evoked potentials and blink reflex in multiple sclerosis. *Neurology (N.Y.)*, **31**, 138–44.

Kiloh, L.G., McComas, A.J., Osselton, J.W., and Upton, A.R.M. (1981). *Clinical Electroencephalography*, fourth edition, Butterworth, London.

Kimura, J. (1983). *Electrodiagnosis in Diseases of Nerve and Muscle: Principles and Practice*, F.A. Davis, Philadelphia.

Luxon, L.M., and Harrison, M.J.G. (1979). Chronic subdural haematoma. *Q. J. Med.*, **48**, 43–53.

McGeorge, A.P. (1981). The electroencephalogram. In: Caird, F.I. (ed.) *Advanced Geriatric Medicine I*, Pitman, London, pp. 80–3.

Masters, C.L., Harris, J.O., Gajdusek, D.C., Gibbs, C.J., Bernouilli, C., and Asher, D.M. (1979). Creutfeldt–Jakob disease: patterns of world-wide occurrence and the significance of familial and sporadic clustering. *Ann. Neurol.*, **5**, 177–88.

Matthews, W.B. (1964). The use and abuse of electroencephalography. *Lancet*, **ii**, 577–9.

Matthews, W.B. (1972). The clinical values of routine electroencephalography. *J. Roy. Coll. Phys.*, **7**, 207–12.

Mills, K.R. (1985). Orthodromic sensory action potentials from palmar stimulation in the diagnosis of the carpal tunnel syndrome. *J. Neurol. Neurosurg. Psychiatry*, **48**, 250–5.

Obrecht, R., Okhomina, F.O.A., and Scott, D.F. (1979). Value of EEG in acute confusional states. *J. Neurol. Neurosurg. Psychiatry*, **42**, 75–7.

Obrist, W.D. (1976). Problems of Ageing. In: Remond, A. (ed.) *Handbook of Electroencephalography and Clinical Neurophysiology*, Vol. 6, Part A, Elsevier, Amsterdam, pp. 275–92.

Ozdemir, C., and Young, R. (1977). The results to be expected from electrical testing in the diagnosis of myasthenia gravis. *Ann. N.Y. Acad. Sci.*, **274**, 203–22.

Peacock, A., Dawkins, K., and Rushworth, G. (1979). Motor neurone disease associated with bronchial carcinoma? *Br. Med. J.*, **ii**, 499–500.

Pond, D.A., and Espir, M.L.E. (1976). Epilepsy. In Raffle, A. (ed.) *Medical Aspects of Fitness to Drive*, HMSO, London, pp. 16–22.

Roberts, M.A., and Caird, F.I. (1982). Investigation of neurological disorders: II Electrophysiology. In Caird, F.I. (ed.) *Neurological Disorders in the Elderly*, Wright, Bristol, pp. 58–9.

Roseman, E., Schmidt, R.P. and Foltz, E.L. (1952). Serial electroencephalopathy in vascular lesion of the brain. *Neurology (Minneap.)*, **2**, 311–31.

Schwartz, M.S., and Scott, D.F. (1971). Isolated petit mal status presenting de novo in middle age. *Lancet*, **ii**, 1399–1401.

Scott, D.F. (1976). *Understanding EEG*, Duckworth, London.

Smaje, J. (1982). Serial stimulation in the diagnosis of carpal tunnel syndrome. *Electroenceph. Clin. Neurophysiol.*, pp. 50P–51P.

Smith, J.S., and Kiloh, L.G. (1981). The investigation of dementia: results in 200 consecutive admissions. *Lancet*, **i**, 824–7.

Stålberg, E. (1980). Clinical electrophysiology in myasthenia gravis. *J. Neurol. Neurosurg. Psychiatry*, **43**, 622–33.

Stålberg, E.E., and Trontelj, J.V. (1979). *Single Fibre Electromyography*, Mirvalle Press, Woking.

Sunderland, S. (1978). *Nerves and Nerve Injuries*, second edition, Churchill Livingstone, London.

Syndulko, K., Hansch, E.C., Cohen, S.N., Pearce, J.W., Goldberg, Z., Tourtelotte, W.W., and Potvin, A.R. (1981). Long latency event related potentials in normal ageing and dementia. In: Courjon, J., Mauguiere, F., and Revol, M. (eds.) *Clinical Applications of Evoked Potentials in Neurology*, Raven Press, New York, pp. 279–86.

Torres, F., Faoro, A., Loewenson, R., and Johnson, E. (1983). The electroencephalogram of elderly subjects revisited. *Electroenceph. Clin. Neurophysiol.*, **56,** 391–8.

Wright, C.E., Harding, G.F.A., and Orwin, A. (1984). Presenile dementia—the use of the flash and pattern VER in diagnosis. *Electroenceph. Clin. Neurophysiol.*, **57,** 405–15.

SECTION TWO

Systematic Neurology

Chapter 8

Cerebrovascular Disease

Peter Humphrey

Consultant Neurologist, Mersey Regional Department of Medical and Surgical Neurology, Walton Hospital, Liverpool and Maelor Hospital, Wrexham

Cerebrovascular disease is one of the commonest causes of death and prolonged disability in the UK. In the elderly it is the most frequent cause of prolonged severe disability. A cerebrovascular accident or stroke is defined by WHO as rapidly developed clinical signs of focal or global (as applied to patients in deep coma and to those with subarachnoid haemorrhage) disturbance of cerebral function lasting more than 24 hours or leading to death, with no apparent other cause than that of vascular origin (Aho *et al.*, 1980). The term reversible ischaemic neurological deficit (RIND) is sometimes used to describe those strokes which last between 24 hours and 3 weeks with full functional recovery. The common term transient ischaemic attack (TIA) describes short-lived events with full recovery. Most authors define these as lasting less than 24 hours, although in some papers they have been described as lasting for different periods of time. Transient ischaemic attacks may also involve the ophthalmic artery and produce episodes of transient visual loss (amaurosis fugax).

INCIDENCE

In the USA stroke is the third commonest cause of death, accounting for 11% of all deaths. From the Framingham study the incidence has been estimated to be approximately 200 per 100 000 of the population (Kannel and Wolf, 1983). In this country, the Oxfordshire Community Stroke Project has shown a similar incidence of 195 per 100 000 per annum (Oxfordshire Community Stroke Project, 1983). Thus, 95 000 patients will suffer a stroke in England and Wales each year. The majority of these will be elderly. Approximately 30% will die in the acute phase; 70% of the remainder will be left with some permanent disability—especially in elderly patients whose recovery tends to be slower and less complete.

Over the last 20 years there has been a clear fall in the incidence of cerebrovascular disease. In England and Wales, Habermann *et al.* (1982) have demonstrated a significant reduction of approximately 20–30% in the mortality rate from cerebrovascular disease at all age groups. This contrasts with the mortality from ischaemic heart disease which has changed little over this same period. The figures from the USA are even more striking. Nicholls and Johansen (1983) have reviewed this fall in cerebrovascular and ischaemic heart disease mortality. In the Rochester study Whisnant (1984) observed a 76% fall in mortality from strokes since 1950. The incidence of both cerebral infarction and haemorrhage has fallen dramatically. There are several reasons for this (Whisnant, 1984; Hachinski, 1984). Part of the change may be related to reclassification of disease. For example, most elderly cases of dementia are now thought to be due to primary degenerative disease and not atherosclerosis as had been previously thought. The more successful treatment of hypertension is likely to be another important factor in the declining incidence of cerebrovascular disease (Whisnant, 1984). However, the incidence of stroke was falling even over the period 1950–60 before the treatment of hypertension became widely practised and there were effective, acceptable hypotensive drugs. It seem unlikely, therefore, that this can explain the whole picture. Hachinski (1984) argues that the reduction in the incidence of rheumatic heart disease and the more effective treatment of transient ischaemic attacks are also likely to be important. It seems improbable, however, that these can explain such a dramatic fall in mortality rate from stroke as that seen in the USA.

There has been a considerable change in our thoughts about the incidence of different types of strokes. It had initially been assumed that the majority of strokes were thrombotic and only a small percentage embolic. It was also difficult to know what percentage of strokes were haemorrhagic until the advent of computed tomographic (CT) scanning, as there was no accurate way of differentiating infarction from haemorrhage, except in those patients who came to post-mortem. Post-mortem data clearly cannot be extrapolated to the community at large. The most comprehensive study in this country has been the Oxfordshire Community Stroke Project (1983) in which either CT scans or post-mortems were obtained on 89% of all strokes occurring over a one-year period. This found that 8% of strokes were due to primary intracerebral haemorrhage, 5% to subarachnoid haemorrhage and 76% to cerebral infarction secondary to thromboembolic disease. It confirmed that clinically differentiating cerebral haemorrhage from thromboembolic disease was inaccurate without CT scanning. Allen (1983) attempted to devise a scoring system to try and improve the clinical differentiation between haemorrhage and thromboembolic disease. Unfortunately there was considerable overlap between these two groups clinically. Furthermore, examination of the cerebrospinal fluid (CSF) is also unreliable as some infarcts become haemorrhagic and some haemorrhages remain entirely intracerebral and do not communicate with the CSF. CT scanning has shown that many small haemorrhages which did not rupture into the subarachnoid space were previously incorrectly characterized as thrombotic. It is equally clear from this and the Oxford-shire Community Stroke Project that CT scanning or post-mortem data are necessary to obtain accurate differentiation for each type of stroke.

What proportion of cerebral infarction is secondary to embolism and what to thrombosis is even less certain. Post-mortem data (Torvik and Jorgensen, 1964; Blackwood *et al.*, 1969) suggest that as many as 50% of cerebral infarcts are secondary to cardiac emboli. However, most clinical studies have put the incidence of cerebral embolic strokes at around 10–20% (Carter 1957; Kurtzke, 1976; Groch *et al.*, 1961); only Gautier and Morelot (1975) have found clinical evidence to suggest that cardiac emboli account for approximately half of all strokes. Clearly, the apparent incidence of embolic strokes will depend on how far investigation is taken to look for a source of emboli. The percentage of artery to artery emboli (e.g. from internal carotid stenosis) is even more difficult to define. It seems likely that the percentage of embolic cerebral infarcts has been severely underestimated in the past. Carotid angiography and more intensive cardiac investigations, including echocardiography, suggest that emboli from the heart and proximal vessels are a common cause of cerebral infarction. Even with our present techniques it is likely that a significant number of embolic strokes are still being missed (Ports *et al.*, 1978; Asinger *et al.*, 1981; Humphrey and Harrison, 1985). Unfortunately the problem is made even more complicated by the fact that vascular disease is a diffuse illness. Most patients for instance who have had a stroke will die a cardiac death rather than from a further stroke. Thus the detection of a cardiac source of emboli does not necessarily mean that embolization has occurred. This is especially so in the elderly where vascular disease at multiple sites is common.

PATHOGENESIS

Stroke

Cerebral thrombosis

Thrombosis usually occurs on an atheromatous plaque. It is most common in the internal carotid and basilar arteries and their branches. Hypertension is the major risk factor for cerebral thrombosis.

In hypertensive patients the extent of the atheroma is increased (Robertson and Strong, 1968). Thrombosis in larger arteries tends to produce large peripheral wedge shaped cortical infarcts (Figure 8.1). When the deep penetrating arteries are involved, small deep lacunar shaped infarcts often follow (Figure 8.2). These particularly affect the deep penetrating arteries of the internal capsule, thalamus and pons where lipohyaline changes in the vessel wall with micro-aneurysm formation occur (Ross Russell, 1963). Miller Fisher has described many different clinical syndromes associated with the small lacunar infarcts (Fisher, 1982). Clinically it was initially thought that these lacunar syndromes could be differentiated from the larger superficial cortical infarcts; however, with the increasing use of CT scanning it has become apparent that there is considerable overlap in the clinical presentation of a superficial cortical infarct and a deep lacunar infarct (Nelson *et al.*, 1980).

Following cerebral infarction, cytotoxic oedema initially develops, with the accumulation of water in glial cells. In addition there is breakdown of the blood–brain barrier and the formation of extracellular (vasogenic) oedema (O'Brien, 1979; Harrison and Ross Russell, 1983). Ischaemic oedema is a mixture of cytotoxic oedema, which occurs within hours of the event, and vasogenic oedema, which reaches a peak after about 3–4 days. These two combine to give cerebral oedema, sometimes associated with herniation and compression of adjacent structures, which may lead to clinical deterioration and drowsiness in the first few days after a cerebral thrombosis.

Cerebral emboli

Cerebral emboli usually come from either the heart or the great vessels in the neck (de Bono, 1983; Harrison and Marshall, 1976) (Table 8.1). The ophthalmic and middle cerebral arteries are common sites for emboli. The resultant infarcts, which may be multiple, can occur in different vascular territories; they are often haemorrhagic.

It is well established that congenital and rheumatic heart disease, mural thrombi following recent myocardial infarction, bacterial endocarditis and

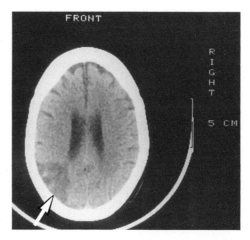

Figure 8.1. CT scan showing superficial cortical infarct.

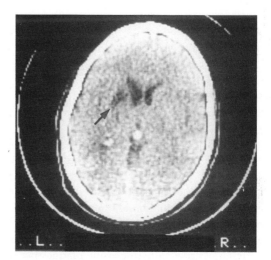

Figure 8.2. CT scan showing deep lacunar infarct in the internal capsule.

arrhythmias, usually atrial fibrillation, are frequent sources of emboli (de Bono, 1983). These are largely composed of fibrin, red cells and platelets. In recent years minor cardiac valvular abnormalities, such as mitral annulus calcification and mitral valve prolapse, have been postulated as sources of emboli. There has been much debate about the significance of these as a source of emboli (Oakley, 1984). Emboli from proximal arteries are also common. The inter-

104

P. Humphrey

TABLE 8.1   CARDIAC SOURCES OF EMBOLI

Left atrium
   thrombus (usually secondary to atrial fibrillation)
   myxoma
   paradoxical embolism

Mitral valve
   rheumatic endocarditis
   infective endocarditis
   marantic endocarditis
   prosthetic valve
   mitral valve prolapse
   mitral annulus calcification

Left ventricle
   thrombus—myocardial infarction, cardiomyopathy
Aortic valve
   rheumatic endocarditis
   infective endocarditis
   marantic endocarditis
   bicuspid valve
   aortic sclerosis and calcification
   prosthetic valve
   syphilitic aortitis

Congenital cardiac disorders

Cardiac surgery
   air embolism
   platelet/fibrin embolism

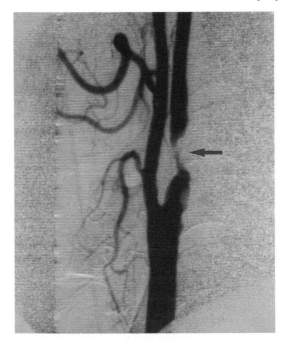

Figure 8.3. Angiogram showing an internal carotid stenosis.

nal carotid artery, where atheromatous narrowing is common, is a particular source of emboli (Figure 8.3). Plaques in this territory tend to ulcerate. Haemorrhage into a plaque is a common phenomenon with the formation of fibrin platelet emboli. On occasions, cholesterol emboli may originate from these plaques presumably due to rupture of lipid into the lumen. As these atherosclerotic plaques become re-endothelialized the emboli cease and the lesion becomes incorporated into the intima of the artery.

Emboli may sometimes be seen on fundoscopy (Fisher, 1959). Platelet emboli are seen only transiently before breaking up and moving on whilst cholesterol emboli often remain in the retinal arteries and are sometimes visible for months after the clinical attack (Figure 8.4). Sometimes emboli from the great vessels or heart valves are calcific. Rarely, fibrin platelet emboli occur on the heart valves in patients with carcinoma, particularly carcinoma of the pancreas, or come from the leg veins having

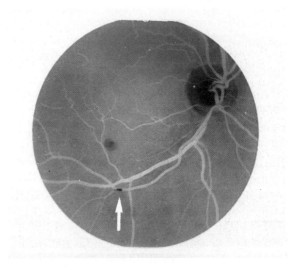

Figure 8.4. Retinal emboli.

passed through an atrial septal defect to enter the cerebral circulation (so-called paradoxical embolus).

Cerebral haemorrhage

There are three main causes of haemorrhage in and around the brain.

(1) Spontaneous intracerebral haemorrhage. This originates from small intracerebral arteries affected by lipohyaline degeneration. It particularly occurs in the basal ganglia, subcortical white matter, cerebellum and pons. Lipohyaline change is caused by plasma permeating into the walls of arterioles which have become weakened through loss of elastic and smooth muscle tissue. This is usually brought about by chronic hypertension. Intracerebral haemorrhage follows rupture of the small microaneurysms (Charcot–Bouchard aneurysms) which form as a result of the vessel wall degeneration. Small lacunar haemorrhages (Figure 8.5) may remain isolated in the cerebral substance or sometimes rupture into the subarachnoid space. Brain swellings, herniation and brain stem compression may follow. If the patient survives, the haemorrhage is usually absorbed leaving a cystic cavity.

(2) Subarachnoid haemorrhage. This usually originates from rupture of berry aneurysms, the latter arising from the large extracerebral vessels around the circle of Willis. These particularly occur at the origin of the anterior cerebral arteries, on the middle cerebral artery and on the posterior communicating artery. They are thought to arise in the wall of these arteries at sites of congenital defects which are aggravated by atheroma and hypertension. Aneurysmal bleeding may extend into the brain substance itself, especially into the frontal lobe if an anterior communicating artery aneurysm ruptures, or into the temporal lobe following rupture of a middle cerebral artery aneurysm. Subarachnoid haemorrhage may cause death from acute raised intracranial pressure with secondary brain stem compression and ischaemia.

(3) Angiomas (arteriovenous malformations). These consist of a mass of tangled arteries and veins which slowly enlarge during adult life. They typically present with either haemorrhage or epileptic seizures. They are usually situated in the cerebral hemispheres but may arise in almost any part of the brain. The bleeding is less profuse and dangerous than from a berry aneurysm.

The other major causes of cerebral haemorrhages are listed in Table 8.2.

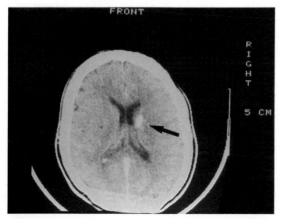

Figure 8.5. CT scan showing a deep lacunar haemorrhage.

TABLE 8.2 COMMON CAUSES OF CEREBRAL HAEMORRHAGE

1. Hypertension
2. Aneurysm
3. Arteriovenous malformation
4. Anticoagulant treatment
5. Bleeding into a primary or secondary tumour
6. Clotting abnormalities/thrombocytopenia

Transient Ischaemic Attacks (TIAs)

Whilst the majority of strokes are thromboembolic and approximately 10% are due to primary intracerebral haemorrhage, transient ischaemic attacks are almost invariably embolic. A few are thought to be haemodynamic.

Carotid

(1) Embolic.

There is a great deal of evidence to support the idea that the majority of TIAs in the carotid territory are embolic. Fisher in 1959 and Ross Russell in 1968 reported seeing emboli passing through the retinal circulation during an attack of amaurosis fugax (Figure 8.4). These are usually platelet emboli which break up and pass on within a few minutes of an attack. Cholesterol emboli may be seen in the retina long after an attack of amaurosis fugax. Furthermore, cholesterol emboli have been found in the brain at autopsy (McDonald, 1967). Angiography and subsequent endarterectomy often show a loose thrombus at the origin of the internal carotid artery in patients having carotid TIAs (Harrison and Marshall, 1977). Fresh ulcerated haemorrhage in the plaque is more likely to be present in patients having recent TIAs.

Symptoms in successive attacks may be similar or sometimes involve different arterial territories; thus a patient may have attacks of amaurosis fugax alternating with weakness or sensory loss down the contralateral arm and leg. Attacks quite frequently cease when the carotid artery occludes. Endarterectomy is often successful in stopping TIAs. These facts leave little doubt that the majority of carotid TIAs are embolic.

(2) Haemodynamic.

A minority of TIAs may have a haemodynamic basis. The first surgical repair to the carotid artery was performed by Eastcott in 1954 (Eastcott *et al.*, 1954). This was on a patient who was having episodes of amaurosis fugax and contralateral limb symptoms which occurred at the time of a tachyarrhythmia. This patient also had a tight internal carotid stenosis. Surgical repair of the stenosis prevented further neurological attacks although the episodes of cardiac arrhythmia continued.

It is unlikely that arrhythmias alone are a common cause of TIAs in patients with normal vascular trees. Brice and colleagues in 1964 showed that blood flow does not fall until the lumen of a vessel is narrowed by at least 75%. TIAs, however, may occur in the presence of only mild stenosis or atheroma alone. Furthermore, Kendall and Marshall in 1963 studied 37 patients with TIAs on a tilt table and lowered the blood pressure with ganglion blocking agents. Diffuse symptoms of syncope were common. These included dizziness, light-headedness and loss of consciousness. Only one patient had a focal TIA similar to his presenting symptom. It seems unlikely, therefore, that hypotension or arrhythmias are a common cause of focal TIAs. The majority of case reports in which haemodynamic factors have been thought to be relevant involved patients with severe multiple vessel disease. Ross Russell and Page in 1983 described four patients with severe widespread occlusive disease who suffered from attacks of visual loss due to transient retinal ischaemia. These attacks were usually provoked by standing or exercise. Stark and Wodak in 1983 described four patients who developed haemodynamic TIAs on standing, some of which resembled focal TIAs; however, these symptoms were often accompanied by dizziness and faintness. Again, all had severe vascular disease.

Unfortunately, it can be very difficult to distinguish between embolic and haemodynamic TIAs clinically. Fisher (1976) described a patient who had frequent TIAs which occurred when hypotensive therapy was begun and which stopped when these drugs were withdrawn. Other factors which may give a clue to the occurrence of haemodynamic TIAs include dizziness and faintness at the onset of these attacks. Haemodynamic TIAs may also be brought on by clear provocative factors such as standing, exercise, straining or even eating (Pantin and Young, 1980). Finally, in many of these cases described in whom a haemodynamic basis was thought to be the cause of the TIAs, the attacks occurred many times a day over a considerable period of time; this is unusual in embolic TIAs. Whilst haemodynamic TIAs are rare compared with embolic TIAs, it is important to identify them if possible, as the approach to treatment will obviously be different.

Vertebrobasilar TIAs

Again, vertebrobasilar TIAs are usually thought to be embolic in nature. However, some are undoubtedly haemodynamic. It is well known that extending the neck is a cause of vertebrobasilar TIAs. This presumably occurs on a haemodynamic basis with kinking of the arterial blood supply (Payne and Spillane, 1957). Sheehan *et al.*, in 1960, demonstrated compression of the vertebral artery by osteophytes in the cervical region when the neck was turned and extended. It is unlikely that this is a common cause of vertebrobasilar TIAs except in patients who also have significant narrowing or occlusion of the carotid arteries so that the cerebral circulation is then dependent on the vertebral arteries for adequate perfusion.

The subclavian steal syndrome is a rare but distinctive cause of haemodynamic vertebrobasilar TIAs. It results from stenosis or occlusion of the subclavian artery, usually on the left. The affected vertebral artery then fills retrogradely from the opposite vertebral artery or the carotid artery via the circle of Willis. Because of the blocked subclavian, blood flow in the relevant arm is dependent on retrograde flow in the vertebral artery. Patients develop symptoms of vertebrobasilar insufficiency when the arm is exercised, since blood is 'stolen' from the brain stem by the arm as it is exercised. It is surprisingly often asymptomatic, however (Hennerici *et al.*, 1981). Furthermore Fields and Lemak (1972), following up a group of 168 cases, found that the risk of major brain stem infarction was very small indeed.

PATHOPHYSIOLOGY

An understanding of the major factors which influence cerebral blood flow is important in the rational management of cerebrovascular disease.

Metabolic Control of Cerebral Blood Flow (CBF)

There is a close link between CBF and metabolic demand. In an atrophic brain the CBF is often low. In most cases this is not because the low CBF has caused the brain to atrophy, but because the reduced metabolic requirement of the atrophic brain is met by a reduced CBF. The reverse is also true. When, for

instance, the cerebral metabolic rate rises considerably during epileptic attacks, there is a marked increase in CBF. This has been beautifully demonstrated using modern CBF techniques, particularly in focal epilepsy. In normal controls, there is a direct relationship between CBF and P_{CO_2}. There is also an inverse relationship between CBF and oxygen saturation (Kety and Schmidt, 1948). This helps to ensure that changes in metabolic demand are matched by adequate oxygen supply to the brain and efficient removal of waste products.

Blood Pressure, Hypertension and CBF

CBF remains constant throughout a normal range of blood pressure by autoregulation. The autoregulatory range extends from approximately 60 to 140 mmHg mean arterial blood pressure; this is roughly equivalent to 80–170 mmHg systolic blood pressure (Lassen, 1959). At blood pressures below this CBF falls and above it CBF rises. In hypertension, autoregulation is maintained, although the whole curve is shifted to the right (Strandgaard *et al.*, 1973) (Figure 8.6). CBF thus begins to fall at a higher mean arterial blood pressure in hypertension than it does in controls. Sudden reduction in blood pressure in hypertensive patients may be sufficient to cause a fall in CBF even though the absolute level to which the blood flow pressure has fallen may not normally be regarded as in the hypotensive range. This is clearly important in the management of chronic hyperten-

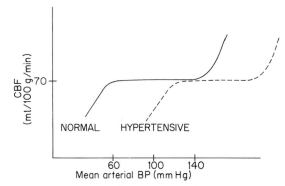

Figure 8.6. Autoregulatory curve of blood pressure (BP) against cerebral blood flow (CBF) in normal and hypertensive patients. (*Reproduced by courtesy of the British Journal of Hospital Medicine.*)

sion. There have been many reports of vascular complications following sudden reduction in blood pressure (Kumar *et al.*, 1976; Cove *et al.*, 1979; Ledingham and Rajagopalan, 1979). Cases of blindness and stroke have been reported immediately following reduction in blood pressure in hypertensive patients who are otherwise well. For instance, Ledingham and Rajagopalan in 1979 described one patient who developed a right hemiplegia with dysphasia after rapid reduction in blood pressure from 240/155 to 140/80. The latter blood pressure would normally be regarded as satisfactory. In a hypertensive patient this value could well have been below the lower limit of autoregulation and therefore resulted in the stroke that followed. Unless the patient has eclampsia, hypertensive encephalopathy, left ventricular failure secondary to hypertension or aortic dissection, there is no need to lower the blood pressure rapidly over a period of minutes to hours. Gentle reduction in blood pressure over a period of days would seem prudent. In hypertension there is evidence that the autoregulatory curve shifts back towards normal after treatment. It would therefore then be reasonable to aim for a more 'normal' blood pressure of 140/90 over a period of days to weeks. This is *not* an argument against treating hypertension, as mortality studies show that this is the major risk factor in all vascular disease, only against abruptly lowering it.

Ischaemia

Infarction follows thrombosis if the collateral circulation is inadequate. Animal studies suggest that there is a central zone of necrosis which occurs when the CBF falls below 10 ml/100 g/min (normal CBF 60–70 ml/100 g/min). Electrical function ceases when CBF falls to 20 ml/100 g/min. Thus between 10 and 20 ml/100 g/min it may be possible to restore electrical function by increasing CBF. Animal experiments suggest that around an ischaemic necrotic centre there may be a penumbra which is viable but functionless (Branston *et al.*, 1977).

CBF tends to be low following an occlusive episode (Fieschi *et al.*, 1966). However, there have been many studies which show that sometimes flow is high compared to the metabolic rate; this has been termed luxury perfusion by Lassen (1966). Positron emission tomography, a technique which measures both CBF and metabolic rate, has recently been used to study cerebral ischaemia in detail. This has shown that ischaemia is common in the early hours after a stroke but that luxury perfusion follows in many cases (Wise *et al.*, 1983). In ischaemia there are two compensatory mechanisms which attempt to maintain metabolic supply. Firstly there is an increase in the cerebral blood volume which helps to maximize the delivery of oxygen and other nutrients to the ischaemic area (Gibbs *et al.*, 1984). Secondly there is an increase in the extraction of oxygen from the blood. Both these compensatory mechanisms occur in cerebral ischaemia and it is only when they are exhausted that necrosis occurs.

Many attempts have been made to find a vasodilator to increase CBF at this time to try and minimize any deficit. Carbon dioxide was an early choice. Unfortunately blood vessels in an ischaemic area are often in a state of vasoparalysis (Paulson, 1970) and lose their ability to respond normally. In stroke patients when carbon dioxide was administered, there was no evidence to suggest that CBF to the ischaemic area rose. In fact if anything the CBF fell. This was because vasodilatation following carbon dioxide occurred in the normal parts of the brain but not in the ischaemic area, with the result that blood was directed away from the ischaemic area towards the rest of the brain—a phenomenon known as intracerebral steal. Vasoparalysis is a common finding following ischaemic episodes. The same phenomenon is seen after the administration of vasodilators and it is therefore not surprising that there is no good evidence to suggest they are beneficial in cerebrovascular disease. Measures directed at improving the viscosity of blood do not suffer from this drawback because a reduction in blood viscosity should improve flow to both normal and ischaemic areas.

The normal autoregulatory response to changes in blood pressure is lost following an ischaemic episode (Paulson, 1970). In this situation there is a direct relationship between CBF and mean arterial blood pressure. This has an important influence on the management of hypertension in acute strokes.

Transient Ischaemic Attacks (TIAs)

There is probably little fundamental difference between a transient ischaemic attack and a stroke with recovery. The belief that TIAs are not associated with structural damage is almost certainly incorrect in some cases. Rees and colleagues in 1970 showed that regional abnormalities in CBF may be present long after a TIA has occurred. In one case the CBF remained low 90 days after the last attack. Furthermore Van der Drift and Kok (1973) demonstrated small infarcts at post-mortem in patients who clinically had only a TIA. It seems reasonable to investigate both strokes with recovery and TIAs in a similar way to prevent a further attack.

RISK FACTORS

Age

Age is the most important predictive factor in cerebrovascular disease. The incidence of stroke is low before the age of 40. It rises from an annual incidence of less than 1 per 100 000 per year to more than 2000 per 100 000 per year by the age of 75 (Kannel and Wolf, 1983).

Hypertension

After age, hypertension is the most powerful risk factor for both haemorrhage and atherosclerotic cerebrovascular disease. Although most physicians pay more attention to diastolic blood pressure, systolic blood pressure more closely reflects the risk of further stroke. Furthermore there is no clear cut-off at which the risk begins to rise. The Framingham study shows that the risk increases with increasing systolic blood pressure even from within the normotensive range (Kannel and Wolf, 1983).

Ross Russell (1963), confirming Charcot and Bouchard's observations, found that hypertensive patients were more likely to have small microaneurysms usually deep within the basal ganglia, cerebellum, pons or subcortical white matter. These may thrombose in lacunar infarcts (Figure 8.2) or

rupture, causing lacunar haemorrhage (Figure 8.5). In addition Robertson and Strong (1968) showed that atherosclerosis in large vessels was more advanced in hypertensive patients.

It used to be widely believed that hypotension, with a resultant fall in CBF, was also a risk factor for stroke. Epidemiological data suggest that this is rare. Occasionally in severe arteriopaths with widespread occlusive disease one may see a worsening of the deficit following treatment with hypotensive therapy. This is, however, the exception rather than the rule. Hypotension tends to produce a different pattern of deficit to that seen in most stroke patients. After a cardiac arrest, for example, diffuse cerebral damage affects the watershed areas.

Transient Ischaemic Attacks

The increased risk of stroke following transient ischaemic attack was reviewed by Brust (1977). The available data showed that the risk of stroke lay between zero and 50% after a TIA. This enormous variance was due largely to different methods of data collection. The large epidemiological studies suggest that the risk of a stroke after a TIA is approximately 30% in the first 5 years. It is greatest in the first year and falls progressively with time elapsing from the TIA (Mohr, 1978; Kannel and Wolf, 1983). The Framingham data suggest that the risk of stroke is increased by at least ten times in the first year after a TIA (Kannel and Wolf, 1983).

Coronary Artery Disease

Atherosclerosis is clearly a widespread disease. Patients with coronary artery disease are at an increased risk of stroke. Cardiac enlargement on the chest X-ray, congestive cardiac failure, ECG abnormalities such as left ventricular enlargement, intravascular conduction disturbances and ST/T wave changes are all associated with an increased risk of cerebrovascular disease (Kannel and Wolf, 1983). Furthermore, the chief cause of death after a TIA or a stroke is not a further stroke but a myocardial infarct or sudden death presumed to be of myocardial origin (Sacco *et al.*, 1982).

Diabetes Mellitus

An elevated blood sugar appears to be an independent risk factor according to the Framingham data (Kannel and Wolf, 1983).

Haematocrit

There is no doubt that polycythaemia rubra vera is associated with an increased risk of cerebrovascular disease. There have been recent data suggesting that a haematocrit in the high normal range may also be an independent risk factor (Kannel and Wolf, 1983).

Other Risk Factors

Other parameters such as cholesterol, smoking, lack of exercise and obesity have been suggested as independent risk factors (Kannel and Wolf, 1983; Bonita *et al.*, 1986). Whilst elevated lipid levels and smoking are definite independent risk factors in the aetiology of coronary artery disease, their role in cerebrovascular disease is much less clear-cut. As a practical policy I think patients should be advised to stop smoking and to alter their diet if they have a markedly elevated cholesterol or triglyceride level. Furthermore because most stroke patients die of coronary artery disease, to divorce coronary and cerebrovascular risk factors into separate groups for management purposes is naïve.

The factors discussed above are relevant to the development of cerebro-atherosclerosis and haemorrhage. Separate from this, there are a large number of other conditions which may present with

TABLE 8.3 OTHER CAUSES OF CEREBRAL INFARCTION

1. Migraine
2. Haematological disorders (see Table 4)
3. Inflammatory arterial disease (see Table 5)
4. Venous thrombosis
5. Trauma to neck
6. Infection
7. Malignancy—neoplastic angioendotheliosis
8. Hypertensive encephalopathy
9. Subarachnoid haemorrhage
10. Post-therapeutic irradiation

TABLE 8.4 HAEMATOLOGICAL DISORDERS CAUSING STROKE

1. Polycythaemia rubra vera
2. Essential thrombocythaemia
3. Sickle cell disease
4. Leukaemia
5. Thrombocytopenia
6. Thrombotic thrombocytopenic purpura
7. Hyperviscosity
   multiple myeloma
   Waldenström's macroglobulinaemia

TABLE 8.5 INFLAMMATORY ARTERIAL DISEASE

1. Giant cell arteritis
2. Polyarteritis nodosa
3. Systemic lupus erythematosus
4. Granulomatous angiitis
5. Wegener's granulomatosis
6. Sarcoid angitis
7. Scleroderma
8. Rheumatoid arthritis
9. Syphilis

ischaemic cerebrovascular disease unrelated to atherosclerosis (Tables 8.3, 8.4 and 8.5).

CLINICAL SYNDROMES

Carotid Territory

Anterior cerebral artery

The anterior cerebral artery passes forwards and over the corpus callosum, supplying the medial part of the cerebral hemisphere. It thus supplies the entire motor and sensory cortex controlling the leg area. The voluntary control of bladder function lies just anterior to the leg area. Ischaemia in the anterior cerebral artery territory may therefore produce urgency of micturition or incontinence. Because this artery also supplies the frontal pole, there may be disturbances of intellect, judgement and emotional control. It also gives off a small branch which supplies the anterior limb of the internal capsule, ischaemia of which results in a hemiplegia.

Middle cerebral artery

The middle cerebral artery supplies most of the lateral surface of the cerebral hemisphere. It also gives off small penetrating branches (lenticulostriate arteries) which pass deep to supply the basal ganglia and internal capsule.

Ischaemia produces a hemiparesis with hemisensory loss affecting mainly the face and arm with the leg being involved to a lesser extent. Sometimes if only a small area is affected there may be only weakness of the hand, in particular finger extensors and interossei. These patients are sometimes mistakenly diagnosed as having a radial nerve palsy. However, the sudden onset of the attack for no clear provocative reason and the presence of weakness of the interossei and finger extensors are usually sufficient to give the clue that this has been a cortical event. There may be a homonymous hemianopia. This can occur in either a small superficial cortical infarct or deep lacunar infarct (see below). If the dominant hemisphere is affected, dysphasia is common. This is usually a mixed receptive and expressive dysphasia. Non-dominant hemisphere lesions produce topographical disorientation with inattention and neglect of the left side; there may also be difficulty with dressing.

Apraxia also occurs in dominant hemisphere lesions, though it may be masked by dysphasia.

Internal carotid artery

This produces a syndrome resembling combined anterior and middle cerebral artery occlusion. Furthermore, the first branch of the internal carotid artery is the ophthalmic artery. Loss of vision to one eye may accompany carotid artery occlusion, particularly if both internal and external carotid arteries are involved. More frequently, however, episodes of fleeting visual loss (amaurosis fugax) occur. These are usually embolic and produce either transient complete unilateral loss of vision or altitudinal field loss if only the upper or lower half of the retina is involved. The patient usually describes a curtain coming down across his vision. Rarely these attacks are haemodynamic in origin; in these cases there are often clear provocative features before each attack

such as standing, exercising, straining at stool, all of which tend to reduce retinal perfusion (Ross Russell and Page, 1983). Haemodynamic episodes of amaurosis fugax are more often described in vague terms—frequently as a blurring of vision. Sometimes patients report an increase in visual contrast, with light objects appearing brighter and dark ones darker.

Because of damage to the sympathetic fibres in the carotid sheath there may be an ipsilateral Horner's syndrome following carotid artery occlusion. There may also be exaggerated pulsation in the branches of the external carotid artery (particularly the superficial temporal artery). Increased collateral blood flow through this artery shunts blood via the orbital vessels into the ophthalmic artery and then into the circle of Willis in an attempt to compensate for the internal carotid occlusion, the patient thus performing his own extracranial–intracranial anastomosis. Sometimes the increased collateral flow is so marked that the superficial temporal artery on the side of the occlusion becomes tender and painful. This can mimic temporal arteritis. It is particularly important in this situation that the temporal artery is not biopsied as a major collateral source of blood will then be obliterated.

Vertebrobasilar Territory

Posterior cerebral artery

These paired vessels are formed by the bifurcation of the basilar trunk. They supply the occipital lobes, the upper part of the brain stem and the medial surface of the temporal lobe. Field defects, usually unilateral, are the principal result of ischaemia of the posterior cerebral artery. Lesions on both sides may produce bilateral visual symptoms which are most frequently manifest by simple visual hallucinations such as flashes of light or zig-zag lines in both visual fields. If severe then cortical blindness can follow. Pupillary responses in this condition are spared as the pupillary fibres travelling to the midbrain are not involved. The patient often confabulates, has hallucinations and little insight, or may even deny his blindness (Anton's syndrome). The confabulation and confusion are thought to be due to ischaemia of the medial part of the temporal lobe. Sometimes transient amnesia may be seen because of isolated ischaemia to the medial aspect of the temporal lobe. The posterior cerebral artery also supplies the upper part of the thalamus. Infarction here produces sensory impairment over the contralateral side of the body which may be accompanied by a very unpleasant pain; this can be spontaneous or induced by light touch of the skin (thalamic syndrome).

Vertebrobasilar ischaemia in the brain stem

The signs following vertebrobasilar ischaemia depend on the level of the lesion in the brain stem (Caplan, 1981). Occlusion of the terminal basilar artery produces signs of posterior cerebral artery occlusion as described above. If midbrain ischaemia occurs, pupillary changes with impaired vertical gaze or ocular motor nerve dysfunction are seen. Damage to the pons produces horizontal gaze palsy with facial weakness or sensory loss. In either case a quadriparesis or hemiparesis may also occur.

A wide range of other syndromes, many of which Fisher (1982) relates to lacunar infarcts, are reported to follow ischaemia of a localized area of the brain stem. The basic pattern is one of ipsilateral cranial nerve palsies combined with contralateral paresis or sensory loss which affects either the arm and leg or face, arm and leg, depending on the level in the brain stem at which it occurs. There may also be ipsilateral cerebellar signs. The most common example is thrombosis of the posterior inferior cerebellar artery. This produces ischaemia of the dorsolateral medulla with palsies affecting cranial nerves V, VI, VII, IX, and X, cerebellar ataxia and a Horner's syndrome on the same side as the lesion with contralateral spinothalamic loss in the arm and leg. Hemiplegia is rare because the pyramidal tracts lying ventrally are spared.

Occlusion of the basilar artery itself is often fatal producing flaccid tetraplegia and loss of brain stem reflexes. Coma often occurs. It is important to distinguish this from the rare 'locked-in' syndrome in which there is ventral ischaemia of the midbrain (Hawkes, 1974). The clinical picture here is similar except that the patient is fully alert. He may appear to be unconscious because he is completely immobile apart from vertical movements of the eyes and occasionally the eyelids. It is important to check for the presence of these eye movements in any 'unconscious' patient before accepting that the patient is truly unconscious.

Positional or postural vertigo is often thought to be due to vertebrobasilar ischaemia. If there is no other evidence of vascular disease or vertebrobasilar ischaemia it is better not to label such cases as vertebrobasilar ischaemia as the symptoms are frequently due to inner ear disease.

Subclavian steal syndrome

The basis of this syndrome is described in the section on vertebrobasilar TIAs (above). Symptoms may occur after exercising the arm, though they may at times be unrelated to arm exercise. Doppler studies, however, have demonstrated that subclavian stenosis and occlusion may often be asymptomatic.

Lacunae

The clinical pictures seen with lacunar infarcts often overlap with those seen in conditions described above. These small microinfarcts described by Fisher are commonly seen in hypertensive patients. Many lacunar syndromes have been described. The four most frequently encountered are detailed in Table 8.6. Sometimes multiple lacunar infarcts (l'état lacunaire) occur. In such cases, there is often, but by no means always, a history of preceding minor stroke. The resulting syndrome is of a pseudobulbar palsy with dementia, dysarthria, small-stepping gait (marche à petits pas), unsteadiness and incontinence.

TABLE 8.6   COMMON LACUNAR INFARCTS

Clinical type	Site of lesion
Pure motor hemiplegia	Internal capsule; pons; cerebral peduncle
Pure hemi-anaesthesia	Thalamus
Ataxic hemiparesis	Pons; internal capsule
Dysarthria/clumsy hand syndrome	Pons; internal capsule

Border Zone Infarcts

The clinical patterns so far described follow occlusion of individual blood vessels. Sometimes there is a generalized reduction in cerebral blood flow (Torvik, 1984). This is most commonly seen after a cardiac arrest of hypoxic damage during cardiac surgery. Ischaemia is then especially marked in the border zone between the territory of individual arteries because here perfusion pressure is least. The parieto-occipital zone is the area most often affected, where border zone infarcts produce visual field defects (often partial and easily missed on routine examination), reading difficulties, visual disorientation and constructional apraxia (Ross Russell and Bharucha, 1978). In the frontal border zone, slowing up, pathological grasp reflexes, gait disturbances and incontinence may occur.

Spinal Cord Disease

Spinal cord ischaemia is rare. It may occur in isolation or may follow aortic aneurysm formation or dissection or sometimes after vascular surgery to the aorta. Complete ischaemia of the cord results in loss of power and sensation below the ischaemic level. Sometimes ischaemia is confined to the anterior spinal artery territory. The posterior spinal artery supplies the dorsal columns whilst the anterior spinal artery supplies the rest of the spinal cord. Ischaemia of the anterior cerebral artery produces complete weakness and loss of pain and temperature sensation below the level of the lesion with intact vibration and joint position sense.

Cerebral Haemorrhage

Subarachnoid haemorrhage

Subarachnoid haemorrhage usually presents with sudden collapse or onset of severe headache, often associated with nausea, vomiting, photophobia and marked neck stiffness. The level of consciousness varies from coma to full alertness, most patients being obtunded and restless. Signs of focal damage, for example a hemiparesis, may be present, especially after rupture of a middle cerebral artery

aneurysm. If haemorrhage is severe and there is a marked rise in intracranial pressure, retinal haemorrhages and papilloedema may be seen. Transient cardiac arrhythmias are common and glycosuria may be found.

Intracerebral haemorrhage

Intracerebral haemorrhage often presents with symptoms similar to infarcts due to thromboembolism. The nature of the symptoms will depend on the site of the intracerebral haemorrhage. Headache tends to be an early feature. It is also more common to see drowsiness and coma in the first 24 hours after a cerebral haemorrhage than after an infarct. If blood spreads into the subarachnoid space, meningism may be present.

Cerebellar haematoma or haemorrhage deserves special mention. This often presents with severe dizziness or unsteadiness followed rapidly by nausea, vomiting, headache and drowsiness. Initially the patient may be alert, but the level of consciousness may deteriorate very rapidly, usually due to acute hydrocephalus (Figure 8.7). Once the patient becomes drowsy, death will occur in the majority of patients due to raised intracranial pressure, unless this is relieved urgently (Heros, 1982; Sandercock *et al.*, 1985). Most neurosurgeons agree that a deteriorating level of consciousness is an indication for

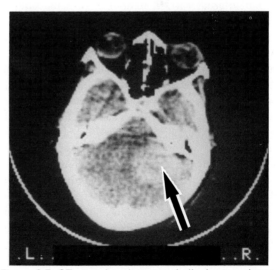

Figure 8.7. CT scan showing a cerebellar haemorrhage.

emergency sub-occipital craniectomy to decompress the haematoma. This is often followed by dramatic improvement with markedly improved level of consciousness and usually full recovery. Whilst there is much debate as to whether intracerebral haemorrhage at other sites warrants surgery at any stage, there is widespread agreement that surgery for cerebellar haemorrhage is useful and may be life-saving.

CLINICAL EXAMINATION

Careful examination of the cardiovascular as well as the nervous system is essential. All peripheral pulses should be checked and any bruits noted. A carotid bruit at the angle of the jaw is the best clinical guide to the presence of an internal carotid stenosis. However, there are many false positives and negatives (Humphrey and Bradbury, 1984). Bruits do not arise from the stenosis itself but are thought to be due to arterial wall vibration resulting from turbulence in the arterial flow distal to a stenosis. Because of this, they may be heard when there is a contralateral or ipsilateral internal carotid occlusion, due to the increased flow in vessels that remain patent. Occasionally, atheroma without stenosis may cause sufficient turbulence to generate a bruit. Finally, though rarely, bruits may originate from external carotid stenosis. There are also false negatives in which internal carotid stenosis is present, but no bruit is heard. This mainly occurs with mild stenosis but more importantly with very tight stenoses. When the stenosis exceeds 90%, reduction in flow may be so marked that there is little turbulence distal to the stenosis and the bruit, therefore, disappears. Whilst a bruit is the best clinical guide to an internal carotid stenosis, attacks of amaurosis fugax combined with contralateral hemiparesis, coexisting intermittent claudication, age over 50 and hypertension all increase the chance of finding a stenosis at angiography (Harrison and Marshall, 1975; Wilson and Ross Russell, 1977).

Examination of the fundus is particularly important as one occasionally sees emboli lodged in the major retinal arteries or at their bifurcations (Figure 8.4). It is important to check the blood pressure in each arm; a difference of more than 15 mmHg

systolic with or without a supraclavicular bruit, suggests a subclavian stenosis or occlusion.

DIFFERENTIAL DIAGNOSIS

Transient Ischaemic Attacks (TIAs)

Attacks similar to TIAs may occur in migraine (Bartleson, 1984). It is important, therefore, to ask about the presence of more typical migrainous attacks and about headache. Headache is rare in TIAs due to emboli. Focal epilepsy may sometimes be mistaken for TIAs, particularly with focal sensory epilepsy when it may be difficult to distinguish numbness in a TIA from tingling in a focal sensory attack. In Norris and Hachinski's (1982) study, the commonest misdiagnosis was an unwitnessed or unrecognized seizure, most of the patients being admitted in a post-ictal state. If there is any suggestion of a progressive defect or raised intracranial pressure then it may be necessary to consider investigation to exclude a tumour. Rarely, tumours present with transient episodes of focal neurological disturbance without epileptic features (Ross, 1983; Loeb, 1979), which may be confused with TIAs.

There are many other causes of symptoms similar to TIAs. These include hypoglycaemia (Meyer and Portnoy, 1958), hyperviscosity states, hyponatraemia (Faris and Poser, 1964), hepatic and renal failure and hypercalcaemia (Longo and Witherspoon, 1980). Chronic subdural haematomas may also present with attacks identical to TIAs (Luxon and Harrison, 1979). Finally giant aneurysms, which particularly occur in the elderly, are often filled with thrombotic material and may occasionally give rise to embolic TIAs (Steel *et al.*, 1982).

Stroke

'Stroke', like TIA, is merely a descriptive term for a set of clinical symptoms and signs. Rarely cerebral tumour, subdural haematoma, encephalitis or abscess may present with a stroke-like picture, particularly if a focal deficit occurs in a stepwise manner or evolves over a matter of hours to days (Luxon and Harrison, 1979). Conversely, a cerebrovascular accident may present subacutely. This is especially likely if there is further propagation of an original thrombus, additional embolism, secondary oedema or haemorrhage.

The difficulty of distinguishing haemorrhage from an infarction on clinical grounds alone has already been noted (Allen, 1983). However, a history of previous TIAs, presence of emboli in the retina, recent myocardial infarction or a clear cardiac source of emboli, all point towards a thromboembolic episode. Early headache and loss of consciousness, persistent drowsiness or unconsciousness 24 hours after admission, vomiting, meningism, bilateral extensor plantars and a markedly elevated diastolic blood pressure (greater than 130 mmHg) suggest haemorrhage.

INVESTIGATION

This is directed at confirming the diagnosis and identifying any risk factors. All patients with stroke TIA should have the tests listed in Table 8.7. Abnormal results may suggest further appropriate investigation. If there is clear evidence of cardiac disease, an echocardiogram may be necessary to delineate this further; M-mode studies provide reliable information about the state of the heart valves but fail to demonstrate mural thrombi, for which two-dimensional (2D) echocardiogram is more useful (Ports *et al.*, 1978; Asinger *et al.*, 1981).

If there is doubt about the diagnosis, CT scanning may be necessary. This will certainly differentiate haemorrhage from infarction and is mandatory if anticoagulants are being considered. Interestingly, it may not always differentiate a tumour from an infarct. In fact Norris and Hachinski (1982) showed

that it was not a substitute for careful clinical assessment; indeed, a CT scan was no better at differentiating tumour from infarction than careful clinical assessment. Some centres do not yet have access to CT scanning and may have to rely on the isotope scan. Following a stroke, the isotope scan becomes positive after a few days. It usually remains positive for about 6–8 weeks before returning to normal. If a tumour is present and the isotope scan is positive then the abnormality will be unchanged or more marked after 6–8 weeks, whereas in the case of a vascular lesion the abnormality will resolve. It is useful therefore to repeat the isotope scan at 6–8 weeks if there is doubt about the diagnosis and CT scanning is not available. The pattern of the abnormality on the isotope scan may also give a clue. It is often wedge shaped in vascular disease but more clearly a discrete mass with a tumour. Furthermore, an isotope scan is very useful for picking out a subdural haematoma which is an important treatable cause of apparent stroke in the elderly.

There is much debate about the role of endarterectomy in patients with TIAs and a carotid stenosis. If the patient is otherwise well, then one needs to consider angiography. In this country this investigation is almost exclusively reserved for carotid TIAs or stroke patients who have made a good recovery and thus have much to lose from a further attack. It is very rarely performed in vertebrobasilar TIAs. In any case, it is indicated only in those who are fit for surgery. It is virtually never indicated for acute stroke, unless there is evidence of subarachnoid haemorrhage and the neurological centre to which one refers is prepared to take patients over the age of 65.

The purpose of angiography is to identify an operable stenosis at the origin of the internal carotid artery (Figure 8.3). Whether one performs angiography will be influenced by the policy of the local vascular surgeon and, in particular, the age up to which he is prepared to perform an endarterectomy. The decision for surgery should depend, in my opinion, more upon the general health of the patient, rather than on chronological age. If patients are otherwise well and have a clear history of carotid TIAs, I would be prepared to investigate them with a view to endarterectomy up to their mid 70s.

TABLE 8.7 ROUTINE INVESTIGATIONS IN STROKE OR TIA PATIENTS

Full blood count (including platelets)
Erythrocyte Sedimentation Rate (ESR)
Urea and electrolytes
Blood glucose
Fasting lipids
Syphilis serology
Sickling test (in at-risk groups)
Urinalysis
Electrocardiograph
Chest X-ray
Skull X-ray

Unfortunately, only 30% of all patients referred to a neurological centre with carotid TIAs have an operable lesion (Humphrey and Marshall, 1981). Thus a considerable number of patients will be exposed to the risk of angiography without further action being taken.

Whilst the risks of the newer imaging methods, such as digital subtraction angiography, are less than those of conventional angiography, there is still a possibility of precipitating a stroke. This has encouraged the development of truly non-invasive methods for detecting carotid bifurcation disease. These are based on two distinct methods (Woodcock, 1981). The first uses Doppler ultrasonography, which is particularly useful in detecting carotid occlusions and carotid stenosis greater than 50% (Hennerici *et al.*, 1981). The second uses B-mode ultrasonic imaging to create an anatomical picture of the vessel wall and is especially helpful in detecting mild to moderate atheroma (Ginsberg and Cebul, 1983). These two methods have been combined in the Duplex scanner, the results of which correlate well with angiography in all grades of atheromatous disease. Duplex scanning, however, is very operator dependent and it needs considerable practice and time to master the techniques and interpret the results. Our own experience with Doppler ultrasonography has confirmed that it is useful in picking up carotid stenoses and occlusions (Humphrey and Bradbury, 1984). It was considerably more reliable than the presence of a carotid bruit alone.

Angiography remains the gold standard for visualizing the vascular tree. As already mentioned, it carries a small risk of stroke. Whilst most would put this risk at about 1%, a prospective study has suggested that when stroke is looked for carefully, the risks may be higher (Steiner *et al.*, 1983). The risk of surgery, like that of angiography, varies markedly from centre to centre and this must account for the widespread variation in the use of angiography in the UK. The UK TIA Study Group (1983) found that while some centres routinely subject patients with carotid TIAs to angiography, others rarely use angiography.

Recently, digital subtraction angiography, with computerized imaging of the cerebral vessels after either intravenous or intra-arterial injection of contrast media, has become available. This is less hazardous than conventional angiography. However, it provides good quality pictures in only about 80% of cases (Little *et al.*, 1982). It is likely that over the next 10 years this will replace conventional angiography in most patients with vascular disease, although it is not yet clear whether the contrast media will need to be given intra-arterially or intravenously to obtain adequate pictures.

MANAGEMENT

Immediate Management

Preservation of the airway, maintaining fluid balance and nursing in the semiprone position are important if the patient is drowsy. Cerebral oedema is a significant factor in large infarcts and may be associated with a deteriorating level of consciousness. Steroids have not been shown to be of any significant use and there is no justification for their routine use (Mulley *et al.*, 1978). Hyperosmolar agents such as glycerol may reduce the degree of cerebral oedema, although as yet the clinical value of these is unclear (Frithz and Werner, 1975; Bayer *et al.*, 1987). Improving cerebral blood flow by giving low molecular weight dextran, which reduces the haematocrit, has not been shown to be of any worthwhile benefit in clinical studies in acute stroke (Matthews *et al.*, 1976; Italian Acute Stroke Study Group, 1988).

There is, as discussed earlier, considerable doubt about the safety of lowering blood pressure immediately after a stroke. The normal autoregulatory response to changes in blood pressure is lost following an ischaemic episode (Paulson, 1970), so that there is then a direct relationship between cerebral blood flow and mean arterial pressure. For this reason, hypertension should not be treated acutely in most patients, unless there is evidence of dissection, hypertensive encephalopathy (Dinsdale, 1982) or a cerebral haemorrhage. It is often difficult to differentiate cerebral haemorrhage from thrombosis without CT scanning. However, intracerebral haemorrhage is comparatively rare, accounting for only about 10% of all strokes. Furthermore, cerebral haemorrhage and hypertensive encephalopathy are much more likely if the diastolic pressure exceeds 130 mmHg. If

CT scanning is not available, a reasonable compromise therefore is to lower blood pressure in the acute situation, if the diastolic is greater than 130 mmHg, to levels of about 100 to 110 mmHg.

It is important to be clear about the difference between management of hypertension in the acute situation, where the primary concern is to maintain cerebral blood flow, and that in the long term where a raised blood pressure is a risk factor for further strokes. Patients who recover from an acute stroke and are found to have a raised blood pressure (diastolic greater than 100–110 mmHg) have a better prognosis if treated with an hypotensive agent. Autoregulation partly returns after a stroke, although it may still be impaired several years later (Waltz, 1970; Symon *et al.*, 1975). Although exact guidelines cannot be given, if the blood pressure remains elevated a month after the acute ischaemic event, it is reasonable to institute hypotensive therapy. It is then safe to lower blood pressure, although prudent to lower it gradually for the reasons already given.

Anticoagulants have no part to play in the management of acute thrombotic stroke. They need to be considered, however, where there is a clear source of emboli and haemorrhage has been excluded on the CT scan. Unfortunately, secondary bleeding into an infarct may occur and this needs to be balanced against the risk of further emboli. In rheumatic heart disease, with or without atrial fibrillation, anticoagulants may be given after one week, although some clinicians delay treatment for 2–3 weeks to minimize the risk of bleeding into the artefact. Although not conclusive, the evidence suggests that if the infarct is not large, the risk of secondary haemorrhage due to anticoagulants is less than the risk of further emboli (Koller, 1982; Furlan *et al.*, 1982). It is mandatory, however, to perform a CT scan prior to anticoagulation to exclude an intracerebral haemorrhage or haemorrhagic infarct. The Oxfordshire Community Stroke Project (1983) has clearly shown that in patients who have a stroke and are in atrial fibrillation, several will have had a haemorrhagic episode and not a thromboembolic one.

The risks of further emboli in lone atrial fibrillation are also substantial (Wolf *et al.*, 1983). Whether long-term anticoagulation is useful in this group is unclear. Many physicians would anticoagulate for at least the 6 month period following a stroke when the risks of further emboli seem greatest. After a myocardial infarction there is a small risk that mural thrombi may become dislodged and enter the cerebral circulation (Bean, 1938). This risk lasts only for a few weeks and short-term anticoagulation for 3–6 months may be necessary. Long-term anticoagulation may be considered if a left ventricular aneurysm is present and surgical correction is not thought justifiable.

Whilst most strokes are of sudden onset and the deficit reaches a maximum in a very short time, they may occasionally occur in a stuttering fashion—a 'stroke in evolution'. Anticoagulants have been advocated for the stuttering or progressive stroke in evolution to prevent further deterioration, even if there is no embolic source (Millikan and McDowell, 1981; Gautier, 1985). This should be considered only if a CT scan is performed to exclude haemorrhage. Cerebrospinal fluid (CSF) examination is not adequate. Short-term anticoagulants may be given for about 3 months to prevent further propagation of the thrombus.

As already mentioned, there is no place for surgery in the management of acute stroke unless there is cerebellar haemorrhage, in which case there is good evidence that decomposition and evacuation of the haematoma may be followed by a dramatic recovery (Heros, 1982). Even if carotid stenosis is known to be present, emergency endarterectomy is not indicated in a stuttering or completed stroke, as risks of surgery are much higher in this situation.

LONG-TERM MANAGEMENT: PROGNOSIS AND REHABILITATION

The level of consciousness is the most important initial prognostic sign. Ninety per cent of those in coma die within a few weeks of admission, compared to only 30% if the patient is alert. Approximately 60% of all those who recover become functionally independent, although many of these will still have a persistent neurological deficit. The prognosis is worst in those with urinary incontinence, complete hemiplegia with severe joint position sense loss, with severe neglect of one side, a gaze palsy or difficulty sitting unaided (Oxbury *et al.*, 1975; Prescott *et al.*, 1982). Most recovery occurs within the first 3 months, although some further slight improvement can occur up to 6–12 months (Wade *et al.*, 1983).

Physiotherapy, occupational therapy and speech therapy are aimed at ensuring that the maximum functional benefit is derived from reversal of deficit or from the use of the remaining intact nervous system. It is clear that, in addition, simple practical advice and a positive, but realistic, attitude on the part of the clinical team and family, will help the patient to come to terms with his disability and make the most of the recovery that has occurred. The role of remedial therapy in the management of stroke patients is discussed in Section 4.

The role of the specialist stroke units has also been much debated (Wade *et al.*, 1985; Norris and Hachinski, 1986). In the majority of cases, they at least ensure a more positive attitude to the management of stroke and make it easier for the various members of the medical and paramedical staff to work together within a coherent framework. Wade *et al.* argued that the quality of the 'human services' and their organization are at least as important as and possibly more important than the 'physical facilities'. With appropriate commitment, this could probably be achieved by concentrating stroke patients on a general medical ward, provided that there is good liaison between nurses, therapists, medical staff and others involved in the patient's care and that a positive but realistic attitude is adopted to the stroke patient.

Advice and treatment regarding any of the risk factors discussed above is required. We have already dealt with the question of treating hypertension in the acute stage following stroke. In the long term, when autoregulation at least partly returns following a stroke, most clinical trials have suggested that the prognosis is improved by appropriate treatment of blood pressure (Johnston *et al.*, 1981). It is prudent to aim for diastolic pressures of around 100 mmHg.

There is insufficient space to do justice to the recent work that has been carried out, by the European Working Party on high blood pressure in the elderly, into the primary prevention of stroke by means of treating mild to moderate hypertension

(Editorial, 1985; Amery *et al.*, 1985). Nevertheless, it is worth noting that the treatment of blood pressure reduced mortality from both cardiac and cerebrovascular causes. There was also reduction in non-fatal cerebrovascular events. Unfortunately, however, overall mortality was not reduced. The level of blood pressure treated in the European study (Amery *et al.*, 1985) was between 90 and 119 mmHg diastolic. Moreover, at least two of the drugs used in the study, triamterene and methyldopa, would not now be used in first line treatment of hypertension.

Long-term follow-up suggests that the risk of a further stroke is smaller than that of death from myocardial infarction (Sacco *et al.*, 1982). This underlines the diffuse nature of vascular disease and the importance of considering risk factors for cardiac and cerebrovascular disease together. It may be as important to treat angina in a stroke patient as it is to deal directly with cerebrovascular problems.

TRANSIENT ISCHAEMIC ATTACKS AND STROKES WITH RECOVERY

Medical Treatment

Following a TIA or complete recovery from a stroke, full investigation needs to be considered. The risk of a further permanent stoke is approximately 5–10% per annum (Brust, 1977). Advice and treatment to correct any risk factors has already been described earlier. Hypertension is far and away the most important risk factor for both cerebral haemorrhage and infarction. Blood pressures in excess of 100 mmHg diastolic should be treated, although it is probably the systolic pressure which is a better prognostic guide to the risk of further stroke. Unfortunately this is much more liable to fluctuate and more difficult to control than the diastolic pressure. It is important to lower blood pressure slowly as the autoregulatory range is higher in hypertension (see Figure 8.6). With treatment the autoregulatory curve probably reverts towards normal (Vorstrup *et al.*, 1984). It is perfectly adequate to lower blood pressure gradually over a period of days to weeks. The patient should be advised to give up smoking. Diabetes should be brought under control. A raised haematocrit (greater than 50) should be lowered by venesection to under 50. If there is a bad family history of cerebrovascular and cardiovascular disease with a marked hyperlipidaemia then dietary advice should also be given. This is not of proven value in cerebrovascular disease; however, there is good evidence that cholesterol is a risk factor for cardiac disease from which the majority of these patients will die.

In the majority of patients with TIAs, surgery is unlikely to be appropriate (see below). The only treatment is medical and the decision lies between whether to use antiplatelet therapy or anticoagulant drugs. There is good evidence that antiplatelet agents are useful in the prevention of stroke. The largest trials (Fields *et al.*, 1977; Canadian Cooperative Study Group, 1978; Bousser *et al.*, 1983; The UK TIA Study Group, 1988; Antiplatelet Trialists' Collaboration, 1988) suggest that aspirin is useful in the prevention of stroke and myocardial infarction after TIA and probably in the prevention of stroke after an initial stroke. The dose of aspirin in most studies has varied between 1300 and 300 mg a day. There is much experimental evidence to suggest that lower doses of aspirin (approximately 60 mg a day), may be equally or more effective (Masotti *et al.*, 1979). One of the ways in which aspirin is thought to act is on prostaglandin synthesis. Prostacyclin (epoprostenol, PGI_2) is produced in the vessel wall and causes vasodilatation and platelet disaggregation—the effects therapy is designed to achieve. Platelets also produce thromboxane A_2 (TXA_2), again a prostaglandin; this causes vasoconstriction and platelet aggregation. High dose aspirin probably blocks both thromboxane A_2 and prostacyclin production. Low dose aspirin, on the other hand, may block thromboxane A_2 synthesis without affecting prostacyclin synthesis. Clearly this is the ideal aim of therapy and it is for this reason that the low dose aspirin has been suggested. Unfortunately, as yet, results are not available from sufficiently large clinical studies to support this. The UK TIA Study (1988) has treated patients with either 1200 mg of aspirin a day, 300 mg of aspirin a day, or placebo. Unfortunately there is no very low dose arm to this trial because it was planned so long ago. The study has shown that 300 mg a day is as effective as 1200 mg.

The value of dipyridamole (Persantin) and sulphinpyrazone (Anturan) is doubtful. There is considerable experimental evidence of their antiplatelet effects, but no convincing proof of their clinical value. The Canadian Cooperative Study Group (1978) found no evidence that sulphinpyrazone was of any value. Bousser and her colleagues in France (1983) also failed to demonstrate that dipyridamole (Persantin) was of any use in patients with TIAs or stroke with recovery. The practice of putting patients routinely on aspirin and Persantin rather than aspirin alone is therefore to be discouraged. There has been only one study showing that Persantin might be of any value and this was in patients with prosthetic heart valves who were already on anticoagulants (Sullivan *et al.*, 1968).

My own practice is to use one adult aspirin (300 mg a day). If there is any past history of indigestion or ulcer or some other contraindication to aspirin then I usually advise the patient to take either 75–150 mg soluble aspirin with a meal or an enteric coated preparation. Very few patients are unable to take low dose aspirin in this way. Sometimes anti-ulcer therapy may be necessary in addition to aspirin. Dipyridamole is reserved for those in whom aspirin cannot be tolerated even in this way, or in whom TIAs continue despite aspirin therapy.

The role of anticoagulants in the management of TIAs without any cardiac source of emboli is controversial (Brust, 1977). There have been no satisfactory trials. The numbers in all published studies are much too small to furnish useful results. If antiplatelet therapy fails to control TIAs, anticoagulants are often considered. However, there is no doubt they are associated with an increased risk of cerebral haemorrhage. As the risk of stroke after a TIA is highest in the first 6 months, anticoagulants are rarely given long term except in those with cardiac emboli.

Long-term anticoagulants are reserved mainly for patients with cardiac emboli due to rheumatic heart disease, with or without atrial fibrillation (Easton and Sherman, 1980). Occasionally heart valve replacement may be necessary where a persistent source of emboli cannot be controlled by anticoagulant and antiplatelet therapy. The place of long-term anticoagulants in those with lone atrial fibrillation is unclear. There have unfortunately been no satisfactory trials in this situation. Some clinicians use the antiplatelet agents, others short-term anticoagulation and yet others long-term anti-coagulation. In patients with mild valvular abnor-malities such as mitral valve prolapse there is also controversy about the risk of cardiac emboli and anticoagulants are not usually given.

Surgical treatment

Internal carotid endarterectomy

Approximately 25% of TIAs in the carotid territory will arise from an operable stenosis at the origin of the internal carotid artery (Harrison and Marshall, 1975; Humphrey and Marshall, 1981). The 5 year risk of a completed stroke after carotid TIAs is approximately 30%. The first reconstruction of the internal carotid artery was performed by Eastcott and colleagues in 1954. Since then the role of endarterectomy to remove a carotid stenosis or atheromatous plaque has become widely accepted. Thompson and Talkington (1976) quoted an opera-tive morbidity and mortality less than 2% for this operation. There have been many similar series. The only controlled study from Fields *et al.* (1970) is difficult to interpret but was used to support the concept that surgery was better than medical treat-ment. Unfortunately not all series produced such good figures. Easton and Sherman (1977) published an operative morbidity and mortality in excess of 20%. Although the same group has since reported considerably better figures, there are now several studies confirming a significant morbidity and mor-tality in many centres. Browse and Ross Russell (1984) have recently reported a morbidity and mortality of around 1% from St Thomas's Hospital, where there is a particular interest in vascular surgery.

In this country, doubts about endarterectomy persist and because of this a multicentre trial was started several years ago. This started in the UK, although there are now many European centres taking part. The study has now recruited approxi-mately 1000 patients, randomized into medical or surgical treatment and then followed up on a regular basis. The results will probably not be available for several years, but as it is the largest randomized study, they will be awaited with interest.

Carotid endarterectomy should be performed only by those who do the operation frequently and have an overall mortality and morbidity of less than 5% for angiography and surgery combined. It is not an operation for the amateur. The biological age of the patient is more important than the chronological age. Provided there is no evidence of widespread vascular disease, it is reasonable to continue to perform endarterectomies on patients up to their early 70s.

The risks of endarterectomy following a stroke are greater than after a TIA even if there has been full recovery (Harrison, 1982). The risks are also greater if there is a contralateral carotid occlusion or stenosis. If there is a non-stenotic ulcerating plaque, it is best to treat these patients medically at first and consider surgery only if the attacks continue despite adequate medical treatment.

The complications of endarterectomy may be due to local vascular problems such as mural thrombosis after the endarterectomy, cessation of blood flow during the operation or embolization at the time of surgery. Other local complications include damage to the hypoglossal curve, the recurrent laryngeal nerve, sympathetic fibres in the carotid sheath, the glossopharyngeal and facial nerves as well as sensory loss to the skin in the neck and around the ear (Dehn and Taylor, 1983). The majority of these local complications are transient and recover in less than 12 months.

Extracranial and intracranial anastomosis

Over the last decade much interest has focused on surgical methods of improving blood flow after a stroke. Many patients have undergone anastomosis operations to divert blood from the extracranial vessels, such as the superficial artery, to the intra-cranial vessels, such as the middle cerebral artery. This is the most widely performed anastomosis and is technically an easy operation. In the USA it has become particularly common but it has also been carried out in many centres in this country.

The indications for such operations were considered to be the following (Marshall, 1982):

(1) Internal carotid occlusion with continuing symptoms or cerebrovascular events.
(2) Intracranial carotid stenosis with continuing TIAs.
(3) Middle cerebral artery stenosis or occlusion.

Barnett has recently reported the result of his International Cooperative Study (The EC–IC Bypass Study Group, 1985). This has demonstrated that in the groups outlined above, there was no benefit from EC–IC anastomosis in a total of 1377 patients. At present, therefore, there seems no indication for this operation to be performed at all.

It is also now clear from ultrasonography and Doppler flow studies that most patients have done their own EC–IC anastomosis after a carotid occlusion (Trockel *et al.*, 1984), flow in the supra-orbital and supratrochlear vessels, which are branches of the superficial temporal artery around the eye, being reversed. This reversal of flow means that blood is now being shunted from the external carotid artery in through the ophthalmic artery to the circle of Willis. This is occasionally seen at angiography following an internal carotid occlusion. However, with Doppler ultrasonography it is observed almost universally. The circle of Willis and the cerebral hemisphere is thus now being supplied from branches of the external carotid artery. There are many other external/internal anastomotic channels which can open up following intracranial artery occlusion and it seems unlikely on these grounds that 'therapeutic' anastomosis will add benefit. An EC–IC anastomosis remains an operation looking for an indication.

ASYMPTOMATIC BRUITS

In the USA prophylactic endarterectomy for asymptomatic internal carotid stenosis has been widely performed. Asymptomatic bruits occur in 7% of subjects over 65. However, the long-term studies suggest that the risk of stroke in such patients is in fact quite small (approximately 4% per annum). Furthermore, of the strokes that occurred only half were in the territory of the bruit. It is likely, therefore, that asymptomatic bruit is merely an indicator of vascular disease rather than a risk factor operative in a particular arterial territory (Wolf *et al.*, 1981). There seems no indication for surgery for asymptomatic carotid stenosis.

MULTI-INFARCT DEMENTIA (see also Chapter 27)

Multi-infarct dementia is commonly associated with hypertension and multiple small deep infarcts. There is often a history of stepwise progression although at times deterioration may be gradual. This used to be thought the commonest cause of dementia, but CT scanning has shown that most dementias are due to primary degenerative disease such as Alzheimer's disease and not to multiple infarcts. The presentation of multi-infarct dementia depends on the areas of the brain involved. There may be a history and signs of a pseudobulbar palsy with focal neurological disturbance or dysarthria, dysphasia or dyspraxia. Frontal lobe involvement may give rise to incontinence and a slow shuffling gait (marche à petits pas), which accompanies the intellectual deterioration. Unfortunately, there is no specific treatment for multi-infarct dementia other than dealing with the risk factors described already under the treatment of TIAs. Often vascular disease and primary degenerative dementia coexist. Unless there is a history of small discrete stroke-like episodes in the past or CT scanning shows multiple infarcts, the majority of these patients will in fact turn out to have a primary Alzheimer type of degenerative dementia rather than a multi-infarct dementia (Brust, 1983).

It may be difficult to distinguish multi-infarct dementia from normal pressure hydrocephalus, especially if there is no clear history of preceding 'strokes'. Normal pressure hydrocephalus presents with the clinical triad of dementia, a gait disorder similar to an apraxia and urgency with urinary incontinence. It may follow many years after subarachnoid haemorrhage, meningitis or head injury. It is important because it is one of the few treatable causes of dementia and may respond to shunting which relieves the hydrocephalus (Adams *et al.*, 1965; Milne Anderson, 1986). CT scanning and, if necessary, CSF pressure monitoring may help to distinguish these two conditions.

A rare form of dementia due to white matter disease may also be seen in hypertensive or arteriosclerotic patients (Loizou *et al.*, 1981). This is known as Binswanger's disease (subcortical arteriosclerotic encephalopathy) and presents with dementia, pyramidal, extrapyramidal and cerebellar signs. The onset may be stuttering. The CT scan shows extensive subcortical white matter with low attenuation rather than discrete infarcts. There is no specific treatment.

REFERENCES

Adams, R.D., Fisher, C.M., Harim, S., Ojemann, R.G., and Sweet, W.H. (1965). Symptomatic occult hydrocephalus with "normal" cerebrospinal-fluid pressure: A treatable syndrome. *N. Engl. J. Med.*, **273**, 117–26.

Aho, K., Harmsen, P., Hatano, S., Marquardsen, J., Smirnov, V.E., and Strasser, T. (1980). Cerebrovascular disease in the community. Results of a WHO collaborative study. *Bull. WHO*, **58**, 113–30.

Allen, C.M.C. (1983). Clinical diagnosis of the acute stroke syndrome, *Q. J. Med.*, **52**, 515–23.

Amery, A., Birkenhager, W., Brixko, P., Bulpitt, C., Clement, D., Deruyttere, M., De Shaepdryver, A., Dollery, C., Fagard, R., Forette, F., Forte, J., Hamdy, R., Henry, J.F., Joossens, J.V., Leonett, G., Lund-Johansen, P., O'Malley, K., Petrie, J., Strasser, T., Tuomilehto, J., and Williams, B. (1985). Mortality and morbidity results from the European Working Party on High Blood Pressure in the Elderly Trial. *Lancet*, **i**, 1349–54.

Antiplatelet Trialists' Collaboration (1988). Secondary prevention of vascular disease by prolonged antiplatelet agent. *Br. Med. J.*, **i**, 320–31.

Asinger, R.W., Mikell, F.L., Sharma, B., and Hodges, M. (1981). Observations on detecting left ventricular thrombus with two-dimensional echocardiography. *Am. J. Cardiol.*, **47**, 145–56.

Bartleson, J.D. (1984). Transient and persistent neurological manifestations of migraine. *Stroke*, **15**, 383–6.

Bayer, A.J., Pathy, M.S.J., and Newcombe, R. (1987). Double-blind randomised trial of intravenous glycerol in acute stroke. *Lancet*, **i**, 405–9.

Bean, W.B. (1938). Infarction of heart III: Clinical course and morphological findings. *Ann. Intern. Med.*, **12**, 71–94.

Blackwood, W., Hallpike, J.F., Kocen, R.S., and Mair, W.G.P. (1969). Atheromatous disease of the carotid arterial system and embolism from the heart in cerebral infarction: A morbid anatomical study. *Brain*, **92**, 897–910.

Bonita, R., Scragg, R., Stewart, A., Jackson, R., and

Beaglehole, R. (1986). Cigarette smoking and risk of premature stroke in men and women. *Br. Med. J.*, **293**, 6–8.

Bousser, M.G., Eschwege, E., Haguenau, M., Lefaucconier, J.M., Thibult, N., and Touboul, P.J. (1983). 'AICLA' controlled trial of aspirin and dipyridamole in the secondary prevention of athero-thrombotic cerebral ischaemia. *Stroke*, **14**, 5–14.

Branston, N.M., Strong, A.J., and Symon, L. (1977). Extracellular potassium activity, evoked potential and tissue blood flow. *J. Neurol. Sci.*, **32**, 305–21.

Brice, J.G., Dowsett, D.J., and Lowe, R.D. (1964). Haemodynamic effects of carotid artery stenosis. *Br. Med. J.*, **ii**, 1363–6.

Browse, N.L., and Ross Russell, R. (1984). Carotid endarterectomy and the Javid shunt: The early results of 215 consecutive operations for transient ischaemic attacks. *Br. J. Surg.*, **71**, 53–7.

Brust, J.C.M. (1977). Transient ischaemic attacks: natural history and anticoagulation. *Neurology*, **27**, 701–7.

Brust, J.C.M. (1983). Vascular dementia—still overdiagnosed. *Stroke*, **14**, 298–300.

Canadian Cooperative Study Group. (1978). A randomised trial of aspirin and sulfinpyrazone in threatened stroke. *N. Engl. J. Med.*, **299**, 53–9.

Caplan, L.R. (1981). Vertebrobasilar disease. *Stroke*, **12**, 111–14.

Carter, A.B. (1957). The immediate treatment of cerebral embolism. *Q. J. Med.*, **50**, 335–48.

Cove, D.H., Seddon, M., Fletcher, R.F., and Duke, D.C. (1979). Blindness after treatment for malignant hypertension. *Br. Med. J.*, **ii**, 245–6.

de Bono, D.P. (1983). Cardiac causes of stroke. In: Ross Russell, R.W. (ed.) *Cerebral Arterial Disease*, Churchill Livingstone, Edinburgh, pp. 324–36.

Dehn, T.C.B., and Taylor, G.W. (1983). Local neurological complications following carotid endarterectomy. In: Greenhalgh, R.M., and Clifford Rose, F. (eds.) *Progress in Stroke Research 2*, Pitman, London, pp. 484–91.

Dinsdale, H.B. (1982). Hypertensive encephalopathy. *Stroke*, **13**, 717–19.

Eastcott, H.H.G., Pickering, G.W., and Rob, C. (1954). Reconstruction of internal carotid artery in a patient with intermittent attacks of hemiplegia. *Lancet*, **ii**, 994–6.

Easton, J.D., and Sherman, D.G. (1977). Stroke and mortality rate in carotid endarterectomy: 228 consecutive operations. *Stroke*, **8**, 565–8.

Easton, J.D., and Sherman, D.G. (1980). Management of cerebral embolism of cardiac origin. *Stroke*, **11**, 433–42.

Editorial. (1985). Treatment of hypertension: The 1985 results. *Lancet*, **ii**, 645–7.

Faris, A.A., and Poser, C.M. (1964). Experimental production of focal neurological deficit by systemic hyponatraemia. *Neurology (Minneapolis)*, **14**, 206–11.

Fields, W.S., Maslenikov, V., Meyer, J.S., Haas, W.K.,

Remington, R.D., and Macdonald, M.C. (1970). Joint study of extracranial arterial occlusion. V. Progress report of prognosis following surgery or non-surgical treatment for transient cerebral ischaemic attacks and cervical carotid artery lesions. *J.A.M.A.*, **211**, 1993–2003.

Fields, W.S., and Lemak, N.A. (1972). Subclavian steal—a review of 168 cases. *J.A.M.A.*, **222**, 1139–43.

Fields, W.S., Lemak, N.A., Frankowski, R.F., and Hardy, R.J. (1977). Controlled trial of aspirin in cerebral ischaemia. *Stroke*, **8**, 301–14.

Fieschi, C., Agnoli, A., Battistini, N., and Bossao, L. (1966). Regional cerebral blood flow in patients with brain infarcts. *Arch. Neurol.*, **15**, 653–63.

Fisher, C.M. (1959). Observations of the fundus oculi in transient monocular blindness. *Neurology (Minneapolis)*, **9**, 333–47.

Fisher, C.M. (1976). In: Scheinberg, P. (ed.) *Cerebrovascular disease—Tenth Princeton Conference*, Raven Press, New York, pp. 50–3.

Fisher, C.M. (1982). Lacunar strokes and infarcts: A review. *Neurology*, **32**, 871–6.

Frithz, G., and Werner, I. (1975). The effect of glycerol infusion in acute cerebral infarction. *Acta Med. Scand.*, **198**, 287–9.

Furlan, A.J., Cavalier, S.J., Hobbs, R.E., Weinsten, M.A., and Modic, M.T. (1982). Haemorrhage and anticoagulation after non-septic embolic brain infarction. *Neurology*, **32**, 280–2.

Gautier, J.C. (1985). Stroke-in-progression. *Stroke*, **16**, 729–33.

Gautier, J.C., and Morelot, D. (1975). Infarctus cerebraux. *Nouv. Presse Med.*, **4**, 2575–80.

Gibbs, J.M., Wise, R.J.S., Leenders, K.L., and Jones, T. (1984). Evaluation of cerebral perfusion reserve in patients with carotid artery occlusion. *Lancet*, **i**, 182–6.

Ginsberg, M.D., and Cebul, R.D. (1983). Non-invasive diagnosis of carotid artery disease. In: Harrison, M.J.G., and Dyken, M.L. (eds.) *Cerebral Vascular Disease*, Butterworths International Medical Reviews, London, Vol. 3, 215–53.

Groch, S., McDevitt, E., and Wright, I.S. (1961). A long term study of cerebral vascular disease. *Ann. Intern. Med.*, **55**, 358–67.

Habermann, S., Capildeo, R., and Clifford-Rose, F. (1982). Diverging trends in cerebrovascular disease and ischaemic heart diseases mortality. *Stroke*, **13**, 582–9.

Hachinski, V. (1984). Decreased incidence and mortality of stroke. *Stroke*, **15**, 376–8.

Harrison, M.J.G. (1982). Carotid endarterectomy. In: Rice Edwards, J.M. (ed.) *Topical Reviews in Neurosurgery*, Vol. 1, John Wright P.S.G., Bristol, pp. 57–80.

Harrison, M.J.G., and Marshall, J. (1975). Indications for angiography and surgery in carotid artery disease. *Br. Med. J.*, **i**, 616–18.

Harrison, M.J.G., and Marshall, J. (1976). Angiographic appearance of carotid bifurcation in patients with completed stroke, transient ischaemic attacks and cerebral tumour. *Br. Med. J.*, **i**, 205–7.

Harrison, M.J.G., and Marshall, J. (1977). The findings of thrombus at carotid endarterectomy and its relationship to the timing of surgery. *Br. J. Surg.*, **64**, 511–12.

Harrison, M.J.G., and Ross Russell, R.W. (1983). Medical treatment. In: Harrison, M.J.G., and Dyken, M.L. (eds.) *Cerebral Vascular Disease*, Butterworths, International Medical Reviews, London, Vol. 3, 254–83.

Hawkes, C.H. (1974). 'Locked-In' syndrome: Report of 7 cases. *Br. Med. J.*, **iv**, 379–82.

Hennerici, M., Aulich, A., Sandmann, W., and Freund, H.J. (1981). Incidence of asymptomatic extracranial arterial disease. *Stroke*, **12**, 750–8.

Heros, R.C. (1982). Cerebellar haemorrhage and infarction. *Stroke*, **13**, 106–9.

Humphrey, P.R.D., and Bradbury, P.G. (1984). Continuous wave Doppler ultrasonography in the detection of carotid stenosis and occlusion. *J. Neurol. Neurosurg. Psychiatry*, **47**, 1128–30.

Humphrey, P.R.D., and Harrison, M.J.G. (1985). How often can an embolic stroke be diagnosed clinically?: A clinicopathological correlation. *Postgrad. Med. J.*, **61**, 1039–42.

Humphrey, P.R.D., and Marshall, J. (1981). Transient ischaemic attacks and strokes with recovery: Prognosis and investigation. *Stroke*, **12**, 765–9.

Italian Acute Stroke Study Group (1988). Haemodilution in acute stroke. Results of the Italian Haemodilution Trial. *Lancet*, **i**, 318–21.

Johnston, J.H., Beevers, D.G., Dunn, P.G., Larkin, H., and Titterington, D.M. (1981). The importance of good blood pressure control in the prevention of stroke recurrence in hypertensive patients. *Postgrad. Med. J.*, **57**, 690–3.

Kannel, W.B., and Wolf, P.A. (1983). Epidemiology of cerebrovascular disease. In: Ross Russell, R.W. (ed.) *Vascular Disease of the Central Nervous System*, Churchill Livingstone, Edinburgh, pp. 1–24.

Kendall, B.E., and Marshall, J. (1963). Role of hypotension in the genesis of transient focal cerebral ischaemic attacks. *Br. Med. J.* **ii**, 344–8.

Kety, S.S., and Schmidt, C.F. (1948). The nitrous oxide method for the quantitative determination of cerebral blood flow in man. *J. Clin. Invest.*, **27**, 484–92.

Koller, R.L. (1982). Recurrent embolic cerebral infarction and anticoagulation. *Neurology*, **32**, 283–5.

Kumar, G.K., Lastoor, F.C., Robago, J.R., and Rassaque, M.A. (1976). Side effects of diazoxide. *J.A.M.A.*, **235**, 275–6.

Kurtzke, J.F. (1976). An introduction to the epidemiology of cerebrovascular disease. In: Scheinberg, P. (ed.) *Cerebrovascular Disease—Tenth Princeton Conference*, Raven Press, New York, p. 239.

Lassen, N.A. (1959). Cerebral blood flow and oxygen consumption in man. *Physiol. Rev.*, **36**, 183–238.

Lassen, N.A. (1966). The luxury perfusion syndrome and its possible relation to acute metabolic acidosis localized within the brain. *Lancet*, **ii**, 1113–15.

Ledingham, J.G.G., and Rajagopalan, B. (1979). Cerebral complications in the treatment of accelerated hypertension. *Q. J. Med.*, **48**, 25–41.

Little, J.R., Furlan, A.J., Modic, M.T., and Weinstein, M.A. (1982). Digital subtraction angiography by cerebrovascular disease. *Stroke*, **13**, 557–66.

Loeb, C. (1979). In: Goldstein, M.L., Bolis, L., Fieschi, C., Gorini, S., and Millikan, C.H. (eds.) *Advances in Neurology*, Vol. 25, Raven Press, New York, pp. 141–8.

Loizou, L., Kendall, B.E., and Marshall, J. (1981). Subcortical arteriosclerotic encephalopathy: A clinical and radiological investigation. *J. Neurol. Neurosurg. Psychiatry*, **44**, 294–304.

Longo, D.L., and Witherspoon, J.M. (1980). Focal neurological symptoms in hypercalcaemia. *Neurology (Minneapolis)*, **30**, 200–1.

Luxon, L.M., and Harrison, M.J.G. (1979). Chronic subdural haematoma. *Q. J. Med.*, **48**, 43–53.

McDonald, W.I. (1967). Recurrent cholesterol embolism as a cause of fluctuating cerebral symptoms. *J. Neurol. Neurosurg. Psychiatry*, **30**, 489–95.

Marshall, J. (1982). Indications for extracranial-intracranial anastomosis. In: Rice Edwards, J.M. (ed.) *Topical Reviews in Neurosurgery*, Vol. 1, John Wright/P.G.S., Bristol, pp. 81–92.

Masotti, G., Galanti, G., Poggesi, L., Abbate, R., and Neri Serneri, G.G. (1979). Differential inhibition of prostacyclin production and platelet aggregation by aspirin. *Lancet*, **ii**, 1213–16.

Matthews, W.B., Oxbury, J.M., Grainger, K.M.R., and Greenhall, R.C.D. (1976). A blind controlled trial of dextran 40 in the treatment of ischaemic stroke. *Brain*, **99**, 193–206.

Meyer, J.S., and Portnoy, H.S. (1958). Localised cerebral hypoglycaemia simulating stroke. *Neurology (Minneapolis)*, **8**, 601–14.

Millikan, C.H., and McDowell, F.H. (1981). Treatment of progressing stroke. *Stroke*, **12**, 397–409.

Milne Anderson, J. (1986). Normal pressure hydrocephalus. *Br. Med. J.*, **293**, 837–8.

Mohr, J.P. (1978). Transient ischaemic attacks and the prevention of stroke. *N. Engl. J. Med.*, **299**, 93–5.

Mulley, G., Wilcox, R.G., and Mitchell, J.R.A. (1978). Dexamethasone in acute stroke. *Br. Med. J.*, **ii**, 994–6.

Nelson, R.F., Pullicino, P., Kendall, B.E., and Marshall, J. (1980). Computed tomography in patients presenting with lacunar syndrome. *Stroke*, **11**, 256–61.

Nicholls, E., and Johnansen, H. (1983). Implications of changing trends in cerebrovascular and cardiovascular disease mortality. *Stroke*, **14**, 153–6.

Norris, J.W., and Hachinski, V.C. (1982). Misdiagnosis of stroke. *Lancet*, **1**, 328–31.

Norris, J.W., and Hachinski, V.C. (1986). Stroke units of stroke centres 1986. *Stroke*, **17**, 360–2.

Oakley, C.M. (1984). Mitral valve prolapse: harbinger of death or variant of normal? *Br. Med. J.*, **i**, 1853–4.

O'Brien, M.D. (1979). Ischaemic cerebral oedema. *Stroke*, **10**, 623–8.

Oxbury, J.M., Greenhall, R.C.D., and Grainger, K.M.R. (1975). Predicting the outcome of stroke: acute stage after cerebral infarction. *Br. Med. J.*, **ii**, 125–7.

Oxfordshire Community Stroke Project (1983). Incidence of stroke in Oxfordshire: first year's experience of a Community Stroke Register. *Br. Med. J.*, **ii**, 713–16.

Pantin, C.F.A., and Young, R.A.L. (1980). Post prandial blindness. *Br. Med. J.*, **ii**, 1686.

Paulson, C.B. (1970). Regional cerebral blood flow in apoplexy due to occlusion of the middle cerebral artery. *Neurology*, **20**, 63–77.

Payne, E.E., and Spillane, J.D. (1957). The cervical spine. An anatomico-pathological study of 70 specimens with particular reference to the problem of cervical spondylosis. *Brain*, **80**, 571–96.

Ports, T.A., Cogan, J., Schiller, N.B., and Rapaport, E. (1978). Echocardiography of left ventricular masses. *Circulation*, **58**, 528–36.

Prescott, R.J., Garraway, W.M., and Akhtar, A.J. (1982). Predicting functional outcome following acute stroke using a standard clinical examination. *Stroke*, **13**, 641–7.

Rees, J.E., du Boulay, G.H., Bull, J.W.D., Marshall, J., Ross Russell, R.W., and Symon, L. (1970). Regional cerebral blood flow in transient attacks. *Lancet*, **ii**, 1210–13.

Robertson, W.B., and Strong, J.P. (1968). Atherosclerosis in persons with hypertension and diabetes mellitus. *Lab. Invest.*, **18**, 538–51.

Ross, R.T. (1983). Transient tumour attacks. *Arch. Neurol.*, **40**, 633–6.

Ross Russell, R.W. (1963). Observations on intracerebral aneurysms. *Brain*, **86**, 425–42.

Ross Russell, R.W. (1968). The source of retinal emboli. *Lancet*, **ii**, 789–92.

Ross Russell, R.W., and Bharucha, N. (1978). The recognition and prevention of border zone cerebral ischaemia during cardiac surgery. *Q. J. Med.*, **47**, 303–23.

Ross Russell, R.W., and Page, N.G.R. (1983). Critical perfusion of brain and retina. *Brain*, **106**, 419–34.

Sacco, R.L., Wolf, P.A., Kannel, W.B., and McNamara, P. (1982). Survival and recurrence following stroke: the Framingham study. *Stroke*, **13**, 290–5.

Sandercock, P., Molyneux, A., and Warlow, C. (1985). Value of computed tomography in patients with stroke. Oxford Community Stroke Project. *Br. Med. J.*, **290**, 193–7.

Sheehan, S., Bauer, R.B., and Meyer, J.S. (1960). Vertebral artery compression in cervical spondylosis. *Neurology (Minneapolis)*, **10**, 968–86.

Stark, R.J., and Wodak, J. (1983). Primary orthostatic cerebral ischaemia. *J. Neurol. Neurosurg. Psychiatry*, **46**, 883–91.

Steel, J.G., Thomas, H.A., and Strollo, P.J. (1982). Fusiform basilar aneurysm as a cause of embolic stroke. *Stroke*, **13**, 712–16.

Steiner, T.J., McIvor, J., Perkin, G.D., Greenhalgh, R.M., and Rose, F.C. (1983). Morbidity of arch and carotid angiography: prospective survey. In: Greenhalgh, R.M., and Rose, F.C. (eds.) *Progress in Stroke Research 2*, Pitman, London, pp. 136–53.

Strandgaard, S., Olesen, J., Skinhoj, E., and Lassen, N.A. (1973). Autoregulation of brain circulation in severe arterial hypertension. *Br. Med. J.*, **i**, 507–10.

Sullivan, J.M., Harken, O.E., and Gorlin, R. (1968). Pharmacologic control of thrombo-embolic complications of cardiac valve replacement: a preliminary report. *N. Engl. J. Med.*, **279**, 576–80.

Symon, L., Branston, N.M., and Strong, A.J. (1976). Autoregulation in acute focal ischaemia. *Stroke*, **7**, 547–54.

Symon, L., Crockard, H.A., Dorsch, N.W.C., Branston, N.M., and Juhasz, J. (1975). Local cerebral blood flow and vascular reactivity in a chronic stable stroke in baboons. *Stroke*, **6**, 482–92.

The EC–IC Bypass Study Group. (1985). Failure of extracranial/intracranial arterial bypass to reduce the risk of ischaemic stroke. The results of an international randomised trial, 1985. *N. Engl. J. Med.*, **313**, 1191–1200.

Thompson, J.E., and Talkington, C.M. (1976). Carotid endarterectomy. *Ann. Surg.*, **184**, 1–15.

Torvik, A. (1984). The pathogenesis of watershed infarcts in the brain. *Stroke*, **15**, 221–3.

Torvik, A., and Jorgensen, L. (1964). Thrombotic and embolic occlusions of the carotid arteries in an autopsy material. *J. Neurol. Sci.*, **1**, 24–39.

Trockel, U., Hennerici, M., Aulich, A., and Sandmann, W. (1984). The superiority of combined continuous wave Doppler examination over periorbital Doppler for the detection of extracranial carotid disease. *J. Neurol. Neurosurg. Psychiatry*, **47**, 43–50.

UK TIA Study Group (1983). Variation in the use of angiography and carotid endarterectomy by neurologists in the U.K.–T.I.A. aspirin trial. *Br. Med. J.*, **i**, 514–17.

UK TIA Study Group (1988). United Kingdom transient ischaemic attack (UK TIA) aspirin trial: interim results. *Br. Med. J.*, **i**, 316–20.

Van der Drift, J.H.A., and Kok, N.K.D. (1972). In: Meyer, J.S., Lechner, H., Reivich, M., and Eichorn, O. (eds.) *Cerebrovascular Disease*, Sixth International Conference, Salzburg (1973), Thieme, Stuttgart.

Vorstrup, S., Barry, D.I., Jarden, J.O., Svendsen, U.G., Braendstrup, O., Graham, D.I., and Strandgaard, S. (1984). Chronic antihypertensive treatment in the rat reverses hypertension-induced changes in cerebral blood flow autoregulation. *Stroke*, **15**, 312–18.

Wade, D.T., Langton Hewer, R., Wood, V.A., Skilbeck, C.E., and Ismail, H.M. (1983). The hemiplegic arm after stroke: measurement and recovery. *J. Neurol. Neurosurg. Psychiatry*, **46**, 521–4.

Wade, D.T., Langton Hewer, R., Skilbeck, C.E., and David, R.M. (1985). In: *Stroke—A Critical Approach to Diagnosis, Treatment and Management*, Chapman and Hall, London, pp. 300–22.

Waltz, A.G. (1970). Effect of $PaCO_2$ on blood flow and micro-vasculature of ischaemic and non-ischaemic cerebral cortex. *Stroke*, **1**, 27–37.

Whisnant, J.P. (1984). The decline of stroke. *Stroke*, **15**, 160–8.

Wilson, L.A., and Ross Russell, R.W. (1977). Amaurosis fugax and carotid artery disease: indications for angiography. *Br. Med. J.*, **ii**, 435–7.

Wise, R.J.S., Bernardi, S., Frackowiak, R.S.J., Legg, N.J., and Jones, T. (1983). Serial observations on the pathophysiology of acute stroke. *Brain*, **106**, 197–222.

Wolf, P.A., Kannel, W.B., Sorlie, P., and McNamara, P. (1981). Asymptomatic carotid bruit and the risk of stroke. *J.A.M.A.*, **245**, 1442–5.

Wolf, P.A., Kannel, W.B., McGee, D.L., Meeks, S.L., Bharucha, N.E., and McNamara, P.M. (1983). Duration of atrial fibrillation and imminence of stroke: the Framingham study. *Stroke*, **14**, 664–7.

Woodcock, J.P. (1981). Special ultrasonic methods for the assessment and imaging of systemic arterial disease. *Br. J. Anaesth.*, **53**, 719–73.

Yatsu, F.M., and Hart, R.G. (1983). Symptomatic carotid bruit and stenosis: a reappraisal. *Stroke*, **14**, 301–4.

The Clinical Neurology of Old Age
Edited by R. Tallis
© 1989 John Wiley & Sons Ltd

Chapter 9

Parkinson's Disease and other Parkinsonian Syndromes

Jeremy Playfer

Consultant Geriatrician, Royal Liverpool Hospital, Liverpool, UK

INTRODUCTION

Parkinson's disease is typical of many conditions treated by geriatricians. It is a disorder of movement resulting in immobility. The onset is in late life, being rare below 50 years, although the disease results from pathological processes which have started much earlier. The condition is chronic, engendering increasing disability with increasing age. Although the condition is degenerative, it can respond well to drug treatment; drug therapy, however, is complicated by age-related pharmacological changes and the presence of other disease. Parkinsonism may be induced by drugs, and side-effects to anti-Parkinson treatment are common, so that iatrogenic factors are of clinical importance. The diagnosis is exclusively clinical, and presentation may be atypical in extreme old age. Rehabilitation and the provision of social support are often important factors in the management of the individual patient.

DEFINITIONS AND CLASSIFICATION

Parkinson's disease is a chronic progressive disorder of the central nervous system characterized by three cardinal signs: bradykinesia, muscular rigidity and resting tremor. The disease itself is idiopathic, and corresponds to paralysis agitans or 'the shaking palsy', originally described by Parkinson in 1817. Symptoms resembling the disease may result from defined causes such as drugs, viral infections, or neurotoxins, in which case the term 'parkinsonism' is used. A disparate group of rare disorders have 'parkinsonism' as a central feature with additional signs of degenerative changes in the central nervous system—the so-called parkinsonism-plus syndromes. They include progressive supranuclear palsy, Shy–Drager syndrome, variants of Alzheimer and Jakob–Creutzfeld dementias, and striatonigral degeneration. The parkinsonian syndrome is a synonym for the simpler and preferable term parkinsonism. Parkinsonism can be classified only partially according to aetiology (see Table 9.1).

TABLE 9.1   CLASSIFICATION OF PARKINSON'S DISEASE

Idiopathic Parkinson's disease
Drug-induced parkinsonism
Neurotoxic parkinsonism
Parkinsonism-plus (multisystem degeneration)
Supranuclear palsy
Shy–Drager syndrome
Olivopontocerebellar degeneration
Striatonigral degeneration
Cerebrovascular associated parkinsonism

EPIDEMIOLOGY AND NATURAL HISTORY OF PARKINSONISM

For a condition which has been recognized for over 150 years, we have an incomplete picture of where the disease occurs, who it affects, and what its normal course is. In a chronic disease of insidious onset, the incidence (the number of new cases emerging in unit time) is almost impossible to determine accurately. The prevalence (the total number of cases per unit of population at a given time) is easier to determine. Comparison between different epidemiological studies is fraught with difficulty—methodology of ascertainment of cases varies, diagnostic criteria are not uniform and, the distinction between parkinsonism and Parkinson's disease is not always made. The study of Kurland and his co-workers in Rochester, Minnesota, is methodologically exact, and the records go back to 1935. A recent report of a 13 year study from 1967 to 1979 showed that there has been little change in annual incidence (Rajput *et al.*, 1984). There were no new cases under the age of 30 years, and the peak incidence was between 75 and 84 years of age. Prevalence rate was 187 per 100 000 population. Comparable surveys in the UK, Iceland and Japan give slightly lower although similar figures, ranging from 66 to 166 per 100 000 (Brewis *et al.*, 1966; Gudmundsson, 1967; Mutch, 1985; Harada, 1983). Although the age breakdown in these studies is often incomplete, the overall prevalence is less than 100 per 100 000 under the age of 60, and over 1000 per 100 000 over that age.

In England and Wales in 1982 there were 2030 deaths due to Parkinson's disease, and just over 11 000 admissions to hospital. The majority of these were among the geriatric age group (Peach and Kellar, 1984). It is estimated that there are 80 000 cases of Parkinson's disease in the UK. As many as 8% of these require institutional care.

Men are slightly more likely to develop Parkinson's disease than women, although the age-related incidence means that more women are afflicted with the disease than men. As mentioned above, there is no evidence that the incidence of Parkinson's disease is changing with time. Apparent increases in prevalence are probably due to changes in the age structure of the population, and better diagnosis,

rather than any fundamental shift in the pattern of the disease. Post-encephalitic parkinsonism, however, is now extremely rare, and survivors from the 1916 epidemic are few and far between. The disease is not socially selective, but there appears to be some inter-racial variation, the condition being less common in Negroes. The disease appears more common in advanced Western nations, but this is probably due to age structure and the greater availability of diagnostic medical services.

Parkinsonian patients are more likely to suffer from psychiatric illness, particularly depression. They tend to have low blood pressures, and it is also claimed that there is a lower incidence of malignancy in this group of patients. This is particularly true of carcinoma of the bronchus and other smoking-related diseases. It has therefore been suggested that smoking might protect against Parkinson's disease. This hypothesis was critically examined by Godwin-Austin *et al.* in 1982, and original epidemiological data were presented by Haack *et al.* in 1981. The theory remains controversial. The importance of epidemiological studies becomes very clear when the aetiology of the condition is considered, and especially when it is appreciated that environmental factors are almost certainly of prime importance in developing the disease (see below).

The natural history of Parkinson's disease has been modified by the introduction of levodopa therapy. Patients survive longer, and the increased expectation of life is demonstrated in all age groups (Kessler, 1972; Sweet and McDowell, 1975; Rinne, 1978; Birkmayer *et al.*, 1974). The standardized mortality ratio, at presentation, for patients who respond to levodopa is close to unity, indicating a normal expectation of life when compared with their peers (Zumstein and Siegfried, 1976; Shaw *et al.*, 1980). Later in the disease the mortality ratio rises and there is a considerable burden of disability; over 50% of sufferers from Parkinson's disease are considered to be moderately or severely disabled.

AETIOLOGY

Although Parkinson's disease must still be regarded as idiopathic, there are many theories as to its causation.

Viruses

Parkinsonism is a late complication of encephalitis lethargica of which the last major epidemic was in 1926. The viral agent causing this condition was never clearly characterized, and the epidemics tended to coincide with influenza epidemics. It has been suggested that the influenza virus might be a cause of Parkinson's disease (Marttila, 1980). Other viruses have been known to produce extrapyramidal syndromes (Hoehm, 1971). Marmot and others have suggested that Parkinson's disease may be a very late result of a viral infection, and have cited supporting evidence from cohort analysis (Marmot, 1981). There is, however, no corroborative evidence from immunology to support such hypotheses.

Premature Ageing

The postural changes and slowing of movement seen in Parkinson's disease often appear to be a caricature of the results of normal ageing on the central nervous system. This has led to the suggestion that Parkinson's disease could be a natural consequence of ageing of the central nervous system, some individuals being selected out by accelerated ageing in the basal ganglion. A number of the pathological changes seen in Parkinson's disease do occur with normal ageing of the nervous system, i.e. loss of neurones, the accumulation of pigments in cells, and the reduction of tyrosine-hydroxylase activity. After the age of 55 the prevalence of Parkinson's disease has an almost exponential relationship with age. The theory that Parkinson's disease is due to premature ageing has been critically appraised by Calne (1981).

Inheritance

Nearly one in five cases of Parkinson's disease report affected relatives and there often appear to be clusters of cases within families. Similar disorders of movement, such as essential tremor and olivopontocerebellar atrophy, have well-defined mendelian inheritance. The twin studies undertaken by Duvoisin and colleagues, however, have shown that the concordance rate for Parkinson's disease among identical twins is negligible, and does not signifi-cantly differ from that among fraternal twins. This study is very strong evidence that heredity plays no significant part in the aetiology of Parkinson's disease (Duvoisin, 1984).

Neurotoxins

It has long been known that chemical agents such as manganese and carbon monoxide can cause extrapyramidal effects. Neuroleptic drugs produce parkinsonism by blockading striatal dopamine receptors. Observations such as these have led to the hypothesis that Parkinson's disease is caused by as yet unidentified neurotoxins within the environment. The discovery of the neurotoxic effects of MPTP (1-methyl, 4-phenyl, 1,2,3,6-tetrahydropyridine) by Langston and others in 1983 has focused an intense research effort into the study of the aetiology of Parkinson's disease. MPTP is an analogue of pethidine used by drug-abusers and it causes a syndrome which is virtually identical to classical Parkinson's disease, responding to anti-parkinsonian therapy in a similar way to Parkinson's disease, but exhibiting a more rapid progression. Primate models have shown that the pathological changes induced by MPTP are similar to those occurring in the naturally occurring disease (Burns *et al.*, 1984). Its toxicity raises the possibility that other foreign compounds may cause similar damage, possibly acting over a longer period, and in smaller amounts. The biotransformation of MPTP suggests that it causes neuronal damage by the production of a free radical MPP^+ during its biotransformation within the neuronal cells of the basal ganglia. The idea of free radicals causing neuronal damage links neatly with some biological theories of ageing which suggest that free radical damage to biomacromolecules is an important cause of deleterious changes associated with ageing.

NEUROPATHOLOGY

The classical pathological findings in Parkinson's disease are degeneration and loss of pigmented neurones in the pars compacta of the substantia nigra, the locus coeruleus and the dorsal motor nucleus of the vagus (den Hartog Jager and Bethlem,

1960). Characteristic changes include reactive gliosis and the accumulation of melanin which may be contained in macrophages or free in the stroma. Lewy bodies are intracellular, eosinophilic inclusions found particularly in the dorsal motor nucleus of the vagus and the substantia innominata. Although these were originally thought to be pathognomonic of Parkinson's disease, they have now been described in both Alzheimer's disease and in the normal elderly brain (Okama and Ghuta, 1976).

The key observation to the understanding of Parkinson's disease was made by Ehringer and Hornykiewicz in 1960, who linked the loss of pigmented cells from the substantia nigra with depletion of the monoamine neurotransmitter dopamine. Further studies by the same team showed that the degree of depletion of dopamine correlated with the severity of the clinical features of Parkinson's disease. Dopamine had to be reduced to about one-fifth of its normal levels for any clinical manifestations to appear. The loss of dopamine is associated with loss of tyrosine hydroxylase activity, the rate limiting enzyme for dopamine synthesis and a marker of cell loss (Riederer *et al.*, 1981; Finch, 1973).

The fact that clinical features arise only when 80% of the dopamine producing capacity has been lost can be explained by two compensatory mechanisms. Firstly, when less dopamine is produced, it turns over faster, as is shown by the changing ratio between dopamine and its main metabolite, homovanillic acid (Williams, 1981). Secondly, postsynaptic dopamine receptors exhibit denervation supersensitivity, associated with an increased number of receptor sites, as demonstrated by radioligand studies (Quinn *et al.*, 1982).

Dopamine present in other areas of the brain, such as the cerebral cortex (the paraolfactory gyrus), the nucleus accumbens and the hypothalamus, shows equivalent reductions in cases of Parkinson's disease (Agid *et al.*, 1984).

Although dopamine is the principal neurotransmitter affected by Parkinson's disease, changes have been described in other neurotransmitters; for example both noradrenaline and serotonin are significantly decreased (Farley *et al.*, 1976). The cholinergic system appears to have enhanced activity in Parkinson's disease, which is consistent with the role of the dopamine pathway in inhibiting responses transmitted by acetylcholine and aspartate. Choline acetyltransferase levels are decreased in Parkinson patients with dementia (Perry *et al.*, 1983). There is decreased gamma-aminobutryic acid (GABA) synthesis and an apparent reduction in the number of GABA binding sites in the substantia nigra. GABA is known to have motor effects, but the significance of this observation is unclear. The levels of several peptide neurotransmitters, in particular methencephalin, substance P and cholecystokinin, have been shown to be decreased (McGeer *et al.*, 1984). The significance of these changes is at present ill-understood.

CLINICAL FEATURES

Classical Parkinson's Disease—The Symptoms and Signs

Tremor is the presenting feature in 70% of cases. It characteristically affects mainly the hands, producing a 'pill-rolling' movement of the fingers and thumb, accompanied by flexion and extension at the wrist. The tremor is characteristically present at rest, but may be aggravated by emotional disturbance or tiredness. It tends to disappear during sleep. In younger patients it is often unilateral, but in the older age groups it is almost invariably bilateral, and may spread to affect other parts of the body, including the head and neck. It has a slow frequency of four to eight cycles per second. Findley and his colleagues have used spectral analysis to analyse the components of the tremor and their techniques may eventually form a more objective basis for the diagnosis of Parkinson's disease (Findley *et al.*, 1981).

Muscular rigidity, one of the main causes of immobility in this condition, is due to generalized hypertonia, involving opposing muscle groups equally and throughout the range of movement. If there is no tremor, this may present as a uniform resistance to movement (leadpipe rigidity); with an established tremor, the response to passive movement is ratchet like (cogwheel rigidity). In severe cases, there is imbalance in tone, leading to the characteristically abnormal flexed posture (McLennan, 1981).

Movements are noticeably slowed in parkinsonian patients (bradykinesia) and some normally spontaneous movements are diminished or abolished (akinesia). Loss of arm swing, and lack of facial expression and blinking, are examples. Patients find it particularly difficult to initiate or stop movement. This is best seen in the gait, which typically consists of small hesitant steps, which then break into a series of rapid small steps, in order to prevent falling forward (festination). Walking is slow, with shuffling steps; the arms flexed, and adducted with little swing. The trunk is bent slightly forward. When walking the patient tends to freeze, and have difficulty setting himself in motion. If the patient is pushed forward or backward, the posture will become unstable (propulsion or retropulsion). The combination of rigidity and bradykinesia may particularly affect speech and writing. The speech is reduced in volume, has a low pitch and loses its rhythmical variation. Micrographia is common.

There is often evidence of autonomic disorder; in particular there is excessive salivation, and, with the mouth held slightly open, saliva may drool from the corners of the mouth. The skin can be greasy, due to excessive sebum secretion. Blood pressure may be low and postural hypotension is not infrequent. Bladder problems are common, and may be due to neurogenic features (Porter and Bors, 1971). Gut mobility is disordered, constipation is common and dysphagia can be troublesome in the later stages of the disease (Broe, 1982).

Psychiatric disturbances are common in parkinsonian patients. Depression is the commonest feature, closely followed by dementia. There seems to be a flattening of affect and a slowing of thought processes (bradyphrenia, Pearce, 1974). Personality disorders have been described. Confusion may complicate drug therapy.

Diagnostic Criteria in the Elderly

The diagnosis of Parkinson's disease is purely clinical. The elderly patient presents particular diagnostic problems as some of the features of Parkinson's disease, particularly slowness of movement and flexed posture, may overlap with age-related neurological changes. Most tremors appearing in old age tend to be attributed to Parkinson's disease, whereas in fact essential familial tremor often presents late in life and is commoner than Parkinson's disease. Familial tremor is distinguished by being an action tremor which is often improved by alcohol, or beta blockers (Jefferson *et al.*, 1979). Presentation of parkinsonism is rarely typical in the elderly. Recurrent falls, inability to transfer in and out of a chair, or difficulty in moving or getting in and out of bed, are very common presentations, though they may be caused by other common illnesses in the elderly, such as depression, dementia, myxoedema, all of which have other features in common with Parkinson's disease.

Although classical cases of Parkinson's disease are seen in extreme old age, more often the disease is complicated by the ageing process and the presence of other diseases. The diagnostic criteria are therefore blurred, and it is difficult to decide whether one is dealing with Parkinson's disease or conditions comparable to the other group of conditions earlier classified as parkinsonism-plus. Several of these entities can be clearly distinguished from Parkinson's disease. In postencephalitic parkinsonism, oculogyric crises, and dyskinesias are very much more common and the condition is associated with dementia and autonomic disturbances. In progressive supranuclear palsy (Steele–Richardson–Olszewski syndrome—Steele *et al.*, 1964) there is difficulty with vertical gaze. In the Shy–Drager syndrome postural hypotension and other autonomic features are marked.

The relationship of dementia with Parkinson's disease is complex and was reviewed by Quinn *et al.* in 1986. The prevalence of dementia in Parkinson's disease represents an increased risk over age- and sex-matched controls of 10–15%. This finding may be explained by one of three hypotheses: firstly, that these patients have a higher risk of developing Alzheimer's disease (though once arteriosclerotic pseudo-Parkinsonism is excluded, multi-infarct dementia is rare in Parkinson's disease); secondly, that the dementia of Parkinson's disease is neuropathologically distinct; and, thirdly, that the co-incidental pathologies of Alzheimer dementia and Parkinson's disease lower the threshold at which dementia is expressed. At present the evidence is inconclusive, though Perry *et al.* (1986) have demonstrated distinct neurochemical changes in the brains of parkinsonian patients who died with dementia. The presence of dementia is often associated with a poor response to drug treatment (Turnbull and Aitken, 1983).

Geriatricians seem to be presented with a range of syndromes giving rise to akinetic rigidity and clinical methods are insufficiently sensitive to discriminate between them. It is sometimes necessary to resort to a clinical trial of levodopa. Those patients responding to the drug are then classified as suffering from parkinsonism, and those not responding are diagnosed as suffering from diffuse degeneration of the nervous system. This method of classification is hardly scientific or elegant, and is an area which seems much in need of research. Within this group of disorders two nosological entities have been picked out. The first entity, arteriosclerotic Parkinson's disease, was elegantly described 50 years ago by McDonald Critchley, and recently rechristened by him arteriosclerotic pseudo-Parkinson's disease (Critchley, 1981). He distinguished parkinsonian cases who had no tremor, had evidence of coexistent pyramidal tract damage, were emotionally labile, and whose progression was stepwise and often determined by cardiovascular events. They do not respond to levodopa and at post-mortem have multiple lacunae often affecting the basal ganglia. This is a well-recognized entity on geriatric wards, but is probably quite distinct from Parkinson's disease. The second entity is senile parkinsonism described by Broe (1982) and is said to be distinguishable from classical Parkinson's disease by virtue of its late onset. Tremor is rare, and posture and balance are affected disproportionately, as is autonomic function. The condition is associated with an early and progressive dementia and while there is a positive response to levodopa, side-effects such as on–off phenomena and dyskinesias are relatively rare. I feel that the entity of senile parkinsonism is difficult to sustain, although there is no doubt that Parkinson's disease is modified by the ageing process.

Drug-induced parkinsonism is probably the most important differential diagnosis of Parkinson's disease and its importance has been increasingly recognized. Williamson and his co-workers found that out of 95 new cases of parkinsonism referred to a geriatric clinic 51% could be attributed to drugs (Stephen and Williamson, 1984). While the clinical features of parkinsonism resolved in two-thirds of the cases on withdrawing the offending drug, recovery was slow, taking on average 2 months. Five of the patients who initially recovered later developed idiopathic Parkinson's disease. Prochlorperazine (Stemetil) was responsible for over half the cases of drug-induced parkinsonism in this series. Many neuroleptic drugs (especially the phenothiazines) bind strongly with dopamine receptors, and in animal experiments have been detected in the brain of rats up to 3 months after a single dosage. Williamson's study (Stephen and Williamson, 1984) indicates that the earlier discontinuance of offending drugs is associated with a good prognosis.

TREATMENT: DRUG THERAPY

Levodopa

The loss of dopamine in the substantia nigra releases the excitatory cholinergic pathways from its inhibitory effect. Therapy is directed to correcting the dopamine deficiency or moderating the excessive cholinergic effect. Dopamine itself cannot be used as a therapeutic agent, as it fails to cross the blood–brain barrier. Birkmayer and Hornykiewicz in 1961 demonstrated that intravenous levodopa reduced the akinesia in Parkinson's disease. In 1967 Cotzias and his co-workers established the clinical effectiveness of oral levodopa, and since 1969 levodopa has been the mainstay of drug treatment in Parkinson's disease.

The use of levodopa alone was associated with a high prevalence of nausea and vomiting due to the peripherally formed dopamine stimulating the chemoreceptor trigger zone in the medulla. In addition, postural hypotension and cardiac dysrhythmias are problems. Peripheral side-effects have now been reduced by combining levodopa with an inhibitor of the enzyme peripheral dopa decarboxylase. Two inhibitors are in common use; benserazide and carbidopa, giving rise to the two preparations Madopar (ratio 4:1 for benserazide) and Sinemet (ratio 10:1 for carbidopa). A minimum quantity of peripheral decarboxylase inhibitor is required to prevent side-effects (Ward *et al.*, 1984) and for this reason, when small doses of Sinemet are used, a relatively increased amount of carbidopa is required, as in 'Sinemet plus' (Tourtellotte *et al.*, 1980). There appears to be little difference between the two combinations in terms of anti-parkinsonian effects, but double-blind randomized cross-over studies do show minor variations in the numbers of side-effects (Diamond *et al.*, 1978; Rinne and Molsa, 1979). The use of peripheral inhibitors increases the efficiency of absorption and allows lower doses of levodopa to be used than previously.

The pharmacokinetics of levodopa are affected by ageing. The two parameters most affected are the area under the curve and the half-life, indicating that the action of the drug is more sustained in the elderly than the young (Evans *et al.*, 1980; Yokochi, 1979). The absorption of levodopa from the bowel is by active transport, and the compound is affected by competition from other amino acids such as tyramine. Absorption is improved by low-protein diets or when taken in the fasting state (Mena and Cotzias, 1975; Nutt *et al.*, 1984). Levodopa is completely metabolized by the liver (Morgan *et al.*, 1971). Peak concentrations are in the order of 0.25 to 2.5 μg/ml, occurring between half an hour and 2 hours after an oral dosage of 1 g of levodopa. The half-life is between 1 and 2 hours, and is unaffected by the presence of a decarboxylase inhibitor (Marsden *et al.*, 1973). It has been difficult to establish a clear relationship between plasma levels and clinical effectiveness of the drug.

Although levodopa has revolutionized the treatment of Parkinson's disease, with chronic long-term usage the majority of patients either experience fluctuations in response to the drug or major side-effects. The drug exhibits tachyphylaxis. The dosage, therefore, has to be increased with time to maintain the therapeutic effect. The threshold at which side-effects occur remains much the same, and with increasing dosage, postural hypotension, psychiatric disturbances, dyskinesias and fluctuations of the disability become almost universal. The normal progression of a patient following the introduction of levodopa has been characterized by Parkes in 1984. After an initially favourable response the patient

experiences predictable end of dose deterioration (wearing off). While the wearing off effects are at first gradual, the switches become increasingly rapid, and the patient exhibits 'on/off phenomena'. At this stage there appears to be an all or none response to levodopa, good periods where mobility is maintained, alternating with other periods where there is freezing. This problem can sometimes be helped by giving frequent smaller doses (Rinne *et al.*, 1973). Almost invariably, however, the clinical response becomes less and less predictable, and the cost of abolishing off periods by increasing dosage is paid for with an increase in dyskinesias, and psychiatric side-effects. (The long-term limitations of the use of levodopa have been recently reviewed by Yahr, 1984.)

Abnormal involuntary movements are a major problem in the elderly parkinsonian patient. The orofacial manifestations—with jaw and tongue movements, and fly catcher tongue—are commoner in older subjects, whereas choreiform limb movements commonly occur more in the young (Fahn and Bressman, 1984). Initially, abnormal movements reflect levodopa levels (peak dose dyskinesias) but once established, dyskinesias often persist, and are associated more with periods of activity than drug dosage ('square wave dyskinesias'). Eventually, the dyskinetic phenomena and on–off phenomena become completely unpredictable (yo-yoing). Lhermitte (1978) has described diphasic dyskinesias which occur at the beginning and end of dose phases. These dyskinesias can be violent and traumatic, but are rare in the older patient.

Psychiatric side-effects are also more likely to occur in elderly subjects. Depression commonly coexists with parkinsonism and contrary to widely held belief is not helped by levodopa (Marsh and Markham, 1983). Levodopa is associated with nightmares and vivid dreams. Visual hallucinations are often Lilliputian, patients seeing small people or animals. Libido may rarely be increased on levodopa, and lead to sexual misdemeanours in elderly men. Psychiatric complications are common when levodopa is combined with other drugs, such as anticholinergic agents or amantadine.

After nearly 20 years of usage, we are still not clear as to the best way to use levodopa. Controversy still rages as to whether levodopa should be introduced early or late and at what dosage (Muenter, 1984; Fahn and Bressman, 1984). It is known that 79% of patients will have adverse affects on levodopa after 5 years' therapy. The suggestion has been made by Mann and Yates (1982) that chronic use of levodopa may accelerate the neuropathological changes occurring in Parkinson's disease, by the production of free-radical metabolites. For this, and other reasons, many clinicians delay the introduction of levodopa. This may mean, however, that effective treatment by levodopa will not be offered until the patient already has disabilities severe enough to affect his physical independence and social life. Others believe that there is no evidence that levodopa is harmful. Studies with positron emission tomography have shown that introduction of levodopa increases markedly the amount of dopamine storage in the brain. Markham and Diamond (1981) demonstrated similar disability scores, irrespective of the duration of levodopa therapy, in patients matched for disease duration, suggesting that there was no advantage in delaying the introduction of the drug. Lees and his co-workers (1981) found that lower doses of levodopa are associated with lower incidence of peak-dose dyskinesias, and this trend to lower doses of levodopa fits in with basic principles of geriatric prescribing, i.e. that drugs should be introduced gradually in the lowest possible dosage, that increases in dosage should be made slowly, and that the simplest possible regimen should be used.

Anticholinergic Drugs and Amantadine

Hyoscine was the first effective drug used in Parkinson's disease by Charcot in the nineteenth century. Subsequently, synthetic anticholinergic drugs have been widely used. Anticholinergics reduce rigidity and tremor marginally and hardly affect akinesia at all. Their side-effects are prohibitive in the elderly; in particular, organic confusional states are the rule rather than the exception. Dryness of the mouth, constipation, dizziness, anxiety all cause distress. Blurring of the vision occurs and there is a real risk of precipitating narrow-angle glaucoma due to pupillary dilatation (Friedman and Neumann, 1972).

Urinary retention may occur in elderly males with prostatic enlargement. Caution has to be observed withdrawing these drugs acutely as rebound deterioration has been described (Hughes *et al.*, 1971).

The chance finding by Schwab and colleagues that the antiviral agent, amantadine, had beneficial effects in Parkinson's disease led to its widespread use (Schwab, 1969). The drug works by increasing presynaptic synthesis and release of dopamine (Stromberg and Svensson, 1971). Tolerance is rapidly developed to the drug, however, and at this stage it is difficult to withdraw. Side-effects—livedo-reticularis, peripheral oedema, and confusional states—occur particularly in women (Shealy *et al.*, 1970). The drug is synergistic with levodopa and may be a useful supplement at times of increased activity (holidays, etc.) (Parkes *et al.*, 1970).

Direct Acting Dopamine Agonists

Levodopa is dependent for its action on its biotransformation to dopamine in striatal cells, which are damaged in Parkinson's disease. Logically, therefore, drugs which mimic dopamine, and act directly on postsynaptic receptor have a theoretical advantage. Bromocriptine is the only dopamine agonist in widespread clinical usage. It is an ergot alkaloid, and has a much longer duration of action than levodopa. The peak benefit is between 2 and 4 hours, and improvement is often maintained for up to 10 hours. Most clinical experience in the use of the drug has been in combination with levodopa, in an attempt to improve wearing off and end of dose phenomena (Grimes *et al.*, 1983; Calne *et al.*, 1984). The doses used have varied from as little as 2.5 mg a day to up to 300 mg a day. More recently Teychenne *et al.* (1982) have advocated low doses titrated with great care, up to about 15 mg a day. In elderly patients the total daily dose should probably be kept below 20 mg. Studies have consistently shown that when patients fail to respond to levodopa it is unlikely that they will respond to bromocriptine. There have been few good studies of using bromocriptine 'de novo'. Lees and Stern (1981) used a mean dosage of 70 mg of bromocriptine per day and found that 28 out of 50 patients responded after a year's treatment. There were many withdrawals due to side-effects but, interestingly, dyskinesias and end of dose deterioration were much less marked.

Bromocriptine is a difficult drug to use as the dose has to be titrated carefully in the individual case. It also has side-effects due to peripheral activity, though these can be blocked by domperidone (Quinn *et al.*, 1981). Nausea and vomiting, psychiatric complications, particularly hallucinations, postural hypotension, erythromelalgia, digitovasospasm, galactorrhoea, nasal stuffiness, and disturbances of liver functions have all been described (Eisler *et al.*, 1981; Duvoisin, 1976).

Several new dopamine agonists have been introduced but none is in widespread clinical usage. Lergotrile, lysuride and pergolide are all ergot derivatives, with very similar side-effects and pharmacological profiles to bromocriptine. No advantage has yet been shown with these drugs as compared with bromocriptine, though their slightly different lengths of action may be useful in individual cases. Lysuride can be given by continuous subcutaneous infusion. Piribedil and apomorphine are non-ergot derivatives, with anti-parkinsonian activity. Both, however, are limited by the severe nausea which they induce.

Selegiline Hydrochloride (Deprenyl)

Selegiline is a selective monoamino oxidase type B inhibitor, which has been available since 1982. By slowing the breakdown of dopamine, selegiline potentiates the effects of levodopa, increasing its duration of action (Lees *et al.*, 1977). Birkmayer *et al.* (1975) demonstrated the action of the drug following intravenous dosage. Subsequently it has been introduced in oral form. Clinical studies have shown its benefit in patients who are beginning to lose their response to levodopa. The drug has a long biological half-life, and single dosages of 5 or 10 mg are effective. It is necessary to reduce the dose of levodopa by approximately one-third on introduction of selegiline. Birkmayer has claimed improvements in akinesia, freezing, on–off phenomena, and fluctuations of disability and rigidity. He claims that the response to levodopa is smoothed out by the use of this drug.

Recent work by Langston (1985) has shown that selegiline may prevent the neurotoxic effects of MPTP. If a monoamine oxidase is implicated in the production of other free radicals likely to damage dopaminergic cells, then it is possible that early use of selegiline as a first line treatment may modify the progression and course of the disease.

Future Possibilities for Drug Treatment

Dopa is a precursor of noradrenaline and can be given in a rather analogous way to levodopa to correct the already identified deficiency in noradrenaline. Early suggestions that this drug may have dramatic effects on freezing phenomena have not been substantiated in the recent study by Quinn *et al.* (1984). The use of COMT inhibitors (catechol-O-methyltransferase) and dopamine beta-hydroxylase inhibitors to modify the metabolites of levodopa is presently undergoing trials, but it is too early to judge likely benefit.

Continuous intravenous infusion of levodopa can abolish variations in response to levodopa (Hardie *et al.*, 1984). Trials are at present being undertaken using slow-release forms of levodopa which mimic continuous intravenous usage. These, however, have not as yet been shown to be successful.

Drug Holidays

Another mechanism for trying to get more out of levodopa therapy is the institution of drug holidays (Kofman, 1984). It is claimed that on chronic levodopa dosages, the postsynaptic cell within the striatum loses its sensitivity to dopamine, and by withdrawing treatment for a period of a week to 10 days sensitivity may be re-established and a lower dose of levodopa may be necessary for periods up to 6 months. There are considerable dangers in this manoeuvre, as elderly patients may become akinetic and develop hypostatic pneumonias, when suddenly withdrawn from levodopa therapy. I feel the practice cannot be recommended within geriatric medicine.

BRAIN GRAFTS

Since idiopathic Parkinson's disease can be considered as being due essentially to loss of dopaminergic cells from the basal ganglia, a logical method of treatment would be grafting healthy cells into the diseased area. Such cerebral implant studies have been successful in animals. Intracerebral transplantation of adrenal tissue in two cases of Parkinson's disease in humans has been successful (Bjorklund *et al.*, 1982). Experiments continue and fetal cells from aborted material may be grafted in the near future.

TREATMENT OF PARKINSON'S DISEASE: NON-DRUG TREATMENT

Because of the importance of drugs in the management of Parkinson's disease, it is often forgotten that the drugs are merely an aid to rehabilitation, and that the patient must be seen in a wider context. It is more difficult to assess the impact of physiotherapy, occupational therapy or speech therapy than that of drug treatment. Nevertheless, Professor Caird has produced studies of occupational therapy and speech therapy which are highly impressive (Caird, 1986).

Physiotherapy attempts to maximize the benefit of drugs by maintaining and correcting posture, encouraging mobility and improving gait pattern (Franklyn and Stern, 1981; Steiner and Flewitt, 1981; Flewitt, 1981). Truncal and rotational movements are particularly difficult for patients with Parkinson's disease, and improve as a consequence of repeated exercises. Parkinsonian patients lose the normal heel strike on walking. As the heel of the foot is used as a brake and the toes as an accelerator in normal walking, reversal of this pattern leads to postural instability and inefficiency. Long-standing parkinsonian patients have shortening of the Achilles tendon which may limit effective rehabilitation.

Occupational therapy has been assessed by clinical trials (Gibberd *et al.*, 1981; Beattie and Caird, 1980) and has been shown to reduce the handicap experienced by elderly parkinsonian patients. Patients can often be helped by modified utensils to lessen the effects of tremor; the use of non-slip mats and bath aids are often helpful. Simple modifications to the patient's home such as providing bed and seats of an appropriate height may make all the difference in independent living. Unfortunately inappropriate aids are often given to patients with Parkinson's disease. For example, a zimmer aid may be counter-

productive as it interrupts the flow of movement during walking—which is exactly the opposite of what is required by the parkinsonian patients. A Rollator or Delta aid may be more appropriate.

The speech defects in Parkinson's disease are complex, and have recently been reviewed by Scott and Caird (1981) and Perry *et al.* (1981). Not only is the volume of speech reduced, but also the rhythm or prosodic element is disrupted. The use of the vocalite aid may produce significant improvement in speech.

As Parkinson's disease is a chronic disabling disease, and patients are easily identified by other members of the community by reason of their disability, social support is an essential element in their management. The Parkinson's Disease Society, 36 Portland Place, London W1N 3DG, has a network of branches nationally, and actively promotes knowledge within this field. It has produced a range of booklets which are designed for the sufferer of the disease and has a National Welfare Officer. It is often helpful for patients to be put in contact with the Society. A recent publication by Oxtoby (1981) identified patients' social needs, and also pointed out that the elderly parkinsonian patients frequently do not get help which is available.

REFERENCES

Agid, Y., Javey-Agid, F., and Ruberg, M. (1984). The neurobiochemistry of Parkinson's disease. In: Callaghan, N., and Galvin, R. (eds.) *Recent Research in Neurology*, Pitman, London.

Beattie, A., and Caird, F.I. (1980). The occupational therapist and the patient with Parkinson's disease. *Br. Med. J.*, **280**, 1354–5.

Birkmayer, W., and Hornykiewicz, O. (1961). Der L-3, 4-Dioxyphenylalanine (= DOPA)—Effekt bei der Parkinson-akinese. *Wien. Klin. Wschr.*, **73**, 787–8.

Birkmayer, W., Ambrozi, L., Neumayer, E., and Riederer, P. (1974). Longevity in Parkinson's disease treated with L-dopa. *Clin. Neurol. Neurosurg.*, **1**, 15–19.

Birkmayer, W., Riederer, P., Youdim, M.B.H., and Linauer, W. (1975). The potentiation of the anti-akinetic effect after levodopa treatment by an inhibitor of MAO-B deprenyl. *J. Neural Transmission*, **36**, 303–26.

Bjorklund, A., Stenevi, U., Dunnett, S.B., and Gage, F.H. (1982). Cross-species neural grafting in a rat model of Parkinson's disease. *Nature*, **298**, 652–4.

Brewis, M., Poskanzer, D.C., Rolland, C., and Miller, H. (1966). Neurological disease in an English city. *Acta Neurol. Scand.*, **42** (Suppl. 24), 31–6.

Broe, G.A. (1982). Parkinsonism and related disorders. In: Caird, F.I. (ed.) *Neurological Disorders in the Elderly*, P.S.G./Wright, Bristol, London, Boston, pp. 115–35.

Burns, S., Markey, S.P., Phillips, J.M., and Crush, C.C. (1984). The neurotoxicity of 1 methyl, 4 pheryl, 1236 tetrahydropyridine in monkey and man. *Can. J. Neurol. Sci.*, **11**, 166–8.

Caird, F. (1986). Speech and occupational therapy in Parkinson's disease. *Advanced Geriatric Medicine* 5, Churchill Livingstone, Edinburgh.

Calne, D.B. (1981). Parkinsonism and ageing. In: Arie, T. (ed.) *Health Care of the Elderly*, Croom Helm, London.

Calne, D.B., Plotkin, C., Williams, A.C., Nutt, J.G., Neophytides, A., and Teychenne, P.F. (1978). Long-term treatment of Parkinsonism with bromocriptine. *Lancet*, **1**, 735–8.

Cotzias, G.C., Wan Woert, M.H., and Schiffer, L.M. (1967). Aromatic amino acids and modification of Parkinsonism. *N. Engl. J. Med.*, **276**, 374–9.

Critchley, M. (1981). Arteriosclerotic pseudo-Parkinsonism. In: Rose, F.C., and Capildeo, R. (eds.) *Research Progress in Parkinson's Disease*, Pitman Medical, London.

Den Hartog Jager, W.A., and Bethlem, J. (1960). The distribution of lewy bodies in the central and automatic nervous systems in idiopathic paralysis agitans. *J. Neurol. Neurosurg. Psychiatry*, **23**, 283–90.

Diamond, S.G., Markham, C.H., and Techiokas, L.J. (1978). A double-blind comparison of levodopa, Madopa and Sinemet in Parkinson disease. *Ann. Neurol.*, **3**, 263–72.

Duvoisin, R.C. (1976). Digital vasospasm with bromocriptine. *Lancet*, **ii**, 204.

Duvoisin, R.C. (1984). Is Parkinson's disease acquired or inherited? *Can J. Neurol. Sci.*, **11**, 151–5.

Ehringer, H., and Hornykiewicz, O. (1960). *O. Klein. Warleushur.* **38**, 1238.

Eisler, T., Hall, R.P., Kalavar, K.A.R., and Calne, D.B. (1981). Erythromelalgia-like eruption in Parkinsonian patients treated with bromocriptine. *Neurology*, **31**, 1368–70.

Evans, M.A., Triggs, E.J., Broe, G.A., and Saines, N. (1980). Systemic availability or orally administered L-dopa in the elderly parkinsonian patient. *Eur. J. Clin. Pharmacol.*, **17**, 215–21.

Fahn, S., and Bressman, S.B. (1984). Should Levodopa therapy for Parkinsonism be started early or late? Evidence against early treatment. *Can. J. Neurol. Sci.*, **11**, 200–6.

Farley, I.J., and Hornykiewicz, O. (1976). In: Birkmayer, W., and Hornykiewicz, O. (eds.) *Advances in Parkinsonism*, Roche, Basel, pp. 178–85.

Finch, C. (1973). Parkinson's disease. *Brain Res.*, **52**, 261–7.

Findley, L.J., Gresty, M.A., and Halmagyi, G.M. (1981). Tremor, the cogwheel phenomenon and clonus in Parkinson's disease. *J. Neurol. Neurosurg. Psychiatry*, **44**, 534–46.

Flewitt, B., Capildeo, R., and Rose, F.C. (1981). Physiotherapy and assessment of Parkinson's disease using the polarised light goniometer. In Rose, F.C., and Capildeo, R. (eds.) *Research Progress in Parkinson's Disease*, Pitman Medical, London, pp. 404–13.

Franklyn, S., and Stern, G.M. (1981). Controlled trial of physiotherapy and occupational therapy for Parkinson's disease. *Br. Med. J.*, **282**, 1969–70.

Friedman, Z., and Neumann, E. (1972). Benzhexol-induced blindness in Parkinson's disease. *Br. Med. J.*, **i**, 605.

Garland, M.G. (1952). Parkinsonism. *Br. Med. J.*, **2**, 1373–4.

Gibberd, F.B., Page, N.G.R., Spencer, K.M., Kinnear, E., and Hawksworth, J.B. (1981). Controlled trial of physiotherapy and occupational therapy for Parkinson's disease. *Br. Med. J.*, **282**, 1196.

Godwin-Austen, R.B., Lee, P.N., Marmot, M.G., and Stern, G.M. (1982). Smoking and Parkinson's disease. *J. Neurol. Neurosurg. Psychiatry*, **45** (7), 577–81.

Grimes, J.D., Delgado, M.R., and Gray, P. (1983). Low-dose bromocriptine therapy in "de-novo" Parkinson's disease: Indications, dosage, initial response rate and adverse effects. *Neurology*, **33** (Suppl. 2), 112–14.

Gudmundsson, K.R. (1967). A clinical survey of Parkinsonism in Iceland. *Acta Neurol. Scand.*, **43** (Suppl. 33), 1–61.

Haack, D.G., Baumann, R.J., McKean, H.E., Jameson, H.D., and Turbek, J.A. (1981). Nicotine exposure and Parkinson's disease. *Am. J. Epidemiol.*, **114** (2), 191–200.

Harada, H., Nishikawa, S., and Takahashi, K. (1983). Epidemiology of Parkinson's disease in a Japanese city. *Arch. Neurol.*, **40** (3), 151–4.

Hardie, R.J., Lees, A.J., and Stern, G.M. (1982). On–off syndrome in Parkinson's disease and intravenous Levodopa. *Lancet*, **ii**, 992–3.

Hoehm, M. Epidemiology of Parkinsonism. In: *Monoamines Nayeaux Centraux et Syndrome de Parkinson*, Geary et Cie, Geneva, pp. 281–300.

Hughes, R.C., Polgar, J.G., Weightman, D., and Walton, J.N. (1971). Levodopa in Parkinsonism: The effects of withdrawal of anticholinergic drugs. *Br. Med. J.*, **ii**, 487–91.

Jefferson, D., Jenner, P., and Marsden, C.D. (1979). B-adrenoreceptor antagonists in essential tremor. *J. Neurol. Neurosurg. Psychiatry*, **42**, 904–9.

Kessler, I.I. (1972). Epidemiologic studies of Parkinson's disease. A community-based survey. *Am. J. Epidemiol.*, **96**, 242–54.

Kofman, O.S. (1984). Are Levodopa "drug holidays" justified? *Can. J. Neurol. Sci.*, **11**, 206–10.

Langston, W.J. (1985). *Trends in Pharmacological Science*, **6** (9), 375–8.

Langston, J.W., Ballard, P.A., Tetrud, J.W., and Irwin, I.

(1983). Chronic Parkinsonism in humans due to a product of moperidine-analog synthesis. *Science*, **219**, 979–80.

Lees, A.J., and Stern, G.M. (1981). Sustained bromocriptine therapy in previously untreated patients with Parkinson's disease. *J. Neurol. Neurosurg. Psychiatry*, **44**, 1020–3.

Lees, A.J., Kohout, L.J., Shaw, K.M., Stern, G.M., Elsworth, J.D., and Sandler, M. (1977). Deprenyl in Parkinson's disease. *Lancet*, **ii**, 791–5.

Lhermitte, F., Agid, Y., and Signoret, J.L. (1978). Onset and end of dose levodopa induced dyskinesias. *Arch. Neurol.*, **35**, 261–3.

McGeer, C.G., Stairs, W.A., and McGeer, P.L. (1984). Neurotransmitters in the basal ganglia. *Can. J. Neurol. Sci.*, **II**, 89–100.

McLennan, L. (1981). Rigidity. In: Rose, F.C., and Capildeo, R. (eds.) *Research Progress in Parkinson's Disease*, Pitman Medical, London, pp. 88–98.

Mann, D., and Yates, L. (1982). Pathogenesis of Parkinson's disease. *Arch. Neurol.*, **39**, 545–9.

Markham, C.H., and Diamond, S.G. (1981). Evidence to support early levodopa therapy in Parkinson disease. *Neurology*, **31**, 125–31.

Marmot, M.C. (1981). Mortality and Parkinson's disease. In: Rose, F.C., and Capildeo, R. (eds.) *Research Progress in Parkinson's Disease*, Pitman Medical, London, pp. 9–17.

Marsden, C.D., Parkes, J.D., and Rees, J.E. (1973). Long-term treatment of Parkinson's disease with an extracerebral dopa decarboxylase inhibitor (L-alpha-methylhydrazine MK 486) and levodopa. *Adv. Neurol.*, **3**, 79–93.

Marsh, G.G., and Markham, C.H. (1973). Does levodopa alter depression and psychopathology in Parkinsonism patients? *J. Neurol. Neurosurg. Psychiatry*, **36**, 925–35.

Marttila, R.J. (1980). Aetiology of Parkinson's disease. *Parkinson's Disease*, Elsevier/North Holland Biomedical Press, Amsterdam, New York, pp. 3–15.

Mena, I., and Cotzias, G.C. (1975). Protein uptake and treatment of Parkinson's disease with levodopa. *N. Engl. J. Med.*, **292**, 181–4.

Morgan, J.P., Bianchine, J.R., Spiegal, H.E., Rivera-Calimlim, L., and Hersey, R.M. (1971). Metabolism of levodopa in patients with Parkinson's disease. *Arch. Neurol.*, **25**, 39–43.

Muenter, M.D. (1984). Should levodopa treatment for Parkinsonism be started early or late? *Can. J. Neurol. Sci.*, **11**, 195–200.

Mutch, W.S. (1985). Aberdeen survey of Parkinson's disease. *Clinical Courier*, **3** (3).

Nutt, J.G., Woodward, W.R., Hammerstad, J.P., Carter, J.H., and Anderson, J.L. (1984). The "on-off" phenomenon in Parkinson's disease. Relation to levodopa absorption and transport. *N. Engl. J. Med.*, **310**, 483–8.

Okama, E., and Ghuta, F. (1976). *Acta Neurol. Scand.*, **34**, 1092–4.

Oxtoby, M. (1981). *Parkinson's Disease, Patients and their Social Needs*, Parkinson's Disease Society, London.

Parkes, J.D. (1984). Some recent aspects of Parkinson's disease. In: Callaghan, N., and Galvin, R. (eds.) *Recent Research in Parkinson's Disease*, Pitman Medical, London, pp. 26–34.

Parkes, J.D., Zilkha, K.J., Calver, D.M., and Knill-Jones, R.P. (1970). Controlled trial of amantadine hydrochloride in Parkinson's disease. *Lancet*, **i**, 259–62.

Parkinson, J. (1817). *Essay on the Shaking Palsy*, Sherwood, Neely and Jones, London.

Peach, H., and Kellar, R. (1984). *Epidemiology of Common Diseases*, Heinemann, London, pp. 159–61.

Pearce, J. (1974). Mental changes in Parkinsonism. *Br. Med. J.* **ii**, 445.

Pentland, B., and Sawers, J.S.A. (1980). Galactorrhoea after withdrawal of bromocriptine. *Br. Med. J.*, **ii**, 716–17.

Perry, R.H. (1986). Recent advances in neuropathology. *Br. Med. Bull.*, **42** (1), 86–90.

Perry, A.R., and Das, P.K. (1981). Speech assessment of patients with Parkinson's disease. In: Rose, F.C., and Capildeo, R. (eds.) *Research Progress in Parkinson's Disease*, Pitman Medical, London, pp. 373–83.

Perry, R.H., Tomlinson, B.R., Candy, J.M., Blessed, F., Foster, J.F., and Bloxham, C.A. (1985). Cortical cholinergic deficit in mentally impaired parkinsonian patients. (Letter.) *Lancet*, **ii**, 789–90.

Porter, R.W., and Bors, E. (1971). Neurogenic bladder in Parkinsonism: Effect of thalamotomy. *J. Neurosurg.*, **34**, 27–32.

Quinn, N., Marsden, C.D., and Parkes, J.D. (1982). Complicated response to fluctuations in Parkinson's disease in response to intravenous infusion of Leva Dopa. *Lancet*, **2** (2), 412–15.

Quinn, N.P., Perlnutter, J.S., and Marsden, C.D. (1984). Acute administration of DL Threo DOPS does not affect the freezing phenomenon in Parkinsonian patients. *Neurology*, **34** (Suppl. 1), 149.

Quinn, N.P., Rooser, M.N., and Marsden, C.D. (1986). Dementia and Parkinson's disease. Pathological and Neurochemical considerations. *Br. Med. Bull.*, **42** (1), 86–90.

Quinn, N., Illas, A., Lhermitte, F., and Agid, Y. (1981). Bromocriptine and domperidone in the treatment of Parkinson's disease. *Neurology*, **31**, 662–7.

Rajput, A.H., Offond, K.P., Beard, C.M., and Kurland, L.T. (1984). Epidemiology of Parkinsonism: Incidence classification and mortality. *Am. Neurol.*, **16**, 278–82.

Riederer, P., Reynolds, G.P., and Birkmayer, W. (1981). Neurochemical correlates of symptomatology and drug induced side effects in Parkinson's disease. In: Rose, F.C., and Capildeo, R. (eds.) *Research Progress in Parkin-*

son's Disease, Pitman Medical, London, Vol. 2, pp. 149–59.

Rinne, U.K. (1978). Recent advances in research on Parkinsonism. *Acta Neurol. Scand.*, **57** (Suppl. 67), 77–113.

Rinne, U.K., and Molsa, P. (1979). Levodopa with benserazide or carbidopa in Parkinson disease. *Neurology*, **29**, 1584–9.

Rinne, U.K., Sonninen, V., and Siirtola, T. (1973). Plasma concentration of levodopa in patients with Parkinson's disease. *Eur. Neurol.*, **10**, 301–10.

Schwab, R.S., England, A.C., Poskanzer, D.C., and Young, R.R. (1969). Amantadine in the treatment of Parkinson's disease. *J.A.M.A.*, **208**, 1168–70.

Scott, S., and Caird, F.I. (1981). Speech therapy for patients with Parkinson's disease. *Br. Med. J.*, **280**, 1354–5.

Shaw, K.M., Lees, A.J., and Stern, G.M. (1980). The impact of treatment with levodopa on Parkinson's disease. *Qt. J. Med.*, **49** (195), 283–93.

Shealy, C.N., Weeith, J.B., and Mercier, D. (1970). Livedo reticularis in patients with Parkinsonism receiving amantadine. *J.A.M.A.*, **212**, 1522–3.

Steele, J.C., Richardson, J.C., and Olczewski, S. (1964). Progressive supranuclear palsy. *Arch. Neurol.*, **10**, 333–59.

Steiner, P., and Flewitt, B. (1981). Controlled trial of physiotherapy and occupational therapy for Parkinson's disease. *Br. Med. J.*, **2**, 282.

Stephen, P.J., and Williamson, J. (1984). Drug induced Parkinsonism in the elderly. *Lancet*, **ii**, 1082–3.

Stromberg, U., and Svensson, T.H. (1971). Further studies on the mode of action of amantadine. *Acta Pharmacol. Toxicol.*, **30**, 161–71.

Sweet, R.D., and McDowell, F.H. (1975). Five years treatment of Parkinson's disease with levodopa: Therapeutic results and survival of 100 patients. *Ann. Intern. Med.*, **83**, 456–63.

Teychenne, P.F., Bergsrud, D., Racy, A., Elton, R.L., and Vern, B. (1982). Bromocriptine: Low dose therapy in Parkinson's disease. *Neurology*, **32**, 577–83.

Tourtellotte, W., Syndulko, K., Potvin, A.R., Hirsch, S.B., and Potvin, J.H. (1980). Increased ratio of carbidopa to levodopa in treatment of Parkinson's disease. *Arch. Neurol.*, **37**, 115–23.

Turnbull, C.J., and Aitken, J.A. (1983). Diagnosis and management of Parkinsonism in the elderly. *Age Ageing*, **12**, 309–16.

Ward, C.D., Trombley, I.K., Calne, D.B., and Kopin, I.J. (1984). L-dopa decarboxylation in chronically treated patients. *Neurology*, **34**, 198–201.

Williams, A. (1981). CSF biochemical studies on some extra-pyramidal diseases. In: Rose, F.C., and Capildeo, R. (eds.) *Research in Progress in Parkinson's Disease*, Pitman Medical, London, pp. 170–81.

Yahr, M.B. (1984). Limitations of the long term use of anti-Parkinsonism drugs. *Can. J. Neurol. Sci.*, **11**, 191–5.

Yokochi, M. (1979). Juvenile Parkinson's disease. Part II. Pharmacokinetic study. *Shinkei Shinpo*, **23**, 1060–73.

Zumstein, H., and Siegfried, J. (1976). Mortality among Parkinson patients treated with L-dopa combined with a decarboxylase inhibitor. *Eur. Neurol.*, **14**, 321–7.

Chapter 10

Other Movement Disorders

Lindsay McLellan

Professor of Rehabilitation, Consultant Neurologist, University Rehabilitation Unit, Southampton General Hospital, Southampton, UK

A range of movement disorders occurs in elderly people. There are two principal differences between the treatment of these disorders in younger adults and treatment in the elderly. First, the disorders in themselves may not greatly concern the elderly person whose activities are already restricted by other conditions, so that an explanation and reassurance that the disorder does not affect health may be all that is required. Second, drugs and neurosurgical procedures are poorly tolerated by elderly people so that it is more difficult to alleviate the disorder without causing troublesome unwanted effects.

TREMORS

The most commonly occurring tremor other than that of parkinsonism is idiopathic (formerly benign essential) tremor (Critchley, 1949; Koop, 1986) (Table 10.1). In some elderly patients with a long history, the word benign is misleading since their activities may be significantly curtailed. In all age ranges, the incidence of a positive family history is approximately 50%, though there are no published surveys examining separately the frequency of a family history in old age. Idiopathic tremor can take many clinical forms, the commonest being a regular postural or action tremor of small amplitude and a rate of about 8–10 Hz. This affects the hands when they are held outstretched, or involved in maintaining a posture, as in holding a cup. The amplitude of the tremor can be large enough to impair handwriting, fine tasks such as doing up buttons, and

pouring out drinks. In some cases, the face and head may also be affected and there is an association between this type of tremor and torsion dystonia, which is discussed in more detail below.

Idiopathic tremor in some individuals becomes worse as a target is approached and thus has some

TABLE 10.1 CAUSES OF TREMOR PRESENTING IN ELDERLY PEOPLE

Characteristics	Causes
Tremor at rest (while completely relaxed)	Parkinsonism (bradykinesia also present)
Tremor while maintaining posture	Physiological tremor Anxiety Hyperthyroidism Drugs (β-adrenergic stimulants, lithium, sodium valproate) Alcohol, and alcohol withdrawal Idiopathic tremor Structural brain disease affecting red nucleus or cerebellar connections, or premotor frontal cortex
Intention tremor	Structural brain disease affecting connections in cerebellum or brain stem Alcohol Sedative and anti-convulsant drugs

features of an intention tremor. Some authorities consider that there is a separate entity affecting elderly people which is termed the tremor of old age. This distinction is of theoretical rather than practical interest, since idiopathic tremor itself is of unknown aetiology and has quite a wide variety of clinical forms.

The principal diagnostic dilemma in an elderly person presenting with tremor is to decide whether or not parkinsonism is the cause. The pathognomonic clinical feature of parkinsonism is bradykinesia in the absence of which parkinsonism should not be diagnosed. This rule is easy to apply in young adults, but elderly people may show slowness of movement from other causes and bradykinesia may be difficult to exclude. Thus the standard test of drumming the index and middle fingers as fast as possible, ensuring that one finger extends as the other flexes, may not be well performed in the presence of osteoarthritis, or by people who have ceased to undertake fine tasks on a regular basis. A helpful indication of parkinsonism is that the alternating movements are not only slow, but show a marked tendency for both fingers to move together in the same direction or for each finger to make a succession of taps while the other fails to move. In the upper limbs, associated movements such as swinging of the arms while walking, are lost. Gait disorders in the elderly can present a considerable diagnostic difficulty (Sudarsky and Routhal, 1983), but as a rule, the bradykinesia of parkinsonism is never restricted to the lower limbs so that normal manual dexterity in an untreated subject virtually excludes parkinsonism.

Other causes of action tremor include sympathomimetic drugs, especially beta adrenergic stimulants such as may be prescribed for the treatment of asthma. Tremor may also occur with the anticonvulsant drug sodium valproate, tricyclic antidepressants or with toxic blood levels of phenytoin. A combination of increased muscle tone and intention tremor may occur in hypothyroidism.

Treatment

Once predisposing causes have been excluded, the treatment consists of a careful explanation and discussion with the patient as to the actual impact of the tremor on their way of life. It is important to identify the circumstances in which the tremor is at its worst and at its best. For example, the tremor may be troublesome only when the patient is in unfamiliar company and may be absent or trivial in the quiet of the home. Attention to sources of anxiety can be supplemented by a small dose of benzodiazepine tranquilliser to cover such specific occasions. If the patient notes that the tremor is markedly improved after an alcoholic drink, the diagnosis of idiopathic tremor is confirmed and such patients may show similar improvements with a small dose of phenobarbitone. The alternative of primidone (Findley and Calzetti, 1982) tends to be poorly tolerated in elderly people. In view of their adverse effects and their addictive potential, all tranquillizing drugs must be regarded as potentially hazardous in the elderly.

By no means all cases of idiopathic tremor are improved by alcohol. Idiopathic tremor is a clinical entity that may embrace a number of subgroups. In some cases, a rapid postural tremor is present at 8–12 Hz, resembling physiological tremor, and this is regarded by some authorities as a defined subtype of idiopathic tremor (Marsden and Fahn, 1982). Beta$_2$ adrenergic blockade, for example with propranolol, can be very helpful in such cases. However, these drugs tend to be less well tolerated in elderly people because of their tendency to cause hypotension, fatigue on exercise, accentuation of bronchospasm, brachycardia, hallucinations and vivid dreams.

Other Therapy

Physiotherapy has no role in the suppression of abnormal involuntary movements. In cases in which the tremor does interfere with dexterity, occupational therapists can help the patient considerably by advising on modifications to clothing and the provision of adapted equipment in the kitchen, bathroom or to assist with the person's interests and hobbies. At the time of writing, there is a severe shortage of occupational therapists in the UK; a recent survey (Mutch *et al.*, 1986) has shown that only 25% of people with parkinsonism have ever seen one, despite the evidence of the benefits they can confer when visiting a patient in their own home (Beattie and Caird, 1980; Oxtoby, 1982). Advice on these matters is more likely to help an elderly person with tremor than the prescription of drugs.

CHOREA, SENILE CHOREA AND TARDIVE DYSKINESIA

Chorea (Table 10.2)

Chorea occurs as a result of lesions in the contra-lateral putamen and caudate nucleus. It consists of

TABLE 10.2 CAUSES OF CHOREA PRESENTING IN ELDERLY PEOPLE

Senile chorea (idiopathic)
Drug-induced:
    (a) Dopaminergic drugs: levodopa, bromocriptine, amantadine, apomorphine, selegiline
    (b) Phenothiazines—as part of the syndrome of tardive dyskinesia (see Table 10.3)
    (c) Phenytoin
Huntington's chorea
Lingual–buccal–facial dyskinesia
Torsion dystonia
Cerebral palsy
Biochemical disorders: hypernatraemia, hypoparathyroidism
Focal lesions of the basal ganglia especially the caudate nucleus
Cerebral degenerations

irregular jerking and twitching movements, particularly of the face, head and neck, and distal segments of the limbs. They are not stereotyped as in tics, but constantly changing. Although they appear to be superimposed upon voluntary movement, they can be accommodated remarkably well, even when they occur during complex acts such as drinking a glass of water. Sometimes they appear semi-purposeful and become incorporated into inappropriate acts such as continually moving and replacing spectacles.

When occurring in elderly people without evidence of focal intracerebral disease, these movements may be called 'senile chorea' (Koop, 1986). It is rare for Huntington's chorea to present in the elderly, though presentation of Huntington's chorea beyond the age of 65 is well known to occur. Senile chorea is thus a clinical entity that is probably due to primary degenerative or ischaemic changes in the brain.

Lingual–Buccal–Facial Dyskinesia

A specific entity of lingual–buccal–facial dyskinesia has been described (Weiner and Klawson, 1973) in which degeneration occurred principally in the putamen and additionally in the caudate nucleus. In untreated subjects there were no involuntary movements in the limbs, but the administration of levodopa caused marked chorea of the limbs, implying the presence of a subclinical disease in the areas of the basal ganglia subserving the limbs. It is not known why the symptoms are so much more prominent in the face. The involuntary movements may be continual, severe and disfiguring, consisting of screwing up of the periorbital muscles and cheeks, forcible protrusion of the tongue and chewing movements of the jaws.

Tardive Dyskinesia

A similar pattern of involuntary movement is seen in tardive dyskinesia, a condition associated with phenothiazine, butyrophenone or thioxanthene drug toxicity (Mackay, 1982; Marsden and Fahn, 1982; Marsden *et al.*, 1983, 1975) (Table 10.3). Classically

TABLE 10.3 DRUGS CAUSING TARDIVE DYSKINESIA

Phenothiazines
Butyrophenones
Thioxanthenes
Metoclopramide

the symptoms appear after treatment for many months or years and become worse when the dose is withdrawn or reduced; the more fortunate patients may then experience very slow improvement but for many the dyskinesia is permanent. This complication is much commoner in elderly subjects. For this reason, prolonged treatment with phenothiazines must be avoided except where they are essential, for example in the control of schizophrenia.

Orofacial dyskinesia is by far the most common manifestation of tardive dyskinesia, but a wide variety of other involuntary movements may occur in addition or instead of orofacial dyskinesia. In elderly people, chorea of the limbs is the second most frequent pattern to occur. Athetosis, ballism and dystonia are also seen. Other patterns include akithesia, or an irresistible desire to move the legs repetitively. These movements may either be purposeless rapid rubbing of one leg up and down on the other in an alternating sequence when sitting, or a kind of compulsive walking in which the patient is continually on the move, the gait being rather irregular and stamping and tending to show bizarre trajectories of the limbs. Dopaminergic drugs, phenytoin, tricyclic anti-depressants, amphetamines and lithium can cause dyskinesia which reverts promptly when the dose is lowered, but this is not tardive dyskinesia.

Acute Dystonic Reactions to Neuroleptic Drugs

Some individuals show an idiosyncratic response to small doses of neuroleptic drugs, which is not related to the dose or duration of administration. For example, the administration of a small dose of prochlorperazine to a susceptible individual may be followed within hours by a severe and very uncomfortable dystonia of the limbs and trunk severe enough at times to cause opisthotonos, accompanied by chorea in the limbs and face. The eyes may be forcibly deviated upwards as in an oculogyric crisis. In other cases, severe akithesia may occur (Schiele *et al.*, 1973). The drug responsible must be stopped and the patient warned not to take neuroleptics in the future. Intravenous anticholinergic drugs such as benztropine 0.5 to 1 mg may bring about a rapid dissolution of the symptoms within 1 to 2 hours, but sometimes the movements take several weeks to subside even with continued anticholinergic treatment.

Levodopa-induced Dyskinesia

The commonest cause of chorea in elderly people is levodopa given for the treatment of parkinsonism. Levodopa does not cause dyskinesia in normal people, implying that the dyskinesia occurs in association with subclinical neuronal damage in the basal ganglia as appears to be the case with facial–buccal dyskinesia. The only effective treatment is to reduce the dose of levodopa.

If the dyskinesia occurs in relation to the timing of the dose, for example at 45–90 minutes after each capsule, the administration of the same daily doses in smaller but more frequent amounts can avoid dyskinesia without prejudicing the benefical effects upon bradykinesia.

Treatment of Chorea and Tardive Dyskinesia

The same general comments apply to the treatment of chorea as for idiopathic tremor. Even tardive dyskinesia is well tolerated in most cases and no drug treatment is necessary once the diagnosis has been explained to the patients. In fact, the effects of drug treatment are usually disappointing and are often negated by side-effects.

Neuroleptic drugs such as pimozide can suppress chorea, but they are best avoided because of the long-term risk of provoking tardive dyskinesia. Tetrabenazine is an effective drug that does not cause tardive dyskinesia, but it appears to accumulate over the first 3 to 4 weeks of administration, causing parkinsonism (which can be profound), dysphagia, drowsiness and troublesome depression. The starting dose is 12.5 mg once or twice a day and increases are made cautiously every 2 to 3 weeks to a maximum in elderly people of 25 mg four times a day.

There is no evidence that anticholinergic drugs improve chorea. Promising reports of a useful clinical response to cholinergic drugs (lecithin or choline chloride) have not been borne out by further experience.

Occupational therapists are again the mainstay of supportive treatment, but interference with speech, swallowing or communication are indications for assessment by speech therapists. Advice on the optimum position of the patient's trunk and head while eating, selection of an appropriate diet that the patient can swallow and training in the use of alternative forms of communication can be extremely valuable in patients with severe orofacial dyskinesia.

ATHETOSIS

Athetosis in British terminology refers to involuntary movements of a slower and more sinuous nature than the jerky movements of chorea. The limbs may take up a position of flexion of the elbow and wrist accompanied by hyperextension and splaying of the digits, or alternatively accompanied by closure of the hand with the thumb being protruded between the index and middle fingers—a characteristic sign of basal ganglia disorder. The posture shifts repeatedly between the flexed position and one of hyperextension of the arm with pronation of the forearm and abduction and internal rotation of the shoulder. For practical clinical purposes athetosis has implications similar to chorea (with which it often coexists), occurring after basal ganglia damage, in tardive dyskinesia, in the acute idiosyncratic dystonic response to neuroleptic drugs and as an unwanted effect of levodopa in parkinsonism.

BALLISM

Ballism is a sudden flinging movement involving proximal and distal segments of the limbs, which propels the limb outwards, forwards or backwards with considerable force sufficient to throw the patient off his feet or cause serious injury to the limbs. While occasionally seen in tardive dyskinesia, it classically occurs in hypertensive patients with cerebrovascular disease due to infarction or haemorrhage in the contralateral subthalamic nucleus. Unilateral ballism, the commonest form, is called hemiballismus and when due to cerebrovascular disease, tends to subside gradually whether treatment is given or not over a period of 1 to 3 months.

Sometimes it persists, or in the acute stages is so severe that treatment has to be given to prevent self injury. Tetrabenazine is the most effective drug. The dosage may need to be increased faster than in the schedule described above because of the need to gain control of the disorder quickly. This means that parkinsonism is likely to be induced and the patient should be carefully observed so that the dose of tetrabenazine can be adjusted in good time.

TORSION DYSTONIA

Generalized torsion dystonia is a very rare condition in elderly people. It occurs sporadically or as an autosomal dominant condition, the age of onset usually being in the second or third decade. Occa-

sionally families are encountered where the onset is later, but onset after the age of 65 has not been described.

Generalized dystonia (formerly known as dystonia musculorum deformans) is a disorder of coactivation of most or all the muscle groups in the affected limbs, trunk, neck and face which can pull the body into bizarre and painful postures, with the features already described as characteristic of a basal ganglia disorder (Rothwell *et al.*, 1983). Nevertheless, no consistent pathological abnormalities are found at autopsy.

Symptomatic dystonias may occur contralateral to lesions of the basal ganglia caused by infection, infarction or neoplasm. Some cases of cerebral palsy have patterns of muscular activation and disorders of posture that are typically dystonic, though it is conventional to refer to them as spastic because evidence of an upper motor neurone lesion is also present. Drug treatment with high doses of benztropine or with carbamazepine or clonazepam may be helpful and surgical stereotactic lesions of the basal ganglia may be indicated in severe cases.

In the elderly, dystonia does not usually take this generalized form except in tardive dyskinesia. The focal dystonias are more common, notably spasmodic torticollis and writer's cramp. These will normally have presented in middle life but usually then persist, becoming gradually worse with the passage of time.

Spasmodic Torticollis

Spasmodic torticollis is a condition in which the neck and sometimes the face are subject to dystonic involuntary movements, the head being pulled forcibly to one or other side, rotated, flexed or extended in a way which is distressing, embarrassing and painful for the subject. It interrupts activities in which hand–eye coordination or eye contact are important.

The form of torticollis varies considerably from one patient to another. In some, the movements are slow and tonic in form, the head being forcibly held to one side for minutes at a time. In others, they are jerky and intermittent and may be accompanied by tremor of the head and neck or myoclonus (Couch,

1976). These movements continuing over many years are associated with painful cervical spondylosis and cervical root symptoms.

For reasons that are not understood, a light touch such as the pressure of the index finger on the chin may, at times, be enough to inhibit some of the involuntary contractions. Training in relaxation, assisted by augmented sensory feedback (biofeedback) has been claimed to be successful in improving the patient's degree of voluntary control over the dystonic movements (Cleeland, 1973; Korein *et al.*, 1976), but sympathy and support may be equally effective.

The drug treatment of choice is anticholinergic medication such as benzhexol, but the doses given have to be large to be effective in most cases, being at least 20 mg daily in the middle-aged adult. Only low doses are tolerated in the elderly, especially if there is evidence of coincidental dementia or hesitancy of micturition. Treatment with carbamazepine or a benzodiazepine such as clonazepam may also be helpful in some cases. Surgical treatment involves either denervation of the affected muscles or bilateral thalamotomy. The effects are unpredictable and surgery is rarely recommended over the age of 70 years. Paralysis of the affected muscles with local injections of botulinum toxin (see section on blepharospasm below) is currently being evaluated.

Writer's Cramp

Writer's cramp is another form of focal dystonia affecting the dominant hand which classically becomes apparent only during the act of writing (Sheehy and Marsden, 1982). No treatment has yet been shown to be effective for this condition. If the patient learns to write with the other hand instead, that hand too may become affected within a 2 to 3 year period.

Some cases of writer's cramp are characterized by dystonic posture in the hand and obvious dystonia in the more proximal muscles of the arm during the act of writing (Hughes and McLellan, 1985). A tremor may occur and on close questioning it may become clear that certain other fine tasks such as using a screwdriver or doing up buttons are also affected to a much lesser degree. It is not clear whether such cases represent a more severe form of the condition or

should be regarded as a separate subtype. It has been suggested that the term simple writer's cramp should be applied to cases in which only writing is affected and dystonic writer's cramp to the more severe clinical forms (Sakai *et al.*, 1981).

MYOCLONUS

This is a complex disorder of considerable neurophysiological interest which is rare in elderly people. It may be defined as involuntary 'muscle jerking, irregular or rhythmic, arising in the central nervous system' (Marsden *et al.*, 1982). Myoclonus cannot temporarily be suppressed by an effort of will and this distinguishes it from tics, though the form of tics and myoclonus may be very similar. It is unusual in myoclonus for the same muscle or groups of muscles to be activated repeatedly, but sometimes the movements are more widely varied and dispersed. However, they are briefer, more shocklike and lack the flowing quality of chorea. Thus a patient subject to myoclonus holding a glass of water may drop or empty the glass involuntarily if myoclonus occurs. The differential diagnosis of myoclonus includes degenerative cerebral disease such as Alzheimer's disease, progressive supranuclear palsy, cerebrovascular disease, certain forms of epilepsy, metabolic encephalopathy (notably renal failure, hepatic failure, hyponatraemia and hypo- or hyperglycaemia) and the long-term effects of encephalitis, diffuse head injury, carbon monoxide poisoning or hypoxia. Certain forms can result from spinal cord lesions.

The rigour with which the underlying cause is pursued in an elderly patient depends upon the severity of the symptoms and the relative risks and benefit of treatment for the underlying cause (see Table 10.4). Myoclonus, like dystonia, may be generalized or focal. The best known example of focal myoclonus is palatal myoclonus, which is most often caused by infarction in an area of the brain stem that includes the red nucleus, inferior olivary nucleus, dentate nucleus and their connecting pathways. There may be a delay of several weeks after the infarction before myoclonus is noted. A few patients have responded to clonazepam, 5-hydroxytryptophan (Magnussen *et al.*, 1977; Williams *et al.*, 1978) or carbamazepine (Sakai *et al.*, 1981). For a further

TABLE 10.4 CAUSES OF MYOCLONUS IN ELDERLY PEOPLE

Physiological
    Normal subjects: sleep jerks, hiccough, etc.

Essential
    Familial or sporadic; no other neurological deficits

Epilepsy

Encephalopathies
    Spinocerebellar degenerations
    Wilson's disease
    Torsion dystonia
    Progressive supranuclear palsy
    Huntington's chorea
    Post-hypoxic encephalopathy
    Post-traumatic encephalopathy

Dementias
    Alzheimer's disease
    Creutzfeld–Jakob disease

Metabolic and toxic disorders
    Hepatic failure
    Renal failure
    Hyponatraemia
    Hypoglycaemia
    Heavy metal poisoning

Focal brain disorders
    Stroke
    Post-haematoma

discussion of this complex and rare group of disorders, the reader is referred to the review by Marsden *et al.* (1982).

TICS

A tic is a stereotyped and apparently involuntary contraction of a muscle or group of muscles. The commonest tics are simple twitching movements caused by short-lived bursts of activity in a small muscle in the face or neck. Tics can be suppressed for a short while by a concentrated effort but a sense of tension and frustration builds up which is relieved by re-emergence of the tic.

Simple Tics

Parts of the muscles round the eyes or mouth are most often involved, including muscles of the nose, tongue, lips and larynx. Involvement of swallowing or respiratory muscles is sometimes combined with phonation to produce grunting or noisy snuffling sounds.

Complex Tics

Some patients exhibit more complex tics in which the head and neck are most commonly involved. Tics involving the shoulders or upper limbs are usually accompanied by head or facial movement. The most common lower limb tic consists of compulsive stamping movements.

The diagnosis of tics presents obvious difficulties particularly when they are relatively mild. A careful history and a reasonably prolonged period of observation may be necessary to establish that the patient is not in fact developing a condition such as torticollis or tardive dyskinesia.

The pathogenesis of tics is unknown and very often no treatment other than reassurance is necessary. Like other involuntary movements, tics are worse in situations of emotional stress. Control of anxiety and relaxation training may help. Patients with tics are said to be unusually difficult to hypnotize. The intermittent use of tranquillizers at times of stress may be helpful, but there is no evidence that these drugs have a specific effect upon the tics themselves.

Blepharospasm

Blepharospasm is involuntary, sustained and forcible closure of the eyelids. It may occur spontaneously or in response to continuous stimuli and is sometimes an isolated disorder, though it often accompanies basal ganglia diseases (Jan Kovic and Ford, 1983), notably postencephalitic parkinsonism. Similar spasms may occur as part of a levodopa-induced dyskinesia.

Isolated blepharospasm responds very poorly to drug treatment. Surgical denervation of the muscles in the upper part of the face is reserved for patients whose spasm is so severe that they cannot see enough to take on essential activities. Recently, some success has been achieved by the subcutaneous injection of very small doses of botulinum toxin into the region of the periorbital muscles (Elston and Ross Russell, 1985). This causes paralysis of the muscles lasting

several months and repeated doses may be necessary
to provide adequate relief. Such treatment does of
course need to be given with considerable care
because of the risk of entry of toxin into the
bloodstream which could be followed by paralysis of
the respiratory muscles; it is not yet established as a
standard clinical treatment.

Hemifacial Spasm

Hemifacial spasm starts as recurrent involuntary
contractions of the orbicularis oculi muscle on one
side of the face, which over the course of weeks or
months come to involve the rest of the muscles on
that side. As the disorder progresses, the affected
muscles may show evidence of weakness and denervation.

Hemifacial spasm is commoner in women and
occurs on the left side of the face more frequently
than on the right. This is presumed to result from a
structural lesion at the point at which the facial nerve
leaves the brain stem to cross the cerebellopontine
angle. Pulsatile compression by elongated arterial
loops (notably the posterior inferior cerebellar
artery) is the commonest cause, but many other
kinds of pathology have been described and thus the
syndrome is a non-specific indication of a structural
lesion in this area.

Surgical microvascular decompression (Jannetta,
1982) is now preferred to surgical crushing of the
nerve which tended to replace the spasm by paralysis. This could be another indication for local
injection of botulinum toxin, but this treatment is
still in its research phase. Drugs are of no value,
except to counteract the anxiety and depression that
any facial spasm tends to induce.

CONCLUSION

In conclusion, involuntary movements occur fairly
frequently in elderly people, but fortunately they are
not usually a sign of a serious or life-threatening
disease and their effect upon the patient's life is more
likely to be one of embarrassment than impairment
of physical functions. As with other conditions
occurring in elderly people, the inconvenience and

risks of treatment need to be judged very carefully
against the benefits. Discussion and careful explanation are the cornerstones of management.

REFERENCES

Beattie, A., and Caird, F.I. (1980). The occupational
    therapist and the patient with Parkinson's disease. *Br.
    Med. J.*, **163**, 1354–5.
Cleeland, C.S. (1973). Behavioural technics in the modifi-
    cation of spasmodic torticollis. *Neurology*, **23**, 1241–7.
Couch, J.R. (1976). Dystonia and tremor in spasmodic
    torticollis. In: Eldridge, R., and Fahn, S. (eds.) *Advances
    in Neurology Vol. 14: Dystonias*, Raven Press, New York,
    pp. 245–58.
Critchley, M. (1949). Observations on essential (heredo
    familial) tremor. *Brain*, **72**, 113–39.
Elston, J.S., and Ross Russell, R.W. (1985). Effect of
    treatment with botulinum toxin on neurogenic blephar-
    ospasm. *Br. Med. J.*, **ii**, 1845–59.
Findley, L.J., and Calzetti, S. (1982). Double-blind
    controlled study of primidone in essential tremor:
    preliminary results. *Br. Med. J.*, **285**, 608.
Hughes, M., and McLellan, D.L. (1985). Increased co-
    activation of the upper limb muscles in writer's cramp.
    J. Neurol. Neurosurg. Psychiatry, **48**, 782–7.
Jannetta, P.J. (1982). Surgical approach to hemifacial
    spasm: Microvascular decompression. In: Marsden,
    C.D., and Fahn, S. (eds.) *Movement Disorders*, Butter-
    worth Scientific, London, pp. 330–3.
Jan Kovic, J., and Ford, J. (1983). Blepharospasm of
    orofacial–cervical dystonia: clinical and pharmacologi-
    cal findings in 100 patients. *Ann. Neurol.*, **13**, 402–11.
Koop, H.R. (1986). The effects of ageing. In: Ashbury,
    A.K., McKhann, G.M., and McDonald, W.I. (eds.)
    Diseases of the Nervous System, William Heinemann
    Medical Books, London, pp. 736–45.
Korein, J., Brading, J. *et al.* (1976). Sensory feedback
    therapy of spasmodic torticollis and dystonia: Results in
    treatment of 55 patients. In: Eldridge, R., and Fahn, S.
    (eds.) *Advances in Neurology Vol. 14: Dystonias*, Raven
    Press, New York, pp. 375–402.
Mackay, A.V.P. (1982). Clinical controversies in tardive
    dyskinesia. In: Marsden, C.D., and Fahn, J. (eds.)
    Movement Disorders, Butterworth Scientific, London, pp.
    249–62.
Magnussen, E. *et al.* (1977). Palatal myoclonus treated
    with 5-hydroxytryptophan and a decarboxylase inhibi-
    tor. *Acta Neurol. Scand.*, **55**, 251–3.
Marsden, C.D., and Fahn, S. (1982). Problems in dyskine-
    sias. In: Marsden, C.D., and Fahn, J. (eds.) *Movement
    Disorders*, Butterworth Scientific, London, pp. 192–3.
Marsden, C.D., Hallett, M., and Fahn, S. (1982). The
    nosology and pathophysiology of myoclonus. In: Mars-
    den, C.D., and Fahn, S. (eds.) *Movement Disorders*,

Butterworth Scientific, London, pp. 196–248.

Marsden, C.D., Mindham, R.H.S., and Mackay, A.V.P. (1983). Extrapyramidal movement disorders produced by antipsychotic drugs. In: Bradley, P.B., and Hirsch, S.R. (eds.) *The Pharmacology and Treatment of Schizophrenia*, Oxford University Press.

Marsden, C.D., Tarsey, D., and Baldessarini, R.J. (1975). Spontaneous and drug-induced movement disorders in psychotic patients. In: Benson, D.F., and Blumer, D. (eds.) *Psychiatric Aspects of Neurological Disease*, Grune and Stratton, New York.

Mutch, W.J. *et al.* (1986). Parkinson's disease: disability, review and management. *Br. Med. J.*, **213**, 675–7.

Oxtoby, M. (1982). *Parkinson's Disease, Patients and their Social Needs*. Parkinson's Disease Society, London.

Rothwell, J.C., Obesso, J.A. *et al.* (1983). Pathophysiology of dystonias. In: Demedt, J.E. (ed.) *Motor Control Mechanisms in Health and Disease*, Raven Press, New York.

Sakai, T. *et al.* (1981). Palatal myoclonus responding to carbamazepine. *Ann. Neurol.*, **9**, 199–200.

Schiele, B.C. *et al.* (1973). Neurological syndromes associated with antipsychotic drug use. *Arch. Gen. Psychiatry*, **28**, 463–7.

Sheehy, M.P., and Marsden, C.D. (1982). Writer's cramp—a focal dystonia. *Brain*, **105**, 461–80.

Sudarsky, L., and Routhal, M. (1983). Gait disorders among elderly patients: A study of 50 patients. *Arch. Neurol.*, **40**, 740–3.

Weiner, W.J., and Klawson, H.C. (1973). Lingual-buccal-facial movements in the elderly: Pathophysiology and treatment. *J. Am. Geriatr. Soc.*, **21**, 318–20.

Williams, A. *et al.* (1978). Palatal myoclonus following herpes zoster ameliorated by 5-hydroxytryptophan and carbidopa. *Neurology*, **28**, 358–9.

The Clinical Neurology of Old Age
Edited by R. Tallis
© 1989 John Wiley & Sons Ltd

Chapter 11

Motor Neurone Disease

Paul Newrick

Senior Medical Registrar, Bristol Royal Infirmary, Bristol, UK

Motor neurone disease (MND) is a highly unpleasant and mysterious condition that offers one of the great challenges in neurology to patient, family and doctor. Charcot, in 1865, was the first to differentiate MND from the many other causes of muscular atrophy which had until then been combined. Over the course of 20 years, he described the clinical and pathological features of this nervous system degeneration with great clarity (Charcot and Joffroy, 1869; Charcot, 1886). However, it has subsequently been recognized that the boundaries of MND are not totally distinct. It overlaps with degenerative central nervous system conditions such as dementia (Castaigne *et al.*, 1972), Parkinson's disease (Bonduelle *et al.*, 1968) and other system atrophies with similar features that occur in different age groups. There is also overlap with entities causing disease of motor neurones, such as viruses and toxins. However, there does remain the widely recognized clinical entity corresponding to idiopathic classical MND, otherwise known as amyotrophic lateral sclerosis in North America.

EPIDEMIOLOGY

The epidemiology of MND is remarkably uniform throughout the world except for two regions of high incidence centring around Guam in the Pacific and the Kii Peninsula in South Japan where the incidence is over fifty times greater. Allowing for variations in reporting, availability of diagnostic facilities and differing classifications, the age-adjusted mortality rate for MND is 0.7–1 per 100 000 (Kurland, 1957). Race, city dwelling and latitude appear to have no influence. Most series have found male to female sex ratios of between 1 and 2 to 1. A recent survey of deaths from MND in England and Wales over the years 1959–79 (Buckley *et al.*, 1983) found an age-adjusted death rate of 1.2 per 100 000 initially rising to 1.6 at the end of the survey period. This rise was most apparent in those over 60 and may depend on improved diagnosis and certification. The sex ratio was consistently about 1.6 : 1. There was a tendency to clustering along the South coast which may be partly attributable to migration of retired old people.

AETIOLOGY

The simple statement that the cause of MND is unknown neglects the great efforts that have gone into aetiological research. Unfortunately, there have been a large number of false trails and unfulfilled promises, rather as with research into multiple sclerosis. It is, of course, much more difficult to determine the cause of a degenerative process rather than one signalled by a clear biochemical clue.

Some of the many observations and suggestions made concerning the aetiology of MND are shown in Table 11.1.

A current area of great interest and promise is that related to nucleic acids. Surviving normal motor

TABLE 11.1 FACTORS IMPLICATED IN THE AETIOLOGY OF MND

Observation/suggestion	Comment	Reference
Epidemiological		
M:F excess	Unhelpful	Buckley *et al.* (1983)
Familial cases	Unhelpful	Buckley *et al.* (1983)
Excess in leather workers	Unhelpful	Buckley *et al.* (1983)
Biochemical/toxic		
Abnormal Ca metabolism	Not understood	Mallette *et al.* (1975)
		Patten and Mallette (1976)
Lead and heavy metals in central nervous system	? Secondary	Kurlander and Patten (1979)
		Yoshimasu *et al.* (1980)
Tri-cresyl phosphate	Irrelevant	Senanayake (1981)
Impaired glucose tolerance	? Secondary	Collins and Engel (1968)
		Shahani *et al.* (1971)
Hexosaminidase deficiency	Not understood	Johnson (1982)
Impaired DNA repair	Promising: see text	
Histopathological		
Skin changes	Not specific	Fullmer *et al.* (1966)
Arterial changes		Stortebecker *et al.* (1970)
Antecedent events		
Tonsillectomy	? Significance	Kahle (1956)
Subtotal gastrectomy	Not relevant	Kondo (1979)
Lead exposure	? Significance	Campbell *et al.* (1970)
Animal hide contact	? Significance	Hanisch *et al.* (1976)
Back injury	? Significance	Gawel *et al.* (1983)
Electric shock	? Significance	Gawel *et al.* (1983)
Malignancy	Uncommon, cases atypical	Norris and Engel (1964)
Immunological		
HLA 3 excess	Uncertain	Antel *et al.* (1976)
Myelinotoxic antibodies	? Secondary	Antel *et al.* (1982)
Antibodies inhibiting neuronal sprouting	? Secondary	Antel *et al.* (1982)
Slow viral		
Previous poliomyelitis	? Accelerated ageing	Mulder *et al.* (1972)
Type C oncornavirus	Mice only	Andrews and Gardener (1974)

neurones in MND have up to 40% less RNA, and that abnormal in composition (Davidson and Hartmann, 1981). Wobbler mice suffer a progressive degeneration of cervical cord motor neurones and have decreased RNA content and protein synthesis (Murakami *et al.*, 1981). These findings probably result from impaired DNA transcription which leads inevitably to accumulation of abnormal cell proteins and defective enzyme systems. A variety of neurological conditions have now been shown to have impaired mechanisms for DNA repair, including

Friedreich's ataxia and ataxia telangiectasia (Bradley and Krasin, 1982). Deficiencies in DNA repair might conceivably be present in the nervous system of MND sufferers and lead to slow accumulation of defective DNA and thus eventually to cell death. This theory allows for a long delay before clinical disease appears and also for a very large variety of factors to be instrumental in stressing the motor neurones to the point at which cell death occurs.

Numerous factors have been investigated. It seems likely that most are merely associations or epiphenomena. Possibly a variety of non-specific insults may be able to produce MND through a final common pathway such as that suggested by the DNA hypothesis.

PATHOLOGY

The essential features are the progressive degeneration and loss of anterior horn cells, most marked in the cervical and lumbar cord, and degeneration of the crossed and uncrossed pyramidal tracts. Cranial nerve nuclei in the brain stem show similar changes usually sparing the third, fourth and sixth nuclei. Secondary gliosis is seen but there is no inflammatory infiltrate. Cortical and subcortical neuronal loss occurs which may be diffuse or localized to the motor strip. Neurofibrillary tangles of the Alzheimer type are not seen in cases in this country, but anterior horn cell inclusions have been observed. Muscles show features of neurogenic atrophy. Peripheral nerves show atrophic changes (Dyck *et al.*, 1975), and occasionally degenerative change in sensory pathways in spinal cord has been described (Brownell *et al.*, 1970). These latter changes may be related to the sensory phenomena often experienced by patients early in the course of the disease.

CLINICAL

MND is essentially a disease of older people with a mean age of onset of 56.5 years (Bonduelle *et al.*, 1970). More than a third of cases start after age 60 and a tenth after age 70. The mean duration of survival is around 3 years, being shorter in those with a bulbar onset (Bonduelle and Bouygues, 1971). This figure masks the fact that disease duration is extremely variable with some surviving more than 10 years and a few less than 1 year. In general, the older the patient the shorter and more severe the course of the disease (Rosen, 1978). Ninety-five per cent of all cases of MND are sporadic. The remaining cases are familial or of the Guam type, but tend to have additional clinical and pathological features and may be different entities altogether.

MND encompasses a spectrum. There are three recognizable clinical syndromes but they virtually always overlap and form a continuum of subtypes.

Progressive muscular atrophy is the term used when the anterior horn cells of the spinal cord are most severely affected. The brain stem analogue of this is called progressive bulbar palsy. Both of these atrophies present features of a lower motor neurone lesion. The third type, integrated as amyotrophic lateral sclerosis, adds upper motor neurone signs to the overall picture. This sort of separation is rather artificial because, with time, the majority of patients manifest features of all three.

Initial clinical presentations are variable and often unilateral or asymmetrical. Patients may complain of easy tiring and weakness of a whole or part of a limb. Usually, however, the complaint is of difficulty with particular movements or actions. Thus, a patient may have noticed that his feet slap on the ground, that he trips easily or that he can no longer do up buttons or hold cutlery. If the weakness is proximal he will complain that he cannot rise up from the chair, climb stairs or brush his hair. Fasciculation may be described as muscles 'jumping' or 'bubbling', and muscle wasting (especially in the hands) is often mentioned directly. Prominent sensory symptoms, especially if associated with sensory signs, should make one consider an alternative diagnosis. Nevertheless, a proportion of patients do experience paraesthesiae, burning, formication and vague discomfort in the early stages (Charcot, 1886). If the initial presentation is of bulbar palsy the patient complains indirectly of dysfunction of lips, tongue, pharynx and larynx, that is of having noticed that his speech is slurred, with particular difficulty with consonants, that his tongue is 'clumsy' and food collects in the mouth. Chewing is tiring and initiation of swallowing difficult. He may dribble easily and the voice may have become hoarse, indistinct or nasal in quality. Liquids may precipitate choking or nasal regurgitation. Solid food becomes increasingly difficult to manage. A proportion will notice exertional breathlessness due to diaphragmatic and intercostal muscle weakness.

Pure upper motor neurone disease is rare and in general exists in varying combination with progressive muscular atrophy and progressive bulbar palsy. This clinical picture with a mixture of signs is generally termed amyotrophic lateral sclerosis and accounts for half of the cases at presentation and four-fifths in the terminal phases (Bonduelle *et al.*, 1970). In addition to the above symptoms, patients also often complain of stiffness and cramps. Indeed, these may pre-date all else by several months. Jerking and spasms of the limbs may be provoked by a large variety of non-specific stimuli. Unusual reflexes may become apparent such as the arm–mouth reflex in which elbow flexion and extension elicits mouth opening (Kuroda *et al.*, 1985). Bulbar problems are compounded by defective control of emotion with easily provoked and inappropriate crying and laughing. Intellect and sphincter control are usually maintained right to the end of the illness.

The clinical signs in a classical case of MND are straightforward. Widespread wasting of muscles (distal at first, spreading proximally) in combination with weakness (initially often less than the degree of wasting would suggest), fasciculation (occurring in both normal and affected muscle and frequently missed on the trunk) and altered reflexes, in the absence of sensory loss, make up an unmistakable picture. Reflexes are heightened and limb tone increased (often with clonus) with upper motor neurone involvement but may disappear as lower motor neurone atrophy progresses. Typically, lower motor neurone signs predominate in the arms and upper motor neurone signs in the legs. This leads to a combination of weak wasted arms and weak spastic legs with extensor plantar responses.

Bulbar palsy manifests with weakness and wasting of the tongue, facial and jaw muscles. Fasciculation is often gross in the tongue which is shrivelled. The jaw jerk is absent and gag reflex impaired. The head may droop because of weak sternomastoids and the patient may continually wipe away dribbled saliva. If the patient is given a glass of water to drink he will do so slowly and may choke and splutter, perhaps with nasal regurgitation. The voice is weak and difficulty is experienced initially with 'd' and 't' and later with labial consonants like 'p' and 'f'. Eventually anarthria results. Coughing is weak and bovine sounding and the face may become expressionless.

Pseudobulbar palsy, due to upper motor neurone involvement, is also manifest as a weak face, jaw and tongue but wasting is absent. The tongue tends to be pointed and stiff. The jaw jerk and gag reflex are exaggerated. Dysarthria is prominent and speech tends to be indistinct, monotonous and slow with prolonged gaps between syllables and words. Expert assessment can distinguish the patterns of speech disturbance associated with bulbar, pseudobulbar and mixed cases (Darley *et al.*, 1969) but most clinicians find this difficult and unnecessary. Usually, as in the limbs, a mixed bulbar picture is found with a combination of atrophic and spastic features.

Many patients, at least initially, present a less clear-cut problem. There may be bizarre patterns of wasting involving perhaps a single limb or part of a limb. Wasting may be seen both distally and proximally in a limb with sparing of intervening musculature. Individual muscles may be wasted in a non-classical pattern that is neither segmental nor symmetrical. Sensory symptoms and non-specific tiredness may deflect attention from early upper motor neurone signs, and a subtle disturbance of speech missed or dismissed as being due to loose dentures. Thus, early bulbar signs that would, in conjunction with limb signs, alert one to a diagnosis of MND may be overlooked. In general, however, most patients exhibit diffuse motor neurone signs that with follow-up become upper and lower in type, tend towards a symmetrical pattern and spread to involve both limbs and brain stem.

During the early course of the disease the differential diagnosis is vast, suggesting as it may do numerous pathological processes at many levels of the nervous system. The non-specificity of early symptoms such as tiredness and cramps may lead one to consider depression or non-neurological disease. With time, however, the diagnosis becomes clear. Table 11.2 summarizes possible sources of confusion early on, but few conditions resemble full-blown MND.

Weak wasted arms with spastic legs due to syringomyelia should not be confused if the characteristic sensory loss is looked for. Cervical spondylosis with cord compression can be a difficult differential especially if sensory loss is minimal. The slow progression will usually distinguish it from MND. Cervical disc protrusions will be seen on myelography but can, of course, coexist with MND. Occasionally, the situation does not become clear until after a cervical decompression procedure.

TABLE 11.2 DIFFERENTIAL DIAGNOSES OF MOTOR NEURONE DISEASE

Feature	Possible confusion with
Wasted arms with spastic legs	Syringomyelia Cervical spondylosis with myelopathy
Unilateral hand wasting	T1 root compression Cervical cord tumour Pachymeningitis Ulnar/median nerve lesion
Spastic paraparesis	Demyelination Cord compression Subacute combined degeneration
Distal weakness/ wasting	Peripheral neuropathy
Proximal weakness/ wasting	Polymyositis Carcinomatous myopathy Diabetic amyotrophy Endocrine/metabolic myopathy
Bulbar disturbance	Brain stem stroke/tumour Myasthenia gravis Syringobulbia Thyrotoxicosis
Muscle wasting	Simple atrophy of elderly Poor diet/malabsorption Malignancy
Cramps	Benign Hypothyroidism Electrolyte disturbance

Presentation with unilateral hand wasting should prompt consideration of a cord or root (e.g. cervical rib) lesion. Such wasting may be due to MND but it is important not to miss root or nerve compression, a spinal tumour or syphilitic pachymeningitis. Presentation as isolated spastic paraparesis should normally prompt investigation for cord compression.

Proximal limb weakness and/or wasting can be confused early on with polymyositis or carcinomatous myopathy. Metabolic conditions (such as osteomalacia, alcohol abuse or diabetic amyotrophy) or endocrine conditions (chiefly adrenal or thyroid disease) also need consideration. In MND, weakness rarely remains confined to a proximal distribution

and muscle tenderness is lacking. Distal weakness or wasting may raise the possibility of one of the many peripheral neuropathies. Here, the progressive course of the disease and the absence of sensory loss make the diagnosis clear, although carcinomatous motor neuropathy can be a difficult differential.

Initial presentation with bulbar disturbance might suggest a vascular accident but the progression of symptoms beyond the brain stem will suggest MND. Syringobulbia may be considered but the presence of nystagmus, vertigo and facial sensory loss eases correct diagnosis. Myasthenia gravis is a possible source of error and any hint of variability or eye signs should prompt a Tensilon test. Occasionally, inflammatory myopathy and thyrotoxicosis (often masked in the elderly) manifest initially with bulbar dysfunction.

Muscle wasting is a feature of many diseases such as carcinomas, malabsorption or the simple atrophy and loss of muscle bulk seen in the elderly. Unlike MND these conditions are associated with little or no weakness. Fasciculation is common and can be precipitated by cold (as in many examination rooms), anxiety and cigarettes. It is usually a benign symptom but when seen in conjunction with wasting indicates active denervation. This will often be due to MND but is also seen in thyrotoxicosis and with anticholinesterases, but these should not be confused easily. Muscle cramps are a frequent and early feature of MND but are a common benign phenomenon of all age groups, as well as being seen commonly in the elderly especially if hypothyroid, dehydrated or on diuretics.

INVESTIGATIONS

The amount of investigation will obviously depend on the clinical setting. It is good clinical practice to restrict tests to those required to exclude a treatable condition. This applies especially in the elderly where concurrent pathology or social circumstances may limit the therapeutic options. In general, the possibility of root or cord compression should be pursued with the appropriate bone radiographs and myelography. Syphilis serology and simple screening tests including chest film, full blood count, viscosity, blood glucose, liver function tests, calcium and thyroid function tests are always indicated.

Repeated blood testing through the course of the illness should be avoided. Whether or not to look for the carcinoma which is associated with a few cases is a moot point. There are very few cases in which treatment of the underlying tumour has led to improvement in the neurological state (Norris and Engel, 1965), although chemotherapy of myeloma has benefited a small number of MND patients. Normally, therefore, it is not helpful to hunt for a primary tumour. Electromyography (EMG) is usually performed, although in clear-cut cases, this only serves to demonstrate to patient and family that the problem is being given careful thought. It will be helpful in early cases with asymmetrical presentations to map out areas of motor neurone deficit in clinically uninvolved muscles and thus confirm the presence of a widespread disorder. Typically recordings demonstrate fasciculation, and sometimes fibrillation potentials also. Recordings during voluntary contraction show motor units of increased duration, and reduced patterns at maximum voluntary effort, helping to distinguish the neurogenic atrophy of MND from a primary myopathic process. EMG also helps to exclude MND in a thin old person with benign fasciculation. Sensory nerve conduction velocities remain normal while maximum motor velocities show no more than slight slowing corresponding to progressive fallout of motor neurones as the disease progresses. Somatosensory evoked potentials are said to be slowed in MND (Cosi *et al.*, 1984) but their utility is not yet established, especially in the elderly who may have confounding pathology such as cervical radiculopathy. Creatine phosphokinase (CPK) is mildly elevated in MND while aldolase is normal. This may help to distinguish MND with unusually severe pain from polymyositis, in which the enzymes tend to be grossly raised.

Muscle biopsy early on is normal or shows denervation atrophy only. Later on changes normally associated with myopathy may be seen and in these cases, CPK tends to be higher (Achari and Anderson, 1974). Muscle biopsy should only exceptionally be required. Cerebrospinal fluid (CSF) examination should not be a routine but can conveniently be taken if myelography is performed. Up to one-third of patients show an elevation in total protein, usually less than 1 g/litre (Guiloff *et al.*, 1980).

MANAGEMENT

Management is essentially supportive. This common and rather bleak neurological dictum means that more, rather than less, effort is required from everyone concerned. Above all, management is a joint process involving liaison between medical and paramedical personnel and family members. Many old people are socially isolated and without family. They may still be maintained in the community for long periods with outpatient care and mobilization of the appropriate services. Psychological support is a very important aspect. Maintenance of a positive attitude by patient and family in the face of advancing disability is possible given honest discussion, excellent treatment and a rapid response time to fresh problems as they arise.

A wide variety of treatments designed to halt the disease have been tried without success (Goldblatt, 1977). Particular lines pursued recently include immunosuppression (Norris, 1972), antivirals (Brooke, 1977) and thyrotrophin releasing hormone (Imoto *et al.*, 1984). Anticholinesterases such as neostigmine may be of slight transient benefit (Lambert and Mulder, 1957), especially in bulbar weakness. Drooling can be eased by reduction of salivation with anticholinergic agents such as benzhexol. If necessary, bilateral transtympanic neurectomy (Zalin and Cooney, 1974) will reduce salivation to minimal levels, as will salivary irradiation.

Cramps and troublesome spasticity can be reduced with diazepam (Valium), baclofen (Lioresal) or dantrolene (Dantrium). Doses should be increased slowly so as to avoid a rapid increase in weakness which is a particular problem with dantrolene. In general, drugs have only a small part to play in MND.

Exercise, besides keeping joints mobile and preventing contractures, may also strengthen surviving motor units, and has been claimed to maintain function longer (Sinaki and Mulder, 1978). Even a frail old person can be reassured that activity is beneficial and will not accelerate deterioration.

There are many aids that can help patients when weakness progresses to the point of disability, and the advice and support of an occupational therapist are essential. Weak grip may be improved with the use of a cock-up wrist splint. Clumsy fingers will find Velcro fasteners easier than buttons and large handled cutlery makes meal times simpler. Foot drop causing trips and falls may be helped by a custom-built moulded splint or caliper. A physiotherapist should be available to make up splints and liaise with the occupational therapist about the supply of the appropriate sticks, crutches or walking frames. Eventually a wheelchair becomes necessary. It is vital that careful thought is given to its supply and whether indoor or outdoor models or both are needed. It should be comfortable enough to sit in for long periods with a weight spreading cushion (such as the Roho) and have adequate foot, back and head rests. Ball-bearing arm supports can be fixed to the chair and by taking the weight of the arms give an increase in functional strength. Electrically operated wheelchairs, requiring the use of a variety of controls, are often too difficult for an old person to manoeuvre and only cause frustration. Weak neck muscles causing lolling of the head should be supported with a comfortable collar which needs to be expertly fitted if it is to be worn all day long. A spare should also be provided to allow for washing. A commode and bath aids are very helpful until late on into the illness.

Bulbar disabilities are among the most distressing. They are embarrassing (dribbling), frightening (choking) and frustrating (communication impairment). All these problems can be assuaged with the right advice and treatment. Drooling can be tackled pharmacologically or with salivary denervation or irradiation, but a ready supply of absorbent tissues also helps considerably. Oral candidiasis should be watched for as an aggravating factor. Dysphagia can be helped with simple advice about small frequent meals of soft food with little liquid. If necessary, a liquidizer should be provided so that any food desired can be taken in semisolid form. If oropharyngeal spasticity rather than wasting predominates, dysphagia may be improved by sucking an ice cube just before the meal (Campbell and Enderby, 1984). In this situation, antispasticity drugs or the simple procedure of cricopharyngeal myotomy can be very useful (Loizou *et al.*, 1980). The incidence of choking on food or pooled secretions can be reduced by good positioning and the encouragement of slow relaxed

meal times (Blount *et al.*, 1979). Repeated choking suggests the need for an indwelling micro-bore nasogastric tube which is usually well tolerated. A relative can be trained to use a portable foot-operated sucker at home for repeated choking on secretions.

Speech disturbance requires specialized advice and follow-up from an experienced speech therapist, as four or more different communication aids may be needed as time progresses (Campbell and Enderby, 1984). In the early stages, dysarthria may be improved with a palatal lift prosthesis (Gonzalez and Aronson, 1970). Needs will vary from simple aids such as a notepad or pointing board to sophisticated electronic instruments with a keyboard and visual or printed output of words or pre-programmed messages. Some devices have the additional advantage of a synthesized voice output which is useful for those with poor vision. As the use of the arms is lost, a scanning aid can be employed in which letters or predetermined messages are lit up with a cursor moved by means of an appropriate microswitch (e.g. under the chin). Finally, when all voluntary movements have faded simple communication can be maintained using eye-movements to 'point' out symbols printed on a clear plastic board held by the observer. All these aids require encouragement and persistence if they are to be effective. Old people, especially, may find the more technological devices too difficult and prefer the simpler items.

Finally, in the terminal stages, dedicated nursing assumes the greatest importance, with life spent between a reclining chair and bed. At this stage, frequent holiday relief admissions are much appreciated and by alleviating strain on the family and community nursing services help to keep the patient at home as long as possible.

The foregoing discussion omits some of the less 'neurological' problems that are a reality of life with MND. A recent study (Newrick and Langton Hewer, 1984) identified falls, constipation, leg swelling, sleep disturbance and pain as major symptomatic problems. These can often be at least partially prevented by early advice. Pain occurs in over half of cases including those who are still independent (Newrick and Langton Hewer, 1985) and is difficult or even impossible to control fully. Much of the pain is musculoskeletal or skin pressure related (Saunders *et al.*, 1981) and although frequent repositioning and simple analgesics help, opiates are often required. Poor sleeping is due to a combination of secretions pooling in the throat and inability to change position. Until a patient-operated turning bed is widely available, the load of repetitive turning at night will continue to fall on the family.

Management of a condition such as MND inevitably warrants consideration of the organization involved. Neurology clinics tend to be disliked, especially by the more disabled patients (Newrick and Langton Hewer, 1984). Problems identified include long waits for transport, seeing inexperienced junior staff and being unsure whom to contact if problems arise with aids or benefits. Inadequate provision of aids and home modifications is a particular problem that occurs frequently. The need for aids or adaptations should be forecast and organized before the situation is urgent. Timing is critical in a progressive disorder and it is disheartening in the extreme for a patient to wait for a device only to find he is no longer in a position to use it.

Who should supervise the MND patient? On the one hand there are the logistic difficulties of following severely disabled people in the hospital clinic and, on the other, there is the need for specialized skills and aids not readily available in the community. A great number of highly skilled professionals are an indispensable part of the team working with the doctor engaged in the care of MND sufferers. The primary health care team is unlikely to have all the resources required. One suggestion has been that a key-worker (perhaps a nurse) should be established from existing staff, to act as the patient's first point of contact, and liaise with all the other hospital and community staff involved (Newrick and Langton Hewer, 1984). It is not clear, at present, what care model is best but enthusiasm is an essential component.

ETHICAL CONSIDERATIONS

MND poses many difficult ethical problems. Should tracheostomy, gastrostomy or mechanical ventilation be performed in a tetraparetic patient with weeks to live? Should opiates be prescribed for pain relief in a patient with severe bulbar palsy and risk respiratory depression? What of intercurrent medical and surgical problems? One must try to find the middle way between therapeutic nihilism and overzealous meddling. There are no hard rules about what constitutes prolonging distress. It is well worth reading the reports (Saunders *et al.*, 1981; Norris *et al.*, 1985) of those with experience of large numbers of MND patients as background to any decision one might take.

MND is a devastating condition but one should resist feelings of hopelessness. Much of the misery can be relieved with expert management, anticipation of future problems, intelligent use of aids and full employment of all the resources available to the therapeutic team.

REFERENCES

Achari, A.N., and Anderson, M.S. (1974). Myopathic changes in amyotrophic lateral sclerosis. *Neurology*, **24**, 477–81.

Andrews, J.M., and Gardener, M.B. (1974). Lower motor neurone degeneration associated with type-C RNA virus infection in mice: neuropathological features. *J. Neuropathol. Exp. Neurol.*, **33**, 285–307.

Antel, J., Amason, B., Fuller, T., and Lehrich, J. (1976). Histocompatibility-typing in amyotrophic lateral sclerosis. *Arch. Neurol.*, **33**, 423–5.

Antel, J.P., Naronha, A.B.C., Oger, J.J.-F., and Amason, B.G.W. (1982). Immunology of amyotrophic lateral sclerosis. In: Rowland, L.P. (ed.) *Human Motor Neuron Diseases*, Raven Press, New York, pp. 395–402.

Blount, M., Bratton, C., and Luttrell, N. (1979). The management of the patient with amyotrophic lateral sclerosis. *Nurs. Clin. North Am.*, **77**, 1–3.

Bonduelle, M., and Bouygues, P. (1971). Sclérose latérale amyotrophique (Maladie de Charcot). *Encyclopédie médico-chirurgical. Système Nerveux*, 17, Paris, pp. 1–20.

Bonduelle, M., Bouygues, P., Escourolle, R., and Lomeau, G. (1968). Évolution simultanée d'une sclérose latérale amyotrophique d'un syndrome parkinsonien et d'une démence progressive. A propos de 2 observations anatomo-cliniques. Essai d'interprétation. *J. Neurol. Sci.*, **6**, 315–32.

Bonduelle, M., Bouygues, P., Lormeau, G., and Keller, J. (1970). Étude clinique et évolutive de 125 cas de sclérose latérale amyotrophique. Limites nosographiques et associations morbides. *Presse Méd.*, **78**, 827–32.

Bradley, W.G., and Krasin, E. (1982). A new hypothesis of the aetiology of amyotrophic lateral sclerosis. *Arch. Neurol.*, **39**, 677–80.

Brooke, M.H. (1977). In: *A Clinician's View of Neuromuscular Diseases*, Williams and Wilkins, Baltimore, Md, pp. 44–57.

Brownell, B., Oppenheimer, D.R., and Hughes, J.T. (1970). The central nervous system in motor neuron disease. *J. Neurol. Neurosurg. Psychiatry*, **33**, 338–57.

Buckley, J., Warlow, C., Smith, P., Hilton-Jones, D., Irvine, S., and Tew, J.R. (1983). Motor neurone disease in England and Wales, 1959–1979. *J. Neurol. Neurosurg. Psychiatry*, **46**, 197–205.

Campbell, A.M.G., Williams, E.R., and Barltrop, D. (1970). Motor neurone disease and exposure to lead. *J. Neurol. Neurosurg. Psychiatry*, **33**, 877–85.

Campbell, M.J., and Enderby, P. (1984). Management of motor neurone disease. *J. Neurol. Sci.*, **64**, 65–71.

Castaigne, P., Lhermitte, F., Cambier, J., Escourolle, R., and Le Bigot, P. (1972). Étude neuropathologique de 61 observations de sclérose latérale amyotrophique. Discussion nosologique. *Rev. Neurol. (Paris)*, **127**, 401–14.

Charcot, J.M. (1886). Leçons sur les maladies du Système Nerveux. In: Bourneville, M.M.D. (ed.) *Oeuvres Complètes*, 2, Delahaye and Lecrosnier, Paris, pp. 212–97.

Charcot, J.M., and Joffroy, A. (1869). Deuz cas d'atrophie musculaire progressive avec lesions de la substance grise et des faisceaux antérolatéraux de la moelle épinière. *Arch. Physiol. Neurol. Pathol.*, **2**, 354–67, 744–60.

Collis, W.J., and Engel, W. (1968). Glucose metabolism in five neuromuscular disorders. *Neurology*, **18**, 915–25.

Cosi, V., Poloni, M., Mazzini, L., and Callieco, R. (1984). Somatosensory evoked potentials in amyotrophic lateral sclerosis. *J. Neurol. Neurosurg. Psychiatry*, **47**, 857–61.

Darley, F.L., Aronson, A.E., and Brown, J.R. (1969). Differential diagnostic patterns of dysarthria. *Speech Res.*, **12**, 246–69.

Davidson, T.J., and Hartmann, H.A. (1981). RNA content and volume of motor neurons in amyotrophic lateral sclerosis. *J. Neuropathol. Exp. Neurol.*, **40**, 187–92.

Dyck, P.J., Stevens, J.C., Mulder, D.W., and Espinosa, R.E. (1975). Frequency of nerve fibre degeneration of peripheral motor and sensory neurons in amyotrophic lateral sclerosis. Morphology of deep and superficial peroneal nerves. *Neurology (Minneapolis)*, **25**, 781–5.

Fullmer, H.M., Lazarus, G., Gibson, W.A., Stam, A.C., and Link, C. (1966). Collagenolytic activity of the skin associated with neuromuscular diseases including amyotrophic lateral sclerosis. *Lancet*, **1**, 1007–9.

Gawel, M., Zaiwalla, Z., and Clifford Rose, F. (1983). Antecedent events in motor neurone disease. *J. Neurol. Neurosurg. Psychiatry*, **46**, 1041–3.

Goldblatt, D. (1977). Treatment of amyotrophic lateral sclerosis. In: Griggs, R.C., and Moxley, R.T. (eds.) *Advances in Neurology*, Vol. 17, Raven Press, New York, pp. 265–83.

Gonzalez, J.B., and Aronson, A.E. (1970). Palatal lift prosthesis for treatment of anatomic and neurologic palatopharyngeal insufficiency. *Cleft Palate J.*, **7**, 91–104.

Guiloff, R.J., McGregor, B., Thompson, E., Blackwood, W., and Paul, E. (1980). Motor neurone disease with elevated cerebrospinal fluid protein. *J. Neurol. Neurosurg. Psychiatry*, **43**, 390–6.

Gurney, M.E., Belton, A.C., Cashman, N., and Antel, J.P. (1984). Inhibition of terminal axonal sprouting by serum from patients with amyotrophic lateral sclerosis. *N. Engl. J. Med.*, **311**, 933–9.

Hanisch, R., Dworsky, R.L., and Henderson, B.E. (1976). A search for clues to the cause of amyotrophic lateral sclerosis. *Arch. Neurol.*, **33**, 456–7.

Imoto, K., Saida, K., Iwamura, K., Saida, T., and Nishitani, H. (1984). Amyotrophic lateral sclerosis; a double-blind crossover trial of thyrotrophin-releasing hormone. *J. Neurol. Neurosurg. Psychiatry*, **47**, 1332–4.

Johnson, W.G. (1982). Hexosaminidase deficiency; a cause of recessively inherited motor neuron diseases. In: Rowland, L.P. (ed.) *Human Motor Neuron Diseases*, Raven Press, New York, pp. 317–29.

Kahle, K.W. (1956). Bulbarparalytische verlaufsform der amyotrophischen lateral Sklerose nach tonsillektomie und Tonsillitis. *Dtsch Z. Nervenheilkal.*, **174**, 573–82.

Kondo, K. (1979). Does gastrectomy predispose to amyotrophic lateral sclerosis? *Arch. Neurol.*, **36**, 586–7.

Kurland, L.T. (1957). Epidemiological investigations of amyotrophic lateral sclerosis; III a genetic interpretation of incidence and geographic distribution. *Mayo Clin. Proc.*, **32**, 449–62.

Kurlander, H.M., and Patten, B.M. (1979). Metals in spinal cord tissue of patients dying of motor neurone disease. *Ann. Neurol.*, **16**, 21–4.

Kuroda, K., Oda, K., and Shibasaki H. (1985). The arm mouth reflex in a patient with amyotrophic lateral sclerosis. *J. Neurol. Neurosurg. Psychiatry*, **48**, 385–6.

Lambert, E.H., and Mulder, D.W. (1957). Electromyographic studies in amyotrophic lateral sclerosis. *Mayo Clin. Proc.*, **32**, 441–7.

Loizou, L.A., Small, M., and Dalton, G.A. (1980). Cricopharyngeal myotomy in motor neurone disease. *J. Neurol. Neurosurg. Psychiatry*, **43**, 42–5.

Mallette, L.E., Patten, B.M., and Engel, W.K. (1975). Neuromuscular disease in secondary hyperparathyroidism. *Ann. Intern. Med.*, **82**, 474–83.

Mulder, D.W., Rosenbaum, R.A., and Layton, D.D. (1972). Late progression of poliomyelitis of forme fruste of amyotrophic lateral sclerosis. *Mayo Clin. Proc.*, **27**, 756–61.

Murakami, T., Mastaglia, F.L., and Mann, D.M.A. (1981). Abnormal RNA metabolism in spinal motor neurons in the wobbler mouse. *Muscle Nerve*, **4**, 407–12.

Newrick, P.G., and Langton Hewer, R. (1984). Motor neurone disease: can we do better? A study of 42 patients. *Br. Med. J.*, **289**, 539–42.

Newrick, P.G., and Langton Hewer, R. (1985). Pain in

motor neurone disease. *J. Neurol. Neurosurg. Psychiatry*, **48**, 838–40.

Norris, F.H. (1972). Discussion. *Trans. Am. Neurol. Ass.*, **97**, 22.

Norris, F.H., and Engel, W.K. (1964). Neoplasia in patients with amyotrophic lateral sclerosis. *Trans. Am. Neurol. Ass.*, **89**, 238–40.

Norris, F.H., and Engel, E.K. (1965). Carcinomatous amyotrophic lateral sclerosis. In: Brain, Lord, and Norris, F.H. (eds.) *The Remote Effects of Cancer on the Nervous System*, Grune and Stratton, New York, pp. 24–34.

Norris, F.H., Smith, R.A., and Denys, E.H. (1985). Motor neurone disease: towards better care. *Br. Med. J.*, **291**, 259–62.

Patten, B.M., and Mallette, L.E. (1976). Motor neurone disease: retrospective study of associated abnormalities. *Dis. Nerv. Syst.*, **37**, 288–321.

Rosen, A.D. (1978). Amyotrophic lateral sclerosis: clinical features and prognosis. *Arch. Neurol.*, **35**, 638–42.

Saunders, C., Walsh, T.D., and Smith, M. (1981). Hospice care in motor neurone disease. In: Saunders, C., Summers, D.H., and Teller, N. *The Living Idea*, Edward Arnold, London.

Senanayake, N. (1981). Tri-cresyl phosphate neuropathy in Sri Lanka: a clinical and neurophysiological study with a 3 year follow-up. *J. Neurol. Neurosurg. Psychiatry*, **44**, 775–80.

Shahani, B., Davies-Jones, G.A.B., and Russell, W.R. (1971). Motor neurone disease: further evidence of an abnormality of nerve metabolism. *J. Neurol. Neurosurg. Psychiatry*, **34**, 185–91.

Sinaki, M., and Mulder, D.W. (1978). Rehabilitation techniques for patients with amyotrophic lateral sclerosis. *Mayo Clin. Proc.*, **53**, 173–8.

Stortebecker, P., Nordstrom, G., Pap de Pestery, M., Seeman, T., and Bjorkerud, S. (1970). Vascular and metabolic studies of amyotrophic lateral sclerosis. 1. Angiopathy in biopsy specimens of peripheral arteries. *Neurology (Minneapolis)*, **20**, 1157–60.

Yoshimasu, F., Yasui, M., Yase, Y., Iwata, S., Gajduse, D.C., Gibbs, C.J., and Chen, M. (1980). Studies on amyotrophic lateral sclerosis by neuron activation analysis. 2. Comparative studies of analytical results on Guam Parkinson's Disease and Japanese amyotrophic lateral sclerosis and Alzheimer disease cases. *Folia Psychiatr. Neurol. Jpn*, **34**, 7582.

Zalin, H., and Cooney, T.C. (1974). Chorda tympani neurectomy—a new approach to submandibular salivary obstruction. *Br. J. Surg.*, **61**, 391–4.

Chapter 12

Diseases of Muscle

Peter Hudgson

Consultant and Senior Lecturer in Neurology, Regional Neurological Centre, Newcastle General Hospital, Newcastle upon Tyne, UK

The principles underlying the investigation and treatment of elderly patients with neuromuscular disorders are exactly the same as those governing the management of children and younger adults in a similar predicament. Certainly the *diagnosis* of patients with neuromuscular diseases rests upon the following:

(1) Exhaustive and, if necessary, repeated clinical evaluation.
(2) Serum 'muscle' enzyme activity, particularly serum creatine kinase (CK) (a non-specific but reasonably accurate index of muscle cell necrosis).
(3) Electromyography (EMG) and nerve conduction velocity studies which should be carried out only in a properly equipped laboratory by experienced observers.
(4) Muscle biopsy with routine enzyme histochemical studies and at least preservation of part of the sample for subsequent ultrastructural studies if indicated. It goes without saying that this procedure should be carried out only in properly equipped departments staffed by those with appropriate technical as well as diagnostic expertise. A minority of patients may also require detailed biochemical/metabolic evaluation and this entails the provision of even more sophisticated laboratory facilities and expertise. Accordingly, it should be clear that the detailed

work-up of patients with neuromuscular disorders can be undertaken effectively only in specialized referral centres. However, that is not to say that the likely diagnosis and its therapeutic implications in their widest sense cannot be arrived at by an experienced clinician in a district general hospital.

The spectrum of muscle disease in the elderly differs both qualitatively and quantitatively from that seen in earlier periods of life. Perhaps the most striking difference is the under-representation of genetically determined disorders of the neuromuscular apparatus. Nonetheless there are exceptions, longevity being the rule in most families with hereditary motor-sensory neuropathy (HMSN Type I). In addition, occasional sporadic cases of spinal muscular atrophy present in the seventh decade (Harding and Thomas, 1980) and myotonic dystrophy has a distinct penchant for manifesting in late life with ptosis and only slight frontal baldness but no clinical myotonia. (This emphasizes the extraordinary variability in the phenotypic expression of the abnormal genome.) The writer has seen this phenomenon three times in elderly women who were investigated in the first instance as potential cases of chronic progressive external ophthalmoplegia (CPEO, see below) (Hudgson, 1986). In view of the relative scarcity of patients with genetically determined disorders of neuromuscular structure and function, however, it would seem reasonable to concentrate upon those conditions in which something can be achieved therapeutically, most particularly the inflammatory myopathies.

INFLAMMATORY MUSCLE DISEASE

Polymyalgia Rheumatica

This condition, described originally by Bruce (1888) as 'senile rheumatic gout' and known by a number of alternative sobriquets, is probably the most dramatic 'inflammatory' myopathy seen in clinical practice. To all intents and purposes, it occurs only in elderly subjects, presenting with progressive pain and stiffness but *not* weakness in the limb-girdle musculature. Ultimately the pain and stiffness (always worst on waking in the morning) may be so severe that the patient is immobilized completely. These symptoms are often accompanied by malaise, night sweats and weight loss and occasionally by other manifestations of the giant-cell arteritis of the aged, particularly cranial arteritis. Polymyalgia is in fact one form of this fascinating condition and its expression in muscle is unique insofar as the disorder of muscle function is not accompanied by the vascular abnormalities *in muscle* which are characteristic in other tissues, for example the superficial temporal arteries. In fact Brooke and Kaplan (1972) demonstrated Type IIb fibre atrophy in needle biopsy material from patients with polymyalgia which reverted to normal after treatment with corticosteroids in a serial biopsy study. The Type IIb fibre was presumably a consequence of the patient's immobility and certainly the biopsy material did not show any of the ischaemic changes described by Carpenter *et al.* (1976) in 'vasculitic' polymyositis (although muscle ischaemia would seem an entirely reasonable candidate for the principal pathogenetic factor on *a priori* grounds). However, synovial biopsy demonstrates typical granulomatous inflammation with giant cells in the media of the small arterial channels. Some of these patients have arthralgias or even a frank polyarthritis (Bruk, 1967).

There is no clinical weakness, as will be evident on examination if muscle pain permits sufficient cooperation, serum CK levels are not elevated and the EMG is normal. However, the erythrocyte sedimentation rate is grossly elevated in the vast majority of cases (this is not always so in the closely related condition cranial arteritis), not uncommonly exceeding 100 mm in the first hour. The combination of painful, stiff muscles with a very high ESR should certainly suggest the diagnosis of polymyalgia rheumatica and confirmation will be provided by a rapid resolution of the patient's symptoms on treatment with an oral corticosteroid, usually within 48–72 hours. Prednisone or prednisolone in a starting dose of 60 mg daily has been the regimen of choice in this department for some years. Great care must be taken not to reduce the dose too quickly after the patient's myalgia has settled as this carries a measurable risk of relapse or the emergence of another manifestation of giant-cell arteritis. Equally clearly, the risks of chronic over-treatment must always be borne in mind, particularly the development of a steroid myopathy (see below), aggravation of pre-existing senile osteoporosis, occasionally painless rupture of the Achilles tendon and gastrointestinal irritation. Concurrent administration of an H_2 receptor blocker may reduce the risk of the latter.

Occasional doubts have been expressed about the nosological status of polymyalgia rheumatica. In particular, it has been asserted that the condition is entirely epiphenomenal, being no more than a non-specific tissue response to other disease states, especially malignant neoplasms (Currey and Barnes, 1978). However, the author is unaware of any statistically validated studies confirming such an association. In his experience and that of his colleagues, polymyalgia rheumatica is a nosological entity in its own right with a consistent natural history and a close association with giant-cell arteritis of old age.

Polymyositis and Dermatomyositis

Hudgson and Walton (1979) reviewed the global epidemiology of inflammatory muscle disease in some detail and a reassessment of the situation during the ensuing 8 years has shown no major change in experience locally or elsewhere, including the Third World (although epidemiological data from Africa in particular are arguably less reliable than they were 10 years ago because of local politico-economic difficulties). Certainly the referral patterns for patients of all ages seen in this Centre have not changed appreciably in the last decade and the experience of colleagues in Western Europe, North America and Australasia is similar. However, our estimates of the incidence and prevalence of what many authorities now call 'idiopathic inflammatory myopathy' in the developed world are likely to be 'skewed' by the fact that the majority of cases are seen in so-called 'centres of reference' (Hoffman *et al.*, 1983). Nonetheless, a reasonably clear pattern of the global distribution of the various forms of inflammatory muscle disease has emerged during the last 10 years and it appears to be reasonably reproducible. This pattern is as follows:

(1) 'Myositis' in patients of all ages in the Third World is *infective* in origin, almost without exception. In the majority of cases, *Staphylococcus aureus*, phage Type II, will prove to be the infecting organism (Foster, 1965; Taylor and Henderson, 1972). It has been suggested that many, if not all, cases of 'tropical' *pyo*myositis are complications of underlying parasitic or viral myositis (Leading article, 1978). However, early and effective chemotherapeu-tic-cum-surgical treatment of the pyogenic infection will lead to satisfactory and usually rapid clinical resolution with little or nothing in the way of incapacitating residual deficit.

(2) Viral myositis is unquestionably the commonest form of inflammatory muscle disease seen in the developed world. Myalgia is a regular accompaniment of even trivial infections such as 'gastroenteritis' (Middleton *et al.*, 1970) and reaches its zenith in Bornholm disease, where anterior chest wall pain particularly may be mistaken for that of myocardial infarction. Most cases of Bornholm disease are due to direct invasion of the muscle cell by Coxsackie B5 virus.

It should be noted that *bacterial* myositis is exceedingly uncommon in the West, although occasional cases of gas gangrene due to infection with *Clostridium welchii* still occur, usually in patients sustaining

multiple injuries in road traffic accidents or after major abdominal surgery. In the latter instance, the afflicted individual is most often elderly and infirm.

(3) Polymyositis and dermatomyositis (hereafter referred to as 'idiopathic inflammatory myopathy' or IIM) constitute the commonest *acquired* non-infective myopathies seen in clinical practice in the West. Precise incidence and prevalence data are not available on a wide scale and, most particularly, in patients in the older age groups. Nonetheless, epidemiological studies in Memphis, Tennessee (Medsger *et al.*, 1970) indicate that the incidence of IIM in black females was three to four times higher than that in white females ($P < 0.001$). Similar differences have been determined in patients with systemic lupus erythematosus and progressive systemic sclerosis in the USA and are reflected in comparable epidemiological statistics in the north-east of England (De Vere and Bradley, 1975). The latter study suggested that the prevalence of IIM over a 20 year period up to the time of publication was approximately 8 per 100 000 of what *was* a relatively homogeneous population, although the sex incidence of IIM *reversed* over the age of 55 years, presumably a reflection of male smoking habits at the time—this statistic is almost certainly irrelevant now). It is to be hoped that an ongoing prospective study of the natural history of response to treatment of patients with IIM in the north-east of England (Lane *et al.*, 1982; Emslie-Smith and Hudgson, 1987) will shed further light on what remains a rather epidemiologically confused picture.

As far as the classification of IIM is concerned, it is not the purpose of this chapter to explore in detail the long-running controversy surrounding their precise nature and their relationships to each other and to malignant neoplasms. The reader is referred to Hudgson and Peter (1984) for a reasonably up-to-date review of the situation and to Tables 12.1 and 12.2 which summarize the views of 'lumpers' and 'splitters' respectively. Meanwhile, we should turn our attention to the two forms of 'idiopathic' inflammatory myopathy which occur with any frequency in the elderly: chronic 'pure' polymyositis in the female; and dermatomyositis in both sexes (but

TABLE 12.1 WALTON AND ADAMS' (1958) CLASSIFICATION OF INFLAMMATORY MUSCLE DISORDERS

Group I
'Pure' polymyositis
   This type of inflammatory myopathy may present
   in acute (rhabdomyolytic, myoglobinuric),
   subacute and chronic forms

Group II
Polymyositis with minimal or transient skin
involvement
   The commonest mode of presentation of subacute
   inflammatory muscle disease in young or middle-
   aged adults

Group III
Dermatomyositis and myositis associated with other
autoimmune disease

Group IV
Polymyositis and dermatomyositis in association with
malignant neoplasms

TABLE 12.2   BOHAN AND PETER'S (1975) CLASSIFICATION OF INFLAMMATORY MUSCLE DISORDERS

Group I
Primary 'idiopathic' polymyositis

Group II
Primary 'idiopathic' dermatomyositis

Group III
Dermatomyositis and polymyositis in association
with neoplasia

Group IV
Dermatomyositis or polymyositis with associated
collagen vascular disease ('overlap' syndromes)

---

predominantly the male).

Chronic polymyositis in middle-aged and elderly females without any associations was regarded as 'menopausal' or 'late-life' muscular dystrophy, notwithstanding the fact that inflammatory cell infiltrates had been observed in an early biopsy study of these patients (Nevin, 1936) and that they responded to treatment with ACTH (Shy and McEachern, 1951). Nattrass (1954) in his Presidential Address to the Section of Neurology in the Royal Society of Medicine noted that spontaneous remission, or at least a relapsing and remitting course, was by no means uncommon in these patients, suggesting that a genetically determined primary degeneration of the muscle cell was unlikely. (This was at a time when Ehrlich's doctrine of *horror autotoxicus* still held sway and the concept of autoimmunity was in its earliest infancy.) Since then, it has become clear that this condition is very much a member of the group of 'idiopathic' inflammatory myopathies (or conceivably a point on the spectrum thereof?) and a recent prospective study by Emslie-Smith *et al.* (1987) has shown a remarkably consistent association with autoimmune thyroiditis in these patients. Moreover, long-term immunosuppression with corticosteroids, azathioprine or a combination of the two will produce significant improvement or even remission in the majority (Lane *et al.*, 1982). However, great care has to be exercised with long-term corticosteroid therapy in these patients as they tend to be obese before the initiation of treatment and they develop cushingoid side-effects earlier and more severely than younger females with IIM.

It is always dangerous to apply general rules uncritically to individual cases. However, the risks of a patient over 60 years of age, irrespective of sex, with dermatomyositis harbouring a malignant neoplasm of some kind are so high that 'hunting the primary' is as important a part of patient management as treatment of the presenting problem. Certainly, all patients over the age of 60 years should be screened carefully to exclude epithelial, lymphoproliferative and myeloproliferative neoplasms, if necessary more than once. The often expressed contention that patients with paraneoplastic myopathies do not respond to immunosuppressive therapy is certainly not correct in every case. The writer is aware of several patients with malignant disease including one in the older age group who improved significantly after treatment with corticosteroids. Indeed the oldest patient, a 67 year old male who was wheelchair-bound at the time of presentation with severe subacute dermatomyositis, *walked* back into the clinic after 3 months' treatment with prednisolone when he was anorexic and losing weight with a *visible mass* in the epigastrium (this proved to be a carcinoma of the pyloric antrum). Accordingly, a satisfactory response to immunosuppression does *not* automatically exclude the presence of an occult malignancy of some kind.

In patients with chronic polymyositis and with dermatomyositis, the principles of management are identical. The diagnosis should be confirmed in the usual way, the writer having a marked preference for open biopsy (under local analgesia) in patients with inflammatory muscle disease particularly. If two out of four of the diagnostic criteria laid down by Bohan and Peter (1975) are satisfied, the patients should be treated, in the first instance with prednisolone or prednisolone in a dose of at least 60 mg per day (higher doses may be necessary in acutely ill subjects) for an *adequate* period of time. This will be determined by two factors: the patient's response to therapy clinically (most important) and in terms of laboratory parameters (least reliable); and the development of cushingoid side-effects. Needless to say, one hopes to 'taper' the dose of the corticosteroid employed as soon as possible, although considerable caution has to be exercised in so doing. Certainly unduly hasty steroid withdrawal will almost certainly be followed by relapse which may well be refractory to all treatment modalities (Venables *et al.*, 1982; Lane *et al.*, 1982). However, early and unacceptably severe cushingoid side-effects are likely to plague the management of middle-aged females particularly. In such cases, treatment with a corticosteroid (in more rapidly reducing doses) in combination with azathioprine in a dose of 1.5 mg/kg body weight is the preferred modality and there may be a case for exhibiting azathioprine alone in subjects who are overweight before starting therapy.

In refractory cases, pulsed intravenous methylprednisolone therapy (0.5–1 g daily for up to 4 days) may be helpful in the short term. Other immunosuppressive modalities have been tried in IIM and their value remains uncertain. (These have been reviewed in detail by Lane *et al.*, 1982).

METABOLIC MYOPATHIES (see also Chapter 20)

Corticosteroid Myopathy

Muscle weakness is a well-recognized feature of Cushing's syndrome whether it be due to adrenal cortical hyperplasia, a cortical adenoma or an ACTH-secreting pituitary adenoma. This may be incapacitating in some cases, but almost without exception, it responds quite quickly and usually completely to successful treatment of the underlying endocrinopathy. However, bilateral adrenalectomy for Cushing's *disease* may be followed by the development of hyperpigmentation (Nelson's syndrome) and limb-girdle weakness (Prineas *et al.*, 1968). These features are associated with exceptionally high serum ACTH levels and the myopathy is characterized histopathologically by excessive accumulation of neutral lipid droplets in Type I fibres particularly (Prineas *et al.*, 1968).

The commonest form of corticosteroid myopathy encountered in clinical practice is of course iatrogenic and is one of the commoner management problems in some of the conditions discussed already, notably polymyalgia rheumatica and IIM. In the vast majority of cases, iatrogenic steroid myopathy presents with mild and only gradually progressive weakness of the pelvic girdle muscles particularly. In cases of IIM, it can be very difficult to distinguish this complication from an incomplete response to therapy on clinical grounds and the EMG and serum CK activity are usually unhelpful in this situation (both may be normal). Serial *needle* muscle biopsies have been shown to be of only limited value in monitoring progress in patients with IIM on immunosuppressive regimens (Lane *et al.*, 1982). However, this study did show that *active* IIM was accompanied by a non-specific Type II fibre atrophy. Patients developing a steroid myopathy, on the other hand, had selective Type IIb fibre atrophy (long recognized as the histological/histochemical hallmark of corticosteroid myopathy) in the absence of any evidence of necrobiotic activity—inflammatory cell infiltrates disappear quickly after the institution of therapy. The only treatment of steroid myopathy is withdrawal of the offending drug which has to be accomplished with considerable care as indicated above. Occasional cases of an acute necrobiotic myopathy developing in *younger* patients with severe asthma have been reported after the intravenous administration of large doses of hydrocortisone (see Hudgson, 1988 for a detailed review).

Dysthyroid Myopathies

Muscle weakness has long been recognized as a prominent feature in virtually every case of thyroid overactivity and less frequently in thyroid underactivity (when it may be accompanied by extreme stiffness and painful cramps—Hoffmann's syndrome). In the case of hyperthyroidism, the 'myopathy' remits rapidly with suppression of the metabolic error and, because of this and the need for urgent treatment in many cases, few opportunities have arisen in the past to study the morphological and metabolic changes taking place in the muscle cell in this situation. However, it seems reasonable to assume that T_4 excess influences oxidative metabolism in some way (non-thyroidal hypermetabolism or Luft's disease is a possible analogy) and it certainly increases protein catabolism. Curiously, it *increases* the population of Type II fibres at the expense of Type I fibres and no explanation for this phenomenon has been forthcoming as yet. The observation is reflected in a similar change in experimental hyperthyroidism in rats (Johnson *et al.*, 1980a). Clinically, hyperthyroid myopathy manifests with often rapidly progressive proximal weakness and wasting which may be accompanied by fasciculations. It should always be remembered that myopathy may be the *presenting* manifestation of the disorder in the elderly particularly. The treatment of thyrotoxic myopathy is the treatment of the underlying disease.

Hypothyroid myopathy has received a good deal of attention in the literature although this does not mean that our understanding of the biogenesis of the disorder is any clearer than in hyperthyroidism.

Numerous reports suggest that polysaccharide accumulation is a common feature although its precise relationship to T_4 deficiency remains unclear. Reduced acid maltase activity in muscle has been reported in patients with hypothyroid myopathy (Hurwitz *et al.*, 1970). The levels are approximately the same as those in heterozygote relatives of patients with the disease (Engel and Gomez, 1970).

In this context, it is of particular interest that the histochemical profile of muscles such as quadriceps changes in precisely the opposite direction to that seen in hyperthyroidism; that is to say Type I fibres predominate virtually to the exclusion of Type II fibres (Johnson *et al.*, 1980b). Once again, the explanation for this phenomenon in terms of muscle cell metabolism remains unclear, although the increase in muscle tone may be a contributing factor. Clinically, hypothyroid myopathy presents with generalized weakness (not wasting), increased muscle tone and painful cramps. Satisfactory replacement therapy will be followed by complete remission of the neuromuscular symptoms in all cases.

Dysthyroid Ophthalmopathy (Ophthalmic Graves' Disease, Orbital Myositis)

The link between hyperthyroid and hypothyroid myopathies is the unpredictable affliction of the extra-ocular muscles associated with autoimmune thyroiditis, irrespective of the level of thyroid function at the time. The pathological basis for dysthyroid ophthalmopathy is 'autoimmune' inflammatory infiltration of the extra-ocular muscles with associated oedema and some inflammation of the fat and connective tissue within the orbital cavity. The development of dysthyroid eye disease is associated with circulating antibodies against surface antigens of extra-ocular muscle (Kendall-Taylor *et al.*, 1984) although a clear-cut pathogenetic relationship between these two phenomena has yet to be defined. The diagnosis of 'orbital myositis' can be assisted by computed tomographic (CT) scanning of the orbits which demonstrates enlargement of the extra-ocular muscles (Hudgson, 1988). The treatment of this condition remains problematical. A reasonable response to treatment with steroids or other immuno-suppressives may be anticipated in most cases although surgical decompression of the orbit may still be necessary in that small minority of cases where vision is threatened by raised intra-orbital pressure. Ideally, the situation should never progress that far in the first place.

Diabetes Mellitus and Other Disorders of Carbohydrate Metabolism

There is no firm evidence that diabetes mellitus affects the muscle cell directly, although muscle weakness and wasting are extremely common in the commonly associated disorders of the peripheral nervous system, notably, mononeuritis simplex et multiplex. One example of the genre is worthy of special mention in the elderly, so-called 'diabetic amyotrophy' (Garland, 1955) which is, in fact, a selective ischaemic neuropathy affecting the femoral nerve trunk. This condition may even be the presenting manifestation of maturity onset diabetes, especially in elderly males. It commences with often excruciatingly severe pain in one or both thighs which interferes with sleep and which frequently requires opiates for satisfactory relief. The neuropathy then progresses to weakness and wasting (often gross) of the quadriceps with loss of the relevant knee jerk(s) and little or nothing in the way of sensory loss. Neuralgic amyotrophy is a self-limiting condition which may leave the patient with mild or only minimal incapacity after a few months. Its natural history does not appear to be affected materially by satisfactory control of the associated carbohydrate intolerance.

Endogenous hypoglycaemia is not encountered frequently in the elderly. Its deleterious effects on the *central* nervous system are well recognized in general, although the rare complication of hypoglycaemic neuronopathy may well be overlooked. Described first by Mulder *et al.* (1954), hypoglycaemic neuronopathy is due to chronic hypoglycaemic damage to the anterior horn cells and dorsal root ganglia and it may be mistaken for motor neurone disease. However, clear-cut clinical evidence of sensory involvement should rule out this possibility.

TABLE 12.3 CLINICAL COMPONENTS OF THE KEARNS–SAYRE SYNDROME

1 Chronic progressive external ophthalmoplegia
2 Retinal pigmentation
3 Limb-girdle myopathy (variable, usually mild)
4 Variable degrees of atrioventricular conduction defects, complete heart block and sometimes causing sudden death, usually in *younger* patients
5 Cerebellar ataxia with loss of Purkinje cells
6 Axonal peripheral neuropathy
7 Sensorineural deafness
8 Diabetes mellitus

CHRONIC PROGRESSIVE EXTERNAL OPHTHALMOPLEGIA (CPEO)

Described originally by Hutchinson (1879), CPEO was regarded as a degenerative disorder affecting the oculomotor nuclei until the seminal paper of Kiloh and Nevin (1951) reclassifying it as a primary myopathy with occasional limb-girdle involvement. Since then it has become clear that CPEO may occur in isolation or in variable association with numerous other disorders. These are listed in Table 12.3 and in 'full flower', they constitute what has become known as the Kearns–Sayre syndrome (Kearns and Sayre, 1959). This dramatic constellation can present at any age although CPEO does tend to manifest in isolation in older patients. The majority of cases reported to date have been sporadic, although occasional familial examples have been noted with a pattern suggesting an autosomal recessive mode of inheritance. Detailed morphological studies of limb-girdle muscle biopsies (Johnson *et al.*, 1983) have shown that these patients have a 'mitochondrial myopathy' with 'ragged red' fibres, abnormal mitochondria and patchy loss of cytochrome *c*-oxidase activity (in 'ragged red' fibres and some others). The histochemical abnormality is reflected in reduced enzyme activity on biochemical analysis (not absent as in cases of generalized cytochrome *c*-oxidase deficiency).

CONCLUSION

The above has been no more than an introduction to the myology of old age, although the entities described are those which will be encountered most often in clinical practice. Myasthenia gravis, is discussed in detail in Chapter 25, the Lambert–Eaton syndrome in Chapter 21, and motor neurone disease in Chapter 11. It should be remembered that these disorders may occasionally cause diagnostic confusion with primary muscle cell disease. In the case of myasthenia gravis, myotonic dystrophy and CPEO, both constitute important differential diagnoses and the Lambert–Eaton myasthenic syndrome may be confused or indeed coexist with polymyositis. Some cases of motor neurone disease may be difficult to distinguish from the limb-girdle myopathies, including polymyositis, although the asymmetry of the weakness and wasting in the former is a useful clinical pointer to anterior horn cell dysfunction. In the author's experience, confusion most often arises in elderly patients with motor neurone disease who often look and sound 'myasthenic' in the early stages of their illness.

The importance of early recognition of the inflammatory muscle disorders in the elderly cannot be stressed too strongly. In the particular case of polymyalgia rheumatica, muscle pain and stiffness may be bad enough to immobilize the patient completely with the consequent risk of death from inanition (the author has seen this occasionally in patients living by themselves). In patients with either polymyositis or dermatomyositis, the risk of a coexistent neoplasm, which may not manifest clinically, is sufficiently high to justify 'hunting the primary' in the hope that the neoplasm will be susceptible to surgical or other therapeutic intervention.

ACKNOWLEDGEMENTS

The author wishes to thank all the physicians in the Northern Region whose referrals over the years have formed the basis for the experience recorded above. All personal work referred to above was supported by the Muscular Dystrophy Group of Great Britain. He is also very grateful to Miss M.A. Waugh and Mrs A. Bowe who typed the manuscript.

REFERENCES

Bohan, A., and Peter, J.B. (1975). Polymyositis and dermatomyositis. *N. Engl. J. Med.*, **292**: 344–7, 403–7.

Brooke, M.H., and Kaplan, H. (1972). Muscle pathology in rheumatoid arthritis, polymyalgia rheumatica and polymyositis. *Arch. Pathol.*, **94**, 101–18.

Bruce, W. (1888). Cited by Bruk, 1967.

Bruk, M.E. (1967). Articular and vascular manifestations of polymyalgia rheumatica. *Ann. Rheumatol. Dis.*, **26**, 103–16.

Carpenter, S., Karpati, G., Rothman, S., and Watters, G. (1976). The childhood type of dermatomyositis. *Neurology*, **26**, 952–62.

Currey, H.F.L., and Barnes, H.G. (1978). Complicated polymyalgia. *Br. Med. J.*, **i**, 50.

De Vere, R., and Bradley, W.G. (1975). Polymyositis: Its presentation, morbidity and mortality. *Brain*, **98**, 637–66.

Emslie-Smith, A.M., and Hudgson, P. The association between idiopathic inflammatory myopathy and autoimmune thyroiditis in females. In preparation.

Engel, A.G., and Gomez, M.R. (1970). Acid maltase levels in muscle and in heterozygous acid maltase deficiency and in non-weak and neuromuscular disease controls. *J. Neurol. Neurosurg. Psychiatry*, **33**, 801–4.

Foster, W.D. (1965). The bacteriology of tropical pyomyositis in Uganda. *J. Hygiene (Camb.)*, **63**, 517–24.

Garland, H.G. (1955). Diabetic amyotrophy. *Br. Med. J.*, **ii**, 1287–90.

Harding, A.E., and Thomas, P.K. (1980). Hereditary distal spinal muscular atrophy. A report on 34 cases and a review of the literature. *J. Neurol. Sci.*, **45**, 337–48.

Hoffman, G., Franck, W.A., Raddatz, D.A., and Stallones, L. (1983). Presentation, treatment and prognosis of idiopathic inflammatory muscle disease in a rural hospital. *Am. J. Med.*, **75**, 433–8.

Hudgson, P. (1986). Myopathic disorders. In: Triger, D.R. (ed.) *Advanced Medicine*, 22, Baillière Tindall, London, pp. 385–98.

Hudgson, P. (1988). Endocrine and metabolic myopathies. In: Swash, M., and Oxbury, J.N. (eds.) *Clinical Neurology*, Churchill Livingstone, Edinburgh. In press.

Hudgson, P., and Peter, J.B. (1984). Classification (of inflammatory muscle diseases). *Clin. Rheum. Dis.*, **10**, 3–8.

Hudgson, P., and Walton, J.N. (1979). Polymyositis and other inflammatory myopathies. In: Vinken, P.J., and Bruyn, G.W. (eds.) *Handbook of Clinical Neurology*, North Holland, Amsterdam, pp. 51–93.

Hurwitz, L., McCormick, D., and Allen, I.V. (1970). Reduced muscle L-1, 4-glucosidase (acid maltase) activity in hypothyroid myopathy. *Lancet*, **i**, 67.

Hutchinson, J. (1879). An ophthalmoplegia externa or symmetrical immobility (partial) of the eye with ptosis. *Trans. Med.-Chir. Soc. Edinb.*, **62**, 307.

Johnson, M.A., Mastaglia, F.L., and Montgomery, A. (1980a). The histochemical and contractile properties of hyperthyroid mammalian skeletal muscle. *IRCS: Medical Science*, **8**, 711.

Johnson, M.A., Mastaglia, F.L., Montgomery, A., Pope, B., and Weeds, A.G. (1980b). A neurally-mediated effect of thyroid hormone deficiency on slow twitch skeletal muscle? In: Pette, D. (ed.) *Plasticity of Muscle*, De Gruyter, Berlin, pp. 607–15.

Johnson, M.A., Turnbull, D.M., Dick, D.J., and Sherratt, H.S.A. (1983). A partial deficiency of cytochrome c oxidase in chronic progressive externa ophthalmoplegia. *J. Neurol. Sci*, **60**, 31–53.

Kearns, T.P., and Sayre, G.P. (1959). Retinitis pigmentosa, external ophthalmoplegia and complete heart block. *Arch. Ophthalmol.*, **60**, 280–9.

Kendall-Taylor, P., Atkinson, S., and Holcombe, M. (1984). A specific IgG in Graves' ophthalmopathy and its relation to retro-orbital and thyroid autoimmunity. *Br. Med. J.*, **ii**, 1183–6.

Kiloh, L.G., and Nevin, S. (1951). Progressive dystrophy of external ocular muscles (ocular myopathy). *Brain*, **74**, 115–43.

Lane, R.J., Mosquera, I.E., Nicholson, L.V.B., Johnson, M.A., Hudgson, P., and Walton, J.N. (1982). Clinical, biochemical and histological responses to treatment in polymyositis. A prospective study. *Fifth International Congress on Neuromuscular Diseases*, Marseilles, France (abstract 24.2).

Leading article (1978). *Lancet*, **i**, 862.

Medsger, T.A., Dawson, W.N., and Masi, A.T. (1970). The epidemiology of polymyositis. *Am. J. Med.*, **48**, 715–23.

Middleton, P.J., Alexander, R.M., and Szymanski, M.T. (1970). Severe myositis during recovery from influenza. *Lancet*, **ii**, 533–5.

Mulder, D.W., Bastron, J.A., and Lambert, E.H. (1954). Hyper-insulin neuronopathy. *Neurology*, **27**, 722–82.

Nattrass, F.J. (1954). Recovery from "muscular dystrophy". *Brain*, **77**, 549–70.

Nevin, S. (1936). Two cases of muscular degeneration occurring in late adult life with a review of the recording of late progressive muscular dystrophy (late progressive myopathy). *Q. J. Med.*, **5**, 51–68.

Prineas, J.W., Hall, R., Barwick, D.D., and Watson, A.J. (1968). Myopathy associated with pigmentation following adrenalectomy for Cushing's syndrome. *Q. J. Med.*, **37**, 63–77.

Shy, G.M., and McEachern, D. (1951). The clinical features and response to cortisone of menopausal muscular dystrophy. *J. Neurol. Neurosurg. Psychiatry*, **14**, 101–17.

Taylor, J.F., and Henderson, B.F. (1972). Tropical myositis. In: Shaper, A.G., Kibukamusoke, J.W., and Hutt, M.S.R. (eds.) *Medicine in a Tropical Environment*, British Medical Association, London, pp. 32–44.

Venables, G.S., Bates, D., Cartlidge, N.E.F., and Hudgson, P. (1982). Acute polymyositis with subcutaneous oedema. *J. Neurol. Sci.*, **55**, 161–4.

Chapter 13

Diseases of Peripheral Nerves

R. K. Olney

Assistant Professor, Department of Neurology, University of California, San Francisco, USA

Peripheral nerve function normally declines with advancing age, in that there are age-related changes which are universal, progressive and irreversible (Olney, 1985). The prevalence of peripheral nerve disease also increases with advancing age, at least in part because systemic diseases producing peripheral neuropathy are more common. While the distinction between normal age-related changes and distal axonal polyneuropathy may be challenging, other patterns of peripheral nerve disease are unequivocally pathological at any age, even if mild in severity. This chapter will initially review the classification and diagnostic approach for the clinical patterns of peripheral nerve disease; then, specific disease entities will be discussed, together with their more particular clinical features and management.

CLASSIFICATION

The symptoms and signs of peripheral nerve disease are the result of a limited number of pathophysiological mechanisms and pathological processes. Negative symptoms (loss of sensory or motor function) are the result of structural (axonal degeneration) or functional (conduction block) disruption of nerve conduction between the periphery and central nervous system, whereas positive symptoms (paraesthesias or dysaesthesias) are due to spontaneous discharges in peripheral axons.

Axonal degeneration occurs from pathological changes which may primarily affect the cell body, the middle portion of the axon, or the distal end of the axon. When the disease primarily affects the cell body and leads to its death, the cell body and its axon degenerate together. This type of peripheral nerve disease is termed a neuronopathy and is typically selective for sensory or motor involvement. With other diseases the soma survives, but the distal portion of the axons do not; then, distal axonal degeneration occurs, with the longest axons affected first and most severely. When the middle portion of a peripheral nerve is transected by physical trauma or by infarction, all sensory, motor and autonomic axons distal to the transection undergo wallerian degeneration; a mononeuropathy (or multiple mononeuropathies) results.

Conduction block occurs from demyelination; the pathological process primarily affects either the Schwann cell or the myelin sheath. When the pathogenesis is biochemical or immune-mediated, a generalized demyelinating neuropathy results. Recurrent compression of a nerve leads to the localized demyelination typical of an entrapment neuropathy.

Based on the nature and distribution of pathological involvement, peripheral nerve disease may be classified as shown in Table 13.1, which is a modification of the schema proposed by Spencer and Schaumburg (1980).

TABLE 13.1   CLASSIFICATION OF PERIPHERAL NERVE DISEASE

I. Generalized symmetrical polyneuropathy
    a. length-dependent:
        distal axonal polyneuropathy
    b. non-length dependent:
        1. demyelinating polyneuropathy
            (myelinopathy)
        2. neuronopathy
II. Mononeuropathy or multiple mononeuropathies
    a. axonal degeneration predominant
    b. focal demyelination predominant

CLINICAL PATTERNS OF PRESENTATION, INCLUDING DIFFERENTIAL DIAGNOSIS AND INITIAL DIAGNOSTIC APPROACH

Distal Axonal Polyneuropathy

Toxic, systemic metabolic, genetic or other mechanisms produce alterations in the neurone which cause the neuronal processes most remote from the cell body to degenerate in distal axonal polyneuropathy. The symptoms and signs are therefore manifest in a length-dependent distribution, being most severe initially in the distal lower extremities. The initial symptoms are usually numbness, paraesthesia, or dysaesthesias in the feet. Pain, temperature, light touch, and vibration are diminished in a stocking–glove distribution (but proprioception may be relatively spared). Weakness is first manifest in the intrinsic foot muscles, and then in the anterior compartment and intrinsic hand muscles. Ankle reflexes are typically absent, and other deep tendon reflexes are depressed.

Before the diagnosis of a distal axonal polyneuropathy is made, symptoms and signs must exceed those attributable to normal age-related changes in peripheral nerve function. Diminution of vibratory perception in the feet and at the ankle is consistently observed by the age of 70 years, and is often present by the age of 60 (Potvin *et al.*, 1980). Distal impairment in pain, temperature, and touch are less pronounced, but may also occur; distal paraesthesias and dysaesthesias are neither universal nor clearly more frequent in older than younger populations

(Olney, 1985). While ankle reflexes are absent in one-fifth of active, healthy individuals who are living independently in the community and are older than 70 years, depression of the ankle reflex is nearly universally present by this age (Olney *et al.*, 1983). Other deep tendon reflexes are mildly, but less prominently depressed with advancing age. The bulk and strength of muscles are universally reduced with advancing age, but these changes are not clearly more prominent distally. Thus, although moderate signs of distal sensory (especially for vibration) and reflex impairment may be normal in older individuals, positive sensory symptoms, severe diminution of distal sensory perception, and distally prominent weakness should be considered indicative of polyneuropathy at any age.

If the severity of distal symptoms or signs exceeds these normal limits for age, electromyography (EMG) and nerve conduction studies are obtained to confirm that the pathophysiological abnormalities are primarily those of distal axonal degeneration: nerve conduction studies demonstrate amplitude reduction of compound action potentials (more so than reduced conduction velocity), and EMG evidence for acute or chronic partial denervation is most prominent in distal muscles.

Electrophysiological confirmation of the diagnosis is followed by a search for specific aetiological associations (Table 13.2). A careful history is taken for possible exposure to alcohol and toxins (including prescribed drugs and environmental chemicals) and for a possible familial incidence of polyneuropathy. A fasting blood glucose level (possible to diagnose diabetes mellitus) is one of the initial tests obtained. Particularly if neither alcoholism nor diabetes is found (the two most common causes for distal axonal polyneuropathy) or if the polyneuropathy is severe, further evaluation usually includes testing for other endocrine diseases (especially hypothyroidism), vitamin deficiencies (B12 and folate), monoclonal proteins (serum protein electrophoresis and immunoelectrophoresis of serum and urine), and other diseases (erythrocyte sedimentation rate, urea, creatinine, occult blood in stools, and chest X-ray). Nerve biopsy is not performed unless one of several specific diagnoses, such as vasculitis or amyloidosis, is suspected.

TABLE 13.2 DIFFERENTIAL DIAGNOSIS OF DISTAL AXONAL POLYNEUROPATHY

1. Systemic metabolic and/or endocrine diseases
   a. diabetes mellitus
   b. uraemia
   c. hypothyroidism
   d. other
2. Nutritional and vitamin deficiencies
   a. alcoholism and nutritional deficiency
   b. vitamin B12 deficiency
   c. other
3. Toxic exposures
   a. prescribed medications
   b. environmental chemicals
4. Systemic vascular diseases
   a. collagen-vascular diseases
   b. other
5. Neoplasia
6. Paraproteinaemias
7. Primary systemic amyloidosis
8. Inherited axonal polyneuropathies
9. Idiopathic distal axonal polyneuropathy

Demyelinating Polyneuropathy

Demyelinating neuropathies in later life usually arise from immune-mediated widespread segmental demyelination (myelinopathy), either with or without associated monoclonal proteins. Toxic neuropathies which produce primary demyelination are rare. Demyelinating neuropathies are commonly hereditary only in children and young adults. Clinically, weakness is often more prominent than sensory disturbances, and affects proximal as well as distal muscles. Although diffuse, the severity of weakness is easily recognized as abnormal for age. Tendon reflexes are usually absent diffusely.

Electrophysiological studies reveal severely reduced conduction velocities in several nerves (to less than 60% of the lower tolerance limit of normal) or several areas of conduction block. Further evaluation includes detailed testing for a monoclonal protein by protein electrophoresis and immunoelectrophoresis or immunofixation studies on the serum and urine. A complete blood count with differential, skeletal survey, and sometimes bone marrow biopsy may be necessary to distinguish myelomas and other haematological diseases from ones of less certain significance (so-called benign monoclonal gammo-

pathies). Cerebrospinal fluid analysis, for elevated protein without significant pleocytosis, and sometimes nerve biopsy are performed to further support the presence of chronic inflammatory polyradiculoneuropathies, especially before instituting steroid or immunosuppressive therapy. If spinal fluid pleocytosis is significant, other associated diseases, such as Lyme disease and even the spectrum of human immunodeficiency virus related diseases, may warrant consideration.

Neuronopathy

A syndrome which clinically resembles motor neuronopathy is occasionally associated with paraproteinaemia. In these cases, electrophysiological studies often provide evidence for proximal demyelination. Therefore, most of these rare cases may be classified with the demyelinating polyneuropathies; other cases closely resemble motor neurone disease.

Sensory neuronopathy presents with widespread diminution of sensory functions, especially joint position. Clumsiness of the hands and gait impairment may be so severe that weakness is simulated. However, electrophysiological studies reveal a generalized absence or reduced amplitude of sensory nerve action potentials, while motor nerve conduction and EMG studies are normal. B12 deficiency or malignancy are the aetiologies most frequently established, and pyridoxine intoxication, tabes dorsalis, and collagen-vascular diseases (Sjögren's syndrome in particular) are less common causes. Many cases do not have an identifiable cause, even with long-term follow-up to exclude malignancy.

Autonomic Neuropathy (see also Chapter 14)

Autonomic neuropathy usually presents with orthostatic hypotension; urinary retention or incontinence, impotence, and nocturnal diarrhoea are other common problems. Autonomic neuropathy usually occurs in association with sensorimotor manifestations of a distal axonal (typically diabetic or amyloid) or demyelinating (especially acute inflammatory) polyneuropathy. Rarely, autonomic neuropathy occurs in isolation in idiopathic orthostatic hypotension (Bannister *et al.*, 1981) and pure pandysautonomia (Young *et al.*, 1975). Electrocardio-graphic evaluation of the R-R interval during deep breathing and Valsalva manoeuvre is simple, non-invasive, and useful in documenting the severity of cardiovascular involvement; other types of autono-mic testing are more elaborate (Low, 1984; Niakan *et al.*, 1986).

Mononeuropathy

When sensory and motor symptoms develop focally with or without pain, a mononeuropathy is sus-pected and electrophysiological studies are useful to establish the diagnosis. If the involved nerve has evidence for demyelination at a typical entrapment site and there is no evidence for polyneuropathy, the entrapment syndrome may be treated as discussed below without major concern for more widespread disease; if coexistent polyneuropathy is also found, treatment of the entrapment syndrome may be conservative while the cause of the underlying polyneuropathy is determined and treated. How-ever, if symptoms developed abruptly and axonal degeneration is prominent, causes of nerve infarction should be evaluated, with fasting blood glucose, erythrocyte sedimentation rate, antinuclear anti-body titre, rheumatoid titre, protein electrophoresis, immunoelectrophoresis of blood and urine, quanti-tative cryoglobulin levels, and often nerve biopsy. In a patient with a known tumour, the possibility of metastatic disease must also be considered.

SPECIFIC PERIPHERAL NERVE DISEASE

Peripheral Nerve Disease Secondary to Compression or Entrapment

Peripheral nerve is susceptible to injury by focal mechanical pressures which deform the myelin sheath. Paranodal and segmental demyelination are produced as the mildest manifestation of injury. When mechanical pressure occurs with greater force and/or for a longer duration, axonal degeneration is associated with the focal demyelination; if the pres-sure and/or its duration are even more severe, complete wallerian degeneration of the nerve may result. Peripheral nerve compression, which may

arise from an extrinsic source or from entrapment within a fibrous or fibro-osseous tunnel, is extremely common. In one pathological study of median and ulnar nerves of twelve subjects without known peripheral nerve disease who were undergoing rou-tine autopsy, signs of median nerve entrapment in the carpal tunnel and of compressive injury to the ulnar nerve at the elbow were found in 42% (5/12) of the nerves at each location, and 67% (8/12) of the individuals had one or both of these mononeuro-pathies (Neary *et al.*, 1975). Thus, a majority of elderly subjects may have one of these two focal neuropathies, at least subclinically.

Carpal tunnel syndrome

The clinical symptoms and signs of median nerve entrapment at the wrist comprise the carpal tunnel syndrome, and over one-fourth of the patients in large surgical series have presented between the ages of 60 and 80 years, with women outnumbering men by three to one (Phalen, 1972). Initial symptoms are usually sensory; intermittent paraesthesias and numbness of one hand occur in association with a more diffuse aching pain in that limb, especially with use of the hand or at night. Presentation may, rarely, be with painless wasting and weakness of the thenar muscles; this occurs more often in older individuals.

In the typical cases with sensory complaints, the only abnormality on clinical examination may be a positive Tinel's sign over the median nerve at the wrist; motor and sensory deficits are often absent. In other cases, there are marked sensory and motor deficits in the median distribution. Electrophysiolo-gical studies provide evidence for slowing of sensory and/or motor conduction through the carpal tunnel in over 95% of cases, since demyelination is a prominent part of the pathophysiology. When the neurological deficits are severe (as the painless cases usually are), signs of axonal degeneration are also present. If carpal tunnel syndrome is diagnosed, the possibility of asymptomatic contralateral involve-ment must be considered, since half will be bilateral.

The majority of cases are caused by non-specific flexor tenosynovitis (Dawson *et al.*, 1983a). Still, diabetic polyneuropathy or rheumatoid flexor tenosynovitis will be found in over one-fourth (Phalen, 1972), and the rare patient with hypothyroidism will have long-term benefit from thyroid supplementation.

If the neurological deficit is mild, treatment is conservative, with splinting of the wrist in the neutral position. Although often prescribed, the benefits of oral anti-inflammatory agents are not well documented. Steroid injection into the carpal tunnel provides long-term benefit in only one-fourth of patients (Phalen, 1966). When treatable associated conditions, such as hypothyroidism, are found or when the carpal tunnel syndrome is mild, conservative therapy is quite satisfactory. If the initial neurological deficit is severe (e.g. thenar atrophy), or if conservative treatment fails, surgical decompression of the carpal tunnel is highly effective in relieving pain and in halting further progression of the deficit (Phalen, 1972).

Ulnar neuropathy at the elbow

Ulnar neuropathy at the elbow may equal the frequency of the carpal tunnel syndrome in older individuals (Neary *et al.*, 1975), since prolonged bedrest and arthritis are causes for compression in this region. The most frequent complaints are either numbness and paraesthesias of the fifth digit or weakness of the hand. Pain is much less common and less prominent (Chan *et al.*, 1980).

On examination, altered sensation in the ulnar distribution is present in nearly all patients, and weakness of ulnar intrinsic hand muscles in most. Deforming arthritis at the elbow has been observed in 25% (post-traumatic arthritis in 15%, osteoarthritis in 10%), even when young adults are included in the series (Chan *et al.*, 1980). With electrophysiological studies, the identification of axonal degeneration in the ulnar distribution helps quantify the severity of the deficit, but ulnar neuropathy can be localized only by significant conduction slowing limited to the elbow segment of the nerve.

Ulnar neuropathy at the elbow can be divided into several syndromes based upon associated clinical features (e.g. history of trauma and the presence of arthritis), electrophysiological localization, and operative findings. The major divisions which

influence management decisions are chronic cubital tunnel syndrome, other chronic ulnar neuropathies, and acute ulnar neuropathy. The general indications for surgery on the chronic cases are: (1) a mild motor deficit which has progressed under medical observation, and (2) a moderate motor deficit which is not the result of a single recent traumatic event. Early simple decompression is preferable for the cubital tunnel syndrome (Miller and Hummel, 1980; Chan *et al.*, 1980). The other chronic ulnar neuropathies often require anterior transplantation (Chan *et al.*, 1980). The reduced likelihood of benefit makes surgeons less inclined to operate when the motor deficit is severe, and when the ulnar neuropathy is acute, regardless of severity (Chan *et al.*, 1980). In the case of ulnar neuropathy which develops from acute external compression perioperatively, the long-term outcome is similar irrespective of whether treatment is medical or surgical (Miller and Camp, 1979).

Ulnar neuropathy at or distal to the wrist

Distal ulnar neuropathies are not unusual in patients who use walking frames for significant weight support. These neuropathies commonly present with bilateral hand wasting and weakness. Electrophysiological testing, which includes study of the first dorsal interosseous muscle, is quite helpful in establishing the diagnosis (Olney and Wilbourn, 1985). When the source of extrinsic compression is obvious (as it is in a patient who uses a walker), treatment consists of padding the canal of Guyon region (e.g. bicyclist gloves) and patient education.

Peroneal neuropathy at the fibular head

The most common lower extremity focal neuropathy is the peroneal neuropathy at the fibular head, which presents with a footdrop. If the weakness includes eversion in addition to dorsiflexion, full strength for inversion is helpful in clinically distinguishing a fifth lumbar radiculopathy. Electrophysiological studies are useful to localize the nerve lesion and provide prognostic information, since the presence of demyelination with conduction block and the absence of axonal degeneration indicate a good chance of an excellent long-term outcome. Acute compression is the usual aetiology, and improvement generally occurs without surgical intervention. If the acute compression did not occur perioperatively, educating the patient to avoid tight leg crossing is advisable. If insidiously progressive without known trauma, cysts, tumours and other causes of focal compression may be present and indicate the need for surgical intervention (Dawson et al., 1983b). Treatment also includes bracing the ankle joint to increase stability with walking; a plastic ankle–foot orthosis is usually quite adequate.

Tarsal tunnel syndrome

The tarsal tunnel syndrome consists of intermittent paraesthesias and pain in one or both feet due to entrapment of the tibial nerve at the ankle. These symptoms may develop with prolonged standing or at night. A positive Tinel's sign over the tarsal tunnel region and mild sensory alteration over the plantar surface of the foot are the usual physical signs. However, distal axonal polyneuropathies often present with similar symptoms and signs, so careful electrophysiological distinction of these two possibilities is important (DeLisa and Saeed, 1983). If the diagnosis is clearly established, surgical decompression is often beneficial.

Peripheral Neuropathy Associated with Systemic Metabolic Disease

Diabetes mellitus

The most common peripheral nerve disease in Western society is diabetic neuropathy. Although the estimated prevalence of diabetic neuropathy varies widely depending on the criteria for its diagnosis, there is uniform acceptance that its prevalence increases with the duration of diabetes. In the largest clinical series, 7.5% of diabetics had neuropathy at the time their diabetes was diagnosed, while the prevalence rose to 50% after 25 years (Pirart, 1978). There is no clear evidence that the neuropathies are different in insulin dependent and non-insulin dependent diabetics. Several different clinical patterns of peripheral neuropathy may develop in both types.

The most common peripheral neuropathy of diabetes is the distal axonal polyneuropathy. Elderly patients with non-insulin dependent diabetes sometimes have pronounced distal numbness even at the time diabetes is diagnosed, presumably since undiagnosed diabetes may have been present for months or years. More typically, diabetes has been recognized for years before the patient complains of distal sensory loss, or before the clinician first detects significant distal numbness. When positive symptoms are prominent, presentation is often earlier in the course of the diabetes. Distal weakness does not usually impair walking or manual activities until years after onset of sensory symptoms. Autonomic involvement may be prominent even early in the course of the polyneuropathy and may cause life-threatening complications (Niakan et al., 1986); or autonomic abnormalities may be inconspicuous even when sensory and motor deficits are severe.

There has long been debate concerning the relative contribution of axonal degeneration and segmental demyelination to the pathophysiology of the distal symmetrical polyneuropathy. The initial pathological abnormality in most diabetic nerves is segmental demyelination (Thomas and Lascelles, 1966). However, the severity of symptoms and signs correlates better with the extent of axonal degeneration than with the prominence of segmental demyelination, whether assessed electrophysiologically or pathologically (Behse et al., 1977 and Dyck et al., 1980). Furthermore, recent studies have provided evidence that the axonal degeneration is primary, multifocal, and associated with microvascular disease; these studies imply that the pathogenesis of symptomatic diabetic polyneuropathy involves multifocal nerve infarction and may be less directly related to metabolic factors, such as glucose control (Dyck et al., 1986b, 1986c). Whether an independent process (Behse et al., 1977) or secondary to variable changes in axonal calibré (Dyck et al., 1986c), segmental demyelination seems irrelevant to the pathophysiology and pathogenesis of symptomatic polyneuropathy (Olney, 1986). Therefore the distal symmetrical polyneuropathy of diabetes is now clearly categorized as a distal axonal polyneuropathy.

Polyneuropathy is generally less severe in diabetics with 'good' control than in those with 'poor' control (Pirart, 1978). However, the correlation is not precise, and rigorous control has not produced consistently documentable therapeutic benefit (Service *et al.*, 1983). Aldose reductase inhibitors and supplementation with *myo*-inositol have received extensive study, and multicentre trials using aldose reductase inhibitors are in progress. However, clear evidence of therapeutic response of the neuropathy to these interventions has yet to be shown (Brown and Asbury, 1984). Since the pathogenesis of the polyneuropathy seems closely associated with microvascular disease, therapeutic trials with new agents to improve the microcirculation are likely to be forthcoming. For the present, the only accepted therapeutic intervention for diabetic polyneuropathy is improved glucose control. The rigour of this control is determined case by case, by weighing the severity of the polyneuropathy against the risk of stricter glucose control; a several month trial on insulin therapy is often initiated, if this is not already part of the regimen. Other than improved glucose control, treatment is symptomatic, as will be discussed below.

Diabetics also develop other patterns of peripheral nerve disease, such as symmetrical or asymmetrical proximal motor neuropathy. These two patterns often share the common features of subacute progression of proximal leg weakness, poor glucose control, weight loss, and pain; furthermore, long-standing diabetes and distal axonal polyneuropathy are often part of the background setting for both. Diabetic amyotrophy was initially coined to describe this syndrome when the pattern was asymmetrical (Garland, 1955); in a later pathological study, one case was shown to be caused by ischaemic multiple mononeuropathy (Raff *et al.*, 1968). The pathogenesis of the symmetrical pattern is less clear and may involve similar microvascular disease and/or metabolic factors. Since its aetiology is more controversial, the non-specific term diabetic amyotrophy is now more commonly applied to the symmetrical pattern (Brown and Asbury, 1984). The asymmetrical pattern is almost always painful and evolves more rapidly (the deficit often reaching its peak over days), while the symmetrical variety tends to be less painful and to progress over weeks (Brown and Asbury, 1984). In both, femorally innervated muscles (iliopsoas and quadriceps) have prominent weakness but careful examination can usually identify significant weakness in the obturator and other distributions. By contrast to the distal axonal polyneuropathy, both of these proximal patterns characteristically improve over weeks to several months, usually coincidentally with improved glucose control (Bastron and Thomas, 1981).

Ischaemic mononeuropathy (single or multiple) or radiculopathy may cause thoracic or abdominal pain in association with weight loss. While weakness cannot be demonstrated clinically, a dysaesthetic dermatome and electromyographic evidence for acute radicular denervation are often present (Kikta *et al.*, 1982). The prognosis for recovery is good, so recognition is most important to help prevent an inappropriately pessimistic prognosis and unnecessary evaluation for pulmonary and abdominal malignancy.

Entrapment mononeuropathy or multiple mononeuropathies are also seen in diabetics, usually superimposed on the polyneuropathy. In this setting, conservative treatment with splinting, rest, and anti-inflammatory drugs are tried before surgical therapy under most circumstances.

Hypoglycaemia

Peripheral nerve disease is rarely seen in association with hypoglycaemia. Only 28 cases with islet cell tumours were reported by 1982 (Jaspan *et al.*, 1982), and the relative contribution of hypoglycaemia, hyperinsulinism, or other tumour-related factors is unclear. Although predominantly motor presentations have been reported to resemble motor neurone disease, the cases studied in greatest detail had clear electrophysiological and neuropathological (sural nerve biopsy) evidence of degeneration of sensory and motor axons (Jaspan *et al.*, 1982).

Uraemia

Uraemia has been shown to cause only distal axonal polyneuropathy. The presenting symptoms are distal sensory ones, and may include dysaesthesias, paraesthesias, or numbness. Although distal muscular cramping may occur early, distal weakness insidiously follows the sensory symptoms. Autonomic features are usually inconspicuous. The duration and severity, rather than cause, of the underlying renal failure are important with regard to the pathogenesis of the polyneuropathy, and 60–70% of patients will have at least mild polyneuropathy by the time haemodialysis becomes necessary (Asbury, 1984). Electrophysiologically, reduced amplitude of compound nerve and muscle action potentials is the most prominent abnormality, but conduction velocities are reduced more than expected for the degree of axonal degeneration. This is explained pathologically by segmental demyelination secondary to primary distal axonal atrophy (Dyck *et al.*, 1971). With renal transplantation, complete recovery of the polyneuropathy occurs over 6–12 months; haemodialysis leads to stabilization, improvement, or even recovery (Asbury, 1984). This polyneuropathy is not expected to produce major disability independently, so treatment decisions focus on the underlying renal failure from a broad medical perspective.

Hypothyroidism

Two different types of peripheral nerve disease are recognized to occur with hypothyroidism: distal axonal polyneuropathy and the carpal tunnel syndrome. The latter is the more common, and the clinical features are typical as described earlier; however, treatment is usually conservative with thyroid supplementation, splinting, and analgesics. Although rarely encountered now that thyroid function tests are widely available, hypothyroid polyneuropathy presents with distal sensory symptoms. Electrophysiological and pathological abnormalities are those of distal axonal polyneuropathy (Pollard *et al.*, 1982). The polyneuropathy may be fully or partially reversed with thyroid supplementation therapy.

Hyperthyroidism

Although proximal weakness from thyrotoxic myopathy is well recognized, the possible association of hyperthyroidism and peripheral nerve disease is controversial. The rare case reports with this association have usually included multiple associated diseases (Bastron, 1984), but other series have provided electrophysiological evidence for mild or subclinical distal axonal polyneuropathy (Layzer, 1985). Whether the rare coincidence of inflammatory demyelinating polyneuropathy and hyperthyroidism represents a pathogenetic association or pure chance is also controversial (Feibel and Campa, 1976).

Other systemic metabolic or endocrine diseases

In addition to the well-recognized development of the carpal tunnel syndrome in acromegalics, distal lower extremity sensory symptoms from polyneuropathy are also common. Electrophysiologically, the abnormalities are those typical for distal axonal polyneuropathy, which is also supported pathologically (Low *et al.*, 1974). Surgical release of the carpal tunnel is often beneficial. The polyneuropathy may not be improved by surgical removal or irradiation of the pituitary tumour.

Porphyric neuropathy with acute diffuse axonal degeneration is unlikely to present initially in late life, but it is wise to include it in the differential diagnosis of acute life-threatening peripheral neuropathy, when the Guillain–Barré syndrome is under consideration.

Alcoholism and Nutritional Deficiency Associated with Peripheral Neuropathy
(see also Chapter 20)

Alcoholism and nutritional deficiency

In Western societies, the peripheral neuropathy associated with alcoholism and nutritional deficiency is probably exceeded in prevalence only by diabetic peripheral neuropathy. Although the relative pathogenetic contributions of alcohol as a direct toxin versus the association of nutritional deficiency remain unclear, the clinical presentation is consistently one of a distal axonal polyneuropathy. Distal sensory symptoms, occasionally including burning pain, are typical at the onset, but distally prominent weakness is also detected on examination when the sensory deficit is significant. Electrophysiologically, sensory action potentials are small with reduced conduction velocity, or they are absent; similar motor nerve conduction abnormalities are present in more severe cases. However, segmental demyelination is rarely seen pathologically, and nerve conduction velocities are not reduced sufficiently to provide unequivocal evidence of demyelination, even in advanced cases (Behse and Buchthal, 1977). If the intake of alcohol is discontinued, the prognosis for recovery from the polyneuropathy is good, independent of the patient's age (Hillbom and Wennberg, 1984).

Vitamin B12 deficiency

Vitamin B12 deficiency results from reduced availability of intrinsic factor, which is produced by gastric parietal cells. Pernicious anaemia and subacute combined degeneration of the spinal cord are typically present when peripheral nerve involvement produces a sensory neuronopathy or a distal sensory axonal polyneuropathy. However, the anaemia may be absent, especially if folic acid intake is high. Since transcobalamin II is the only circulating carrier protein responsible for cell delivery of B12 and since this protein has a lower concentration and a higher turnover rate than transcobalamin I, serum B12 levels can be normal for several weeks despite severe neurological symptoms and signs (Donaldson *et al.*, 1977). When B12 deficiency is clinically suspected, a Schilling test should be performed. The paraesthesias and marked loss of vibratory and proprioceptive functions, with sensory ataxia and pseudoathetosis, may be the result of either posterior column or peripheral nerve involvement. Sensory neuropathy is more strongly suggested when tendon reflexes are clinically depressed. Electrophysiologically, sensory nerve action potentials are absent or reduced in amplitude, and somatosensory evoked potentials are abnormal in most cases with neurological signs (Fine and Hallett, 1980; McCombe and McLeod, 1984). Pathologically, degeneration of sensory axons can be demonstrated in sural biopsies (McCombe and McLeod, 1984). If initiated early, improvement occurs with parenteral B12 therapy, 100 μg intramuscularly daily for several days, weekly for one month, and then monthly for the remainder of the

patient's life. However, when symptoms and signs have been chronically present, progression is halted, but little, if any, improvement occurs. Prompt diagnosis is therefore important (Cox-Klazinga and Endtz, 1980; McCombe and McLeod, 1984).

Vitamin E deficiency

Chronic vitamin E deficiency due to intestinal malabsorption, chronic hepatic cholestasis, or abetalipoproteinaemia causes a syndrome in which dysarthria and cerebellar ataxia are associated with prominent proprioceptive loss and depressed or absent tendon reflexes; degeneration of sensory axons has been supported electrophysiologically by low amplitude or absent sensory action potentials (Harding *et al.*, 1982). Although a less homogeneous spectrum of neurological abnormalities has been identified in which degeneration of peripheral sensory axons is not uniform (Satya-Murti *et al.*, 1986), chronic vitamin E deficiency should be included in the differential diagnosis of spinocerebellar degeneration associated with peripheral neuropathy.

Toxic Peripheral Neuropathy

Toxic peripheral neuropathies are usually distal axonal polyneuropathies (Schaumburg and Spencer, 1979; Spencer and Schaumburg, 1980). Furthermore, mixed sensorimotor involvement is most common, though some toxins may occasionally produce predominantly sensory or motor involvement (Tables 13.3 and 13.4). Those with predomin-

TABLE 13.3 TOXIC PERIPHERAL NEUROPATHIES: COMMONLY ASSOCIATED MEDICATIONS

Predominantly sensory axonal	Mixed axonal
cisplatin	amiodarone
metronidazole	disulfiram
misonidazole	ethambutol
pyridoxine	gold salts
Predominantly motor axonal	hydralazine
dapsone	isoniazid
vinca alkaloids	nitrofurantoin
Demyelinating	nitrous oxide
perhexiline	penicillamine
	phenytoin

TABLE 13.4 TOXIC PERIPHERAL NEUROPATH-IES: COMMONLY ASSOCIATED ENVIRONMENTAL CHEMICALS

Predominantly sensory axonal arsenic thallium Predominantly motor axonal lead	Mixed axonal acrylamide monomer benzene carbon disulphide carbon tetrachloride ethylene oxide methyl bromide methyl *N*-butyl ketone *n*-hexane organophosphates trichloroethylene

antly sensory involvement often resemble sensory neuronopathy. More rare still are those with prominent electrophysiological and pathological evidence for demyelination, such as perhexiline or diphtheritic toxin; other toxins such as hexacarbons and heavy metals produce prominent demyelination only for a limited time interval after exposure, usually between several weeks to several months. Whenever peripheral nerve disease is identified, a detailed history of drug and environmental exposure to potential toxins is always advisable. Some drugs and chemicals which are commonly associated with peripheral neuropathy are listed in Tables 13.3 and 13.4.

Peripheral Neuropathy Associated with Systemic Vascular Diseases

Atherosclerosis

Excepting rare cases of mononeuropathy or multiple mononeuropathy produced by emboli to vasa nervorum, a pathogenetic association of atherosclerosis with peripheral neuropathy either is infrequent or is controversial (Daube and Dyck, 1984; Parry, 1985). Acute non-embolic distal limb ischaemia may at least rarely produce ischaemic mononeuropathies, while other distal tissues remain viable (Wilbourn *et al.*, 1983). In severe atherosclerosis without emboli, skin and muscle more often become necrotic before significant axonal degeneration of peripheral nerve occurs.

Collagen-vascular diseases

The characteristic peripheral neuropathy associated with collagen-vascular diseases in general, but especially polyarteritis nodosa, is a mononeuropathy multiplex with axonal degeneration from multifocal nerve infarctions (Conn and Dyck, 1984; Parry, 1985; Bouchet *et al.*, 1986). Patients present after one or more episodes of acute pain occurring in association with a sensorimotor deficit. Occasionally, many such episodes produce confluent deficits that clinically resemble distal axonal polyneuropathy. This presentation is more common for rheumatoid and systemic lupus neuropathies (Parry, 1985). At any point during the course of rheumatoid arthritis, multiple mononeuropathies typically occur in association with severe arthritis, high titres of rheumatoid factor, and systemic arteritis (Conn *et al.*, 1972; Peyronnard *et al.*, 1982).

Electrophysiological studies reveal reduced amplitude of sensory and motor responses in the involved nerve distributions. Nerve biopsy is necessary for pathological confirmation of vasculitis. An electrophysiologically abnormal sural nerve is most often chosen (Wees *et al.*, 1981). The associated systemic signs, the erythrocyte sedimentation rate, and the antinuclear antibody and other titres are necessary for determining the specific type of vasculitic disease. However, the final diagnosis may, not uncommonly, be that of a non-systemic vasculitic multiple mononeuropathy that may be limited to the peripheral nervous system (Dyck *et al.*, 1985a; Kissel *et al.*, 1985). With treatment specific for the underlying collagen-vascular disease, 6 month and 5 year survivals of 80% and 60%, respectively, have been observed, and the neuropathy improves in 86% of surviving patients at 1 year (Chang *et al.*, 1984).

Peripheral Neuropathy Associated with Infectious Diseases

Leprosy

The most common peripheral nerve disease worldwide is leprosy; it is uncommon in the USA and Europe, where immigrants are most often affected. There are two major forms of disease caused by the *Mycobacterium leprae*. In tuberculoid leprosy, the infection is well localized to the region of the cutaneous lesions, which mark the granulomatous cellular immune response against the organism. In lepromatous leprosy, the infection is poorly contained by the host's immune system; while the cutaneous reaction is less intense, the peripheral neuropathy is more diffuse. The peripheral neuropathy is characterized by one or more patches of sensory loss; these are caused by infiltration and degeneration of cutaneous nerve branches in the cooler regions of the body, such as the pinnae of the ears and the dorsal surfaces of the distal extremities. The treatment of choice is dapsone and rifampicin for both forms, with addition of clofazimine for patients with the lepromatous form (World Health Organization Study Group, 1982).

Spirochaetal associated peripheral neuropathy

The multifocal, often demyelinating, peripheral neuropathy which results from infection with the spirochaete *Borrelia burgdorferi* is referred to as tick-borne meningopolyneuritis, or Bannwarth's syndrome, in Europe and as Lyme disease in the USA. In contrast to the Guillain–Barré syndrome, the spinal fluid contains a lymphocytic pleocytosis (27–450 cells/m^3) in addition to a normal or elevated protein, and treatment may include corticosteroids (Reik *et al.*, 1979).

Peripheral neuropathy associated with human immunodeficiency virus

Several patterns of peripheral neuropathy have been described in association with the human immunodeficiency virus (Lipkin *et al.*, 1985). The inflammatory demyelinating polyneuropathies can present either acutely (often in antibody positive patients) or chronically (often in antibody positive or AIDS-related complex), and spinal fluid pleocytosis is common. Later in the course of the disease, sensory neuronopathy or distal axonal polyneuropathy becomes increasingly prevalent.

Acute Inflammatory Demyelinating Polyradiculoneuropathy

Acute inflammatory demyelinating polyradiculo-neuropathy, or the Guillain–Barré syndrome, is an acutely progressive peripheral nerve disease in which generalized weakness and areflexia develop over days in association with only mild sensory loss. However, several clinical variants, with pain and severe sensory loss, may occur (Asbury, 1981). Weakness of proximal limb and respiratory musculature, in addition to distal limb involvement, is helpful in suggesting a demyelinating, rather than the more common distal axonal, polyneuropathy early in the clinical course. The progressive phase of the weakness, during which 10–23% become respirator dependent, should be completed by 4 weeks and is followed by a plateau phase of days to weeks. Then, full recovery occurs over weeks to several months, although 7–22% (usually the ones requiring ventilatory support for months) improve but are left with residual disability; furthermore, 2–5% die during the course of this monophasic illness (Guillain–Barré Syndrome Study Group, 1985).

The cerebrospinal fluid typically has an elevated protein without pleocytosis (cytoalbuminological dissociation) after the first week (Asbury, 1981). Electrophysiological studies provide clear evidence for multifocal demyelination in 40–60%. However, up to 20% of patients may have no clear electrophysiological abnormalities, with the remainder having less specific evidence of demyelination (Eisen and Humphreys, 1974; McLeod, 1981; Albers *et al.*, 1985).

Acute inflammatory demyelinating polyradiculopathy has long been considered a pathogenetic prototype for cell-mediated immunity in neurological disease. Inflammatory lesions are pathologically characterized by demyelination in association with infiltrates of lymphocytes and macrophages; these lesions are scattered throughout the peripheral nervous system and appear quite similar to experimental allergic neuritis (Prineas, 1981). Recent studies have also found evidence for a possible role of the humoral immune system in its pathogenesis. Plasmapheresis has been found to have a therapeutic benefit (Osterman *et al.*, 1984; Guillain–Barré Syndrome Study Group, 1985), and anti-peripheral-nerve-myelin antibodies are present early in the course of the illness and decline with clinical improvement (Koski *et al.*, 1986). Although the Guillain–Barré syndrome is well characterized pathologically, there is no need to obtain sural nerve biopsies routinely for confirmation of the diagnosis.

The mainstay of treatment is supportive care and includes ventilatory assistance, if necessary; the prevention and treatment of respiratory infection and deep vein thrombosis; maintenance of fluid and electrolyte balance; minimization of autonomic failure; provision of adequate nutrition; prevention of contractures and pressure sores; psychological support; finally, rehabilitation. Corticosteroids have not been shown to be beneficial (Hughes *et al.*, 1978) and, furthermore, are relatively contraindicated since they may contribute to more frequent relapses (Hughes *et al.*, 1981). The only effective treatment, in addition to supportive care, is plasmapheresis (Osterman *et al.*, 1984; Guillain–Barré Syndrome Study Group, 1985). While plasmapheresis has been recommended in the initial 2 to 4 weeks for patients with the Guillain–Barré syndrome who are able to walk 5 metres only with a walker or who have greater weakness, the role of this therapy for milder cases is less clear.

Chronic Inflammatory Demyelinating Polyradiculoneuropathy

Chronic inflammatory demyelinating polyradiculoneuropathy is similar to the acute variety in its symptoms, signs, cytoalbuminological dissociation, and abnormalities with electrophysiological and pathological studies. The major differences are the course, prognosis, and treatment (Dyck *et al.*, 1975; Prineas and McLeod, 1976). The chronic course of weakness is either one of slow progression over months-to-years or one of stepwise progression over weeks-to-months with partial remission. Ten per cent of patients die from this disease and 25% become severely disabled despite treatment (Dyck *et al.*, 1975; Prineas and McLeod, 1976). Sural nerve biopsy is commonly obtained in the chronic cases, before initiating long-term treatment; demyelination induced by mononuclear cell infiltration, 'onion bulbs' (hypertrophic myelination), and secondary axonal degeneration are characteristically seen (Dyck *et al.*, 1975; Prineas and McLeod, 1976). By contrast to the acute variety, prednisone improves the course of the chronic disease in a significant number of patients (Dyck *et al.*, 1982). Plasmapheresis also has a beneficial effect on the course of the chronic variety (Dyck *et al.*, 1986a). Despite the lack of clear evidence for benefit, immunosuppression with azathioprine or cyclophosphamide is often recommended for patients with severe motor disability, when progression continues despite the previous therapies or when potential complications (e.g. osteoporosis) dictate the need for withdrawal or avoidance of prednisone (Dalakas and Engel, 1981; Dyck *et al.*, 1985b).

Sarcoid Peripheral Neuropathy

Sarcoid is a systemic disease of unknown cause in which the incidence of neurological involvement has been variably reported from 1% to 66% (Delany, 1977; Matthews, 1984; Challenor *et al.*, 1984). In nearly all series, unilateral or bilateral facial nerve weakness is the most common, and often the only, neurological abnormality (Matthews, 1984). When non-cranial peripheral nerves are involved, multiple mononeuropathies are typical with a subacute fluctuating course and often with unusual truncal areas of sensory loss; onset for this presentation has been reported as late as the eighth decade (Matthews, 1984). Electrophysiological evidence for multiple mononeuropathy has been found in up to 66% of sarcoid patients with normal neurological examination (Challenor *et al.*, 1984), but the incidence of clinically apparent peripheral neuropathy may be closer to 15% (Delany, 1977). Rare reports of distal polyneuropathy are likely to represent examples of confluent multiple mononeuropathies. Pathologically, involved segments of peripheral nerve have non-caseating granulomas (Matthews, 1984). If the peripheral neuropathy does not spontaneously resolve, treatment with prednisone is usually beneficial (Matthews, 1984).

Peripheral Neuropathy Associated with Neoplasia (see also Chapter 21)

Distal axonal polyneuropathy

Although uniformly present late in the course of clinically obvious carcinoma, the incidence of occult carcinoma is not clearly increased when an elderly patient presents with a typical sensorimotor distal axonal polyneuropathy, which has subacute or chronic progression (Hawley *et al.*, 1980; McLeod, 1984). The incidence of distal axonal polyneuropathy in carcinoma is highest for lung primaries, but is still less than 5% even after the lung carcinoma is diagnosed (McLeod, 1984).

Inflammatory demyelinating polyneuropathy

While distal axonal polyneuropathy is less common with lymphoma than carcinoma, lymphomas are associated with an increased incidence of inflammatory demyelinating polyneuropathy (McLeod and Walsh, 1984). The clinical features are the same as the non-neoplasia associated ones, which were discussed earlier; progression of weakness may follow either an acute or chronic course. A few of the subacute cases have preservation of the deep tendon reflexes, so as clinically to resemble a motor neuronopathy (Schold *et al.*, 1979); however, pathological documentation of proximal demylination in these cases suggests that they may be a variation of inflammatory demyelinating polyneuropathy.

Sensory neuronopathy

Sensory neuronopathy has quite distinctive clinical features and, in contrast to distal axonal polyneuropathy, typically precedes the diagnosis of carcinoma by 6–15 months if paraneoplastic in origin (Horwich *et al.*, 1977; McLeod, 1984). Numbness, paraesthesias, or dysthaesias are the usual initial complaint. These often begin distally in the lower extremities, but may also first develop in the face or other more proximal distributions. Sensory ataxia of gait and pseudoathetotic movements of the fingers are also common, due to the proprioceptive loss. Sensory examination reveals diminished perception of all modalities. Deep tendon reflexes are depressed or absent, but weakness is usually mild or absent even when disability is severe. Cerebrospinal fluid may be normal, but often reveals a mild lymphocytic pleocytosis and/or an elevated protein. Electrophysiologically, sensory action potentials are absent (or rarely obtained with marked amplitude reduction), but motor conduction studies are normal, or nearly so

(Horwich *et al.*, 1977; McLeod, 1984). Pathologically, there is inflammation and degeneration of dorsal root ganglia and degeneration of posterior columns and sensory nerves (Horwich *et al.*, 1977; McLeod, 1984). Oat cell carcinoma of the lung is the most frequently associated neoplasm (Horwich *et al.*, 1977). However, idiopathic cases (in which no carcinoma develops even with long-term follow-up) may be more common than the paraneoplastic ones (Mitsumoto *et al.*, 1985; Dalakas, 1986). The differential diagnosis also includes B12 deficiency, pyridoxine toxicity, Sjögren's syndrome and acquired immunodeficiency syndrome. No treatment has been shown to be effective for the paraneoplastic cases.

Mononeuropathy and multiple mononeuropathy

Primary tumours of peripheral nerves present with a mononeuropathy (Brooks, 1984), but metastatic tumours more often present with multiple mononeuropathies in a single limb or with a plexus lesion (McLeod, 1984; McLeod and Walsh, 1984). Less commonly, more widespread metastasis or a paraneoplastic vasculitis may cause a multiple mononeuropathy which affects more than one limb (Johnson *et al.*, 1979).

Paraproteinaemic Peripheral Neuropathy

Over the past decade, major inroads have been made into the category of so-called idiopathic polyneuropathy through recognition of the association between paraproteins and peripheral nerve disease (Kelly, 1985). This new development has particular relevance to the geriatric population, since the prevalence of paraproteinaemic disorders in general, and benign monoclonal gammopathies in particular, increases with advancing age. Across a broad age range, 10% of patients with peripheral neuropathy have monoclonal protein abnormalities (Kelly *et al.*, 1981).

Multiple myeloma

The association between multiple myeloma and a particular type of peripheral neuropathy is most clearly defined for osteosclerotic myeloma and chronic demyelinating polyneuropathy. Osteosclerotic lesions are present in only 3% of multiple myelomas, and these patients are generally younger (usually 40–65 years). However, 50% of such patients have peripheral neuropathy; and, when peripheral neuropathy is present, it is usually the cause for presentation (Kelly *et al.*, 1983). The chief complaint is more often distal paraesthesias than weakness. However, weakness of distal muscles is usually more prominent on examination than is the sensory deficit, and deep tendon reflexes are depressed or absent. Spinal fluid protein is elevated, and nerve conduction velocity is severely reduced into the range typical for demyelination. Serum immunoelectrophoresis identifies a small monoclonal protein in 75% of cases. Although rare, especially over the age of 65 years, recognition is important, since tumoricidal irradiation of solitary lesions usually reverses the polyneuropathy (Kelly *et al.*, 1983).

In the more typical multiple myelomas with osteolytic skeletal lesions, the prevalence of peripheral neuropathy is lower, being clinically evident in 2–13% (Kelly, 1985). The patterns of peripheral neuropathy are less uniform; although a mild distal axonal polyneuropathy is most common, an increased incidence of the more distinctive inflammatory demyelinating neuropathies has also been described, as with lymphomas. The course of the myeloma and the peripheral neuropathy are typically independent, so the causal relationship is often unclear (Kelly, 1985).

Although most cases of multiple myeloma can be distinguished from primary systemic amyloidosis by an increase of plasma cells in the bone marrow (> 15%), by a rise in monoclonal protein in the serum (> 3 g/dl), and by the presence of lytic bone lesions, rarely the two overlap (Kelly *et al.*, 1979). Several cases have been reported in which amyloid deposits have been pathologically demonstrated in multiple myeloma neuropathy (McLeod *et al.*, 1984).

Macroglobulinaemia

Waldenström's macroglobulinaemia is associated with peripheral neuropathy in up to 25% of cases

(McLeod *et al.*, 1984). In most cases, the weight loss, fatigue, anaemia, mucosal bleeding, and other non-neurological signs precede the neuropathy, but the neuropathy may rarely precede the systemic signs by years. The presenting complaint of the peripheral neuropathy is typically distal paraesthesias or numbness, but weakness is often prominent on examination (McLeod *et al.*, 1984). Spinal fluid protein is frequently elevated. Nerve conduction velocities are most often severely reduced into the range typical for demyelination (Kelly, 1985). Remission of the peripheral neuropathy with treatment of the macroglobulinaemia has been reported, but is unusual (McLeod *et al.* 1984).

Benign monoclonal neuropathies

After multiple myeloma, macroglobulinaemia, and primary systemic amyloidosis have been excluded, there remains a significant group of patients with monoclonal proteins and peripheral neuropathy; furthermore, this association is frequently detected in geriatric patients. The prevalence of monoclonal proteins in population-based studies has been less than 1% until after the seventh or eighth decades; over the age of 80 years, the prevalence has been in excess of 5% (Axelsson *et al.*, 1966; Kyle and Bayrd, 1976). In a group of consecutive patients who were referred for electrophysiological studies and who were found to have peripheral neuropathy, 5% had a benign monoclonal gammopathy in one series (Kelly *et al.*, 1981).

Both demyelinating and distal axonal polyneuropathies have been described, with progression usually chronic. The most consistent clinical syndrome seems to be that of a chronically progressive demyelinating polyneuropathy with IgM gammopathies, particularly those with kappa light chains and/or with antibody reactivity to myelin associated glycoprotein, or anti-MAG (Kelly, 1985). IgG gammopathies are more often distal axonal polyneuropathies, but demyelinating ones have also been described in some patients. Distal paraesthesias are the usual presenting complaint. When weakness in proximal muscles is found on examination, nerve conduction studies usually reveal marked slowing into the range typical for demyelination, and segmental demyelination is confirmed pathologically in the sural nerve. Therapeutic benefit has been inconsistently seen with corticosteroids, cytotoxic medications, and plasmapheresis in various combinations, so the drug of choice is far from clear (Kelly, 1985). Since the risks of all potential therapies are significant, treatment is usually deferred unless significant motor disability has developed; one drug or combination of therapies is continued (if tolerated) for 3 to 6 months, before changing the therapeutic regimen if benefit does not result.

Primary Systemic Amyloidosis

Primary systemic amyloidosis is a multisystem disease in which less than a fifth develop peripheral neuropathy; the major manifestations may be renal, cardiac, haematological, or gastrointestinal. However, if present, the peripheral neuropathy is often the cause for presentation (Kelly *et al.*, 1979). Males are more commonly affected than females by a 9:1 ratio, and half are in their seventh or eighth decade. The neuropathic presentation is typically one of a painful distal symmetrical axonal polyneuropathy with prominent autonomic symptoms. Pain and temperature are diminished more than vibration and joint position; distal weakness is often mild and reflexes preserved. Nearly two-thirds of patients have a monoclonal protein in the serum and/or urine with immunoelectrophoresis. Spinal fluid protein is often mildly elevated. Electrophysiologically, sensory action potentials are typically absent, and motor abnormalities are mild. The diagnosis cannot be made without the pathological demonstration of amyloid in some tissue, such as rectal, renal, hepatic, small intestinal or nervous; in cases with neuropathy, amyloid is reliably present around endoneurial vascular structures. Unfortunately, no treatment is known to alter the course of the neuropathy (Kelly *et al.*, 1979).

Inherited Peripheral Neuropathy

Hereditary amyloid

In addition to primary systemic and secondary amyloidosis, there are four varieties of hereditary amyloidosis, all of which are autosomal dominant (Harding and Thomas, 1984; Cohen and Rubinow, 1984). These usually present either (1) in the third or fourth decade with autonomic failure and loss of pain and temperature sense in the distal lower extremities or (2) in middle adult life with carpal tunnel syndrome. These hereditary neuropathies are part of the differential diagnosis for amyloid deposition in peripheral nerve; however, primary systemic amyloidosis and amyloidosis secondary to paraproteinaemia are much more likely to occur in the geriatric population than are the hereditary amyloidoses.

Hereditary motor and sensory neuropathy

The prevalence of hereditary motor and sensory neuropathies (HMSN) in late life is unclear; the hypertrophic HMSN Type I and the neuronal HMSN Type II are the most common ones and are at least compatible with survival into the eighth decade (Dyck, 1984). With intensive evaluation of peripheral neuropathies which remain unclassified at the time of tertiary referral, 42% of 205 patients have had an undiagnosed inherited neuropathy; the most common of these newly diagnosed inherited neuropathies are HMSN Types I and II (Dyck *et al.*, 1981). The prevalence of undiagnosed HMSN may be lower in the seventh and later decades of life, but the detailed inquiry of family history and the examination of family members with suspicious symptoms are warranted.

Hereditary motor neuropathy and hereditary sensory autonomic neuropathy

The prevalence of these disorders is lower than the HMSNs throughout adult life; although all of these are most unlikely to present in late life, a positive family history for a similar disorder would suggest the advisability of examining other family members.

Peripheral neuropathy in association with hereditary multisystem neurological diseases

Peripheral neuropathy may develop as one manifestation of a hereditary multisystem neurological disease, especially early in life. This may be occasionally seen at an advanced age with olivopontocerebellar atrophies and spinocerebellar degenerations, where a mild distal axonal polyneuropathy is associated.

Idiopathic Peripheral Nerve Disease

Even after intensive evaluation of peripheral neuropathies which had been unclassified at the time of tertiary referral, 24% of 205 patients across a broad age range remain undiagnosed (Dyck *et al.*, 1981). These cases are typically distal axonal neuropathies, and may be more common and difficult to distinguish from 'normal' age-related decline in peripheral nerve function over the age of 60 years.

TREATMENT AND REHABILITATION

In the preceding sections, specific treatments which may cure or reverse the underlying pathogenetic mechanism have been discussed. General approaches for the symptomatic treatment of pain and for rehabilitation are also important.

Several drugs may be useful in palliating the pain which sometimes results from peripheral neuropathy, but none is curative (see also Chapter 22). A frank discussion with the patient of this, and of simple approaches to pain control without prescription medications, is a useful initial step. Two aspirin and a 15 minute soak of the feet in cold water before retiring to bed may prove adequate for some patients. If not, the first choice of prescription medication often depends on the type of pain. If burning dysaesthetic pain in the feet is most symptomatic at night, an evening dose of antidepressant (such as amitriptyline) may be helpful. This should start low and be increased gradually. Dry mouth and morning drowsiness become dose limiting. For sharp shooting pain which is most prominent in the daytime, phenytoin or carbamazepine are often more useful. While carbamazepine is usually more beneficial, phenytoin can be more safely administered without frequent blood tests for toxicity. After these three drugs, the next choice is less clear; prazosin and baclofen are sometimes beneficial. For diabetics, pentoxiphylline may improve microcirculation and decrease pain. Occasionally, transcutaneous nerve stimulators provide long-term benefit.

A common sense discussion of activities of daily living is important to help prevent injury and better maintain function. When numbness of the feet is present, soft but protective footware should be worn at all times, and each foot should be visually inspected at least once a day for early detection of sores and injuries. Bathwater and other potential sources for burns should be habitually tested with a body part which has maintained normal thermal sensation. Large handled eating utensils, cups, and tools will help preserve function as manual dexterity and sensation becomes compromised; Velcro straps on shoes and garments and button hooks are also useful for some patients.

Another rehabilitative measure which is often useful for patients with significant weakness is the prescription of orthotic devices. Plastic ankle–foot orthoses are often useful for patients with partial foot drop, as are wrist splints for patients with wrist drop. Prescription of sturdier metal braces is usually less beneficial, since their greater weight places significantly increased demand on the muscles which act on the joint above (and/or below) the braced one.

Treatments are available for some features of autonomic failure (see also Chapter 14). Orthostatic hypotension is often one of the more disabling symptoms. Initially decreasing or discontinuing any antihypertensive medications in use and avoidance of dehydration may be adequate. Elastic stockings (more effective but poorly tolerated if fitted up to the diaphragm) and nocturnal elevation of the head of the bed are sometimes useful. If these measures are not sufficiently effective, fludrocortisone 0.1–0.3 mg per day and other medications are often beneficial (Niakan *et al.*, 1986).

REFERENCES

Albers, J.W., Donofrio, P.D., and McGonagle, T.K. (1985). Sequential electrodiagnostic abnormalities in acute inflammatory demyelinating polyradiculoneuropathy. *Muscle Nerve*, **8**, 528–39.

Asbury, A.K. (1981). Diagnostic considerations in Guillain-Barré syndrome. *Ann. Neurol.*, **9** (Suppl.), 1–5.

Asbury, A.K. (1984). Uremic neuropathy. In: Dyck, P.J., Thomas, P.K., Lambert, E.H., and Bunge, R. (eds.) *Peripheral Neuropathy*, W. B. Saunders, Philadelphia, pp. 1811–25.

Axelsson, U., Bachmann, R., and Hallen, J. (1966). Frequency of pathological proteins (M-components) in 6,995 sera from an adult population. *Acta Med. Scand.*, **179**, 235–47.

Bannister, R., Crowe, R., Eames, R., and Burnstock, G. (1981). Adrenergic innervation in autonomic failure. *Neurology*, **31**, 1501–6.

Bastron, J.A. (1984). Neuropathy in diseases of the thyroid and pituitary glands. In: Dyck, P.J., Thomas, P.K., Lambert, E.H., and Bunge, R. (eds.) *Peripheral Neuropathy*, W. B. Saunders, Philadelphia, pp. 1833–46.

Bastron, J.A., and Thomas, J.E. (1981). Diabetic polyradiculopathy, clinical and electromyographic findings in 105 patients. *Mayo Clin. Proc.*, **56**, 725–32.

Behse, F., and Buchthal, F. (1977). Alcoholic neuropathy: clinical, electrophysiological, and biopsy findings. *Ann. Neurol.*, **2**, 95–110.

Behse, F., Buchthal, F., and Carlsen, F. (1977). Nerve biopsy and conduction studies in diabetic neuropathy. *J. Neurol. Neurosurg. Psychiatry*, **40**, 1072–82.

Bouche, P., Leger, J.M., Travers, M.A., Cathala, H.P., and Castaigne, P. (1986). Peripheral neuropathy in systemic vasculitis: clinical and electrophysiologic study of 22 patients. *Neurology*, **37**, 1598–1602.

Brooks, D. (1984). Clinical presentation and treatment of peripheral nerve tumors. In: Dyck, P.J., Thomas, P.K., Lambert, E.H., and Bunge, R. (eds.) *Peripheral Neuropathy*, W. B. Saunders, Philadelphia, pp. 2236–51.

Brown, M.J. and Asbury, A.K. (1984). Diabetic neuropathy. *Ann. Neurol.*, **15**, 2–12.

Challenor, Y.B., Felton, C.P., and Brust, J.C.M. (1984). Peripheral nerve involvement in sarcoidosis: an electrodiagnostic study. *J. Neurol. Neurosurg. Psychiatry*, **47**, 1219–22.

Chan, R.C., Paine, K.W.E., and Varughese, G. (1980). Ulnar neuropathy at the elbow: comparison of simple decompression and anterior transposition. *Neurosurgery*, **7**, 545–50.

Chang, R.W., Bell, C.L., and Hallett, M. (1984). Clinical characteristics and prognosis of vasculitic mononeuropathy multiplex. *Arch. Neurol.*, **41**, 618–21.

Cohen, A.S., and Rubinow, A. (1984). Amyloid neuropathy. In: Dyck, P.J., Thomas, P.K., Lambert, E.H., and Bunge, R. (eds.), *Peripheral Neuropathy*, W. B. Saunders, Philadelphia, pp. 1866–98.

Conn, D.L., and Dyck, P.J. (1984). Angiopathic neuropathy in connective tissue diseases. In: Dyck, P.J., Thomas, P.K., Lambert, E.H., and Bunge, R. (eds.) *Peripheral Neuropathy*, W. B. Saunders, Philadelphia, pp. 2027–43.

Conn, D.L., McDuffie, F.C., and Dyck, P.J. (1972). Immunopathological study of sural nerves in rheumatoid arthritis. *Arthritis Rheum.*, **15**, 135–43.

Cox-Klazinga, M., and Endtz, L.J. (1980). Peripheral nerve involvement in pernicious anemia. *J. Neurol. Sci.*, **45**, 367–71.

Dalakas, M.C. (1986). Chronic idiopathic ataxic neuropathy. *Ann. Neurol.*, **19**, 545–54.

Dalakas, M.C., and Engel, W.K. (1981). Chronic relapsing (dysimmune) polyneuropathy: pathogenesis and treatment. *Ann. Neurol.*, **9** (Suppl.), 134–45.

Daube, J.R., and Dyck, P.J. (1984). Neuropathy due to peripheral vascular diseases. In: Dyck, P.J., Thomas P.K., Lambert, E.H., and Bunge, R. (eds.) *Peripheral Neuropathy*, W. B. Saunders, Philadelphia, pp. 1458–78.

Dawson, D.M., Hallett, M., and Millender, L.H. (1983a). The carpal tunnel syndrome. In: *Entrapment Neuropathies*, Little, Brown, Boston, pp. 5–59.

Dawson, D.M., Hallet, M., and Millender, L.H. (1983b). Peroneal nerve entrapment. In: *Entrapment Neuropathies*, Little, Brown, Boston, pp. 201–10.

Delaney, P. (1977). Neurologic manifestations in sarcoidosis. *Ann. Intern. Med.*, **87**, 336–45.

Delisa, J.A., and Saeed, M.A. (1983). AAEE Case Report #8: The tarsal tunnel syndrome. *Muscle Nerve*, **6**, 664–70.

Donaldson, R.M., Brand, M., and Serfilippi, D. (1977). Changes in circulating transcobalamin II after injection of cyanocobalamin. *N. Engl. J. Med.*, **296**, 1427–30.

Dyck, P.J. (1984). Inherited neuronal degeneration and atrophy affecting peripheral motor, sensory and autonomic neurons. In: Dyck, P.J., Thomas, P.K., Lambert, E.H., and Bunge, R. (eds.) *Peripheral Neuropathy*, W. B. Saunders, Philadelphia, pp. 1600–55.

Dyck, P.J., Johnson, W.J., Lambert, E.H., and O'Brien, P.C. (1971). Segmental demyelination secondary to axonal degeneration in uremic neuropathy. *Mayo Clin. Proc.*, **46**, 400–31.

Dyck, P.J., Lais, A.C., Ohta, M., Bastron, J.A., Okazaki, H., and Groover, R.V. (1975). Chronic inflammatory polyradiculoneuropathy. *Mayo Clin. Proc.*, **50**, 621–37.

Dyck, P.J., Sherman, W.R., Hallcher, L.M., Service, F.J., O'Brien, P.C., Grina, L.A., Palumbo, P.J., and Swanson, C.J. (1980). Human diabetic endoneurial sorbitol, fructose, and *myo*-inositol related to sural nerve morphometry. *Ann. Neurol.*, **8**, 590–6.

Dyck, P.J., Oviatt, K.F., and Lambert, E.H. (1981). Intensive evaluation of referred unclassified neuropathies yields improved diagnosis. *Ann. Neurol.*, **10**, 222–6.

Dyck, P.J., O'Brien, P.C., Oviatt, K.F., Dinapoli, R.P., Daube, J.R., Bartleson, J.D., Mokri, B., Swift, T., Low, P.A., and Windebank, A.J. (1982). Prednisone improves chronic inflammatory demyelinating polyradiculoneuropathy more than no treatment. *Ann. Neurol.*, **11**, 136–41.

Dyck, P.J., Conn, D., Low, P.A. and Windebank, A. (1985a). Nonsystemic vasculitic multiple mononeuropathy. *Neurology*, **35** (Suppl. 1), 292.

Dyck, P.J., O'Brien, P., Swanson, C., Low, P., and Daube, J. (1985b). Combined azathioprine and prednisone in chronic inflammatory demyelinating polyneuropathy. *Neurology*, **35**, 1173–6.

Dyck, P.J., Daube, J., O'Brien, P., Pinda, A., Low, P.A.,

Windebank, A.J., and Swanson, C. (1986a). Plasma exchange in chronic inflammatory demyelinating polyradiculoneuropathy. *N. Engl. J. Med.*, **314**, 461–5.

Dyck, P.J., Karnes, J.L., O'Brien, P., Okazaki, H., Lais, A., and Englestad, J. (1986b). The spatial distribution of fiber loss in diabetic polyneuropathy suggests ischemia. *Ann. Neurol.*, **19**, 440–9.

Dyck, P.J., Lais, A., Karnes, J.L., O'Brien, P., and Rizza, R. (1986c). Fiber loss is primary and multifocal in sural nerves in diabetic polyneuropathy. *Ann. Neurol.*, **19**, 425–39.

Eisen, A., and Humphreys, P. (1974). The Guillain–Barré Syndrome. A clinical and electrodiagnostic study of 25 cases. *Arch. Neurol.*, **30**, 438–43.

Feibel, J.H., and Campa, J.F. (1976). Thyrotoxic neuropathy (Basedow's paraplegia). *J. Neurol. Neurosurg. Psychiatry*, **39**, 491–7.

Fine, E.J., and Hallett, M. (1980). Neurophysiological study of subacute combined degeneration. *J. Neurol. Sci.*, **45**, 331–6.

Garland, H. (1955). Diabetic amyotrophy. *Br. Med. J.*, **iv**, 1287–90.

Guillain–Barré Syndrome Study Group (1985). Plasmapheresis and acute Guillain–Barré syndrome. *Neurology*, **35**, 1096–1104.

Harding, A.E., and Thomas, P.K. (1984). Genetically determined neuropathies. In: Asbury, A.K., and Gilliatt, R.W. (eds.) *Peripheral Nerve Disorders*, Butterworth, London, pp. 205–42.

Harding, A.E., Muller, D.P.R., Thomas, P.K., and Willison, H.J. (1982). Spinocerebellar degeneration secondary to chronic intestinal malabsorption: a vitamin E deficiency syndrome. *Ann. Neurol.*, **12**, 419–24.

Hawley, R.J., Cohen, M.H., Saini, N., and Armbrustmacher, V.W. (1980). The carcinomatous neuromyopathy of oat cell lung cancer. *Ann. Neurol.*, **7**, 65–72.

Hillbom, M., and Wennberg, A. (1984). Prognosis of alcoholic peripheral neuropathy. *J. Neurol. Neurosurg. Psychiatry*, **47**, 699–703.

Horwich, M.S., Cho, L., Porro, R.S., and Posner, J.B. (1977). Subacute sensory neuropathy: a remote effect of carcinoma. *Ann. Neurol.*, **2**, 7–10.

Hughes, R.A.C., Newson-Davis, J.M., and Perkins, G.D. (1978). Controlled trial of prednisolone in acute polyneuropathy. *Lancet*, **ii**, 1100.

Hughes, R.A.C., Kadlubowski, M., and Hufschmidt, A. (1981). Treatment of acute inflammatory polyneuropathy. *Ann. Neurol.*, **9** (Suppl.), 125–33.

Jaspan, J.B., Wollman, R.L., Bernstein, L., and Rubenstein, A.H. (1982). Hypoglycemic peripheral neuropathy in association with insulinoma: Implication of glucopenia rather than hyperinsulinism. *Medicine*, **61**, 33–44.

Johnson, P.C., Rolak, L.A., Hamilton, R.H., and Laguna, J.F. (1979). Paraneoplastic vasculitis of nerve: a remote effect of cancer. *Ann. Neurol.*, **5**, 437–44.

Kelly, J.J. (1985). Peripheral neuropathies associated with monoclonal proteins: a clinical review. *Muscle Nerve*, **8**, 138–50.

Kelly, J.J., Kyle, R.A., O'Brien, P.C., and Dyck, P.J. (1979). The natural history of peripheral neuropathy in primary systemic amyloidosis. *Ann. Neurol.*, **6**, 1–7.

Kelly, J.J., Kyle, R.A., O'Brien, P.C., and Dyck, P.J., (1981). Prevalance of monoclonal protein in peripheral neuropathy. *Neurology*, **31**, 1480–3.

Kelly, J.J., Kyle, R.A., Miles, J.M., and Dyck, P.J. (1983). Osteosclerotic myeloma and peripheral neuropathy. *Neurology*, **33**, 202–10.

Kikta, D.G., Breuer, A.C., and Wilbourn, A.J. (1982). Thoracic root pain in diabetes: the spectrum of clinical and electromyographic findings. *Ann. Neurol.*, **11**, 80–5.

Kissel, J.T., Slivka, A.P., Warmolts, J.R., and Mendell, J.R. (1985). The clinical spectrum of nectrotizing angiopathy of the peripheral nervous system. *Ann. Neurol.*, **18**, 251–7.

Koski, C.L., Gratz, E., Sutherland, J., and Mayer, R.F. (1986). Clinical correlation with anti-peripheral-nerve myelin antibodies in Guillain-Barré syndrome. *Ann. Neurol.*, **19**, 573–7.

Kyle, R.A., and Bayrd, E.D. (1976). Benign monoclonal gammopathy. In *The Monoclonal Gammopathies*, Charles C. Thomas, Springfield, Illinois, pp. 284–368.

Layzer, R.B. (1985). Endocrine disorders. In *Neuromuscular Manifestations of Systemic Disease*, F. A. Davis, Philadelphia, pp. 79–137.

Lipkin, W.I., Parry, G., Kprov, D., and Abrams, D. (1985). Inflammatory neuropathy in homosexual men with lymphadenopathy. *Neurology*, **35**, 1479–83.

Low, P.A. (1984). Quantitation of autonomic responses. In: Dyck, P.J., Thomas, P.K., Lambert, E.H., and Bunge, R. (eds.), *Peripheral Neuropathy*, W. B. Saunders, Philadelphia, pp. 1139–65.

Low, P.A., McLeod, J.G., Turtle, J.R., Donnelly, P., and Wright, R.G. (1974). Peripheral neuropathy in acromegaly. *Brain*, **97**, 139–52.

McCombe, P.A., and McLeod, J.G. (1984). The peripheral neuropathy of vitamin B12 deficiency. *J. Neurol. Sci.*, **66**, 117–26.

McLeod, J.G. (1981). Electrophysiological studies in the Guillain-Barré syndrome. *Ann. Neurol.*, **9** (Suppl.), 20–7.

McLeod, J.G. (1984). Carcinomatous neuropathy. In: Dyck, P.J., Thomas, P.K., Lambert, E.H., and Bunge, R. (eds.) *Peripheral Neuropathy*, W. B. Saunders, Philadelphia, pp. 2180–91.

McLeod, J.G., and Walsh, J.C. (1984). Peripheral neuropathy associated with lymphoma and other reticuloses. In: Dyck, P.J., Thomas, P.K., Lambert, E.H., and Bunge, R. (eds.) *Peripheral Neuropathy*, W. B. Saunders, Philadelphia, pp. 2192–203.

McLeod, J.G., Walsh, J.C., and Pollard, J.D. (1984). Neuropathies associated with paraproteinemias and dysproteinemias. In: Dyck, P.J., Thomas, P.K., Lambert, E.H., and Bunge, R. (eds.), *Peripheral Neuropathy*, W. B. Saunders, Philadelphia, pp. 1847–65.

Mathews, W.B. (1984). Sarcoid neuropathy. In: Dyck, P.J., Thomas, P.K., Lambert, E.H., and Bunge, R. (eds.) *Peripheral Neuropathy*, W. B. Saunders, Philadelphia, pp. 2018–26.

Miller, R.G., and Camp, P.E. (1979). Postoperative ulnar neuropathy. *J.A.M.A.*, **242**, 1636–9.

Miller, R.G., and Hummel, E.E. (1980). The cubital tunnel syndrome: treatment with simple decompression. *Ann. Neurol.*, **7**, 567–9.

Mitsumoto, H., Wilbourn, A.J., and Massarweh, W. (1985). Acquired "pure" sensory polyneuropathy (APSP): unique clinical features in 30 patients. *Neurology*, **35** (Suppl. 1), 295.

Neary, D., Ochoa, J., and Gilliatt, R.W. (1975). Subclinical entrapment neuropathy in man. *J. Neurol. Sci.*, **24**, 283–98.

Niakan, E., Harati, Y., and Comstock, J.P. (1986). Diabetic autonomic neuropathy. *Metabolism*, **35**, 224–34.

Olney, R.K. (1985). Age-related changes in peripheral nerve function. *Geriatric Medicine Today*, **4**, 76–86.

Olney, R.K. (1986). The pathophysiology of symptomatic diabetic polyneuropathy. *Neurology*, **36** (Suppl. 1), 235.

Olney, R.K., and Wilbourn, A.J. (1985). Ulnar nerve conduction study of the first dorsal interosseous muscle. *Arch. Phys. Med. Rehabil.*, **66**, 16–18.

Olney, R.K., Bromberg, S., and Baumbach, N.J. (1983). Age-related changes in monosynaptic reflex function. *Muscle Nerve*, **6**, 529–30.

Osterman, P.O., Fagius, J., Lundemo, G., Philstedt, P., Pirskanen, R., Siden, A., and Safwenberg, J. (1984). Beneficial effects of plasma exchange in acute inflammatory polyradiculoneuropathy. *Lancet*, **ii**, 1296–8.

Parry, G.J.G. (1985). Mononeuropathy multiplex (AAEE case report #11). *Muscle Nerve*, **8**, 493–8.

Peyronnard, J.-M., Charron, L., Beaudet, F., and Couture, F. (1982). Vasculitic neuropathy in rheumatoid disease and Sjögren syndrome. *Neurology* **32**, 839–45.

Phalen, G.S. (1966). The carpal-tunnel syndrome. *J. Bone Joint Surg.*, **48A**, 211–28.

Phalen, G.S. (1972). The carpal-tunnel syndrome. *Clin. Orthop.*, **83**, 29–40.

Pirart, J. (1978). Diabetes mellitus and its degenerative complications: a prospective study of 4,000 patients observed between 1947 and 1973. *Diabetes Care*, **1**, 168–88 and 252–63.

Pollard, J.D., McLeod, J.G., Angel Honnibal, T.G., and Verheijden, M.A. (1982). Hypothyroid polyneuropathy. *J. Neurol. Sci.*, **53**, 461–71.

Potvin, A.R., Syndulko, K., Tourtellotte, W.W., Lemmon, M.S., and Potvin, J.H. (1980). Human neurologic function and the aging process. *J. Am. Geriatr. Soc.*, **28**, 1–9.

Prineas, J.W. (1981). Pathology of the Guillain-Barré syndrome. *Ann. Neurol.*, 9 (Suppl.), 6–19.

Prineas, J.W., and McLeod, J.G. (1976). Chronic relapsing polyneuritis. *J. Neurol. Sci.*, **27**, 427–58.

Raff, M.C., Sangalang, V., and Asbury, A.K. (1968). Ischemic mononeuropathy multiplex associated with diabetes mellitus. *Arch. Neurol.*, **18**, 487–99.

Reik, L., Steere, A.C., Bartenhagen, N.H., Shope, R.E., and Malawista, S.E. (1979). Neurologic abnormalities of Lyme disease. *Medicine*, **58**, 281–94.

Satya-Murti, S., Howard, L., Krohel, G., and Wolf, B. (1986). The spectrum of neurologic disorder from vitamin E deficiency. *Neurology*, **36**, 917–21.

Schaumburg, H.H., and Spencer, P.S. (1979). Toxic neuropathies. *Neurology*, **29**, 429–31.

Schold, S.C., Cho, E.S., Somasundaram, M., and Posner, J.B. (1979). Subacute motor neuronopathy: a remote effect of lymphoma. *Ann. Neurol.*, **5**, 271–87.

Service, F.J., Daube, J.R., O'Brine, P.C., Zimmerman, B.R., Swanson, C.J., Brennan, M.D., and Dyck, P.J. (1983). Effect of blood glucose control on peripheral nerve function in diabetic patients. *Mayo Clin. Proc.*, **58**, 283–389.

Spencer, P.S., and Schaumburg, H.H. (eds.) (1980). *Experimental and Clinical Neurotoxicology*, Williams & Wilkins, Baltimore, pp. 92–9.

Thomas, P.K., and Lascelles, R.G. (1966). The pathology of diabetic neuropathy. *Q. J. Med.*, **140**, 489–509.

Wees, S.J., Sunwoo, I.N., and Oh, S.J. (1981). Sural nerve biopsy in systemic necrotizing vasculitis. *Am. J. Med.*, **71**, 525–32.

Wilbourn, A.J., Furlan, A.J., Hulley, W., and Ruschhaupt, W. (1983). Ischemic monomelic neuropathy. *Neurology*, **33**, 447–51.

World Health Organization Study Group (1982). Chemotherapy of leprosy for control programmes. *WHO Technical Report Series*, No. 675.

Young, R.R., Asbury, A.K., Corbett, J.L. and Adams, R.D. (1975). Pure pandysautonomia with recovery. *Brain*, **98**, 613–36.

Chapter 14

Autonomic Dysfunction and Abnormal Vascular Reflexes

Michael Lye

Professor of Geriatric Medicine, University Department of Geriatric Medicine, Royal Liverpool Hospital, Liverpool, UK

INTRODUCTION

The autonomic nervous system acts as both the monitor and regulator of the 'milieu intérieur' of Claude Bernard (1865). As the increasingly inefficient maintenance of body homeostasis under stress is one of the hallmarks of 'normal' ageing, it is highly likely that ageing has some direct effect upon the autonomic nervous system. It is, however, extraordinarily difficult to disentangle the effects of ageing from age-related pathological states (neuropathy). Even in relatively young adults in whom the impact of ageing has not had time to become manifest, there is no overall agreement as to the pathology associated with particular clinical syndromes (Bannister, 1983). Syndromes involving the autonomic nervous system show considerable overlap; both clinically and histologically nosological entities are often distinguished only by the relative degree of involvement of different components of the autonomic nervous system.

The autonomic nervous system is intimately involved with other components of the central nervous system, the interactions going both ways (Palkovits, 1980). Thus changes in autonomic function may be secondary to changes, whether ageing or age-related, occurring in the cerebrum, brain stem or spinal cord. Similarly, many autonomic functions act through or in concert with the neuroendocrine system. With improved biochemical and histochemical techniques, investigators have helped our understanding of some of these homeostatic mechanisms, whilst also revealing our ignorance of many other subsystems. Finally, ageing and age-related diseases may impair end organ responsiveness, which may be mistakenly attributed to autonomic nervous system dysfunction.

In this review, the intention is to focus on the effects of ageing and age-related disease upon the autonomic nervous system. In particular, because of its unique importance and the fact that most work has been concentrated in this area, the relationship of the autonomic nervous system to cardiovascular homeostasis will be reviewed. Attention will also be paid to the role of pharmacological agents in both investigating and treating autonomic nervous system dysfunction in the elderly.

MORPHOLOGY AND PHYSIOLOGY

The earlier concept (Myerson, 1938) of the autonomic nervous system being arranged in two separate and opposite acting arms, the sympathetic (adrenergic) and the parasympathetic (cholinergic), has had to be considerably modified. The idea that homeostatic equilibrium was maintained by the opposing effects of excitation and inhibition has proved to be too simplistic. Ahlquist (1948) provided the first insight into the complexities of the autonomic nervous system when he proposed the existence of alpha and beta adrenoceptors within the sympathetic component. Further subdivisions have developed so that we now have the beta$_1$ and beta$_2$ and the alpha$_1$ and alpha$_2$ subsets. The advent of powerful, and to a greater or lesser extent specific, agonists (activators) and antagonists (inhibitors) will allow further exploration and elucidation of this rapidly evolving field.

Techniques are now available for examining specific receptor numbers and affinity and have demonstrated that these parameters are not fixed, but dynamic; in particular, receptors can be down or up regulated, depending on circumstances. Similarly, we now know that neuroendocrine activity (renin, angiotensin, aldosterone and antidiuretic hormone) can markedly influence receptor sensitivity. The autonomic neurotransmitters themselves not only act peripherally, but can modulate autonomic activity within the central nervous system itself.

Table 14.1 provides a summary and functional classification of the organization of the autonomic nervous system. This is necessarily simple and incomplete and no doubt will itself be further modified in the near future. However, as a model, it provides a basis for clinical and pharmacological discussion of the role of the autonomic nervous system in healthy young subjects, the effects of 'normal ageing' and a nosological analysis of pathological lesions. It will be seen that the sympathetic nervous system has its main impact on the peripheral vascular tree while the parasympathetic system mainly affects cardiac and gastrointestinal function. In clinical practice the role of the autonomic nervous system on cardiovascular regulation is crucial. This is not to dismiss autonomic nervous system involvement in other body systems (Table 14.1), but rather it is a reflection of the paucity of knowledge of the autonomic nervous system involvement in extracardiovascular system homeostasis.

At the present time the best assessment and classification of the human autonomic nervous system is pharmacodynamic. So far, most efforts have

looked at alpha and beta adrenoceptor function. Classification of alpha and beta receptors and their various subtypes is based on reactivity of specific receptors to various pharmacological agonist and antagonists (Table 14.2). Alpha$_1$, beta$_1$ and beta$_2$

TABLE 14.1 CLASSIFICATION OF ADRENERGIC RECEPTOR FUNCTION

Alpha$_1$ effects	Skin (vasoconstriction)
	Pupil (mydriasis)
	Intestine (relaxation)
	Liver (glycogenolysis)
Alpha$_2$ effects	Lipolysis (decreased)
	Renin release (reduced)
Beta$_1$ effects	Heart
	(a) Inotropism
	(b) Chronotropism
	(c) Decreased refractory period
Beta$_2$ effects	Muscles (vasodilatation)
	Bronchioles (bronchodilatation)
	Uterus (relaxation)
	Intestine (dilatation)
	Liver (glycogenolysis)

TABLE 14.2 PHARMACOLOGICAL AGENTS USED IN THE ASSESSMENT AND CLASSIFICATION OF RECEPTORS

	Agonist	Antagonist
Adrenergic		
Alpha$_1$	Phenylephrine	Prazosin
Alpha$_2$	Clonidine	Yohimbine
Alpha$_1$+alpha$_2$	Noradrenaline	Phentolamine
Beta$_1$	—	Atenolol
Beta$_2$	Salbutamol	—
Beta$_1$+beta$_2$	Isoprenaline	Propranolol
Cholinergic		
Nicotinic	Nicotine	Hexamethonium
Muscarinic	Muscarine	Atropine

adrenoceptors are all postganglionic sympathetic, whilst alpha$_2$ receptors are presynaptic central sympathetic (Hoffman and Lefkowitz, 1980; Motulsky and Insel, 1982). Alpha$_2$ receptors are largely auto-regulatory with the other receptors acting more as 'effectors' at end organ level.

CARDIOVASCULAR REFLEXES

The function of the cardiovascular system is to provide an adequate supply of oxygen and nutrients to working tissues of the body and to remove the waste products of metabolism. The demands for this service vary from organ to organ and are constantly changing over time and with change induced by stress, either physiological (exercise, posture) or as a result of environmental (temperature, trauma) or pathological conditions. The ability to respond quickly and appropriately to changing conditions is vital to the survival of the organism.

To this end, the cardiovascular system adapts to maintain a constant 'effective plasma volume' (Guyton, 1978). This volume is not a specifically measurable volume on a par with the plasma or blood volume, but in physiological terms is more a hypothetical set-point. The effective plasma volume is constantly monitored by the baroreceptors located in the large vessels and the heart itself which discharge into the brain stem via the glossopharyngeal and carotid sinus nerves (Kirchheim, 1976). Changes in the effective plasma volume cause an increase or decrease in the baroreceptor discharge which activate or inhibit transmission in the efferent side of the autonomic nervous system. The afferents project into the brain stem and, in particular, the nuclei of the tractus solitarius and the paramedian nucleus (Korner, 1970; Miura and Reis, 1972). From the tractus solitarius further afferent fibres project to higher centres. Whilst these centres modulate cardiovascular activity both over the short and long term, their precise location and contribution await further investigation. Efferent fibres project directly into the interomediolateral nucleus of the spinal cord and hence to the preganglionic sympathetic cells of the spinal cord. Postganglionic sympathetic and parasympathetic fibres then radiate outwards to innervate the central and peripheral vascular systems.

The various nuclei and ganglia involved in this complex interconnected autonomic nervous system do not act as simple passive relay stations. The analogy with a 'telephone network' rapidly breaks down and perhaps explains why attempts to model the process by digital computers have been, with present technology, unsuccessful. At all levels from sensor organ to effector organ, synaptic transmission is modulated by neuronal feedback loops and, as is being increasingly recognized, by the neuro-endocrine system (Reis and Fruxe, 1968; Petty and Reid, 1981). As a consequence of this organization, any impairment in one part of the system will activate compensatory feedback loops attenuating the overall damage, but unfortunately, confusing the researcher.

AGEING AND THE AUTONOMIC NERVOUS SYSTEM

Most investigations of the impact of 'normal ageing' upon the autonomic nervous system in both humans and other species have consisted of giving a stimulus and observing an organ response. This is particularly apposite in the evaluation of cardiovascular system reflexes. Unfortunately, if an age-related change in the response is recorded, there has been a tendency to attribute the lesion to the autonomic nervous system. Any evaluation of the autonomic nervous system, however, requires precise location of the impairment within the whole reflex arc including the afferent sensory organ and the effector organ (Lye and Vargas, 1980). The presence of multiple pathology is a feature of human ageing and latent disease is always difficult to exclude in any experimental situation.

It is well documented that the increase in heart rate on standing (Strandell, 1964), during passive tilt (Lee *et al.*, 1966) and active exercise (Cotes *et al.*, 1973) are all markedly attenuated with increasing age in healthy individuals. Similarly, baroreceptor sensitivity (Gribbin *et al.*, 1971), blood pressure maintenance with postural change (Currens, 1948) and sinus arrhythmia (MacLennan and Ritch, 1978; Waddington *et al.*, 1979) are all decreased with increasing years. Because the autonomic nervous system is crucial in all these reflexes, there has been an assumption over the years that it is this system which constitutes a final common pathway of normal homeostatic regulation and that impairment of reflexes is due to degeneration within it (Collins *et al.*, 1980). This may well not be so.

Due consideration has not been taken of age and pathological changes occurring in the end or effector organs (Lye and Vargas, 1980). This is particularly important in relation to cardiovascular autonomic reflexes. For example, the specific age changes occurring in the left atrium and sinoatrial node will impair all those reflexes, whether sympathetic or parasympathetic, that involve changes in heart rate (Davies, 1975). The almost ubiquitous presence of arteriosclerosis in the elderly alters the distensibility of the resistance blood vessels and must play a considerable part in decreased responsiveness to autonomic reflexes (Learoyd and Taylor, 1966; Swales, 1979; Robinson *et al.*, 1983). Changes in elasticity of the carotid vessels will affect the 'sensitivity' of the carotid baroreceptor (Ludbrook *et al.*, 1977). Arteriosclerosis to varying degree is observed in most elderly people and will affect the afferent loop of any pressure mediated reflex. Finally, the elderly often have glucose intolerance and overt diabetes mellitus, a condition which invariably impairs cardiovascular homeostasis to a greater or lesser extent (Ewing *et al.*, 1978; Sundkvist *et al.*, 1979).

Structural Age Changes

Remarkably little is known about morphological age changes in the autonomic nervous system. It is generally agreed that certain neurones in the central nervous system decrease in number with increasing age (Timiras, 1972) though there is considerable debate as to actual fall out rates and their functional significance (Bowen and Davison, 1976). Age changes within post-mitotic cells and in the supporting parenchyma of the nervous system occur in a more predictable fashion, but again, the relevance is obscure (Wilkinson and Davies, 1981). (For a discussion of neural cell changes with age, the reader is referred to Chapter 1.)

Transmission through autonomic ganglia and nerve conduction velocity are slowed with increasing age, mainly due to segmental Schwann cell disruption and breakages within the myelin sheath (Ochoa and Mair, 1969). The number of impulses that autonomic ganglia are able to generate decreases due to a decline in intrinsic excitability. Frolkis (1968) found that a higher current was required in older rats to reduce heart rate via the vagus nerve compared with young rats. Within the gut it has been found that autonomic innervation decreases in humans with age (Isvailov *et al.*, 1978). This phenomenon is similar to, though less pronounced than, the changes seen in splanchnic nerves in diabetics with overt peripheral neuropathy (Low *et al.*, 1975). On the basis of this scant evidence, it seems that some degree of autonomic denervation does occur with increasing age in healthy individuals (Collins, 1983).

Physiological Age Changes

Receptors

As yet cholinergic receptors have not been studied in relation to 'normal ageing' (Tasch and Stoetling, 1986). Little more is known about ageing and alpha adrenergic function, but more studies have been reported for beta adrenergic function. Unfortunately, clear conclusions cannot be drawn mainly because of differences between different studies.

There is little conclusive evidence that ageing affects alpha adrenoceptor activity in any consistent manner (Motulsky and Insel, 1982). There is one report that the dose of phenylephrine needed to elevate blood pressure is higher in elderly subjects than in younger ones (Elliot *et al.*, 1982). These authors concluded that age reduced $alpha_1$ receptor activity, but ignored possible (and probable) changes in vascular wall mechanisms due to arteriosclerosis. Similarly, aortic contractility following noradrenaline may be decreased in the elderly, but again, mechanical factors were not considered, so that few conclusions about $alpha_2$ receptor function and ageing can be drawn (Finch, 1977). Studies of human platelet $alpha_2$ receptors have found inconsistent or variable changes with increasing age (Elliot *et al.*, 1981; Motulsky and Insel, 1982; Scott, 1982).

The relationship of beta adrenoceptor function to ageing has been studied in many tissues and species. Results obtained in different species and in different tissues tend to be contradictory and it is unsafe to extrapolate from results in one tissue to other tissues or species. It has long been known that the cardiac response to the beta agonist, isoprenaline, is markedly attenuated by age in humans (Yin *et al.*, 1976). Initially, this was interpreted as being a direct effect of sympathetic denervation. By blocking parasympathetic function with atropine, Yin and colleagues (1979) confirmed that the lesion was on the sympathetic arm of the reflex arc. This work was subsequently confirmed by others (London *et al.*, 1976; Vestal *et al.*, 1979). Similar conclusions were reached by workers using specific beta adrenoceptor blocking agents, particularly propranolol (Conway *et al.*, 1971; Vestal *et al.*, 1979; Yin *et al.*, 1978).

Following on from these studies, the hypothesis that the number of adrenoceptors was decreased by increasing age was investigated. The results are almost impossible to interpret. Many workers found decreased numbers of receptors (Motulsky and Insel, 1982; Vestal *et al.*, 1979; Schocken and Roth, 1977). Others have found no change in receptor numbers with increasing age (McDevitt *et al.*, 1976; Van Brummelen *et al.*, 1981; Lakatta, 1979). However, the number of active receptors in tissues is not fixed: they are subject to up- and down-regulation depending upon the general sympathetic tone (Tasch and Stoetling, 1986). There is some evidence that the ability to up-regulate receptors is diminished by increasing age, whereas down-regulation is unaltered (Weiss *et al.*, 1979; Hui and Connolly, 1981). This result requires to be confirmed in other species; Weiss and colleagues used rats and the situation may be different in humans.

Finally, the function of adrenoceptors, as assessed by ligand affinity and ability to stimulate adenylate cyclase activity, has been studied. Many workers report that beta receptor affinity is decreased by increasing age (Kostis *et al.*, 1982; Elliot *et al.*, 1981, 1982; Dillon *et al.*, 1980; Krall *et al.*, 1981). As would be anticipated, other workers have found no effect of increasing age on receptor affinity (Weiss *et al.*, 1979; Vestal *et al.*, 1979; Schocken and Roth, 1977). An intriguing possibility, however, has been raised by

the observation that age decreases the responsiveness of adenylate cyclase to noradrenaline in many tissues and that cAMP dependent protein kinase—the final common pathway at cellular level of sympathetic activity—is less active in the elderly (Weiss *et al.*, 1979). This observation is similar to the age-decreased activity of arginine vasopressin (antidiuretic hormone) on renal tubular function (Davies *et al.*, 1986; Kirkland *et al.*, 1984).

Neurotransmitters

In clinical practice, the measurement of plasma noradrenaline concentration is widely used as a measure of sympathetic activity (Rowe and Troen, 1980; Young *et al.*, 1980). Plasma noradrenaline represents a small and somewhat variable 'overspill' from that portion released at nerve endings (Kopin, 1964). There is overwhelming evidence that plasma levels of noradrenaline, both at rest and during stress (tilt, exercise), are higher in healthy elderly subjects than in the young (Prinz *et al.*, 1979; Pedersen and Christensen, 1975; Ziegler *et al.*, 1976; Palmer *et al.*, 1978; Sever *et al.*, 1977; Rubin *et al.*, 1982). Careful selection of subjects and precise evaluation have confirmed that the raised plasma levels are not due to age-related decreases in blood flow, renal clearance or decreased breakdown by catecholamine-*o*-methyltransferase (Bhagat, 1979; Rubin *et al.*, 1982). Whilst clearance is affected by age (Esler *et al.*, 1981a), it is insufficient to account for the raised plasma levels reported (Esler *et al.*, 1981b). Similarly, the measured spillover rates and plasma levels correlate well with haemodynamic measures of sympathetic activity (Yamaguchi *et al.*, 1975; Esler *et al.*, 1977).

The general consensus is that basal levels of noradrenaline rise in healthy humans and in most other mammalian species with increasing age (Christensen, 1973; Lake *et al.*, 1976; 1977; Coulombe *et al.*, 1977; Sever *et al.*, 1977; Bertel *et al.*, 1980; Messerli *et al.*, 1981; Prinz *et al.*, 1984; Veith *et al.*, 1986; Lehman and Keul, 1986), though a few workers have been unable to demonstrate an age difference in young and old humans (De Champlain and Cousineau, 1977; Cryer *et al.*, 1978; Jones *et al.*, 1978; Messerli *et al.*, 1983). This inconsistency may be due to subject selection, or to the conditions under which measurements were made. Thus Jones and colleagues (1978) found an age-associated relationship in Caucasian males but not in females and non-Caucasians. Messerli and colleagues (1983) found no relationship with age in hypertensive patients, confirming the earlier results of De Champlain and Cousineau (1977). Saar and Gordon (1979) reported that the age effect was eliminated if the subjects were maintained supine for up to 9 hours before samples were obtained. Overall, it must be concluded that increasing age is associated with increasing basal plasma noradrenaline levels, though differences are reduced if subjects with apparent or latent diseases are excluded and a proper period of acclimatization is allowed (Docherty and O'Malley, 1985).

The age-associated increase in plasma noradrenaline levels is real and not due to a grossly reduced clearance (Rubin *et al.*, 1982; Hoeldtke and Cilmi, 1985; Docherty and O'Malley, 1985), though renal clearance, especially in the presence of renal disease, must be taken into account in assessing individual plasma noradrenaline levels (Esler *et al.*, 1981a). There is some evidence that raised levels are due to enhanced activity of dopamine beta hydroxylase (Banerji *et al.*, 1984; Freedman *et al.*, 1972) which is a part of the synthetic pathway for catecholamines (Tasch and Stoetling, 1986). There is a positive, but not precise, relationship between blood pressure in young hypertensives and plasma noradrenaline levels (Messerli *et al.*, 1981). This, however, is not the case in the elderly (Rubin *et al.*, 1982).

An interesting report that plasma noradrenaline levels are higher in females than in males (Jones *et al.*, 1978), subsequently confirmed by Davidson and colleagues (1984), led to suggestions that age-associated changes in body composition (increase in proportion of body fat) may underlie the mechanism by which plasma noradrenaline levels are increased in the elderly (Veith *et al.*, 1986). Another intriguing correlation is that of plasma noradrenaline levels with sleep and ageing (Prinz *et al.*, 1984). It is as yet unknown which is cause and which is effect—do old people sleep less because their sympathetic tone (as indicated by plasma noradrenaline levels) is high or does broken sleep increase sympathetic activity?

POSTURAL HYPOTENSION IN THE ELDERLY

The syndrome of postural hypotension encompasses a number of conditions, aetiologies and physiopathological states, the end result of which is a reduction in cerebral perfusion on changing from the supine to the erect position leading to often vague symptoms of global cerebral dysfunction. In clinical practice the condition is diagnosed and monitored by measuring blood pressure changes, but it must be remembered that the relationship between blood pressure changes and central nervous system symptoms is extremely variable both between subjects and within subjects over time. Some individuals develop symptoms only whilst exercising in the erect position, whilst others may be unable even to sit upright.

Prevalence

Numerous studies over the years have shown that the prevalence in young and middle-aged individuals is very low—probably less than 1% (Currens, 1948; Norris *et al.*, 1953). Beyond middle age, however, the frequency increases dramatically such that up to 18% of people over the age of 65 years show significant (> 20 mmHg) falls in systolic blood pressure on standing (Rodstein and Zeman, 1957; Johnson *et al.*, 1965; Caird *et al.*, 1973). Approximately 5% of over 65 year olds demonstrate falls in systolic blood pressure of more than 40 mmHg. There is one isolated report suggesting that there is no age-related increase in prevalence of postural hypotension (Myers *et al.*, 1978). Unfortunately that study is difficult to interpret because the subjects were supine for only 5 minutes before standing. At least 20 minutes supine is required before the cardiovascular system reaches a stable level (Vargas and Lye, 1982).

Aetiology

The aetiology of postural hypotension in the elderly, especially if the condition is symptomatic, is invariably multifactorial (Lye and Vargas, 1985). The condition is usually a combination of age-related defects in homeostatic regulatory activity and extrinsic precipitating and/or potentiating factors. In practice it is rare for the clinician to find a single neurological cause of postural hypotension in elderly patients. Neurological lesions are important, but even in the context of *The Clinical Neurology of Old Age* it is appropriate to consider non-neurological aspects. Immobility from whatever cause, including the relative immobility of space flight, is a potent factor in the development of postural hypotension (Fareeduddin and Abelmann, 1969; Hamilton *et al.*, 1982; Malorta and Murthy, 1977). Whilst immobility causes a de-tuning of cardiovascular reflexes at all ages, it is particularly frequent in the elderly (Campbell and Reinken, 1985). Unfortunately, the elderly take longer to recover following mobilization and during this period falls may lead to loss of confidence or to trauma, further reinforcing the desire of the patient to cease activity. This vicious circle cannot be treated entirely by the physician; it requires the full support of a rehabilitation team of physiotherapists, rehabilitation nurses, etc.

Environmental factors may be important (Table 14.3). The combination of a hot bed and a cold bedroom is quite dangerous for the elderly if they are afflicted with the common problem of nocturia (Lukash *et al.*, 1964; Lyle *et al.*, 1961). Climbing out of a hot bath often involves a partial Valsalva manoeuvre reducing venous return and precipitating a marked fall in blood pressure (Salih *et al.*, 1985). Simple advice to avoid sudden posture change in these circumstances leads to relief of symptoms. Defecation syncope in constipated elderly patients (Pathy, 1978) and cough syncope (Sharpey-Schafer, 1953) in chronic bronchitic patients can usually be identified by a careful history of the circumstances surrounding the event. Detailed questioning is needed as elderly patients may not make the association.

The elderly are subject to polypharmacy and numerous drugs have been found to lead directly or indirectly to postural hypotension (Table 14.4). Antihypertensive agents, by their very nature, are prone to produce postural symptoms (Jackson *et al.*, 1976; O'Donnell, 1959; Page, 1980). Unfortunately, the newer agents, initially thought to be safer, including calcium channel blocking agents (Murphy *et al.*, 1983) and angiotensin-converting enzyme inhibitors (Cleland *et al.*, 1985; Coulshed *et al.*, 1985),

TABLE 14.3 PRECIPITATING FACTORS RELATING TO THE SYNDROME OF POSTURAL HYPOTENSION IN THE ELDERLY

Environmental:
Immobility/recumbency
Hot weather/bath/bed
Exercise
Post-prandial
Altitude

Cardiovascular:
Myocardial infarction
Arrhythmias
Mitral valve prolapse
Aortic stenosis
Myxoma
Alcohol

Blood volume:
Dehydration
Hyponatraemia
Hypokalaemia
Varicose veins
Haemorrhage
Anaemia (B12)

Physiological:
Cough
Micturition
Defecation
Isometric exercise
Rectal examination
Pyrexia

Metabolic:
Diabetes mellitus
Hypopituitarism
Addison's disease
Thyrotoxicosis/myxoedema
Porphyria
Hyperbradykinism

have proved in practice to be no better than the older agents. Whilst diuretics used in the treatment of cardiac failure do not seem to cause postural hypotension, they do so in elderly hypertensives (Myers *et al.*, 1978; Tidieksaar, 1979). Of particular concern are drugs used in the management of Parkinson's disease. Both levodopa (Godwin-Austin *et al.*, 1971) and bromocriptine (Van Loon, 1979) have produced disabling postural symptoms, though with the former drug, combination with high dose carbidopa

TABLE 14.4 DRUGS ASSOCIATED WITH POSTURAL HYPOTENSION

Antihypertensives:
Ganglion-blocking agents
Diuretics, especially loop agents
Alpha-methyldopa
Beta-blocking agents
Calcium channel antagonists
Angiotensin-coverting enzyme inhibitors
Reserpine
Glyceryl trinitrate
Prazosin

'Sedatives':
Phenothiazines
Tranquillizers
Barbiturates
Tricyclic antidepressants
Antihistamines

Others:
Insulin
Anti-parkinsonian agents
Alcohol

TABLE 14.5 NEUROLOGICAL LESIONS ASSOCIATED WITH POSTURAL HYPOTENSION

Central:
Cerebrovascular disease
Acute stroke
Parkinson's disease
Cerebral hypoxia
Wernicke's encephalopathy
Space-occupying lesions
Olivopontocerebellar degeneration

Peripheral:
Diabetes mellitus
Carcinoma (especially bronchial/pancreatic)
Guillain–Barré neuropathy
Alcoholism
Haemodialysis
Amyloid
Rheumatoid arthritis
Syringomyelia
Cervical myelopathy
Transverse myelitis
Porphyria
Tabes dorsalis
Thiamine deficiency
Riley–Day syndrome
Multiple sclerosis
Holmes–Adie syndrome
Rodenticide poisoning

Idiopathic orthostatic hypotension:
Multisystem atrophy (Shy–Drager)
Parkinsonian idiopathic orthostatic hypotension

may alleviate the postural response (Watanabe *et al.*, 1971). Tricyclic antidepressants have proved to be a particularly severe problem in elderly depressed patients (Glassman, 1979).

The neurological causes of postural hypotension are legion (Table 14.5). In many of the neurological syndromes postural hypotension is a relatively minor problem since the disability produced by motor and sensory deficits may immobilize the patient to such an extent that he cannot stand. In others, however, the postural hypotension itself produces the disability. Most causes of postural hypotension in young people may manifest in old age, especially if potentiated by other factors (Table 14.3). Other conditions, however, are seen solely or mainly in the elderly and are worthy of further discussion.

Acute stroke and acute cerebrovascular disease commonly precipitate postural hypotension in the elderly (Gross, 1970; Johnson *et al.*, 1965). The astute clinician seeing his elderly stroke patient half slumped in a chair semiconscious or confused soon measures the blood pressure in that position. Whilst remobilization of elderly stroke patients at an early stage is laudable, it should not be at the expense of

cerebral blood flow. In some stroke patients there is evidence of damage to the sympathetic vasomotor centre itself (Lye and Vargas, 1985). In these individuals plasma noradrenaline levels fail to rise on head-up tilt and the postural hypotension tends to persist. In others postural symptoms are associated only with an acute stroke and tend to remit over the course of a few days. In these patients there is a transitory failure of cerebral autoregulation associated with peripheral arteriosclerosis (Tohmek *et al.*, 1979; Wollner *et al.*, 1979). In both cases the symptoms are worsened by dehydration, usually secondary to poor nursing care (Himmelstein *et al.*, 1983).

The term idiopathic orthostatic hypotension (IOH) encompasses a number of neurological syndromes. The aetiology of these degenerative syndromes is unknown. Clinically there are two main varieties, though there is some overlap. Shy and Drager (1960) described their eponymous syndrome of autonomic failure associated with multisystem atrophy, though the syndrome had been previously described by Bradbury and Eggleston (1925). In this condition there is selective degeneration of brain stem cells, pigmented melanin nuclei and of cells in the dorsal vagal nuclei (Bannister and Oppenheimer, 1972). The variety of neurological disturbances is wide and includes cerebellar ataxia, bulbar palsy and parkinsonism which may precede or follow the autonomic failure. These patients have normal supine levels of noradrenaline which fail to increase on head-up tilt, suggesting a preganglionic lesion (Bannister *et al.*, 1977; Polinsky *et al.*, 1981).

In older patients IOH tends to be more benign and autonomic failure occurs in isolation or only combined with parkinsonian features (Bannister and Oppenheimer, 1972). Multisystem atrophy and cerebellar lesions do not occur. Supine noradrenaline levels are low and fail to rise on standing, indicating a peripheral (postganglionic) sympathetic denervation (Bannister *et al.*, 1977). In both types of IOH, other problems involving bladder and bowel sphincter function, sweating and impotence are common (Thomas *et al.*, 1981). Patients with IOH often die from cerebral ischaemic episodes, presumably related to hypotensive crises. Death occurs on average 7 to 8 years after the appearance of symptoms and some 4 years after the onset of neurological signs.

MANAGEMENT OF POSTURAL HYPOTENSION: INVESTIGATION

The most important aspect of the management of old people with postural symptoms is to obtain a detailed history of the immediate circumstances surrounding the episodes. This may be difficult with patients who may be confused and are certainly overwhelmed by the effects of a decrease in cerebral blood flow (Wollner *et al.*, 1979). The symptoms of postural hypotension are so vague that a high index of suspicion is necessary if cases are to be recognized. The episodic nature of the symptoms related to

change in posture, often with a diurnal variation, or to exercise, should alert the clinician to a possible diagnosis (Hoffbrand, 1982).

If the diagnosis is suspected, measurement of blood pressure will confirm the suspicion. Unfortunately, the patient's blood pressure may be elevated by the presence of the doctor or the visit to hospital, thus masking any falls in blood pressure. The patient needs to be settled, supine for at least 20 minutes, before measurements are made (Tuckman and Shillingford, 1966; Vargas, 1983). The consulting room needs to be warm and quiet—a shivering patient will have a raised blood pressure. Patients should then try to replicate the precise manoeuvre which brings on symptoms in his usual circumstances. The blood pressure should be recorded at the onset of symptoms or at 2 and 5 minutes after changing posture (Bradshaw and Edwards, 1986). The measurements require to be repeated at different times of the day, and, before excluding the diagnosis, over a period of several days (Lye and Vargas, 1985). Inconvenient though it may be for the investigator, measuring blood pressure changes when the patient first rises in the morning often reveals a large fall which may not be apparent during the rest of the day.

A fall of 20 mmHg or more in systolic blood pressure, whether or not accompanied by symptoms, establishes that the patient, however old, has impairment of postural blood pressure control (Caird *et al.*, 1973, Hickler *et al.*, 1960; Johnson *et al.*, 1965; Rodstein and Zeman, 1957). Smaller falls in blood pressure are probably significant if they are accompanied in a predictable manner by symptoms. Unfortunately the relation, in elderly subjects, between the fall in blood pressure and symptoms is tenuous with some individuals showing falls of more than 40 mmHg and no symptoms whilst others are prostrated by falls of 10 mmHg. The differences are presumably related to age changes in cerebral autoregulation (Patri, 1985; Warren *et al.*, 1985). Much further work is, however, required in this area.

Having established the presence of postural hypotension, the next stage is a detailed search for precipitating or potentiating factors (Table 14.3). All drugs being taken by the patient should be carefully reviewed (Table 14.4). It is important not to forget that the patient may be taking non-prescribed drugs, such as those belonging to a relative, or purchasing 'over the counter' drugs. Often the elderly have been taking drugs for many years and may omit to inform the doctor, even on direct questioning. Reference should be made to the patient's general practitioner, close relative, or better still, a visit to the patient's home should be carried out. Some elderly patients' bathroom cabinets would put a retail chemist's stockroom to shame! Where patients require essential drugs, changing to a different category or altering time of administration may prove to be a simple remedy.

Laboratory Investigations

Minimal baseline investigations include full blood count, plasma electrolytes, urea, creatinine and blood sugar measurements (Bradshaw and Edwards, 1986). A chest X-ray is mandatory—very small bronchial carcinomas may give rise to severe postural hypotension (Park *et al.*, 1972). An ordinary 12-lead ECG may reveal potential arrhythmias suggesting the value of 24 hour or stress (tilt) monitoring (Seda *et al.*, 1980). A serum vitamin B12 measurement may reveal deficiency prior to the development of changes in other haematological indices (White *et al.*, 1981). In elderly patients especially a case for routine thyroid function testing can be made and tests should certainly be performed in patients with postural hypotension (Bhum *et al.*, 1980). Thyrotoxicosis in the elderly is often very atypical and easily overlooked. Other more specific investigations will depend on findings from clinical history, examination and baseline investigations. In elderly patients with postural hypotension it is not safe to attribute aetiology to the first abnormality discovered as so often the syndrome is multifactorial in origin (Caird *et al.*, 1973).

Specific Tests

Detailed tests of cardiovascular reflexes and autonomic function in elderly patients with postural hypotension are, as yet, usually unjustified in clinical practice as they do not influence management (Lye and Vargas, 1985). The problems of multiple patho-logy, polypharmacy and latent disease in elderly patients make their interpretation problematical in the extreme. Even in younger subjects, detailed assessment of cardiovascular reflexes helps little with management as specific therapies are not as yet available for any specific lesions which may be identified (Baum *et al.*, 1981; Clarke and Ewing, 1982; Fisher *et al.*, 1985; Weiling *et al.*, 1983).

In the elderly, even a simple measurement of heart rate acceleration during posture changes is of little value as so many older patients are in chronic atrial fibrillation, are taking digoxin or maintain a persistent tachycardia because of coexisting cardiovascular decompensation (Bradshaw and Edwards, 1986; Webb and Impallomeni, 1987). The measurement of plasma noradrenaline before and after tilt or standing does help to differentiate between multisystem atrophy of the Shy–Drager variety and idiopathic orthostatic hypotension, which is useful for prognostic purposes (Bannister *et al.*, 1977; Brown, 1983; Cryer *et al.*, 1978; Lake *et al.*, 1976; Vargas *et al.*, 1984).

In specialized research environments there has been much interest in the investigation of postural reflexes and 'normal ranges' for many of the stress tests used have been established for the elderly (Clark and Mapstone, 1986; Collins *et al.*, 1980; Kaijiser and Sachs, 1985; Parnati *et al.*, 1985; Pfeifer *et al.*, 1983; Smith, 1984; Smith and Fasler, 1983; Vargas *et al.*, 1984). Whilst some workers believe specific tests assess the integrity of specific reflexes (Henrich, 1982; Kalbfeisch *et al.*, 1977), it is preferable to employ a battery of different tests to gain an overall assessment of the autonomic nervous system (Clarke and Mapstone, 1986; Ewing and Clarke, 1982). In the not too distant future this research activity may provide detailed insights into the physiopathology of postural hypotension leading to precise location of lesion(s) and further, to provide a rational basis for therapy (Lye and Vargas, 1980).

TREATMENT OF POSTURAL HYPOTENSION

The very multiplicity of treatments used in both young and old patients with postural hypotension testifies to their lack of effectiveness (Lye and Vargas, 1985). The most important step is the identification and removal of any precipitating or potentiating factors (Table 14.3). Following this, drugs should be reviewed (Table 14.4). Any drug taken by an old patient should be implicated and if in doubt should be withdrawn or changed whilst monitoring the change in postural blood pressure symptoms. Such a therapeutic trial often produces surprisingly beneficial results.

Physical approaches

It may be impossible to correct the patient's homeostatic reflexes, but it is always possible to modify the patient's external environment. Thus, a hand-held shower may be safer than a bath. The provision of a bath seat may allow the patient to change from supine to standing via an intermediate stage of sitting. Patients should be advised to rise from bed in stages—sitting upright in bed for 5 minutes, then 5 minutes with legs over the side of the bed before standing will often prevent the more serious falls following a night's recumbency (Bradshaw and Edwards, 1986).

The requirements of the aerospace industry have led to the development of extremely effective anti-gravity suits (Rosehamer and Thornstrand, 1973). Unfortunately, their cumbersome nature precludes their use in more down to earth settings (Lye and Vargas, 1985). A compromise, using elastic hosiery, especially if extended to waist level is effective (Ibrahim *et al.*, 1975; Lorentz, 1974; Sheps, 1976). Whilst many elderly patients may initially profess great difficulty in using these garments, it is well worth persisting. They must, however, be fitted correctly and the best size chosen. A surgical appliance officer is necessary for this. If needs be, the garments can be put on by a district nurse and left in situ for up to 3 days. The suggestion that they may worsen postural hypotension (Bannister, 1979) is not borne out by experience.

It has been known for many years that the symptoms of postural hypotension can be alleviated by sleeping with the head of the bed raised (Maclean and Allen, 1940). It is not exactly clear how this works. Certainly head-up tilt at night reduces nocturnal diuresis with the implication that this will restore a depleted effective plasma volume (Bannis-

ter *et al.*, 1969; Wilson *et al.*, 1969). Volume changes, however, have not been measured using this manoeuvre. Alternatively, or additionally, head-up tilt, by reducing renal artery (afferent) pressure stimulates renin and the angiotensin–aldosterone axis (Love *et al.*, 1971).

Another hypothesis would be that this posture 'down-regulates' cerebral autoregulation adapting the brain to a lower perfusion pressure (Lye and Vargas, 1985). This is the picture one sees in elderly patients where the manoeuvre often relieves the symptoms, but has little effect on the blood pressure changes. The degree of head-up tilt should be gradually increased at weekly intervals, starting from 10° and reaching 20° before concluding that the method is not going to work (Bradshaw and Edwards, 1986). Bricks or sand-filled paint tins should be used to elevate the bed head. If the bed 'crashes' in the middle of the night, this will undoubtedly increase noradrenaline release, but this is not sustained long enough to be of benefit! A recent review concluded that this was the single most efficacious manoeuvre in treating postural hypotension (Watson, 1987). I would concur.

Fixed atrial tachypacing has been used with some success in individual patients (Hiltbold, 1980; Moss *et al.*, 1980). Unfortunately, this approach works only in a very small minority of patients and should be reserved perhaps for those patients with posturally induced bradyarrhythmias. The ability to maintain blood pressure by an increase in heart rate will always be limited. The dangers of pacemaker-induced arrhythmias in the elderly are not to be ignored. Polinsky and colleagues (1983) described the use of an automated infuser of noradrenaline which was driven by change in blood pressure. As yet, this device has been used only for short periods (hours), but should prove useful in intensive care and during spinal anaesthesia where postural hypotension may be a particularly serious problem (Bergenwold *et al.*, 1981).

Drugs

The list of drugs used in the treatment of postural hypotension is as long as the list of drugs causing the syndrome. Indeed, some drugs have (had) a place in both lists! All the older drugs act by a straight-forward effect in elevating the blood pressure. Unfortunately, this produces a conflict—maintaining an acceptable level of blood pressure in the erect posture inevitably leads to a level which is too high in the supine position. It should always be borne in mind that many of the impaired reflexes in postural hypotension also impair mechanisms which lower blood pressure in, for example, the supine position.

Vitamins and minerals

Occasionally, pernicious anaemia may present with a peripheral neuropathy and postural hypotension (White *et al.*, 1981). The postural symptoms respond gratifyingly to replacement therapy. Malnutrition in the elderly rarely manifests as postural hypotension in the absence of severe anaemia or B12 deficiency (Bradshaw and Edwards, 1986; Lye and Vargas, 1985). Sodium deficiency, as revealed by hyponatraemia, rarely gives rise to postural hypotension as there is no association with volume depletion in this syndrome (Lye, 1984). The exception would be the sodium depletion associated with Addison's disease (Spingarn and Hitzig, 1942) and primary hyperaldosteronism (Biglierri and McLlroy, 1966). Wernicke's encephalopathy producing postural hypotension will respond to thiamine replacement (Birchfield, 1964; Gravallese and Vicor, 1957). Hormone replacement in elderly patients with pan-hypopituitarism effectively relieves postural symptoms (Belchetz, 1985).

Sympathomimetic amines

These agents have been used for many years in the management of postural hypotension (Ghrist and Brown, 1928; Barnett and Wagner, 1958). They act either directly upon vascular smooth muscle to produce vasoconstriction even in the presence of denervation or, alternatively, they increase output of or decrease re-uptake of noradrenaline at the sympathetic terminal. Drugs acting by the former mechanism will include noradrenaline itself, phenylephrine, midodrine and prenalterol (Davies *et al.*, 1980b; Goovaerts *et al.*, 1984; Schirger *et al.*, 1981). Examples of the latter group of drugs will

include amphetamines, methylphenidate and *p*-tyramine combined with a monoamine oxidase inhibitor (Nanda *et al.*, 1976; Parks *et al.*, 1961; Davies *et al.*, 1978a). All these drugs, however, suffer from two major drawbacks. Whilst usually effective in raising the blood pressure in the erect position, supine hypertension is almost invariable and may even occur without alleviating the postural fall (Davies *et al.*, 1978a). Secondly, they are all arrhythmogenic (Goovaerts *et al.*, 1984). These adverse effects preclude their use in the elderly (Lye and Vargas, 1985).

Dihydroergotamine

This agent is an alpha adrenergic agonist acting on vascular receptors, especially those located in capacitance veins (Mellander and Nordenfelt, 1970; Aellig, 1974). It may also increase vasoconstrictor prostaglandins leading to arteriolar and venous constriction (Bradshaw and Edwards, 1986). Several studies have reported on its variable effectiveness (Bajada, 1979; Bevegard *et al.*, 1974; Benowitz *et al.*, 1980; Jennings *et al.*, 1979; Sturmer, 1976). Again, supine hypertension is a problem and peripheral gangrene has occurred (Bevegard *et al.*, 1974; Bradshaw and Edwards, 1986; Fouad *et al.*, 1981). Supine hypertension seems to be a particular problem in the elderly (Bobik *et al.*, 1981). The oral bioavailability of the drug is very poor (Bobick *et al.*, 1981; Oliver 1980), though this is less apparent in the elderly who may have reduced first pass hepatic metabolism.

The use of dihydroergotamine in the long-term treatment of postural hypotension in the elderly cannot be recommended (Lye and Vargas, 1985). Parenteral administration for short-term maintenance of blood pressure is safe and effective (Bergenwold *et al.*, 1972). Its efficacy and safety have been confirmed in aged individuals during surgery and has allowed spinal anaesthesia in otherwise very frail elderly patients (Bergenwold *et al.*, 1981).

Mineralocorticoids

Corticosteroids have been advocated for the treatment of postural hypotension for nearly 30 years (Hickler *et al.*, 1959). The reasoning behind their use depends on the assumption that postural hypotension is often due to salt and water depletion. The most popular agent has been 9-alpha fludrocortisone, a potent mineralocorticoid with a relatively low glucocorticoid effect (Bannister *et al.*, 1969; Campbell *et al.*, 1976; Davies *et al.*, 1978b; 1979; Decaux, 1979). However, it should be appreciated that the majority of patients with postural hypotension are not salt or water depleted in the absence of specific endocrine diseases (Lye and Vargas, 1985) and, further, any increase in blood volume induced by mineralocorticoid is but temporary (Chobanion *et al.*, 1979). There is good evidence that their long-term effect is via increasing sensitivity of peripheral blood vessels to endogenous vasoconstrictors (Davies *et al.*, 1978b; 1979; Shear, 1968; Schatz *et al.*, 1976).

Mineralocorticoids tend to be limited by their severe side-effects. Fluid retention is a particular problem in the early stages for elderly patients (Lye and Vargas, 1985), though the problem may be reduced by starting treatment with low dose (0.1 mg/day) fludrocortisone (Bradshaw and Edwards, 1986; Schatz *et al.*, 1976). Supine hypertension occurs and is particularly dangerous in the elderly (Chobanion *et al.*, 1979). Electrolyte imbalance, particularly hypokalaemia requiring potassium replacement, is common (Thomas *et al.*, 1981). Attempts have been made, not always successfully, to reduce the incidence of adverse effects by combining fludrocortisone with prostaglandin synthetase inhibitors (Perkins and Lee, 1978; Watt *et al.*, 1981).

Prostaglandin synthetase inhibitors

The idea that vasodilating prostaglandins were involved in either the initiation or the maintenance of postural hypotension (Smythies and Russell, 1974) provided a rationale for the use of prostaglandin synthetase inhibitors in treatment. Most experience has been obtained with indomethacin, a potent inhibitor of the synthesis of PGE_1 and PGI_2 (Abate *et al.*, 1979; Bannister *et al.*, 1978; Davies *et al.*, 1980a; Kochar and Itskovitz, 1978; Sutcliffe, 1980). Indomethacin may increase sensitivity of peripheral vessels to endogenous vasoconstrictors, though this effect is less than that produced by mineralocorticoids (Davies *et al.*, 1980a; Imaizumi *et al.*, 1984).

The side-effect profile of indomethacin is such that its use cannot be recommended in the elderly (De Jong, 1985; Puddey *et al.*, 1985; Zimran *et al.*, 1985). Other non-steroidal anti-inflammatory agents with prostaglandin synthetase inhibitory activity have been employed. Foremost amongst these is flurbiprofen, a potent inhibitor, but of only questionable efficacy in the management of postural hypotension (Perkins and Lee, 1978; Watt *et al.*, 1981). Its efficacy has been enhanced by combining it with low dose fludrocortisone (Bradshaw and Edwards, 1986; Lye and Vargas, 1985). It is, however, unlikely that any non-steroidal anti-inflammatory agent will be safe enough to use in elderly patients with renal impairment—an almost universal consequence of ageing (Adams *et al.*, 1986; Caradoc-Davies, 1984; Langman *et al.*, 1985; Levy and Lye, 1987).

Adrenergic agents

Propranolol has been used to counter orthostatic tachycardia (Miller *et al.*, 1977) in autonomic failure as a sole agent in the Shy–Drager and IOH syndromes (Breretti *et al.*, 1979; 1981) and to counteract the supine hypertension produced by other agents (Lye and Vargas, 1985). The limiting factor, especially in the elderly, is the precipitation of cardiac failure. Drugs with high intrinsic sympathomimetic activity (ISA) which act as agonists when sympathetic tone is low and as antagonists when the tone is high would be useful. Initially pindolol was thought to be effective (Frewin *et al.*, 1980; Man in't Veld and Schalekamp, 1981), but the initial enthusiasm was dampened particularly by the development of cardiac failure in many patients so treated (Davidson and Smith, 1981; Davies *et al.*, 1981). Xamaterol is an adrenergic agent with very high ISA and initial reports of benefit are encouraging (Mehlsen and Trap-Jensen, 1986; Yamashita, 1987). Much more experience is required before its place in therapy can be adequately assessed. Much is promised by newer adrenergic agents but, as yet, little has been delivered.

Miscellaneous drugs

An adrenergic vasodilator (clonidine) has been used successfully to treat postural hypotension, but this unlikely therapy has not been followed up (Robertson *et al.*, 1983). Dopamine antagonists (metoclopramide) theoretically could benefit patients with impaired postural reflexes who have developed dopamine excess (Thorburn and Sowton, 1973) and there is some anecdotal evidence to support this (Kuchel *et al.*, 1980; Bessa *et al.*, 1984). Side-effects, particularly involving the extrapyramidal system (Bateman *et al.*, 1985), limit the use of dopamine antagonists, especially in the elderly (Orme and Tallis, 1984).

Arginine vasopressin (human antidiuretic hormone, AVP) has been shown to reverse some of the consequences of postural hypotension, in particular nocturnal diuresis and morning hypotension (Mathias *et al.*, 1986; Mohring, 1980; Williams *et al.*, 1986). Long-term results with intranasal synthetic analogues of AVP are awaited with interest (Watson, 1987).

A Practical Approach

The first and most important step in the management of postural hypotension in old people is the identification and removal of precipitating or potentiating factors (Table 14.3). Other—often multiple—problems apart from postural hypotension must also be treated. Any increase in general 'physical fitness' is beneficial. Restoring the confidence of patients who may have suffered repeated trauma from multiple falls is essential. Training (or 'conditioning') patients to avoid potential precipitating movements sometimes is helpful, though cooperation may be less than ideal.

Provision of elastic support garments and encouragement in their use is safe and effective. Sleeping with the bed in the head-up position would be the next stage. In the few remaining patients in whom these measures have not completely alleviated the symptoms, if not the postural changes in blood pressure, drugs may be considered as a last resort if the symptoms are severely disabling. Low dose fludrocortisone with adequate monitoring of supine blood pressure and plasma electrolytes would be the first choice for elderly patients. Low dose flurbiprofen could be added subsequently. There are no other safe effective drugs generally available. Xamaterol

and synthetic AVP analogues hold some hope for the future. Much further basic research is needed to be pursued in order to characterize the precise lesions involved and to exploit pharmacological advances in receptor dynamics in this serious and disabling condition.

REFERENCES

Abate, G., Polimeni, R.M., Cuccuvullo, F., Puddu, P., and Linzi, S. (1979). Effects of indomethacin on postural hypotension in Parkinsonism. *Br. Med. J.*, **ii**, 1466–68.

Adams, D.H., Howie, A.J., Michael, J., McConkey, B., Bacon, P.A., and Adu, D. (1986). Non-steroidal anti-inflammatory drugs and renal failure. *Lancet*, **i**, 57–60.

Aellig, W.H. (1974). Venoconstrictor effect of dihydroergotamine in superficial hand veins. *Eur. J. Clin. Pharmacol.*, **7**, 137–9.

Ahlquist, R.P. (1948). A study of adrenotropic receptors. *Am. J. Physiol.*, **153**, 586–600.

Bajada, S. (1979). Dihydroergotamine therapy in symptomatic postural hypotension. *Aust. N.Z. J. Med.*, **9**, 709–12.

Banerji, T.K., Parkening, T.A., and Collins, T.J. (1984). Adrenomedullary catecholaminergic activity increases with age in male laboratory rodents. *J. Gerontol.*, **39**, 264–8.

Bannister, R. (1979). Chronic autonomic failure with postural hypotension. *Lancet*, **ii**, 404–6.

Bannister, R. (1983). Introduction and classification. In: Bannister, R. (ed.) *Autonomic Failure*, Oxford, New York, pp. 1–13.

Bannister, R., Ardill, L., and Fentem, P. (1969). An assessment of various methods of treatment of idiopathic orthostatic hypotension. *Q.J. Med.*, **38**, 377–95.

Bannister, R., Davies, B., and Sever, P. (1978). Indomethacin for Shy–Drager syndrome. *Lancet*, **i**, 1312.

Bannister, R., and Oppenheimer, D.R. (1972). Degenerative disease of the nervous system associated with autonomic failure. *Brain*, **95**, 457–74.

Bannister, R., Sever, P., and Gross, M. (1977). Cardiovascular reflexes and biochemical responses in progressive autonomic failure. *Brain*, **100**, 327–44.

Barnett, A.J., and Wagner, G.R. (1958). Severe orthostatic hypotension: Case report and description of response to sympathomimetic drugs. *Am. Heart J.*, **56**, 412–24.

Bateman, D.N., Rawlins, M.D., and Simpson, J.M. (1985). Extrapyramidal reactions with metoclopramide. *Br. Med. J.*, **291**, 930–2.

Baum, W.B., Jackson, A., Patton, R.W., and Raven, P.B. (1981). Comparison of heart rate measurement protocols used during autonomic function tests. *J. Appl. Physiol.* **51**, 516–19.

Belchetz, P.E. (1985). Idiopathic hypopituitarism in the elderly. *Br. Med. J.*, **291**, 247–8.

Benowitz, N.L., Byrd, R., Schambelan, M., Rosenberg, J., and Roizen, M.F. (1980). Dihydroergotamine treatment for orthostatic hypotension from vacor rodenticide. *Ann. Intern. Med.*, **92**, 387–8.

Bergenwold, L., Eklund, B., Kaijiser, L., Klingenstrom, P., and Westermark, L. (1972). Haemodynamic effects of dihydroergotamine during spinal anaesthesia in man. *Acta Anaesth. Scand.*, **16**, 235–9.

Bergenwold, L., Freyschuss, U., Kaijiser, L., and Westermark, L. (1981). Cardiovascular response to spinal anaesthesia in elderly men: Effects of head-up tilt and dihydroergotamine administration. *Clin. Physiol.*, **1**, 453–60.

Bernard, C. (1865). *Introduction à l'Étude de la Médecine Expérimentale*. Ballière, Paris.

Bertel, O., Buhler, F.R., Kiowski, W., and Lutold, B.E. (1980). Decreased beta-adrenergic responsiveness as related to age, blood pressure and plasma catecholamines in patients with essential hypertension. *Hypertension*, **2**, 130–8.

Bessa, A.M., Zanella, H.T., Saragoca, M.A., Mulineri, R.A., Czepielewski, M., Ribiero, A.B., and Ramos, O.L. (1984). Acute haemodynamic and humoral effects of metoclopramide on blood pressure control. Improvement in subjects with diabetic orthostatic hypotension. *Clin. Pharmacol. Ther.*, **36**, 738–44.

Bevegard, S., Castenfors, J., and Lindblad, L.E. (1974). Haemodynamic effects of dihydroergotamine in patients with postural hypotension. *Acta Med. Scand.*, **196**, 473–7.

Bhagat, B.D. (1979). *Mode of Action of Autonomic Drugs*, Graceway Publishers, Flushing, New York.

Bhum, I., Barkan, A., and Yeshuran, D. (1980). Thyrotoxicosis presenting as orthostatic hypotension. *Postgrad. Med. J.*, **56**, 425–6.

Biglierri, E.G., and McLlroy, M.B. (1966). Abnormalities of renal function and circulating reflexes in primary aldosteronism. *Circulation*, **33**, 80–6.

Birchfield, R.I. (1964). Postural hypotension in Wernicke's disease: a manifestation of autonomic nervous system involvement. *Am. J. Med.*, **36**, 404–11.

Bobik, A., Jennings, G., Skews, H., Esler, M., and McLean, A. (1981). Low oral bioavailability of dihydroergotamine and first pass extraction in patients with orthostatic hypotension. *Clin. Pharmacol. Ther.*, **30**, 673–9.

Bowen, D.M., and Davison, A.N. (1976). Biochemistry of brain degeneration. In: Davison, A.N. (ed.) *Biochemistry and Neurological Disease*, Blackwell, Oxford, pp. 2–51.

Bradbury, S., and Eggleston, C. (1925). Postural hypotension: A report of three cases. *Am. Heart J.*, **1**, 73–86.

Bradshaw, M.J., and Edwards, R.T.M. (1986). Postural hypotension—pathophysiology and management. *Q. J. Med.*, **60**, 643–57.

Breretti, G., Chiarietto, M., Lavecchia, G., and Rengo, F. (1979). Effects of propranolol in a case of orthostatic hypotension. *Br. Heart J.*, **41**, 245.

Breretti, G., Chiarietto, M., Guidise, P., De Michelle, G., Mansi, D., and Campanella, G. (1981). Effective treatment of orthostatic hypotension by propranolol in the Shy–Drager syndrome. *Am. Heart J.*, **102**, 5938–41.

Brown, M.J. (1983). Catecholamine measurements in clinical medicine. *Postgrad. Med. J.*, **59**, 479–82.

Caird, F.I., Andrews, G.R., and Kennedy, R.D. (1973). Effect of posture on blood pressure in the elderly. *Br. Heart J.*, **35**, 527–30.

Campbell, A.J., and Reinken, J. (1985). Postural hypotension in old age: Prevalence, association and prognosis. *J. Clin. Exp. Gerontol*, **7**, 163–75.

Campbell, I.W., Ewing, D.J., and Clarke, B.F. (1976). Therapeutic experience with fludrocortisone in diabetic postural hypotension. *Br. Med. J.*, **1**, 872–4.

Caradoc-Davies, T.H. (1984). Nonsteroidal anti-inflammatory drugs, arthritis and gastrointestinal bleeding in elderly inpatients. *Age Ageing*, **13**, 295–8.

Chobanion, A.V., Volicer, L., Fifft, C.P., Garvas, M., Liang, C.S., and Faxon, D. (1979). Mineralocorticoid-induced hypertension in patients with orthostatic hypotension. *N. Engl. J. Med.*, **301**, 68–73.

Christensen, N.J. (1973). Plasma noradrenaline and adrenaline in patients with thyrotoxicosis and myxoedema. *Clin. Sci. Mol. Med.*, **45**, 163–71.

Clark, C.V., and Mapstone, R. (1986). Age-adjusted normal tolerance limits for cardiovascular autonomic function assessment in the elderly. *Age Ageing*, **15**, 221–9.

Clarke, B.F., and Ewing, D.J. (1982). Cardiovascular reflex tests in the natural history of diabetic autonomic neuropathy. *N.Y. State J. Med.*, **82**, 903–8.

Cleland, J.G.F., Dargie, H.J., McAlpine, H., Ball, S.G., Morton, J.J., Robertson, J.I.S., and Ford, I. (1985). Severe hypotension after first dose of enalapril in heart failure. *Br. Med. J.*, **291**, 1309–12.

Collins, K.J. (1983). Autonomic failure in the elderly. In: Bannister, R. (ed.) *Autonomic Failure*, Oxford University Press, Oxford, pp. 489–507.

Collins, K.J., Exton-Smith, A.N., James, M.H., and Oliver, D.J. (1980). Functional changes in autonomic nervous responses with ageing. *Age Ageing*, **9**, 17–24.

Conway, J., Wheeler, R., and Sannerstedt, R. (1971). Sympathetic nervous activity during exercise in relation to age. *Cardiovascular. Res.*, **5**, 577.

Cotes, J.E., Hall, A.M., Johnson, G.R., Jones, P.R.M., and Knibbs, A.V. (1973). Decline with age of cardiac frequency during submaximal exercise in healthy women. *Proc. Physiol. Soc.*, **263**, 24–5.

Coulombe, P., Dussault, J.H., and Walker, P. (1977). Catecholamine metabolism in thyroid disease II. Norepinephrine secretion rate in hyperthyroidism and hypothyroidism. *J. Clin. Endocrinol. Metab.*, **44**, 1185–9.

Coulshed, N.J., Davies, S.J., and Turney, J.H. (1985).

Prolonged hypotension after fever during enalapril treatment. *Lancet*, **i**, 222.

Cryer, P.E., Silverberg, A.B., Santiago, J.V., and Shah, S.D. (1978). Plasma catecholamines in diabetes: The syndromes of hypoadrenergic and hyperadrenergic postural hypotension. *Am. J. Med.*, **64**, 407–19.

Currens, J.H. (1948). A comparison of the blood pressure in the lying and standing position: A study of 500 men and 500 women. *Am. Heart J.*, **35**, 646–54.

Davidson, A.C., and Smith, S.E. (1981). Pindolol in orthostatic hypotension. *Br. Med. J.*, **282**, 1704.

Davidson, L., Vandongen, R., Rouse, I.L., Beilin, L.J., and Tunney, A. (1984). Sex-related differences in resting and stimulated plasma noradrenaline and adrenaline. *Clin. Sci.*, **67**, 347–52.

Davies, B., Bannister, R., and Sever, P. (1978a). Pressor amines and monoamine oxidase inhibitors for treatment of postural hypotension in autonomic failure: Limitations and hazards. *Lancet*, **i**, 172–5.

Davies, B., Bannister, R., and Sever, P. (1980a). Indomethacin treatment of postural hypotension in autonomic failure. *Br. Med. J.*, **280**, 1229.

Davies, B., Bannister, R., Sever, P., and Wilcox, C.S. (1979). The pressor action of noradrenaline, angiotensin II and saralasin in chronic autonomic failure treated with fludrocortisone. *Br. J. Clin. Pharmacol.*, **8**, 253–60.

Davies, B., Bannister, R., Mathias, C., and Sever, P. (1981). Pindolol in postural hypotension: The case for caution. *Lancet*, **ii**, 982–3.

Davies, H.E. (1975). Respiratory change in heart rate. Sinus arrhythmia in the elderly. *Gerontol. Clin.*, **17**, 96–100.

Davies, I., Goddard, C., and Fotheringham, A.P. (1986). The effect of age on the control of water conservation in the laboratory mouse—metabolic studies. *Exp. Gerontol.*, **20**, 53–60.

Davies, I.B., Bannister, R., Sever, P.S., and Wilcox, C.S. (1978b). Fludrocortisone in the treatment of postural hypotension: Altered sensitivity to pressor agents. *Br. J. Clin. Pharmacol*, **6**, 444–5.

Davies, I.B., Bannister, R., Hensby, C., and Sever, P.S. (1980b). The pressor actions of noradrenaline and angiotensin II in chronic autonomic failure treated with indomethacin. *Br. J. Clin. Pharmacol.*, **10**, 223–9.

De Champlain, J., and Cousineau, D. (1977). Lack of correlation between age and circulatory catecholamines in hypertensive patients. *N. Engl. J. Med.*, **297**, 672.

De Jong, P.E. (1985). Incidence of hyperkalaemia induced by indomethacin. *Br. Med. J.*, **291**, 1047.

Decaux, G. (1979). Fludrocortisone in orthostatic hypotension. *N. Engl. J. Med.*, **301**, 1121–2.

Dillon, N., Chung, S., Kelly, J., and O'Malley, K. (1980). Age and beta adrenoreceptor-mediated function. *Clin. Pharmacol. Ther.*, **27**, 769–72.

Docherty, J.R., and O'Malley, K. (1985). Ageing and

alpha-adrenoceptors. *Clin. Sci.*, **68** (Suppl. 10), 1335–65.

Elliot, H.L., Rubin, P.C., Scott, P.J., and Reid, J.L. (1981). Vascular alpha receptors and age. *Eur. J. Clin. Invest.*, **11**, 9.

Elliot, H.L., Sumner, D.J., McLean, K., and Reid, J.L. (1982). Effect of age on the responsiveness of vascular alpha-adrenoceptors in man. *J. Cardiovasc. Pharmacol.*, **4**, 388–92.

Esler, M., Zweifler, A., Randall, O., Julius, S., and De Quattro, V. (1977). Agreement between three different indices of sympathetic nervous system activity in essential hypertension. *Mayo Clin. Proc.*, **52**, 379–82.

Esler, M., Skews, M., Leonard, P., Jackman, G., Bobik, A., and Korner, P. (1981a). Age-dependence of noradrenaline kinetics in normal subjects. *Clin. Sci.*, **60**, 217–19.

Esler, M., Jackman, G., Bobik, A., Leonard, P., Kelleher, D., Skews, H., Jennings, G., and Korner, P. (1981b). Norepinephrine kinetics in essential hypertension. Defective neuronal uptake of norepinephrine in some patients. *Hypertension*, **3**, 40–4.

Ewing, D.J., and Clarke, B.F. (1982). Diagnosis and management of diabetic autonomic neuropathy. *Br. Med. J.*, **285**, 916–18.

Ewing, D.J., Campbell, I.W., Murray, A., Neilson, J.M., and Clarke, B.F. (1978). Immediate heart rate response to standing: Simple test for autonomic neuropathy in diabetes. *Br. Med. J.*, **1**, 145–7.

Fareeduddin, K., and Abelmann, W.H. (1969). Impaired orthostatic tolerance after bed rest in patients with myocardial infarction. *N. Engl. J. Med.*, **280**, 345–50.

Finch, C.E. (1977). Neuroendocrine and autonomic aspects of ageing. In: Finch, C.E., and Hayflick, L. (eds.) *Handbook of the Biology of Ageing*, Van Nostrand Reinhold, Cincinnati, pp. 262–80.

Fisher, B.M., Henderson, E., and Frier, B.M. (1985). Diagnostic yield of screening tests of autonomic neuropathy in asymptomatic diabetics. *Clin. Sci.*, **68** (Suppl. 11), 15P.

Fouad, F.M., Tarazi, R.C., and Bravo, E.L. (1981). Dihydroergotamine in idiopathic orthostatic hypotension. Short-term intramuscular and long-term oral therapy. *Clin. Pharmacol. Ther.*, **30**, 782–9.

Freedman, L.S., Chuchi, T., Goldstein, M., Axelrod, R., Fish, I., and Davies, J. (1972). Changes in human serum dopamine beta-hydroxylase activity with age. *Nature*, **236**, 310–11.

Frewin, D.B., Leonello, P.P., Penhall, R.K., and Harding, P.E. (1980). Pindolol in orthostatic hypotension: Possible therapy? *Med. J. Aust.*, **1**, 128.

Frolkis, V.V. (1968). The autonomic nervous system in the ageing organism. *Triangle*, **8**, 322–8.

Ghrist, D.G., and Brown, G.E. (1928). Postural hypotension with syncope: Its successful treatment with ephedrin. *Am. J. Med.*, **175**, 336–49.

Glassman, A.H. (1979). Clinical characteristics of imipramine-induced orthostatic hypotension. *Lancet*, **1**, 468–72.

Godwin-Austin, R.B., Frears, C.C., and Bergman, S. (1971). Incidence of side-effects from levo-dopa during the introduction of treatment. *Br. Med. J.*, **1**, 267–8.

Goovaerts, J., Verfaillie, C., Fagard, R., and Knockaert, D. (1984). Effect of prenalterol on orthostatic hypertension in the Shy–Drager syndrome. *Br. Med. J.*, **288**, 817–18.

Gravallese, M.A.J.R., and Vicor, M. (1957). Circulatory studies in Wernicke's encephalopathy with special reference to the occurrence of a state of high cardiac output and postural hypotension. *Circulation*, **15**, 836–44.

Gribbin, B., Pickering, T.G., Sleight, P., and Peto, R. (1971). Effect of age and high blood pressure on baroreflex sensitivity in man. *Circulation Res.*, **29**, 424–31.

Gross, M. (1970). The effect of posture on subjects with cerebrovascular disease. *Q. J. Med.*, **39**, 485–91.

Guyton, A.C. (1978). Essential cardiovascular regulation—The control linkage between bodily needs and circulatory function. In: Dickinson, C.J., and Marks, J. (eds.) *Developments in Cardiovascular Medicine*, MTP Press, London, pp. 265–302.

Hamilton, B.H., Devoshia, C., and Levin, B.E. (1982). Physiological effects of bed rest. *Lancet*, **1**, 51.

Henrich, W.L. (1982). Autonomic insufficiency. *Arch. Intern. Med.*, **142**, 339–44.

Hickler, R.B., Hoskins, R.G., and Hamlin, J.T. (1960). The clinical evaluation of faulty orthostatic mechanisms. *Med. Clin. North Am.*, **44**, 1237–50.

Hickler, R.B., Thompson, G.R., Fox, L.M., and Hamlin, J.T. (1959). Successful treatment of orthostatic hypotension with 9 alpha fluorohydrocortisone. *N. Engl. J. Med.*, **261**, 788–91.

Hiltbold, P. (1980). Atrial tachypacing for primary orthostatic hypotension. *N. Engl. J. Med.*, **303**, 885.

Himmelstein, D.U., Jones, A.A., and Woolhandler, S. (1983). Hypernatraemic dehydration in nursing home patients: An indicator of neglect. *J. Am. Geriatr. Soc.*, **31**, 466–71.

Hoeldtke, R.D., and Cilmi, K.M. (1985). Effects of ageing on catecholamine metabolism. *J. Clin. Endocrinol. Metab.*, **60**, 479–84.

Hoffbrand, B.I. (1982). Postexertional hypotension: A valuable physical sign. *Br. Med. J.*, **285**, 1242.

Hoffman, B.B., and Lefkowitz, R.J. (1980). Alpha-adrenergic receptors in man. *N. Engl. J. Med.*, **302**, 1390–6.

Hui, K.K.P., and Connolly, M.E. (1981). Increased numbers of beta-receptors in orthostatic hypotension due to autonomic dysfunction. *N. Engl. J. Med.*, **304**, 1473–5.

Ibrahim, M.M., Tarzi, R.C., and Dustan, H.P. (1975). Orthostatic hypotension: mechanisms and management. *Am. Heart J.*, **90**, 513–20.

Imaizumi, T., Takeshita, A., Ashihara, T., Nakamura, M., Tsuji, S., and Shibazaki, H. (1984). Increase in reflex vasoconstriction with indomethacin in patients with orthostatic hypotension and CNS involvement. *Br. Heart J.*, **52**, 581–4.

Isvailov, B., Mairov, V.N., and Soloviov, N.A. (1978). Morphometric features of changes in the neurones of the jejunum in the ageing body. *Arkh. Anat. Histol. Embryol.*, **75**, 53–6.

Jackson, G., Pierscianowski, T.A., Mahon, W. and Condon, J. (1976). Inappropriate antihypertensive therapy in the elderly. *Lancet*, **ii**, 1317–18.

Jennings, G., Esler, M., and Holmes, R. (1979). Treatment of orthostatic hypotension with dihydroergotamine. *Br. Med. J.*, **ii**, 307.

Johnson, R.H., Smith, A.C., Spalding, J.M.K., and Wollner, L. (1965). Effect of posture on blood pressure in elderly patients. *Lancet*, **i**, 731–3.

Jones, D.H., Hamilton, C.A., and Reid, J.L. (1978). Plasma noradrenaline, age and blood pressure: A population study. *Clin. Sci. Mol. Med.*, **55**, 735–55.

Kaijiser, L., and Sachs, C. (1985). Autonomic cardiovascular responses in old age. *Clin. Physiol.*, **5**, 347–57.

Kalbfeisch, J.H., Reinke, J.A., Porth, C.J., and Thomas, J.E. (1977). Effect of age on circulatory response to postural and Valsalva tests. *Proc. Soc. Exp. Biol. Med.*, **156**, 100–3.

Kirchheim, M.R. (1976). Systemic arterial baroreceptor reflexes. *Physiol. Rev.*, **56**, 100–76.

Kirkland, J.L., Lye, M., Goddard, C., Vargas, E., and Davies, I. (1984). Plasma arginine vasopressin in dehydrated elderly patients. *Clin. Endocrinol.*, **20**, 451–6.

Kochar, M.S., and Itskovitz, M.D. (1978). Treatment of idopathic orthostatic hypotension (Shy–Drager syndrome) with indomethacin. *Lancet*, **i**, 1011–14.

Kopin, I.J. (1964). Storage and metabolism of catecholamines, the role of monoamine oxidase. *Pharmacol. Rev.*, **16**, 179–91.

Korner, P.I. (1970). Central nervous control of autonomic function—possible implications in the pathogenesis of hypertension. *Circ. Res.*, **11**, 159–68.

Kostis, J.B., Moreyra, A.E., Amendo, M.T., Di Pietro, J., Cosgrove, N., and Kuo, P.T. (1982). The effect of age on heart rate in subjects free of heart disease. *Circulation*, **65**, 141–5.

Krall, J.F., Connolly, M., Weishart, R., and Tuck, M.L. (1981). Age related elevation of plasma catecholamine concentration and reduced responsiveness of lymphocyte adenylate cyclase. *J. Clin. Endocrinol. Metab.*, **52**, 863–7.

Kuchel, O., Buu, N.T., Gutkowska, J., and Genest, J. (1980). Treatment of severe orthostatic hypotension by metoclopramide. *Ann. Intern. Med.*, **93**, 841–3.

Lakatta, E.G. (1979). Alterations in the cardiovascular system that occur in advanced age. *Fed. Proc.*, **38**, 163–7.

Lake, C.R., Ziegler, M.G., and Kopin, I.J. (1976). Use of plasma norepinephrine for evaluation of sympathetic neuronal function in man. *Life Sci.*, **18**, 1315–26.

Lake, C.R., Ziegler, M.G., Coleman, M.D., and Kopin, I.J. (1977). Age-adjusted plasma norepinephrine levels are similar in normotensive and hypertensive subjects. *N. Engl. J. Med.*, **296**, 208–9.

Langman, M.J.S., Morgan, L., and Worrall, A. (1985). Use of anti-inflammatory drugs by patients admitted with small or large bowel perforation. *Br. Med. J.*, **290**, 347–9.

Learoyd, B.M., and Taylor, M.G. (1966). Alterations with age in the visco-elastic properties of human arterial walls. *Circulation Research*, **18**, 278–92.

Lee, T.D., Lindeman, R.D., Yiengst, M.J., and Shock, N.W. (1966). Influence of age on the cardiovascular and renal response to tilting. *J. Appl. Physiol.*, **21**, 55–61.

Lehman, M., and Keul, J. (1986). Age-associated changes of exercise-induced plasma catecholamine responses. *Eur. J. Appl. Physiol. Occ. Physiol.*, **55**, 302–6.

Levy, D.W., and Lye, M. (1987). Diuretics and potassium in the elderly. *J. Roy. Coll. Phys. (London)*, **21**, 148–52.

London, G.M., Safar, M.D., Weiss, Y.A., and Milliez, P.L. (1976). Isoproterenol sensitivity and total body clearance of propranolol in hypertensive patients. *J. Clin. Pharmacol.*, **16**, 174–82.

Lorentz, I.T. (1974). Postural hypotension. *Med. J. Aust.*, **2**, 816–18.

Love, D.R., Brown, J.J., Chinn, R.H., Johnson, R.H., Lever, A.F., Park, D.M., and Robertson, J.I.S. (1971). Plasma renin concentration in idiopathic postural hypotension: Differential response in subjects with probable afferent and efferent autonomic failure. *Clin. Sci.*, **41**, 289–99.

Low, P.A., Walsh, J.C., Huang, C.Y., and McLeod, J.G. (1975). Sympathetic nervous system in diabetic neuropathy—a clinical and pathological study. *Brain*, **98**, 341–56.

Ludbrook, J., Mancia, G., Ferrari, A., and Zanchetti, A. (1977). The variable-pressure neck-chamber for studying the carotid baroreflex in man. *Clin. Sci. Mol. Med.*, **53**, 165–71.

Lukash, W.M., Sawyer, G.T., and Davies, J.E. (1964). Micturition syncope produced by orthostasis and bladder distension. *N. Engl. J. Med.*, **270**, 341–4.

Lye, M. (1984). Electrolyte disorders in the elderly. *Clin. Endocrinol. Metab.*, **13**, 377–98.

Lye, M., and Vargas, E. (1980). The assessment of autonomic function in the elderly. *Age Ageing*, **9**, 210–14.

Lye, M., and Vargas, E. (1985). Postural hypotension. In: Coodley, E.L. (ed.) *Geriatric Heart Disease*, PSG Publishing, Littleton, Massachusetts, pp. 189–200.

Lyle, C.B., Monroe, J.T., Flinn, D.E., and Lamb, L.E. (1961). Micturition syncope: Report of 24 cases. *N. Engl. J. Med.*, **265**, 982–6.

McDevitt, D.G., Frisk-Holmberg, M., Hollifield, J.W., and Shand, D.G. (1976). Plasma binding and the affinity of propranolol for a beta-receptor in man. *Clin.*

Pharmacol. Ther., **20**, 152–9.

MacLennan, W.J., and Ritch, A.E.S. (1978). Heart rate response to standing as a test for autonomic neuropathy. *Br. Med. J.*, **1**, 505.

Maclean, A.R., and Allen, E.V. (1940). Orthostatic hypotension and orthostatic tachycardia. Treatment with "head-up" tilt. *J.A.M.A.*, **115**, 2162–7.

Malkotra, M.S., and Murthy, W.S. (1977). Changes in orthostatic tolerance in man at an altitude of 3500 metres. *Aviation Space and Environmental Medicine*, **48**, 125–8.

Man in't Veld, A.J., and Schalekamp, M.A.D.H. (1981). Pindolol acts as a beta-adrenoreceptor agonist in orthostatic hypotension: Therapeutic implications. *Br. Med. J.*, **282**, 929–31.

Mathias, C.J., Fosbraey, P., Da Costa, D.F., Thornley, A., and Bannister, R. (1986). The effect of desmopressin on nocturnal polyuria, overnight weight loss and morning postural hypotension in patients with autonomic failure. *Br. Med. J.*, **293**, 353–4.

Mehlsen, J., and Trap-Jensen, J. (1986). Xamaterol, a new selective Beta-1-adrenoceptor partial agonist in the treatment of postural hypotension. *Acta Med. Scand.*, **219**, 173–7.

Mellander, S., and Nordenfelt, I. (1970). Comparative effects of dihydroergotamine and noradrenaline on resistance exchange and capacitance functions in the peripheral circulation. *Clin. Sci.*, **39**, 183–201.

Messerli, F.H., Frohlich, E.D., and Suarez, D.H. (1981). Borderline hypertension: Relationship between age, haemodynamics and circulatory catecholamines. *Circulation*, **64**, 760–4.

Messerli, F.H., Sundgaard-Riise, K., Ventura, H.O., Dunn, F.G., Glade, L.B., and Frohlich, E.D. (1983). Essential hypertension in the elderly: Haemodynamics, intravascular volume, plasma renin activity and circulating catecholamine levels. *Lancet*, **ii**, 983–6.

Miller, A.J., Cohen, C.H., and Glick, S. (1977). Propranolol in the treatment of orthostatic tachycardia associated with orthostatic hypotension. *Am. Heart J.*, **88**, 493–5.

Miura, M., and Reis, D.J. (1972). Role of the solitary and paramedian reticular nuclei in mediating cardiovascular reflex responses from carotid baro- and chemo-receptors. *J. Physiol. (London)*, **223**, 525–8.

Mohring, D. (1980). Greatly enhanced pressor response to antidiuretic hormone in patients with impaired cardiovascular reflexes due to idiopathic orthostatic hypotension. *J. Cardiovasc. Pharmacol.*, **2**, 367–76.

Moss, A.J., Glaser, W., and Topol, E. (1980). Atrial tachypacing in the treatment of a patient with primary orthostatic hypotension. *N. Engl. J. Med.*, **302**, 1456–7.

Motulsky, J.H., and Insel, P.A. (1982). Adrenergic receptors in man. *N. Engl. J. Med.*, **307**, 18–29.

Murphy, M.B., Scriven, A.J.I., and Dollery, C.T. (1983). Role of nifedipine in treatment of hypertension. *Br. Med. J.*, **287**, 257–9.

Myers, M.G., Kearns, P.M., Kennedy, D.S., and Fisher, R.H. (1978). Postural hypotension and diuretic therapy in the elderly. *Can. Med. Assoc. J.*, **119**, 581–5.

Myerson, A. (1938). Human autonomic pharmacology. *J.A.M.A.*, **110**, 101–3.

Nanda, R.N., Johnson, R.H., and Keogh, H.J. (1976). Treatment of neurogenic orthostatic hypotension with a mono-amine oxidase inhibitor and tyramine. *Lancet*, **ii**, 1164–7.

Norris, A.H., Shock, N.W., and Yiengst, M.J. (1953). Age changes in heart rate and blood pressure responses to tilting and standardised exercise. *Circulation*, **8**, 521–6.

Ochoa, J., and Mair, W.C.P. (1969). The normal sural nerve in man. Part 2: Changes in the axons and Schwann cells due to ageing. *Acta Neuropathol. (Berlin)*, **13**, 217–39.

O'Donnell, T.V. (1959). Studies in postural hypotension following ganglion blocking drugs. *Clin. Sci.*, **18**, 237–49.

Oliver, I.N., Jennings, G.L., Bobik, A., and Esler, M. (1980). Low bioavailability as a cause of apparent failure of dihydroergotamine in orthostatic hypotension. *Br. Med. J.*, **281**, 275–6.

Orme, M.L.'E., and Tallis, R.C. (1984). Metoclopramide and tardive dyskinesia in the elderly. *Br. Med. J.*, **289**, 397–8.

Page, I.H. (1980). Severe hypotension during febrile episodes in patients taking antihypertensives. *N. Engl. J. Med.*, **302**, 865.

Palkovits, M. (1980). The anatomy of central cardiovascular neurones. In: Fruxe, K., Goldstein, M., Hokfelt, T., and Hokfelt, B. (eds.) *Central Adrenaline Neurones*, Pergamon Press, Oxford, pp. 3–17.

Palmer, G.T., Ziegler, M.G., and Lake, C.R. (1978). Response of norepinephrine and blood pressure to stress increases with age. *Gerontology*, **33**, 482–8.

Park, D.M., Johnson, R.H., Crean, G.P., and Robinson, J.F. (1972). Orthostatic hypotension in bronchial carcinoma. *Br. Med. J.*, **3**, 510–11.

Parks, V.J., Sandison, A.G., Skinner, S.L., and Whelan, R.F. (1961). Sympathomimetic drugs in orthostatic hypotension. *Lancet*, **i**, 1133–6.

Parnati, G., Pomidossi, G., Ramirez, A., Cesana, B., and Mancia, G. (1985). Variability of the haemodynamic responses to laboratory tests employed in assessment of neural cardiovascular regulation in the elderly. *Clin. Sci.*, **69**, 533–40.

Pathy, M.S. (1978). Defaecation syncope. *Age Ageing*, **7**, 233–6.

Patri, B. (1985). L'hypotension artérielle orthostatique du sujet âge. *Therapie*, **40**, 41–4.

Pedersen, E.B., and Christensen, N.J. (1975). Catecholamines in plasma and urine in patients with essential hypertension determined by double-isotope derivative techniques. *Acta Med. Scand.*, **198**, 373–7.

Perkins, C.M., and Lee, M.R. (1978). Flurbiprofen and fludrocortisone in severe autonomic neuropathy. *Lancet*, **ii**, 1058.

Petty, M.A., and Reid, J.L. (1981). Opiate analogues, substance P and baroreceptor reflexes in the rabbit. *Hypertension*, **3** (Suppl. 1), 142–7.

Pfeifer, M.A., Weinberg, C.R., and Cook, D. (1983). Differential changes of autonomic nervous system function with age in man. *Am. J. Med.*, **75**, 249–58.

Polinsky, R.J., Samaras, G.M., and Kopin, I.J. (1983). Sympathetic neural prosthesis for managing orthostatic hypotension. *Lancet*, **1**, 901–4.

Polinsky, R.J., Kopin, I.J., Ebert, M.H., and Weise, V. (1981). Pharmacologic distinction of different orthostatic hypotension syndromes. *Neurology*, **31**, 1–7.

Prinz, P.N., Vitiello, M.V., and Smallwood, R.G. (1984). Plasma norepinephrine in normal young and aged men: Relationship with sleep. *J. Gerontol.*, **39**, 561–7.

Prinz, P.N., Halter, J., Benedetti, C., and Raskind, M. (1979). Circadian variation of plasma catecholamines in young and old men: Relation to rapid eye movement and slow wave sleep. *J. Clin. Endocrinol. Metab.*, **49**, 300–4.

Puddey, I.B., Beilin, L.J., Vandongen, R., Banks, R., and Rouse, I. (1985). Differential effects of sulindac and indomethacin on blood pressure in treated essential hypertensive subjects. *Clin. Sci.*, **69**, 327–36.

Reis, D.J., and Fruxe, K. (1968). Adrenergic innervation of the carotid sinus. *Am. J. Physiol.*, **215**, 1054–7.

Robertson, D., Goldberg, M.R., Hollister, A.S., Wade, D., and Robertson, R.M. (1983). Clonidine raises blood pressure in severe idiopathic orthostatic hypotension. *Am. J. Med.*, **74**, 193–200.

Robinson, B.J., Johnson, R.H., Lambie, D.G., and Palmer, K.T. (1983). Do elderly patients with an excessive fall in blood pressure on standing have evidence of autonomic failure? *Clin. Sci.*, **64**, 587–91.

Rodstein, M., and Zeman, F.D. (1957). Postural blood pressure changes in the elderly. *J. Chron. Dis.*, **6**, 581–8.

Rosehamer, G., and Thornstrand, C. (1973). Effect of G-suit in treatment of postural hypotension. *Acta Med. Scand.*, **193**, 277–80.

Rowe, J.W., and Troen, B.R. (1980). Sympathetic nervous system and ageing in man. *Endocrine Rev.*, **1**, 167–78.

Rubin, P.C., Scott, P.J., McLean, K., and Reid, J. (1982). Noradrenaline release and clearance in relation to age and blood pressure in man. *Eur. J. Clin. Invest.*, **12**, 121–5.

Saar, N., and Gordon, R.D. (1979). Variability of plasma catecholamine levels: Age, duration of posture and time of day. *Br. J. Clin. Pharmacol.*, **8**, 353–8.

Salih, M.M., Weissberg, P., and Littler, W.A. (1985). The effect of idiopathic orthostatic hypotension on Valsalva responses. *Clin. Sci.*, **69**, 54P.

Schatz, I.J., Miller, M.J., and Frame, B. (1976). Corticosteroids in the management of orthostatic hypotension. *Cardiology (Basel)*, **61**, 271–9.

Schirger, A., Sheps, S.G., Thomas, J.E., and Fealy, R.D. (1981). Midodrine—a new agent in the management of idiopathic orthostatic hypotension and Shy–Drager syndrome. *Mayo Clin. Proc.*, **56**, 429–33.

Schocken, D.D., and Roth, G.S. (1977). Reduced beta-adrenergic receptor concentrations in ageing man. *Nature*, **267**, 856–8.

Scott, P.J. (1982). The effect of age on the responses of human isolated arteries to noradrenaline. *Br. J. Clin. Pharmacol.*, **13**, 237–9.

Seda, P.E., McAnulty, J.H., and Anderson, C.J. (1980). Postural heart block. *Br. Heart J.*, **44**, 221–3.

Sever, P.S., Osukowska, B., Birch, M., and Tunbridge, R.D.G. (1977). Plasma noradrenaline in essential hypertension. *Lancet*, **i**, 1078.

Sharpey-Schafer, E.P. (1953). The mechanism of syncope after coughing. *Br. Med. J.*, **ii**, 860–3.

Shear, L. (1968). Orthostatic hypotension. *Arch. Intern. Med.*, **122**, 467–71.

Sheps, S.G. (1976). Use of an elastic garment in the treatment of orthostatic hypotension. *Cardiology*, **61** (Suppl. 1), 271–9.

Shy, G.M., and Drager, G.A. (1960). A neurological syndrome with orthostatic hypotension. *Arch. Neurol.*, **2**, 511–27.

Smith, S.A. (1984). Diagnostic value of the Valsalva ratio reduction in diabetic autonomic neuropathy: Use of an age-related normal range. *Diabet. Med.*, **1**, 295–7.

Smith, S.A., and Fasler, J.J. (1983). Age-related changes in autonomic function: Relationship with postural hypotension. *Age Ageing*, **12**, 206–10.

Smythies, J.R., and Russell, R.O. (1974). Possible role of prostaglandins in idiopathic postural hypotension. *Lancet*, **ii**, 963.

Spingarn, C.L., and Hitzig, W.M. (1942). Orthostatic circulatory insufficiency: Its occurrence in tabes dorsalis and Addison's disease. *Arch. Intern. Med.*, **69**, 23–40.

Strandell, T. (1964). Circulatory studies in healthy old men. *Acta Med. Scand.*, **175** (Suppl. 414), 1–44.

Sturmer, E. (1976). Pharmacological basis of the treatment of orthostatic disorders with ergot alkaloids. *Cardiology (Basel)*, **61**, 290–301.

Sundkvist, G., Almer, L.-O., and Lilja, B. (1979). Respiratory influence on heart rate in diabetes mellitus. *Br. Med. J.*, **i**, 924–5.

Sutcliffe, R.L.G. (1980). Indomethacin treatment of postural hypotension. *Br. Med. J.*, **1**, 1229.

Swales, J.D. (1979). Pathophysiology of blood pressure in the elderly. *Age Ageing*, **8**, 104–9.

Tasch, M.D., and Stoetling, R.K. (1986). The autonomic nervous system. In: Stephens, C.R., and Assaf, R.A.E. (eds.) *Geriatric Anaesthesia*, Butterworths, Boston, pp. 115–34.

Thomas, J.E., Schinger, A., Fealy, R.D., and Sheps, S.G. (1981). Orthostatic hypotension. *Mayo Clin. Proc.*, **56**, 117–25.

Thorburn, C.W., and Sowton, E. (1973). The haemo-dynamic effects of metoclopramide. *Postgrad. Med. J.*, **49**, 22–5.

Tidieksaar, R. (1979). Postural hypotension and diuretic therapy in the elderly. *Can. Med. Assoc. J.*, **120**, 13.

Timiras, P.S. (1972). *Developmental Physiology and Ageing*, Macmillan, New York.

Tohmek, J.F., Shah, S.D., and Cryer, P.E. (1979). The pathogenesis of hyperadrenergic postural hypotension in diabetic patients. *Am. J. Med.*, **67**, 772–8.

Tuckman, J., and Shillingford, J. (1966). Effect of different degrees of tilt on cardiac ouput, heart rate and blood pressure in normal man. *Br. Heart J.*, **28**, 33–9.

Van Brummelen, P., Buhler, F.R., Kiowski, W., and Amann, F.W. (1981). Age related decrease in cardiac and peripheral vascular responsiveness to isoprenaline. *Clin. Sci.*, **60**, 571–7.

Van Loon, G.R. (1979). Bromocriptine-induced orthostatic hypotension. *Clin. Invest. Med.*, **2**, 131–4.

Vargas, E. (1983). *Cardiovascular mechanisms in the elderly*, PhD Thesis, University of Manchester, Manchester, England.

Vargas, E., and Lye, M. (1982). Physiological responses to posture change in young and old healthy individuals. *Exp. Gerontol.*, **17**, 445–52.

Vargas, E., Rothwell, C., Weinkove, C., and Lye, M. (1984). The measurement of plasma noradrenaline before and after tilt in young and old healthy subjects. *Gerontology*, **30**, 253–60.

Veith, R.C., Featherstone, J.A., Livares, O.A., and Halter, J.B. (1986). Age differences in plasma norepinephrine kinetics in humans. *J. Gerontol.*, **41**, 319–24.

Vestal, R.E., Wood, A.J.J., and Shand, D.G. (1979). Reduced beta-adrenoceptor sensitivity in the elderly. *Clin. Pharmacol. Ther.*, **26**, 181–5.

Waddington, J.L., MacCulloch, M.S., and Sambrooks, J.E. (1979). Resting heart rate variability in man declines with age. *Experientia*, **35**, 1197–8.

Warren, L.R., Butler, R.W., Katholi, C.R., and Halsey, J.H. (1985). Age differences in cerebral blood flow during rest and during mental activation measurements with and without monetary incentive. *J. Gerontol.*, **40**, 53–9.

Watanabe, A.M., Parks, L.C., and Kopin, I.J. (1971). Modification of the cardiovascular effects of L-dopa by decarboxylase inhibitors. *J. Clin. Invest.*, **50**, 1322–8.

Watson, R.D.S. (1987). Treating postural hypotension. *Br. Med. J.*, **294**, 390–1.

Watt, S.J., Tooke, J.E., Perkins, C.M., and Lee, M.R. (1981). The treatment of idopathic orthostatic hypotension: A combination of fludrocortisone and flurbiprofen. *Q.J. Med.*, **198**, 205–12.

Webb, G.C., and Impallomeni, M.G. (1987). Heart failure in the elderly. *Q.J. Med.*, **244**, 641–50.

Weiling, W., Borst, C., Van Brederode, J.F.M., Van Dongen Tormans, M.A., Van Montrans, G.A., and

Dunning, A.J. (1983). Testing for autonomic neuropathy: Heart rate changes after orthostatic manoeuvres and static muscle contractions. *Clin. Sci.*, **64**, 581–6.

Weiss, B., Greenberg, L., and Cantor, E. (1979). Age-related alterations in the development of adrenergic denervation supersensitivity. *Fed. Proc.*, **38**, 1915–19.

White, W.B., Reik, L., and Cutlip, D.E. (1981). Pernicious anaemia seen initially as orthostatic hypotension. *Arch. Intern. Med.*, **141**, 1543–4.

Wilkinson, A., and Davies, I. (1981). The influence of age on hypothalamo-neurohypophyseal system of the mouse: A qualitative ultrastructural analysis of the posterior pituitary. *Mech. Ageing Devel.*, **15**, 129–39.

Williams, T.D.M., Da Costa, D., Mathias, C.J., Bannister, R., and Hightman, G.L. (1986). Pressor effect of arginine vasopressin in progressive autonomic failure. *Clin. Sci.*, **71**, 173–8.

Wilson, R.J., Mills, I.H., and De Bono, E. (1969). Cardiovascular reflexes and the control of aldosterone production and sodium excretion. *Proc. Roy. Soc. Med.*, **62**, 1257–8.

Wollner, L., McCarthy, S.T., Soper, N.D.W., and Macy, D.J. (1979). Failure of cerebral auto-regulation as a cause of brain dysfunction in the elderly. *Br. Med. J.*, **1**, 117–18.

Yamaguchi, N., De Champlain, J., and Nardeau, R.A. (1975). Correlation between the response of the heart to sympathetic stimulation and the release of endogenous catecholamines into the coronary sinus of the dog. *Circ. Res.*, **36**, 662–8.

Yamashita, M. (1987). Treatment of idiopathic orthostatic hypotension with Xamaterol. *Lancet*, **i**, 1431–2.

Yin, F.C.P., Spurgeon, M.A., Raizes, G.S., Greene, M.L., and Shock, N.W. (1976). Age-associated decrease in chronotropic response to isoproterenol. *Circulation*, **54**, 167–72.

Yin, F.C.P., Spurgeon, H.A., Greene, M.L., Lakatta, E.G., and Weisfeldt, M.L. (1979). Age-associated decrease in heart rate response to isoproterenol in dogs. *Mech. Ageing Devel.*, **10**, 17–25.

Yin, R.C.P., Raizes, G.S., Guarnieri, T., Spurgeon, M.A., Lakatta, E.G., Fortini, N.J., and Weisfeldt, M.L. (1978). Age-associated decrease in ventricular response to haemodynamic stress during beta-adrenergic blockade. *Br. Heart J.*, **40**, 1349–55.

Young, J.B., Rowe, J.W., Pallotta, J.A., Sparrow, D., and Landsberg, L. (1980). Enhanced plasma norepinephrine response to upright posture and oral glucose administration in elderly human subjects. *Metabolism*, **29**, 532–9.

Ziegler, M.G., Lake, C.R., and Kopin, I.J. (1976). Plasma noradrenaline increases with age. *Nature*, **261**, 333–5.

Zimran, A., Kramer, M., Plaskin, M., and Hershko, C. (1985). Incidence of hyperkalaemia induced by indomethacin in a hospital population. *Br. Med. J.*, **291**, 107–8.

Chapter 15

Epilepsy

Raymond Tallis

Professor of Geriatric Medicine, Hope Hospital Department of Geriatric Medicine, University of Manchester, Salford, UK

Epilepsy no longer carries the stigma that used to be associated with it and very few epileptic patients feel stigmatized (Ryan *et al.*, 1980). Nevertheless, the psychological impact of an epileptic fit may be profound. In many respects, the problem of epilepsy is comparable to that of recurrent falls: although the condition is episodic, the anxiety it causes may be constant. An elderly person may worry, and not without reason, that future fits may lead to injury— to road traffic accidents, fractures, burns, etc. Moreover, discontinuity of consciousness undermines self-confidence at the deepest level; to an elderly person, a fit may seem a harbinger of death. For these reasons, the management of epilepsy must include reassurance, though without adequate control of fits this may seem somewhat hollow.

The general principles of the management of epilepsy in the elderly patient are essentially the same as in younger patients. The first step is to determine whether or not the episodes are epileptic. The next is to consider the possibility that seizures are symptomatic of an underlying cause. This is highly likely when epilepsy occurs for the first time in old age. If an underlying cause is identified, this may require treatment in its own right. The next step will be control of the fits, usually by drug treatment. Explanation and reassurance to a patient or relative who may, not unreasonably, have been alarmed by the episode(s) is almost as important as drug treatment. Finally, it will be necessary to monitor control of fits, to watch for the emergence of new clues as to

any underlying cause that may need treatment and to ensure that the patient is not disabled by adverse drug reactions.

DEFINITION

'Epilepsy' refers to a continuing tendency to epileptic seizures. For epidemiological purposes, the term is used where a patient has suffered from more than one non-febrile seizure of any type. A single event, such as a fit occurring during an episode of anoxia, would not count as epilepsy. Seizures are defined pathophysiologically as being due to paroxysmal discharges of cerebral activity, in which a critical mass of neurones fires synchronously.

EPIDEMIOLOGY

More than 5% of the population have at least one afebrile seizure during their lives (Hauser and Kurland, 1975). One would expect that the proportion of the population with epileptic fits would rise with age, each age carrying the cumulative prevalence of previous ages. However, epilepsy tends to remit, as indicated by the fact that the overall prevalence rates for active epilepsy have been given variously as 4–6/1000 (Zielinskii, 1982), 3–6/1000 (Hauser, 1978) or 4.3/1000 (Wagner, 1983).

The elderly population will include 'graduate' epileptic patients. With better treatment, and consequently longer survival, of patients with epilepsy, this contribution may be expected to increase. In addition, however, the incidence of new cases rises steeply with age above 50. Hauser and Kurland (1975) found that the annual incidence of epileptic seizures between 1965 and 1967 rose from 11.9 per 100 000 in the 40–59 age range to 82.0 in those over 60. A recent Danish study (Luhdorf *et al.*, 1986) included all patients over 60 in a well-defined population who developed epilepsy during a 5 year period. The incidence of definite epilepsy was 77 per 100 000 new cases per year. There was a significant excess of male patients. Estimates of prevalence are, for the reasons discussed by Hauser and Kurland, often unreliable. Nevertheless, their study showed a rise in older subjects, prevalence increasing from 7.3 per 1000 in the 40–59 age range to 10.2 for those over 60.

THE DIAGNOSIS OF EPILEPSY

Diagnosing epilepsy will imply finding answers to several related but distinct questions:

1. Are the episodes seizures or not?
2. What type of seizures are they?
3. What is the underlying cause?

The answers to questions 2 and 3 will obviously be closely related; for example, a focal seizure will be associated with focal neurological pathology.

Seizures or Not?

The commonest feature of epilepsy at any age is transient impairment or loss of consciousness. In such cases, it is not always easy to distinguish a seizure from other causes of impaired consciousness. If the disturbance of consciousness is forgotten and the patient reports only a fall, then the diagnostic problem is even greater, for the differential diagnosis will include other causes of falls and these may be legion (see Chapter 28). Epilepsy should be considered in all cases where falls are not associated with obvious environmental causes and where orthopaedic, cardiovascular or non-epileptic neurological explanations are not forthcoming.

In those cases where there is a clear story, either from the patient or a witness, of loss of consciousness, the differential diagnosis will include transient hypoglycaemic episodes and syncopal attacks due to a temporary impairment of cerebral circulation.

Hypoglycaemic episodes are usually suggested by the characteristic initial features due to excessive adrenergic activity—tremulousness, anxiety, profuse sweating and palpitations. Cerebral dysfunction follows with behavioural disturbance leading on to clouding of consciousness and coma. There will generally be an obvious predisposing cause, such as hypoglycaemic medication. It must be remembered, however, that the elderly may not always experience the autonomic features associated with hypoglycaemia (see Chapter 20) and that many hypoglycaemic attacks occur at night. Moreover, severe hypoglycaemia may precipitate epileptic seizures in as many as 10–20% of adult cases (Mulder and Rushton, 1959).

The commonest diagnostic dilemma, however, is 'Fit or Faint?' A well-defined aura, clear progression from a tonic to a clonic phase, tongue-biting, incontinence or focal neurological features during an attack, and stupor or prolonged confusion, headache and transient neurological signs after the event are especially helpful discriminating features. Where there is no eye-witness the history will be necessarily incomplete. Nevertheless, post-event confusion and headache are extremely useful historical pointers. It must be remembered, however, that cerebral anoxia, for example in carotid sinus syncope, may cause convulsions.

Transient loss of consciousness due to temporary impairment of cerebral circulation is a particularly important differential diagnosis because there are so many possible causes in the elderly. These include: paroxysmal tachyarrhythmias; Stokes–Adams attacks; carotid sinus syncope; exertional syncope associated with other causes of low cardiac output; cough and micturition syncope; vertebrobasilar ischaemia; transient ischaemic attacks; and postural hypotension. The presence of pallor and sweating, a gradual onset preceded by palpitations, or an association with the assumption of the erect posture, voiding or neck turning, and medication known to cause postural hypotension may help to point to the correct diagnosis. It must not be forgotten, however, that temporal lobe attacks may present with autonomic features.

Patients with cardiac arrhythmias may have symptoms resulting from impaired cerebral perfusion. In addition to syncope, there may be transient confusion, abnormal behaviour and psychoses that may misleadingly suggest a primary cerebral cause. Recurrent cardiac arrhythmias may masquerade as epilepsy. Schott *et al.* (1977) report that 20% of patients referred to a neurological department during a 6 month period with a diagnosis of idiopathic epilepsy were subsequently found to have cardiac arrhythmias that caused or significantly contributed to their symptoms. Most of their patients were young but one would expect the incidence of cardiac arrhythmias to be even higher in an elderly 'epileptic' population. In some cases, arrhythmias were associated with prolonged periods of unconsciousness and convulsions. Hashan and Jameson (1973) described a 60 year old patient with repeated loss of consciousness followed by convulsive movements due to Stokes–Adams attacks. The episodes were heralded by a 'queer feeling' or 'a feeling of heaviness' in the chest.

Separating the contributions of heart and head to a patient's transient cerebral symptoms may prove extremely difficult. Ambulatory ECG and EEG are sometimes useful but they are time-consuming and expensive and may raise more questions than they answer (Blumhardt, 1986). Cardiac arrhythmias recorded on a 24 hour tape may not be clearly related to symptoms (Santos and Lye, 1980); and the same applies to paroxysmal EEG abnormalities. In many cases, episodes do not occur during the period of recording; conversely, the patient may have the symptoms in the absence of recorded abnormalities. There is the additional problem that an arrhythmia coinciding with symptoms may not be the primary cause of the symptoms as, for example, in those cases where seizures precipitate cardiac arrhythmias. In summary, in the case of many 'funny do's' it is often not possible to be sure whether they originate from the heart or the head even after intensive investigation and sophisticated monitoring.

What Type of Fits Are They?

The type of fit may indicate whether or not the epilepsy is primary or secondary. In the vast majority of cases, epilepsy beginning in old age will be secondary, due usually to a structural neurological lesion (see below).

The manifestations of epilepsy are protean and the standard methods of classifying seizures correspondingly complex. In 1969, the International League Against Epilepsy (ILAE) published a scheme for classifying seizures (Gastaut, 1970). This was an attempt to place epileptology on a scientific basis and correlate seizure types with the underlying electrophysiology. Although it was not entirely successful—because it is difficult to match clinical phenomena with electrical features—it did lift the science above lepidopterology. Since the 1969 classification was published, objective and sophisticated methods of studying seizures have become more widely available and in 1981 the ILAE published a proposal for a revised classification (Commission on the Classification and Terminology of the International League Against Epilepsy, 1981). The revised scheme correlates clinical seizure types with ictal and inter-ictal electroencephalographic features (see Table 15.1 for the parts of the table relevant to the elderly).

The ILAE classification takes account of the patterns of electrical discharges during seizures and in inter-ictal records. Partial seizures are those in which the *first* changes suggest activation of neurones limited to part of one cerebral hemisphere. When consciousness is not impaired, a partial seizure is classified as simple; when it is impaired, the seizure is classified as complex. Impairment of consciousness in a partial seizure usually implies bilateral spread of seizure activity. Spread or generalization of electrical activity may lead to secondarily generalized convulsive seizures. Clinically this will manifest as loss of consciousness and tonic–clonic features supervening on initially focal symptoms.

Primary generalized seizures are those in which the first clinical events suggest involvement of both hemispheres from the outset. Ictal EEG patterns are also bilateral from the outset and this presumably reflects neuronal activity which is widespread in both hemispheres. Generalized seizures may be convulsive or non-convulsive. In the former case motor manifestations are initially bilateral. In non-convulsive seizures, there is impairment or interruption of consciousness without motor manifestations.

TABLE 15.1 CLASSIFICATION OF SEIZURES

I. PARTIAL (FOCAL, LOCAL)

A. Simple partial seizures (consciousness not impaired)
1. With motor signs (focal motor with or without march; versive; postural; vocalization)
2. With somatosensory or special-sensory symptoms (somatosensory; visual; auditory; olfactory; gustatory; vertiginous)
3. With autonomic symptoms or signs (epigastric sensation, pallor, sweating, flushing, piloerection, pupillary dilatation)
4. With disturbances of higher cerebral function (dysphasic; dysmnesic; cognitive; affective)
5. Illusions, e.g. macropsia
6. Structured hallucinations, e.g. music, scenes

B. Complex partial seizures (with impairment of consciousness; sometimes beginning with simple symptoms)
1. Simple partial seizure followed by impairment of consciousness or automatisms
2. Impairment of consciousness at the outset, with or without automatisms

C. Partial seizures evolving to secondarily generalized seizures (with convulsive manifestations)

II. GENERALIZED SEIZURES (CONVULSIVE OR NON-CONVULSIVE)

A.1. Absence seizures
a. Impairment of consciousness only
b. With mild clonic components
c. With atonic components
d. With automatisms
e. With autonomic components

A.2. Atypical absences (changes in tone may be more pronounced and onset/cessation less abrupt than in A.1)

B. Myoclonic seizures
Multiple or single myoclonic jerks

C. Clonic seizures

D. Tonic seizures

E. Tonic–clonic seizures

F. Atonic seizures

III. UNCLASSIFIED EPILEPTIC SEIZURES

Impairment of consciousness may be the first event in a convulsive seizure.

It may be helpful to map parts of the new classification on to the traditional terminology, which was based purely on clinical rather than electroencephalographic features. Primary generalized convulsive seizures correspond roughly to the classical 'grand mal' attack without a preceding aura. A grand mal attack preceded by an aura or other focal features corresponds to 'partial seizures evolving to secondarily generalised seizures'. 'Minor' or 'focal' epilepsy covers simple and complex partial seizures; most of the latter were previously included under the heading 'temporal lobe epilepsy', as, amongst the focal seizures, it is those originating in the temporal lobes that are most likely to be associated with impairment of consciousness. Some temporal lobe attacks correspond to simple partial seizures with autonomic or psychic symptoms.

The diagnosis of epilepsy will depend largely on the history. As indicated already, the latter may range from a clear-cut account of a full-blown tonic–clonic seizure, through more subtle manifestations such as absences or transient confusional states to fits that reveal themselves only through their sequelae—such as morning headache after a nocturnal seizure or unexplained falls which are in fact secondary to brief absences.

Focal or secondarily generalized seizures usually imply focal neurological damage, whereas primarily generalized seizures may be idiopathic, due to a constitutionally low seizure threshold, or to a metabolic disturbance lowering the seizure threshold. In an elderly patient, of course, a metabolic disturbance may trigger off a discharge in a focus of pre-existing neurological damage. Whereas the type of fit may be clear from the history, as when, for example, there is a story of a jacksonian march or recurrent stereotyped hallucinations, its precise characterization will often depend on investigations.

What are the relative proportions of the different types of epilepsy? Goodridge and Shorvon (1983) looked at the pattern of epilepsy in the community by surveying 6000 patients on the list of a single general practice: 122 patients were identified with a history of non-febrile seizures; 61% had generalized seizures, 19% had complex partial seizures and the remainder had a combination of partial and general seizures. Interestingly, only one patient had a simple partial seizure, confirming one's impression that focal fits without impairment of consciousness are fairly rare. This study included only 27 epileptic patients over the age of 60 but it does give some idea of the pattern of seizure type in the general population. Gastaut and co-workers (1975) classified 6000 epileptic patients from the Timone Hospital. Out of this enormous series, 2978 were over the age of 15; 81% were classified and the remainder could not be classified. Table 15.2 shows the relative frequencies of the different types of seizures that could be classified (I have modified the headings to conform to the more recent ILAE scheme).

TABLE 15.2   RELATIVE FREQUENCIES OF DIFFERENT TYPES OF EPILEPSY

Type	%
Generalized	20.4
Tonic–clonic	12.0
Absence	2.8
Myoclonic	4.4
Other clonic	0.8
Partial	78.9
Simple	12.3
Complex	55.9
Evolving to secondarily generalized seizures	9.4

From Gastaut *et al.* (1975).

The very high proportion of partial seizures in Gastaut's series may be a reflection of the fact that the Timone is a neurological referral centre. Wagner (1983) in a survey of patients with epilepsy in a region of Denmark found that of 1054 cases, 25% had complex partial seizures, 18% simple partial seizures, 32% primary generalized seizures, and 8% were unclassified. A further 16% were classified as 'heredo-familial'.

Hildick-Smith (1974) has pointed out that series originating from neuromedical centres may have a bias. One such bias is likely to be the under-representation of the elderly; and certainly of the unfit elderly encountered by geriatricians. In Hildick-Smith's own series of 50 patients (mean age 79), 28 had grand mal attacks, twelve had focal attacks and seven had both (the ILAE classification was not used and EEG findings were not reported). Roberts *et al.* (1982) studied 81 patients over 65 and classified their fits as either grand mal or partial, without EEG correlation. Sixty-five per cent had grand mal seizures; 25% only partial seizures (24 motor, two sensory, and one psychomotor); one was unclassifiable. Two patients had both grand mal and partial seizures.

Although these two geriatric series give a lower percentage of focal seizures than Gastaut, this difference may be an artefact, arising out of the lack of EEG information. As already mentioned, the focal origin of a fit that generalizes rapidly may be missed without EEG. This point is well illustrated by the excellent survey of Luhdorf *et al.* (1986) who identified 163 elderly patients in their 5 year study who had not been previously treated. Of these 84 (51%) had grand mal seizures, 69 (42%) had partial or secondarily generalized seizures and ten (6%) were unclassified. Of those with grand mal seizures, however, 32 (38%) had focal abnormalities on the EEG.

Certain features of epilepsy may cause diagnostic problems (see Godfrey *et al.*, 1982 for a discussion of some of these). Foremost are neuropsychiatric presentations. Simple partial seizures associated with disturbances of higher cerebral function or, more particularly, complex partial seizures with or without automatisms, may be labelled as non-specific confusional states or, where there are affective or cognitive features or hallucinations, as manifestations of functional psychiatric illnesses. This is particularly likely in patients with non-convulsive epileptic status (e.g. Drake and Coffey, 1983). Most studies of the psychiatric manifestations of partial seizures have focused on the young (e.g. Rodin *et al.*, 1976) whose fits may be part of a response to extensive brain injury and whose neuropsychiatric symptoms may be more florid. Ellis and Lee (1978) described six patients between the ages of 42 and 69 who presented with acute behavioural changes—withdrawal, mutism, delusional ideas, paranoia and vivid hallucinations. All six had generalized spike and wave discharges. In none was there a previous history of seizures and all responded well to phenytoin or phenobarbitone.

There is a tendency to call this condition 'petit mal status' (e.g. Thompson and Greenhouse, 1968) but this usage should be deprecated. 'Petit mal' should be reserved for non-convulsive epilepsy occurring in childhood and associated with 3/second spike and wave discharges and no ictal or inter-ictal focal features. True petit mal is extremely rare in adult life and although there is a record of one patient who continued to have petit mal until his late seventies (Gibberd, 1972), the vast majority of sufferers have either converted to grand mal or have become fit-free by the time they are 30. In only three of Gibberd's cases did petit mal begin after 30 and none of these was elderly. Andermann and Robb (1972) recommend the term 'absence status' for patients such as those described by Ellis and Lee. This is not merely a matter of nomenclature: the EEG may show focal features with secondary generalization in the inter-ictal record.

Godfrey *et al.* (1982) draw attention to the fact that post-ictal confusion may be very prolonged in the elderly. At least 14% of their patients suffered a confusional state lasting 24 hours or more. In some cases, it could persist as long as a week. This did not seem to depend on a previous history of confusion or evidence of focal neurological disease. Post-ictal paresis, or Todd's palsy, was seen in 16% of these patients. Todd's palsy is especially liable to occur in patients with post-stroke epilepsy, as Fine (1966, 1967) has pointed out, when it may be confused with a further stroke. Post-ictal hemiparesis was the commonest cause for erroneous referral to a stroke unit in Norris and Hachinski's (1982) study of the misdiagnosis of stroke. The susceptibility of the elderly to post-ictal phenomena is easy to understand if one considers the increased metabolic requirements of the brain during a fit, the reduction of oxygen supply and the reduced ability to respond to increased demand.

Post-stroke nightmares, presumed to be ictal in nature because they responded to phenytoin, have been described (Boller *et al.*, 1975).

Somatosensory epilepsy is rare, being present in only 1.42% of Maguiere and Courjon's (1978) series of 8938 patients presenting to an EEG department. Most of the patients have simple paraesthesiae of short duration, usually of the hand and upper limb. Two of the patients of Godfrey *et al.* had episodic pain which responded to anticonvulsants. Sensory epilepsy could easily be confused with transient ischaemic attacks or, as Godfrey points out, other causes of post-hemiplegic pain.

Very localized motor status (epilepsia partialis continua) may be misdiagnosed as an extrapyramidal movement disorder. Thomas *et al.* (1977) noted that the condition tended to be of sudden onset. It may be highly variable in the same patient, sometimes affecting the face followed by the face and the arm or sometimes taking the form of minor clonic jerks of the arm or even of the finger or thumb in isolation. It may affect the tongue alone. There are focal EEG discharges; in some instances a spike may precede each jerk.

Epileptic dizziness, consisting of a sensation of disequilibrium, often with a sense of rotation, has been discussed by Kogeorgos *et al.* (1983). They excluded elderly patients from their survey—presumably because of the difficulty of picking out epilepsy from other causes of dizziness—but there is no reason to assume this does not occur in geriatric patients. In all 30 patients, dizziness occurred in brief episodes, each lasting no more than a few seconds. Nausea was often experienced in the recovery phase. Attack frequency ranged from one per week to several daily. A quarter of the patients had also had generalized convulsions by the time of referral; half of the patients had suffered brief absences. Less commonly there were other temporal lobe features. In all but two patients the inter-ictal EEG showed focal abnormalities in one or both temporal regions. Anticonvulsant treatment was effective in nearly all cases.

What is the Underlying Cause? (see Table 15.3)

The traditional teaching used to be that late onset epilepsy implied a space-occupying lesion. This is not supported by the facts: computed tomographic (CT) scanning has confirmed what experienced practi-

TABLE 15.3 CAUSES OF SEIZURES IN THE ELDERLY

Cerebral disease
  Cerebrovascular disease
  Neoplasia—primary and secondary
  Alzheimer's disease and other non-vascular causes
    of cerebral degeneration
  Subdural haematoma
  Post-traumatic
  Infective or post-infective (meningitis, encephalitis, abscess)

Cardiovascular disease
  Tachyarrhythmias
  Stokes–Adams attacks

Metabolic
  Renal failure
  Hepatic failure
  Hypoglycaemia
  Hyperosmolar diabetes
  Hypocalcaemia
  Water and electrolyte disturbance
  Myxoedema
  Hypoxia
  Hypercapnia

Toxic
  Drugs and drug withdrawal (see Table 15.4)
  Alcohol and alcohol withdrawal

Idiopathic

tioners outside of specialized (and in particular neurosurgical) centres have known for a long time—that cerebrovascular disease is by far the commonest cause.

Cerebrovascular disease

Schold *et al.* (1977) reported cerebrovascular disease in 30% of their cases and nearly 60% of those in whom a cause was found. For Godfrey *et al.* (1982) the corresponding figures were 44% and 52% respectively; and for Hildick-Smith (1974), who did not have access to CT scanning, 42% and 48% respectively. Feuerstein *et al.* (1970) found even higher proportions: 52% and 65%. Luhdorf *et al.* (1986) attributed only 32% of their new cases to cerebrovascular disease but relatively few patients had CT scans.

The relation between epilepsy and cerebrovascu-

lar disease has been studied the other way round. Webster *et al.* (1956) reported epilepsy in 5%, and Marquardsen (1969) and Hildick-Smith (1974) in 8%, of hemiplegic stroke patients. Cocito *et al.* (1982) investigated 141 patients with angiographically proven carotid or middle cerebral artery (MCA) occlusive disease and found that fits occurred some time during the clinical disease in 17.3% of carotid patients and 10.8% of MCA patients. Most seizures were partial motor attacks.

Shorvon *et al.* (1984) carried out an interesting study in which they compared the CT scan appearances of 74 patients with late onset epilepsy and no evidence of cerebral tumours with those of age- and sex-matched controls for evidence of cerebrovascular disease. There was no difference in the degree of cerebral atrophy as judged by enlarged ventricles and cortical sulci but there was an excess of ischaemic lesions in epileptic patients: discrete areas of infarction and attenuation of periventricular white matter. In half of the epileptic patients who were found to have CT evidence of vascular disease, clinical examination was normal.

Shinton *et al.* (1987) found an excess of previous epilepsy in patients admitted to hospital with an acute stroke compared with controls. They interpreted their findings to support the idea that clinically undetectable cerebrovascular disease may present with seizures and that these can be a warning sign of a future stroke.

Other cerebral causes

Hildick-Smith (1974) and Roberts *et al.* (1982) found cerebral tumours in 10% and 12% respectively of their cases. A much lower figure of 2% was found by Schold *et al.* (1977) but they had a very high proportion (50%) of cases in which no cause was found. Luhdorf *et al.* (1986) found tumours in 14%. Of these, all but one were either metastases or inoperable gliomas. Most of the tumour cases in Roberts' series had partial seizures. The rare epilepsia partialis continua (Thomas *et al.*, 1977) and sensory epilepsy (Maguiere and Courjon, 1978) are associated with a higher incidence of tumours. (The relation between epilepsy and different types of tumours is also discussed in Chapter 16.)

The percentage of seizures associated with non-vascular cerebral degeneration is uncertain and will remain so until large series with uniform access to CT scanning facilities are reported. Hildick-Smith attributed 14% of her cases to 'senile dementia (?)' and Roberts *et al.* and Luhdorf *et al.* respectively 7% and 1.3% to cerebral atrophy.

Subdural haematoma is an important remediable cause of epilepsy in the elderly, who are prone to this condition because of cerebral atrophy. It may occur after a relatively trivial head injury and the diagnosis may be missed. Head injury itself is relatively uncommon as a cause of epilepsy in the elderly. Four per cent of Luhdorf's (1986) cases were post-traumatic.

Epileptic fits may occur in severe cerebral infections—meningitis, encephalitis or cerebral abscess—or following recovery from such infections, due to scarring.

Toxic and metabolic causes

Epileptic fits are attributed to toxic or metabolic causes in 12% of Hildick-Smith's cases, 10% of Schold's and 6% of those of Roberts *et al.* Twelve per cent of Luhdorf's cases were attributed to drugs, alcohol or metabolic disturbances. In 25% of patients in a recent series of late onset epilepsy (Dam, 1985) alcohol or alcohol withdrawal was the main cause. Alcohol misuse or alcohol withdrawal appeared to be the sole precipitating factor in 20% of the cases of status epilepticus of Pilke *et al.* (1984). As alcohol abuse is becoming increasingly prevalent amongst the elderly (especially females) this will continue to be a major aetiological factor.

A wide range of metabolic disturbances may precipitate fits in an elderly person; these include uraemia, hepatic failure, myxoedema, hypoxia, hypercapnia, hypoglycaemia, hypocalcaemia, hyponatraemia and water intoxication. Amongst these, uraemia seems to be the commonest in most series.

Drug-induced epilepsy (Chadwick, 1981)

More than 70 different drugs have been suspected of causing convulsions. These include anaesthetic agents, analgesics, steroids, antibiotics, hypnotics, tranquillizers and antidepressants. As Chadwick points out, it is very difficult to prove that a given drug caused the convulsions in a particular case but in certain drugs the probability of a causal relationship seems high. The drugs most likely to be epileptogenic are listed in Table 15.4.

TABLE 15.4 DRUGS WHICH MAY BE EPILEPTOGENIC

Antibiotics
  Benzylpenicillin
  Oxacillin
  Carbenicillin
  Isoniazid
  Cycloserine
Hormones
  Insulin
  Oral hypoglycaemics
  Prednisone
Local anaesthetics/antiarrhythmics
  Lignocaine
  Procaine
  Disopyramide
  Anticholinergics in overdose
Psychotropic drugs
  Chlorpromazine
  Other phenothiazines
  Tricyclic antidepressants
  Lithium
Analeptic drugs
  Aminophylline
  Doxapram
Anaesthetic agents
  Ether
  Methohexitone
  Ketamine
  Halothane
  Althesin
Radiographic contrast media (intrathecally)
  Meglumine iothalamate
  Meglumine iocarmate
  Metrizamide (very rare)
Withdrawal fits
  Benzodiazepines
  Alcohol

Based on Chadwick, 1981

Drug-induced seizures are most likely to occur when the drug is given in high dosage, parenterally or in patients with impaired drug handling. Aminophylline, which has a narrow therapeutic index, and whose disposition may be inhibited by cigarette smoking, is particularly prone to cause generalized seizures. Intravenous aminophylline may cause focal seizures which then generalize (Yarnell and Chu, 1975). These can occur in a neurologically asymptomatic patient and may be prolonged and associated with a poor outcome. Other drugs, notably the benzodiazepines, may cause epilepsy when withdrawn.

Idiopathic

Finally, it must not be forgotten that some patients apparently presenting with epilepsy for the first time in old age will in fact be suffering from a recurrence of earlier epilepsy. In addition, one encounters the occasional patient who has had a lifelong history of epilepsy which has not been recognized or at least adequately treated.

INVESTIGATIONS

The traditional emphasis on remediable structural underlying causes may be inappropriate in many elderly patients. It is based on an exaggerated estimate of the frequency with which tumours are the cause of late onset epilepsy, the percentage of such tumours that are benign or amenable to neurosurgical removal and an underestimate of the importance of other neurological. or, more significantly, metabolic causes. Against this must be offset the relative benignity of modern methods of neurological investigation, in particular imaging techniques, and the often underestimated benefits of having a precise diagnosis of the underlying cause even where this may not be amenable to definitive treatment. The desire of the patient or relative to know what is amiss is not unreasonable; in particular reassurance that fits are not caused by a brain tumour is especially valuable.

General Investigations

Investigation will be guided by the history and findings on examination and by a consideration of the likely causes. Metabolic causes must be ruled out. An estimate of gamma glutamyl transferase may be a useful marker of alcohol consumption. Diabetic patients on treatment should have their control reviewed, especially in the case of nocturnal seizures in patients on oral hypoglycaemic agents. If it is suspected that the fits are secondary to syncope, carotid sinus massage and ambulatory ECG recording may be considered. Lumbar puncture should not be carried out unless there are pointers to infectious disease of the nervous system. The possibility of neurosyphilis can be pursued in the first instance by serum testing, lumbar puncture being indicated only where serology is positive. The yield is usually very low. A chest X-ray may reveal a relevant primary neoplasm and a skull X-ray show evidence of raised intracranial pressure, intracranial calcification or other evidence of an intracerebral neoplasm.

Electroencephalography

The role of the EEG in the management of the epileptic patient is discussed in Chapter 7. It is sufficient here to reiterate certain points:

1. A routine EEG may support the diagnosis of epilepsy, especially if clear-cut paroxysmal discharges are observed.
2. The absence of epileptogenic activity on a routine recording does not rule out the diagnosis of epilepsy.
3. The range of normal increases with age so that discriminating normal from abnormal becomes more difficult. Moreover, non-specific abnormalities are more common.
4. A focal abnormality on the EEG may support the diagnosis of a focal origin for fits and suggest a local neurological cause. In those fits where there is an inadequate history or where the focal phase is too brief to be observed clinically, the suggestion of a focal origin may be raised for the first time. This may guide further investigation.

In summary, the EEG may provide invaluable supporting evidence for the diagnosis and suggest the need for further examination but it should rarely overrule the clinical diagnosis. As is pointed out in

Chapter 7, an EEG cannot determine the need for treatment in a newly diagnosed case, establish the adequacy of treatment or predict the safety of discontinuing therapy.

Neuroradiology (see also Chapter 6)

Which patients should be referred for brain scanning and what are the respective roles of isotope scanning and computed tomography? Scanning may be indicated where there is suspicion of a structural lesion raised by clinical or EEG evidence that the fits are focal in origin. Since this is true of the vast majority of seizures in the elderly, relying on this alone would result in an enormous demand for scanning services. The presence of focal neurological signs and the absence of evidence of a metabolic or toxic cause or a history of head injury will strengthen the case for a scan, particularly if general health is good. This will be especially strong in patients who have progressive neurological signs or features suggestive of raised intracranial pressure. The threshold for scanning will depend at least in part on the available resources. As suggested earlier, scanning should not necessarily be ruled out simply on the grounds that the chances of finding an operable lesion are slim: a patient with as worrying a condition as epilepsy should not be denied a complete diagnosis if this can be obtained without too much discomfort.

The role of the isotope scan has become less clear since the advent of computed tomography. Unlike the CT scan, it has a low pick up rate for infratentorial tumours (though these less commonly give rise to epilepsy). Moreover, a single scan cannot usually distinguish between vascular and neoplastic lesions. It is not uncommon for repeated scanning to be required to differentiate a vascular lesion, in which the abnormality usually resolves, from a neoplastic one, which will or will not get worse. Isotope scanning is often used as a screening procedure to identify those patients who warrant CT scanning. The requirement that an elderly patient earn his CT scan by producing evidence of non-resolving focal lesions on both an isotope scan and an EEG may not, however, represent the best option for the individual patient or the most economical use of resources.

The diagnostic yield of CT scanning in the management of epilepsy has been the subject of many recent studies (e.g. Ramirez-Lassepas *et al.*, 1984; Gastaut and Gastaut, 1976; Young *et al.*, 1982). The largest of these series is that of Gastaut and Gastaut (1976) who scanned 401 out of 500 successive patients in an epilepsy clinic. They found that scanning increased the rate of diagnosis of an organic lesion from 30% to 55%. In 20% of the patients the organic diagnosis had been missed by other methods. More relevant to the elderly is the study of Ramirez-Lassepas *et al.* (1984) who reported on 148 patients studied within 30 days of a first fit. Patients with known tumours, craniotomy, open skull fracture and a history of alcoholism were excluded. A cause for the seizure was found in 48% of cases and a structural lesion was established by CT scanning in 37% of the total series. The authors reported a marked rise in abnormal scans with age— from 30% for patients between 40 and 50 to 60% for those between 70 and 90. As might be expected, there was a much higher percentage of positive scans in patients with focal seizures (36/59) than in those with generalized fits (13/67). Interestingly, many of the positive scans were seen in patients with no focal features or findings and generalized, rather than focal, abnormalities on the EEG.

It is clear, then, that CT scanning may increase the precision with which the diagnosis of the underlying cause of epilepsy can be made. Some authors have questioned the value of this information. Young *et al.* (1982) scanned 220 consecutive patients with epilepsy or isolated seizures. Abnormalities were more likely to be found in patients with focal seizures or focal abnormalities on the EEG than in patients without such features who had normal scans in 94% cases. They pointed out, however, that only a quarter of the abnormalities detected were potentially treatable by surgery and less than 10% of patients had their management changed as a result of CT scanning. In addition, three out of the eleven patients with tumours had initially normal scans. They conclude that routine scanning is inappropriate, that it should be reserved for patients with focal features and that a negative scan should not be sought for reassurance. One could interpret these data quite differently, however, and conclude that

CT scanning was a very powerful way of arriving at an accurate diagnosis; that it produced remarkably few false negatives for tumours (three out of 220 patients); and that having a precise diagnosis is always helpful in planning treatment, in talking to relatives and patients, irrespective of whether it leads to specific, curative treatment. Here, as so often in medicine, decisions reflect personal judgement.

THE TREATMENT OF EPILEPSY

General Measures

Hopkins and Scambler (1977) were sharply critical of the care patients actually receive. They reported unnecessary hospital referrals, unnecessary EEGs, inadequate medication and follow-up supervision that appeared to bear no relation to actual need, with little correlation between the severity of the epilepsy and the frequency of follow-up. In many cases, patients had not had the diagnosis explained to them.

Management, in this, to the patient, most inexplicable and terrifying condition, must begin with an explanation of the events themselves and a reassurance that, in the vast majority of cases, the seizures themselves are unpleasant rather than dangerous. The patient needs to know that the fits can be controlled and that this will require taking medication on a regular basis for an indefinite period of time, possibly for the rest of his or her life.

Many patients will want to know whether fits are brought on by any particular activity and whether for this reason activity should be restricted. The advice in this age group will be the same as in any other: avoid only those activities which would mean immediate danger if a fit occurred. A patient can become more adventurous once the fits are under control or a pattern of infrequent fits is established. Factors which are known to precipitate fits—sleep deprivation, excess alcohol intake and sudden alcohol withdrawal in heavy drinkers—should be avoided. The patient should be warned that the side-effects of anticonvulsant drugs will be increased by alcohol. A tactful prompt from the patient may prevent the doctor from inadvertently prescribing a drug which has a convulsant effect or an antagonistic effect on anticonvulsant therapy.

The patient will also need to be advised of the regulations regarding driving. After a first fit, driving must be stopped, irrespective of whether the fit occurred during sleep. The patient must hand in his driving licence to the driving authorities and notify the Driving and Vehicle Licensing Centre in Swansea. Driving is forbidden for 6 months or a year after a single fit. Those patients who have had more than one fit and whose licences have been withdrawn may reapply for a driving licence in accordance with the regulations that came into force in 1982 (Espir, 1983):

1. No attacks while awake for 2 years.
2. Attacks have occurred only while asleep for 3 years.
3. Driving is not likely to be a source of danger to the public.

Patients on anticonvulsants will be granted a licence for 1, 2, or 3 years but not a full licence. Elderly patients under the age of 70 have to renew their licence when they reach 70 years of age.

Withdrawal of a driving licence will not usually mean loss of a job, as most elderly patients will have retired, but it may mean a serious restriction in mobility. Many elderly patients for this reason feel understandably aggrieved at what they consider to be an unfair ruling, citing friends who have heart conditions or have survived strokes and who represent, in their opinion, a much greater threat to the general public. They may be right. A study from the Netherlands (van der Lugt, 1975) showed that only about 1 in 10 000 road traffic accidents could be attributed with certainty to epilepsy over a 10 year period. They were less likely to occur in built up areas where the level of vigilance was perhaps higher and they rarely involved other vehicles. This figure—which may reflect compliance with medication and good seizure control—is much less than that due to alcohol. Whereas one might expect it to be higher in the elderly, who are more likely to have associated organic brain damage and to suffer from the side-effects of treatment, the Dutch study showed that most of the accidents occurred in the 20–29 age group and that the elderly acounted for fewer than 3% of epilepsy associated accidents.

For these reasons, the management of an elderly

patient who has had a single fit is difficult. If there is no clinical or EEG evidence of an underlying cerebral cause and the fit seems to have been precipitated by exceptional circumstances, the patient may be permitted to drive again in 6 months (Raffle, 1976).

DRUG TREATMENT

The mainstay of treatment is anticonvulsant therapy. This enormous topic will be dealt with under several headings.

When Should Epilepsy be Treated?

The current practice of most neurologists is not to treat a single grand mal seizure, on the basis that only a third of patients will go on to have a second seizure. This estimate, however, is probably optimistic. Elwes *et al.* (1984) followed 133 patients presenting to a neurology outpatient department with a single tonic–clonic seizure unrelated to alcohol withdrawal, drugs, acute metabolic disturbance or fever. The cumulative probability of seizure recurrence was 20% by one month and 62% by a year. One would expect this figure to be even greater in elderly patients in whom there is a higher proportion of symptomatic cases. Since the risks attending an epileptic fit are increased in this age group, there would appear to be a case for treating a first tonic–clonic seizure. Since untreated fits may themselves predispose to more fits, there is an additional reason for early control in the hope of reducing the recurrence rate and improving subsequent prognosis.

There is no information regarding the prognosis for an untreated minor seizure. Since, however, the problems associated with treatment are greater in the elderly, it may be reasonable to wait and see, unless there is clear clinical or CT scanning evidence of a focal lesion.

Monotherapy or Polytherapy?

Guelen *et al.* (1975) showed, in a study of 11 700 epileptic patients, that they were receiving on average 3.2 drugs, of which 84% were anticonvulsants. Over the last 15 years, however, Reynolds and his co-workers have mounted a persuasive case for the use of a single drug in the control of seizures. As a result of

their advocacy of a rational approach, fewer patients are likely to be placed on subtherapeutic doses of a multitude of adversely interacting anticonvulsants. Reynolds *et al.* (1981) summarize the disadvantages of polytherapy as follows:

1. Chronic toxicity is proportional to the number of anticonvulsant drugs.
2. Drug interactions are more likely to occur.
3. The value of individual drugs cannot be assessed;
4. A multiplicity of drugs, leading to intoxication, may exacerbate seizures.

The advantages of monotherapy for elderly patients who may also be on other medication are self-evident.

Reynolds *et al.* (1981) showed that 80% of 31 previously untreated patients with grand mal and/or partial seizures could be rendered seizure-free on phenytoin during a mean follow-up period of 42 months. Twelve per cent out of the 20% who were not properly controlled had non-optimum phenytoin levels due to poor compliance. Only three patients with adequate phenytoin treatment were not controlled and these had additional neuropsychiatric handicaps. Few of the patients in this study were elderly but there is no reason to assume that the conclusions do not apply to the aged, especially as many of the patients in the series had partial epilepsy. Monotherapy with carbamazepine has also been shown to be effective (Callaghan *et al.*, 1978; Andersen *et al.*, 1983).

Where monotherapy has failed, there is little evidence that the introduction of a second drug contributes anything to the management of the patient other than the increased risk of side-effects. Shorvon and Reynolds (1977) found that the addition of a second drug in 50 chronic epileptic patients improved seizure control at a rate not greater than that expected by a placebo. The same authors (1979) also showed that withdrawal of a second drug improved seizure control in a proportion of patients on polypharmacy. The habit of automatically proceeding to a second drug may reflect a failure to appreciate that some types of epilepsy are unresponsive to any anticonvulsant. The outcome for the patient will be the burden of chronic toxicity added to that of epilepsy.

The Choice of Drug

The guidelines for the choice of drug are now less rigid and careful matching of drug to clinical or electrical type of epilepsy is now a thing of the past. The main drugs to consider in the elderly are phenytoin, carbamazepine and sodium valproate, which are all broad spectrum anticonvulsants. (Medication in status epilepticus will be discussed separately.)

The studies cited above have demonstrated the effectiveness of phenytoin monotherapy in most cases. Unfortunately this is a drug with many side-effects and although these may be reduced by careful serum monitoring, they can still be troublesome in the elderly. For example, minor cerebellar side-effects may be more important in an elderly person who already has reasons for being unsteady. Carbamazepine is also effective in most forms of epilepsy that are seen in the elderly. A small double-blind cross-over study (Kosteljanetz *et al.*, 1979) comparing phenytoin and carbamazepine in patients with grand mal and focal motor seizures showed no significant difference between these two drugs in terms of seizure control or side-effects. A point in favour of phenytoin, however, is that the therapeutic range is better defined for this drug than for carbamazepine.

One of the most interesting developments in recent years has been the use of sodium valproate, originally introduced for primary generalized epilepsy, in partial and secondarily generalized fits. Turnbull *et al.* (1985) randomized 140 previously untreated patients with tonic–clonic or partial seizures to receive either phenytoin or sodium valproate. There was no difference in the efficacy of the two drugs, irrespective of the type of seizures the patients suffered, during a follow-up period for 2 to 4 years. Toxic reactions were more frequent in patients on phenytoin, although the difference did not reach statistical significance. Since, in addition to gross toxic reactions, there may be minor impairments of cognitive function with phenytoin, sodium valproate may be the first drug of choice for most seizures in this age group. Chadwick and Turnbull (1985), in their recent comparative review of the efficacy of anticonvulsants, point out that there are large deficits in the literature and that the strong feelings clinicians have about the choice of first-line drugs are not based on adequate information. In view of the comparable efficacy of the three first-line drugs, choice should probably be based on comparative toxicity and, perhaps, cost.

The drugs of first choice in myoclonic epilepsy are probably sodium valproate or clonazepam (Davidson, 1983).

Dosage and Frequency

The time-honoured frequency for anticonvulsant drugs is three times a day. This may not always be rational and may present particular difficulties for elderly patients. Phenytoin is relatively slowly and incompletely absorbed and has a long half-life of 24–48 hours (Woodbury, 1982). For this reason, it is not surprising that it is possible to maintain steady-state levels of this drug with a single daily dose (Buchanan *et al.*, 1972). O'Driscoll *et al.* (1985) compared a single daily dose and divided doses of phenytoin in 46 outpatients in a randomized cross-over study in which each arm of the trial lasted 6 months. There were no differences in seizure frequency, adverse reactions, the results of psychometric tests, compliance or serum plasma concentrations.

As yet, no comparable studies have been carried out with carbamazepine or sodium valproate. The plasma half-life of carbamazepine is very variable, ranging from 18 to 60 hours; it may be reduced on repeated dosages, due to enzyme induction. Towards the end of the first month of therapy, plasma levels fall by about 25%. A smaller autoinduction effect occurs each time the dose is increased. At present two to four daily divided doses are recommended. The half-life of sodium valproate ranges from 9 to 21 hours, with a mean of 12–13 hours. It does not enhance its own metabolism, so that the half-life does not reduce with repeated dose. Even so, it seems unlikely that a single daily dose will provide 24 hour cover. Loiseau (1984) recommends a three times a day schedule, though he suggests that it may be reasonable to start with a single daily dose and then, if this is not successful, to try increasing the frequency.

TABLE 15.5   RECOMMENDED DOSES OF ANTICONVULSANTS

Anticonvulsant	Starting dose	Total daily maintenance dose	Daily frequency
Carbamazepine	100 mg twice a day	300–1600 mg	3–4 times
Phenytoin	200 mg at night	150–500 mg	Once
Sodium valproate	200 mg twice a day	400–2500 mg	Twice

The recommended dosage schedules for the first-line anticonvulsants are given in Table 15.5

The rate of phenytoin metabolism is decreased to such an extent in patients aged between 60 and 79 that they would require 21% less phenytoin to maintain the same steady state concentration (Bauer and Blouin, 1982). On the basis of this, it has been suggested that a lower starting dose (say 200 mg total daily dose) should be employed. Further information on the age dependency of kinetics is required.

Individual variation in kinetics implies that the dose should be individually tailored. The best guide to optimal dosage is the clinical response and the anticonvulsant levels. The case for measuring levels was strongly supported by the observation made by Lascelles *et al.* (1970) that only 45% patients on phenytoin had adequate serum levels. Without monitoring levels, failure to respond to treatment may lead to an inappropriate or premature change of medication. Moreover, the therapeutic ratio is very narrow and phenytoin has concentration dependent kinetics; there is therefore an increased chance of straying outside the therapeutic range. In the case of phenytoin at any rate, free drug level correlates with total drug concentration There is very little variability in protein binding in epileptic patients except in hepatic and renal disease.

There is a clear relation between phenytoin levels and both therapeutic effect and toxicity. These relations are less clear-cut for sodium valproate. It is not possible to define a therapeutic range for carbamazepine, as a wide range of levels is associated with efficacy and side-effects (Callaghan *et al.*, 1978).

The saturation kinetics of phenytoin means that the relationship between the dose and the steady state is not linear. As serum levels near the optimum range, liver enzymes responsible for metabolism become saturated. For this reason, smaller dosage increments, e.g. 25 mg (Mawer *et al.*, 1974), are recommended. Increments of 50 or 100 mg may result in a swing from a subtherapeutic to a toxic dose.

The optimal serum levels of anticonvulsants have not yet been studied separately for the elderly. In view of the incidence of brain damage and age-related changes in the elderly epileptic population, one might expect increased pharmacodynamic sensitivity. This may indicate that the upper limit of the therapeutic range may have to be revised downwards.

Side-effects

Neuropsychiatric

The most important side-effects of anticonvulsant medication are neuropsychiatric. These have recently been comprehensively reviewed by Trimble and Reynolds (1983) who emphasize that they may be overlooked where there are other possible explanations of an insidious deterioration in cognitive function. This is, of course, particularly likely to occur in elderly patients.

The most obvious neurological side-effects of phenytoin—ataxia, dysarthria and nystagmus—are due to cerebellar dysfunction. These, along with blurred vision, are signs of overdosage. Irreversible cerebellar dysfunction occurs only very rarely and then only after many years of chronic intoxication (Reynolds, 1975). Reversible blurring and doubling of vision, dizziness and unsteadiness occur with carbamazepine and are dose related. Tolerance rapidly occurs, allowing much higher concentrations to be achieved subsequently without overt sedation. Over the last decade or so, there have been several clinical and electrophysiological studies of periph-eral neuropathy associated with anticonvulsants (Shorvon and Reynolds, 1982). These have sug-gested that phenytoin, but not carbamazepine or sodium valproate, may be associated with mild neuropathy. It is not clear how much of this is due to folate deficiency (see below). There have been several reports of reversible involuntary movement disorders with different anticonvulsants (e.g. Dravet *et al.*, 1983). Phenytoin, in particular, has been incriminated as producing reversible dyskinesias, involving the face, trunk and limbs similar to those produced by neuroleptics. These usually occur shortly after commencing therapy and are often related to overdosage. Phenytoin, carbamazepine and sodium valproate may all cause asterixis in high dose. Sodium valproate may produce a mild postural or rest tremor (Davidson, 1983). It is often not appreciated that overdosage with anticonvulsants may cause an exacerbation of seizures. Phenytoin may cause headache and insomnia.

Drowsiness is by far the most common neurologi-cal side-effect of anticonvulsants and it would be anticipated that this would be more important in the elderly. Sodium valproate and carbamazepine are superior in this respect to other commonly used anticonvulsants. Minor cognitive impairment short of drowsiness, affecting memory, concentration, memory speed and motor speed, have been well documented (e.g. Thompson and Trimble, 1981). In this regard the adverse impact of phenytoin seems to be much greater than that of carbamazepine or sodium valproate. In view of the evidence reported earlier indicating approximately equal efficacy of all three first-line drugs in controlling most types of seizures, the final choice of medication may be influenced by the frequency of neuropsychiatric side-effects.

Other

Gastrointestinal side-effects are associated with all three drugs. Nausea, vomiting, constipation and gastric irritation occur most commonly with pheny-toin. Sodium valproate may cause increased appetite and weight gain in younger patients, though there is no evidence regarding this in the elderly.

Although osteomalacia has been described with other anticonvulsants, it appears to most commonly associated with phenytoin. Phenytoin-induced metabolizing enzymes in the liver accelerate catabo-lism of vitamin D. Ashworth and Horn (1977) noted biochemical evidence of osteomalacia in 22% of patients on anticonvulsants for over 10 years and nearly half of these had histological evidence of osteomalacia on bone biopsy. Recent studies (Gough *et al.*, 1986) have shown that sodium valproate, unlike phenytoin and carbamazepine, does not cause hypocalcaemia or reduced 25-hydroxyvitamin D levels. Offerman *et al.* (1979) found that the low serum calcium and 25-hydroxyvitamin D in patients on anticonvulsants could be reversed by low dose vitamin D supplementation. Since osteomalacia is more likely to occur in elderly patients whose poor dietary intake of vitamin D and reduced exposure to sunlight already put them at risk, there may be a case for prophylactic vitamin D supplementation, as suggested by Rodbro *et al.* (1974).

Blood dyscrasias may occur with all three drugs. These include thrombocytopenia, granulocytope-nia, agranulocytosis and pancytopenia. With the exception of reversible thrombocytopenia in patients receiving sodium valproate—particularly in high doses—these are very rare. In addition to reducing platelet numbers, sodium valproate may impair aggregation. Platelets should be checked before starting sodium valproate. Patients on phenytoin may develop megaloblastic anaemia due to folate deficiency, this in turn being the consequence of accelerated folate metabolism following the induc-tion of hepatic enzymes.

Hepatic dysfunction may occur on treatment with all three drugs but this has been a matter of particular concern with valproate as it may rarely lead to hepatic failure. For this reason, valproate is usually avoided in patients with liver dysfunction. It is recommended that liver function tests should be carried out before commencing sodium valproate and repeated at 2-monthly intervals during the first 6 months of treatment and that the drug should be discontinued if liver function tests show impairment. Since hepatic failure has been described mainly in very young children who may have metabolic defects, this advice may be over-cautious in the elderly, especially as impaired liver function tests may not predict hepatic failure. It would be a pity if an appropriate drug were underused because of minor impairments of conventional liver function tests. Further research is needed here, however, before the recommendation to avoid valproate in the presence of hepatic dysfunction can be revised. Sodium valproate may also be associated with pancreatitis.

Cutaneous side-effects may occur. Exanthematous rashes are common with phenytoin. More serious skin reactions include lupus erythematosus, erythema multiforme and bullous, exfoliative or purpuric rashes. It is not known how often coarse facies, hirsutism and painful hypertrophied gums occur in epileptic patients who commence therapy for the first time in old age; these features are certainly seen in elderly 'graduate' epileptics. Generalized erythematous rashes, which may be severe, occur in about 3% of patients given carbamezepine. Photosensitivity reactions, urticaria, exfoliative dermatitis, erythema multiforme and the Stevens–Johnson syndrome and lupus erythematosus have also been reported. Transient hair loss—with regrowth of curly hair—has been reported with sodium valproate.

Cardiac failure may rarely be precipitated in elderly patients on carbamazepine due to its antidiuretic hormone stimulating effect.

Drug Interactions

There are numerous interactions between anticonvulsants and other drugs. The important ones are listed in Table 15.6, for which the main source of information was Appendix 1 of the *British National Formulary* Number 12 (1986).

When Can Anticonvulsants be Stopped?

Should all epileptic patients started on treatment be committed to a lifetime of drug therapy? The toxic effects of anticonvulsants and the possibility that an elderly patient will be taking other medication, so that dosage determination is difficult and compliance uncertain, make permanent anticonvulsant treatment unattractive. There have been a few

studies undertaken to determine the success of anticonvulsant withdrawal, and the factors which identify which patients are likely to remain fit free. These are summarized in Chadwick (1983). Juul-Jensen (1964) found that of a series of patients who had been seizure free for 2 years or more, 40% relapsed in 2–5 years after withdrawal from treatment. The chance of relapse was reduced by a slower rate of withdrawal. Those with an onset of epilepsy before 30 had a better prognosis for anticonvulsant withdrawal. As expected, the severity of epilepsy, as judged by the number and frequency of seizures prior to remission, was directly related to the likelihood of relapse. Partial seizures—which are, of course, more common in the elderly—carry a particularly high risk of relapse (Oller-Daurella et al., 1976; Thurston et al., 1982). This correlated with the fact that the presence of known cerebral pathology increased the rate of relapse. A normal EEG prior to withdrawal favours a successful withdrawal but it is dangerous to rely on the EEG alone.

In summary, the evidence suggests that up to 50% of patients who become seizure free for 2 or more years will relapse when medication is reduced or withdrawn. Since late onset, symptomatic epilepsy is more likely to be associated with relapse, one has reluctantly to concede that withdrawal of therapy should not be attempted in most elderly patients who have a good reason to be placed on anticonvulsants in the first place. Whether the epileptic patient in good remission can be maintained on a lower, even subtherapeutic dose of anticonvulsant, is something that will need clarifying. It is certainly worthwhile exploring.

STATUS EPILEPTICUS

The definition of status epilepticus varies. The ILAE (1981) classification proposes that the term should be used whenever a seizure persists for a sufficient length of time or is repeated frequently enough that recovery between attacks does not occur. Another definition is of 'a seizure lasting for at least 30 minutes or repeated frequently enough to produce a fixed and enduring epileptic condition lasting at least 30 minutes' (Celesia et al., 1972).

TABLE 15.6 INTERACTIONS OF FIRST-LINE BROAD SPECTRUM ANTICONVULSANTS

Drug affected	Drug interacting	Effect
1. Drugs that affect anticonvulsants		
All anticonvulsants	Antidepressants	Antagonism
	Phenothiazines	Antagonism
Carbamazepine	Cimetidine	Potentiation
	Dextropropoxyphene	
	Erythromycin	
	Isoniazid	
	Verapamil	
	Viloxazine	
	Diltiazem	
Phenytoin	Amiodarone	Potentiation
	Azapropazone	
	Chloramphenicol	
	Cimetidine	
	Co-trimoxazole	
	Diazepam	
	Disulfiram	
	Influenza vaccine	
	Isoniazid	
	Ketoconazole	
	Miconazole	
	Phenylbutazone	
	Sulphinpyrazone	
	Viloxazine	
	Aspirin	Transient potentiation
	Sodium valproate	
	Folic acid	Occasionally reduces plasma phenytoin
	Rifampicin	Reduces plasma phenytoin
	Sucralfate	Reduced absorption of phenytoin
Sodium valproate	Carbamazepine	Reduced plasma concentrations of valproate
	Phenobarbitone	
	Phenytoin	
	Primidone	
Clonazepam	Cimetidine	Potentiation
2. Drugs affected by anticonvulsants		
Flecainide	Phenytoin	Reduced plasma concentrations
Mexiletine		
Warfarin and nicoumalone	Carbamazepine	Inhibition
	Phenytoin	Both potentiation and inhibition reported
Theophylline	Carbamazepine	Plasma theophylline
	Phenytoin	may be reduced
Haloperidol	Carbamazepine	Reduced plasma haloperidol
Lithium	Carbamazepine	Neurotoxicity may occur
	Phenytoin	without increased plasma concentrations
Tricyclic antidepressants	Antiepileptics	Reduced plasma levels of tricyclics
Doxycycline	Carbamazepine	Reduced plasma concentrations
	Phenytoin	
Ketoconazole	Phenytoin	Reduced plasma ketoconazole
Thyroxine	Carbamazepine	Increased thyroxine metabolism and may increase
	Phenytoin	requirements in primary hypothyroidism
Cortisone	Carbamazepine	Reduced effect
Dexamethasone	Phenytoin	
Hydrocortisone		
Prednisolone		
Prednisone		
Cyclosporin	Phenytoin	Reduced plasma concentration cyclosporin
Methotrexate	Antiepileptics	Increased anti-folate effect

Main Source: *British National Formulary* (1986).

Status epilepticus may be partial, as in jacksonian status, or generalized, as in tonic–clonic status or absence status. Very localized motor status is termed 'epilepsia partialis continua'. An alternative classification is given below:

Convulsive:
    Generalized: tonic–clonic
    Localized: e.g. jacksonian
    Very localized: epilepsia partialis continua
Non-convulsive:
    Absence
    Psychomotor
      Recurrent with inter-ictal confusion
      Confusional state clinically
      indistinguishable from absence status

Tonic–clonic or grand mal status is highly dangerous and, according to Janz (1959), occurs in 1–5% of the epileptic population. This is an old figure and may indicate a higher incidence than is currently the case. Nevertheless, since it is six times as common in symptomatic as in idiopathic epilepsy, one might expect it to be commoner in the elderly epileptic population. In a study of 'tardive status epilepticus' (Celesia *et al.*, 1972) only three patients out of seventeen had idiopathic epilepsy. Stroke, head injury and brain tumour accounted for most of the rest. Sudden unheralded status ('lone status epilepticus') was associated in one small series with a high proportion of, mainly frontal, cerebral tumours (Oxbury and Whitty, 1971).

Despite a frequent association with significant structural lesions, status epilepticus is often preventable. In a study of 98 patients with grand mal status (defined as '2 or more seizures without recovery of consciousness between attacks') (Aminoff and Simon, 1980), half of the patients had not had previous seizures. Of those patients who had had a previous seizure, the commonest single cause was non-compliance with drug therapy (53% cases). Alcohol withdrawal was another important precipitating cause. The recent series of Pilke *et al.* (1984) confirmed the importance of alcohol abuse (implicated in over half the male cases) and changes in, or irregularity of, anticonvulsant therapy (sixteen out of 82 cases).

Convulsive status epilepticus is easily recognized but the protean manifestations of non-convulsive status may be misleading, as already discussed. Complex partial status, in particular, may simulate psychogenic symptoms. Drake and Coffey (1983) describe a patient alternating between unresponsiveness and incomplete or inappropriate responses with grimacing, head posturing and plucking at the bedclothes. During the period of unresponsiveness, continuous epileptic activity was recorded on the EEG.

Convulsive status epilepticus is a serious medical emergency that demands immediate recognition and prompt treatment. Delayed or inadequate treatment may mean death or permanent neurological deficit due to anoxic brain damage. Aminoff's series was associated with a 2.5% mortality and a 12.5% morbidity (Aminoff and Simon, 1980). The picture may be confused by a rise in temperature due to the hypermetabolic state, a peripheral leucocytosis and a status induced cerebrospinal fluid pleocytosis suggesting CNS infection.

Treatment has recently been usefully reviewed by Ward (1987). The initial aims are immediate control of fits, adequate oxygenation and maintaining or restoring biochemical homeostasis. The drug of first choice is still intravenous diazepam which should arrest the seizures in most cases. A typical dose would be 10 mg in 2 ml given over several minutes. It may cause respiratory depression. If this does not abort the fits, an intravenous infusion of diazepam containing 200 mg/l should be initiated. Infusion rates over 40 mg/hour are not recommended. A very large accumulative dose of diazepam, even as much as several hundred milligrams over a 24 hour period, may be necessary to keep the fits under control. In such cases, the patient should be closely monitored for hypotension and occasionally respiratory depression. Clonazepam has no clear advantage over diazepam. Phenytoin may be effective where the patient has not been receiving chronic therapy with this drug. The recommended loading doses are in the region of 15–18 mg/kg. It may cause severe cardiac bradyarrhythmias and cardiac monitoring should be carried out during the period of infusion. Where it is distinctly possible that the patient has not been complying with current phenytoin therapy, there is nothing to be lost by giving a loading dose of this drug. Paraldehyde or chlormethiazole may be effective. Since their effect is transient, they will need to be followed up by oral or intravenous phenytoin. If all else fails, intubation and ventilation may be required and thiopentone may then be used.

Non-convulsive status may respond to an intravenous bolus of diazepam. Clonazepam is said to be especially effective in minor motor status, especially epilepsia partialis continua. Unfortunately it may produce severe drowsiness and this effect may be expected to be more marked in the elderly.

DEATH IN EPILEPSY

Hauser *et al.* (1980) found that the standard mortality ratio was increased in epileptic patients. The increase was less marked, however, in those diagnosed over 60 years of age (1.6 for the first 5 years, 1.8 for the next 5 years) than for those diagnosed in youth or middle age (2.5 for those aged 20–59). Mortality from heart disease was increased in epileptic subjects over the age of 65 in the Minnesota study (Hauser and Kurland, 1975) but the increase appeared to be confined to those in whom the seizures were symptomatic of cerebrovascular disease. The prevalence of heart disease was not related to anticonvulsant status and did not therefore appear to be a side-effect of medication. In a study by Terrence *et al.* (1975) of 37 cases of sudden, unexplained death in epileptic patients, all but two were poorly controlled, having more than one seizure per month. In only three patients was the blood level of anticonvulsants in the therapeutic range. They concluded that inadequate anticonvulsant therapy due to poor compliance was the most important cause of death in patients in whom the fits were not due to a fatal underlying cause.

CONCLUSION

Epilepsy in the elderly is a common problem and the principles of management are similar to those in younger patients. Differentiating epilepsy from other causes of episodic impairment of consciousness may be more difficult. The commonest underlying cause is cerebrovascular disease and investigations aimed at finding a remediable structural cause may

not be very fruitful. Metabolic and toxic causes, especially alcohol abuse, are important. While drug treatment may control fits satisfactorily, dose optimization may be more difficult. There are many unanswered questions in relation to the choice of first-line therapy, and the dynamics, as well as the kinetics, of anticonvulsants in the biologically aged patient have been insufficiently studied. The map of epilepsy in old age, as with so many other neurological diseases in the elderly, has many white spaces.

REFERENCES

Aminoff, M.J., and Simon, R.P. (1980). Status epilepticus. Causes, clinical features and consequences in 98 patients. *Am. J. Med.*, **69** (5), 657–66.

Andermann, F., and Robb, J.P. (1972). Absence status—a reappraisal following review of 38 patients. *Epilepsia*, **13**, 17.

Andersen, E.B., Philbert, A., and Klee, J.G. (1983). Carbamazepine monotherapy in epileptic out-patients. *Acta Neurol. Scand. (Suppl.)*, **94**, 29–34.

Ashworth, B., and Horn, D.B. (1977). Evidence of osteomalacia in an outpatient group of adult epileptics. *Epilepsia*, **18** (1), 37–43.

Bauer, L.A., and Blouin, R.A. (1982). Age and phenytoin kinetics in adult epileptics. *Clin. Pharmacol. Ther.*, **31** (3), 301–4.

Blumhardt, L.D. (1986). Ambulatory ECG and EEG monitoring of patients with blackouts. *Br. J. Hosp. Med.*, **36** (5), 354–60.

Boller, F., Wright, D.G., Cavalieri, R., and Mitsumoto, H. (1975). Paroxysmal "nightmares". Sequel of a stroke responsive to diphenylhydantoin. *Neurology (Minneapolis)*, **25** (11), 1026–8.

Buchanan, R.A., Kinkel, A.W., Gailett, R.J., and Smith, T.C. (1972). Metabolism of diphenylhydantoin following once daily administration. *Neurology*, **22**, 126–30.

Callaghan, N., O'Callaghan, M., Duggan, B., and Feely, M. (1978). Carbamazepine as a single drug in the treatment of epilepsy: A prospective study of serum levels and seizure control. *J. Neurol. Neurosurg. Psychiatry*, **41** (10), 907–12.

Celesia, G.G., Messer, T.B., and Murphy, M.J. (1972). Status epilepticus of late adult onset. *Neurology (Minneapolis)*, **22** (10), 1047–55.

Chadwick, D.W. (1981). Convulsions associated with drug therapy. *Adverse Drug Reaction Bulletin*, **87**, 316–19.

Chadwick, D. (1983). When can anti-convulsant drugs be stopped? In: Warlow, C., and Garfield, J. (eds.) *Dilemmas in the Management of the Neurological Patient*, Churchill Livingstone, Edinburgh.

Chadwick, D., and Turnbull, D.M. (1985). The comparative efficacy of antiepileptic drugs for partial and tonic-clonic seizures. *J. Neurol. Neurosurg. Psychiat.*, **48**, 1073–7.

Cocito, L., Favale, E., and Reni, L. (1982). Epileptic seizures in cerebral arterial occlusive disease. *Stroke*, **13** (2), 189–95.

Commission on the Classification and Terminology of the International League Against Epilepsy (1981). Proposal for revised clinical and electro-encephalographic classification and epileptic seizures. *Epilepsia*, **22**, 489–501.

Dam, A.M. (1985). Late onset epilepsy, etiologies, types of seizure and value of clinical investigation, EEG and CT Scan. *Epilepsia*, **26**, 227–31.

Davidson, D.L.W. (1983). Anti-convulsant drugs. *Br. Med. J.*, **286**, 2043–5.

Drake, M.E., and Coffey, C.E. (1983). Complex partial status epilepticus simulating psychogenic unresponsiveness. *Am. J. Psychiatry*, **140** (6), 800–1.

Dravet, C., Dalla, B.B., Mesdjiane, E., Galland, M.C., and Roger, J. (1983). Phenytoin-induced paroxysmal dyskinesias. In: Oxley, J., Jaanz, D., and Meinardi, H. (eds.) *Chronic Toxicity of Anti-epileptic Drugs*, Raven Press, New York, pp. 229–35.

Ellis, J.M., and Lee, S.I. (1978). Acute prolonged confusion in later life as an ictal state. *Epilepsia*, **19** (2), 119–28.

Elwes, R.D., Johnson, A.L., Shorvon, S.D., and Reynolds, E.H. (1984). The prognosis for seizure control in newly diagnosed epilepsy. *N. Engl. J. Med.*, **311** (15), 944–7.

Espir, M.L.E. (1983). Fitness to drive: Additional guidance on 2. Epilepsy. *Health Trends*, **15**, 46–7.

Feuerstein, J., Weber, M., Kurtz, D., and Rohmer, F. (1970). Étude statistique des crises épileptiques apparaissant après l'âge de 60 ans. *Sem. Hôp. Paris*, **46**, 3125–8.

Fine, W. (1966). Epileptic syndromes in the elderly. *Clin. Gerontol.*, **8**, 21–33.

Fine, W. (1967). Post hemiplegic epilepsy in the elderly. *Br. Med. J.*, **1**, 199–201.

Gastaut, H. (1970). Clinical and electro-encephalographic classification of epileptic seizures. *Epilepsia*, **11**, 102.

Gastaut, H., and Gastaut, J.L. (1976). Computerised transverse axial tomography in epilepsy. *Epilepsia*, **17** (3), 326–36.

Gastaut, H., Gastaut, J.L., Goncalves, A., Silva, G.E., and Fernandez, S.G.R. (1975). Relative frequency of different types of epilepsy: A study employing the classification of the International League Against Epilepsy. *Epilepsia*, **16**, 457.

Gibberd, F.B. (1972). The prognosis of petit mal in adults. *Epilepsia*, **13** (1), 171–5.

Godfrey, J.W., Roberts, M.A., and Caird, F.I. (1982). Epileptic seizures in the elderly: 2 Diagnostic problems. *Age Ageing*, **11**, 29–34.

Goodridge, D.N.G., and Shorvon, S.D. (1983). Epileptic seizures in a population of 6000: I Demography, diagnosis and classification and role of the hospital services. *Br. Med. J.*, **287**, 641–4.

Gough, H., Goggin, T., Bissessar, A., Baker, M., Crowley, M., and Callaghan, N. (1986). A comparative study of the relative influence of different anticonvulsants, UV exposure and diet on vitamin D and calcium metabolism in out-patients with epilepsy. *Q. J. Med.*, **59**, 569–77.

Guelen, P.J.M., van der Kleijn, E., Woudstrau, J., Schneider, H., and Janz, D. (1975). In: Gardner-Thorpe, C., Meinardi, H., and Sherwin, A.L. (eds.) *Clinical Pharmacology of Anti-epileptic Drugs*, Springer Verlag, Berlin, pp. 2–10.

Hashan, R.H.A., and Jameson, H.D. (1973). Cardiac standstill simulating repeated epileptic attacks. *J.A.M.A.*, **224** (6), 887–8.

Hauser, W.A. (1978). Epidemiology of epilepsy. *Adv. Neurol.*, **19**, 313–39.

Hauser, W.A., Annegers, J.F., and Elveback, L.R. (1980). Mortality in patients with epilepsy. *Epilepsia*, **21** (4), 399–412.

Hauser, A., and Kurland, L.T. (1975). The epidemiology of epilepsy in Rochester, Minnesota, 1935 through 1967. *Epilepsia*, **16** (1), 1–66.

Hildick-Smith, M. (1974). Epilepsy in the elderly. *Age Ageing*, **3**, 203–8.

Hopkins, A., and Scambler, G. (1977). How doctors deal with epilepsy. *Lancet*, **i**, 183–6.

Jaanz, D. (1959). Conditions and causes of status epilepticus. *Epilepsia*, **1**, 162–88.

Juul-Jensen, P. (1964). Frequency of recurrence after discontinuance of anti-convulsive therapy in patients with epileptic seizures. A new follow-up study after five years. *Epilepsia*, **9**, 11–16.

Kogeorgos, J., Scott, D.F., and Swash, M. (1981). Epileptic dizziness. *Br. Med. J.* **282**, 687–9.

Kosteljanetz, M., Christiansen, J., Dam, A.M., Hansen, B.S., Lyon, B.B., and Pedersen, H. (1979). Carbamazepine versus phenytoin. A controlled clinical trial in focal motor and generalised epilepsy. *Arch. Neurol.*, **36** (1), 22–4.

Lascelles, P.T., Kocen, R.S., and Reynold, E.H. (1970). The distribution of plasma phenytoin levels in epileptic patients. *J. Neurol. Neurosurg. Psychiatry*, **33**, 501–9.

Loiseau, P. (1984). Rational use of valproate: Indications and drug regimen in epilepsy. *Epilepsia*, **25** (Suppl. 1), 65–72.

Luhdorf, K., Jensen, L.K., and Plesner, A. (1986). Etiology of seizures in the elderly. *Epilepsia*, **27** (4), 458–63.

Maguiere, F., and Coujon, J. (1978). Somatosensory epilepsy. A review of 127 cases. *Brain*, **101**, 307–32.

Marquardsen, J. (1969). The natural history of acute cerebrovascular disease. A retrospective study of 769 patients. *Acta Neurol. Scand.*, **45** (Suppl. 38), 150–2.

Mawer, G.E., Mullen, P.W., Rodgers, M., Robins, A.J.,

and Lucas, S.B. (1974). Phenytoin adjustment in epileptic patients. *Br. J. Clin. Pharmacol.*, **1**, 163–8.

Mulder, D.W., and Rushton, T. (1959). Hyper-insulinism: A rare cause of epilepsy. *Neurology*, **9**, 288–9.

Norris, J.W., and Hachinski, V.C. (1982). Mis-diagnosis of stroke. *Lancet*, **1**, 328–31.

O'Driscoll, K., Ghadiali, Crawford, P., and Chadwick, D. (1985). A comparison of single daily dose and divided dose of phenytoin in epileptic outpatients. *Acta Ther.*, **11**, 375–85.

Offermann, G., Pinto, V., and Kruse, R. (1979). Antiepileptic drugs and vitamin D supplementation. *Epilepsia*, **20** (1), 3–15.

Oller-Daurella, L., Pamies, R., and Oller, L. (1976). In: Jaanz, D. (ed.) Reduction or discontinuance of antiepileptic drugs in patients seizure-free for more than five years. *Epileptology*, Thieme-Verlag, Stuttgart, pp. 218–27.

Oxbury, J.M., and Whitty, C.W. (1971). The syndome of isolated status epilepticus. *J. Neurol. Neurosurg. Psychiatry*, **34** (2), 182–4.

Pilke, A., Partinen, M., and Kovanen, J. (1984). Status epilepticus and alcohol abuse: An analysis of 82 status epilepticus admissions. *Acta Neurol. Scand.*, **70** (6), 443–50.

Raffle, A. (ed.) (1976). *Medical Aspects of Fitness to Drive*, third edition, Medical Commission on Accident Prevention, London.

Ramirez-Lassepas, M., Cipolle, R.J., Morillo, L.R., and Gumnit, R.J. (1984). Value of computed tomography scan in the evaluation of adult patients after their first seizure. *Ann. Neurol.*, **15** (6), 436–43.

Reynolds, E.H. (1975). Chronic anti-epileptic toxicity: A review. *Epilepsia*, **16**, 319–52.

Reynolds, E.H., Shorvon, S.D., Galbraith, A.W., Chadwick, D., Dellaportas, C.I., and Vydelingum, L. (1981). Phenytoin mono-therapy for epilepsy: A long-term prospective study, assisted by serum level monitoring, in previously untreated patients. *Epilepsia*, **22** (4), 475–88.

Roberts, M.A., Godfrey, J.W., and Caird, F.I. (1982). Epileptic seizures in the elderly: 1 Aetiology and type of seizure. *Age Ageing*, **11**, 24–8.

Rodbro, P., Christiansen, C., and Lund, M. (1974). Subjective symptoms in epileptic patients on anticonvulsant drugs. A controlled therapeutic trial of the effect of vitamin D. *Acta Neurol. Scand.*, **52** (2), 87–93.

Rodin, E.A., Katz, M., and Lennox, K. (1976). Differences between patients with temporal lobe seizures and those with other forms of epileptic attacks. *Epilepsia*, **17** (3), 313–20.

Ryan, R., Kempner, K., and Emlen, A.C. (1980). The stigma of epilepsy as a self-concept. *Epilepsia*, **21** (4), 433–44.

Santos, A.G.R. dos, and Lye, M.D.W. (1980). Transient cardiac arrhythmias in healthy elderly individuals: how relevant are they? *J. Clin. Exp. Gerontol.*, **2** (4), 245–58.

Schold, C., Warnell, P.R., and Earnest, N.P. (1977). Origin of seizures in elderly patients. *J.A.M.A.*, **238**, 1177–8.

Schott, G.D., Macleod, A.A., and Jewitt, E.D. (1977). Cardiac arrhythmias that masquerade as epilepsy. *Br. Med. J.*, **i**, 1454–7.

Shinton, R.A., Gill, J.S., Zezulk, A.V., and Beevers, D.J. (1987). The frequency of epilepsy preceding stroke. *Lancet*, **i**, 11–13.

Shorvon, S.D., and Reynolds, E.H. (1977). Unnecessary polypharmacy for epilepsy. *Br. Med. J.*, **1**, 1635–7.

Shorvon, S.D., and Reynolds, E.H. (1979). Reduction of polypharmacy for epilepsy. *Br. Med. J.*, **2**, 1023–5.

Shorvon, S.D., and Reynolds, E.H. (1982). Anti-convulsant peripheral neuropathy: A clinical and electrophysiological study of patients on single drug treatment with phenytoin, carbamazepine or barbiturates. *J. Neurol. Neurosurg. Psychiatry*, **45**, 620–6.

Shorvon, S.D., Gilliatt, R.W., Cox, T.C., and Yu, Y.L. (1984). Evidence of vascular disease from CT scanning in late onset epilepsy. *J. Neurol. Neurosurg. Psychiatry*, **47** (3), 225–30.

Terrence, C.F., Wisotzkey, H.M., and Perper, J.A. (1975). Unexpected, unexplained death in epileptic patients. *Neurology (Minneapolis)*, **25** (6), 594–8.

Thomas, J.E., Reagan, T.J., and Klass, D.W. (1977). Epilepsia partialis continua. A review of 32 cases. *Arch. Neurol.*, **34** (5), 266–75.

Thompson, P.J., and Trimble, M.R. (1981). Sodium valproate and cognitive functioning in normal volunteers. *Br. J. Clin. Pharmacol.*, **12**, 819–24.

Thompson, S.W., and Greenhouse, A.H. (1968). Petit mal status in adults. *Ann. Intern. Med.*, **68**, 1271–9.

Thurston, J.H., Thurston, D.L., Hixon, B.B., and Keller, A.J. (1982). Prognosis in childhood epilepsy. *N. Engl. J. Med.*, **306**, 831–6.

Trimble, M.R., and Reynolds, E.H. (1983). Neuropsychiatric toxicity of anticonvulsant drugs. In: Matthews, W.B. and Glaser, G.H. (eds.) *Recent Advances in Clinical Neurology*, Vol. 4, Churchill Livingstone, Edinburgh, London.

Turnbull, D.M., Howell, D., Rawlins, M.D., Weightman, D., and Chadwick, D.W. (1985). Which drug for the adult patient with epilepsy: phenytoin or valproate? *Br. Med. J.*, **290**, 815–19.

van der Lugt, P.J. (1975). Traffic accidents caused by epilepsy. *Epilepsia*, **15** (5), 50–1.

Wagner, A.L. (1983). A clinical and epidemiological study of adult patients with epilepsy. *Acta Neurol. Scand.*, **94** (Suppl.), 63–72.

Ward, C. (1987). Status epilepticus. *Hospital Update*, **13** (3), 190–202.

Webster, J.E., Gurdjian, E.S., and Martin, F.A. (1956). Carotid artery occlusion. *Neurology (Minneapolis)*, **6**, 491–502.

Woodbury, D.M. (1982). Diphenylhydantoin: Absorption, distribution and excretion. In: Woodbury, D.M., Penry, J.K., and Pippinger, C.E. (eds.) *Antiepileptic Drugs*, Raven Press, New York, p. 191.

Yarnell, P.R., and Chu, N.S. (1975). Focal seizures and aminophylline. *Neurology (Minneapolis)*, **25** (9), 819–22.

Young, A.C., Costanzi, J.B., Mohr, P.D., and Forbes, W.S. (1982). Is routine computerised axial tomography in epilepsy worthwhile? *Lancet*, **ii,** 1446–7.

Zielinskii, J.J. (1982). Epidemiology. In: Laidlaw, J., and Richens, A., (eds.) *A Textbook of Epilepsy*, second edition, Churchill Livingstone, Edinburgh, pp. 16–33.

The Clinical Neurology of Old Age
Edited by R. Tallis
© 1989 John Wiley & Sons Ltd

Chapter 16

Tumours of the Nervous System

Michael Sharr

Regional Neurosurgical Unit, Brook General Hospital, Woolwich, London, UK

INTRODUCTION

The ageing nervous system is no more or less likely to undergo neoplastic change than that of a younger individual. Nevertheless, some tumours are age-related; for example, although they are occasionally found in adults, it is very rare for a medulloblastoma to occur after childhood. Conversely, spinal meningiomas are very rare in childhood and tend to occur in middle-aged and elderly females. The commonest brain tumour, the malignant glioma, usually occurs in adults and presentation after the sixth decade is far from rare: almost 25% of Salcman's (1982) patients were aged 61 to 80 and a similar proportion of Pennybacker's (1968) patients had malignant gliomas. These and other figures would seem to refute Cushing's (1932) claim that less than 5% of intracranial tumours occurred in patients greater than 60 years of age. In all probability this was more a reflection of the diagnosis being made only on patients reaching neurosurgical centres. Even so, it is still wise to remember that neurosurgical neoplastic disease in old people is rare and only 0.9% of all admissions in Twomey's series (1978) proved to have an intracranial tumour.

Tumour site may also be age-related, the majority of astrocytomas in children being below the tentorium, whereas the majority in adults (and certainly in elderly patients) arise in the hemispheres. Metastatic tumours occur approximately as frequently as malignant gliomas according to some authorities (Pennybacker, 1968; Twomey, 1978) or slightly less

(Salcman, 1982; Friedman and Odom, 1972). Metastatic tumours may be underreported in neurosurgical series as many patients with metastatic disease would not be transferred to a specialist unit. Presentation may differ between age groups and this may be related to the inevitable cerebral atrophy that will exist in an older patient, delaying the onset of raised intracranial pressure. The co-presence of other diseases common in the elderly and the effect of drug therapy may also modify presentation.

INTRACRANIAL TUMOURS

Classification

The tumours likely to occur in elderly people are shown in Table 16.1. This list is not exhaustive but includes the commoner lesions and excludes rarer lesions that are more likely to be of pathological, rather than clinical, relevance.

Pathology

Supratentorial

The important tumours are the gliomas (i.e. tumours of the glia, a type of 'connective tissue') of which the commonest is the astrocytoma. A low grade ('benign') astrocytoma of the hemisphere is exceedingly rare in old people, and the commonest tumours are malignant gliomas.

TABLE 16.1 SOME INTRACRANIAL TUMOURS OF THE ELDERLY

Supratentorial	Infratentorial
Glioma (astrocytoma Grades 3–4)	Cerebellar metastasis haemangioblastoma
Metastasis	Fourth ventricle
Meningioma	ependymoma
Pituitary adenoma	choroid plexus papilloma
	Cerebellopontine angle acoustic neuroma meningioma
Craniopharyngioma	Brain stem glioma

Pituitary tumours are uncommon in elderly people but this may relate to bias against the elderly in terms of neurosurgical referrals. Certainly the incidence was very low in the series of Twomey (1978) and Friedman and Odom (1972) and Salcman (1982), though it was surprisingly high in that of Cooney and Solitare (1972). The commonest pituitary tumour is a non-secreting chromophobe adenoma that may produce both endocrine and systemic disturbances as well as compressive effects especially on the optic nerves and chiasm. The very rare craniopharyngioma cannot on clinical grounds alone be distinguished from a pituitary tumour although presentation with dementia (Bartlett 1971), usually associated with hydrocephalus, is commoner in an older person and more likely to produce such a problem than a pituitary tumour. It is still difficult to understand how what is thought to be a developmental lesion could present as late as the sixth or seventh decade or even beyond.

The meningioma is the classical benign intracranial tumour and its incidence is usually well below that of glioma and metastatic tumour. However, in the elderly the incidence tends to increase and in Salcman's (1982) series it was the commonest tumour. It is more common in females. The various cell types are not of any great clinical significance except that the so-called angioblastic meningioma has a greater tendency to recur. Site is an important influence on recurrence and the common parasagittal, falx, basal and sphenoid wing tumours may not

be totally removable so that recurrence may occur. This, however, is less likely in old age since life expectancy in elderly patients is much less than that of younger ones. Convexity tumours can be totally removed along with their dural attachment and recurrence is therefore less likely.

The usual primary sites for an intracranial metastasis are lung, breast, melanoma, and gastrointestinal tract. 'Site unknown' still forms a significant percentage in some series (Sharr, 1979).

Infratentorial

A metastatic tumour may occur in the vermis or cerebellar hemispheres. An infratentorial glioma will arise in the brain stem, but such a tumour in the elderly must be extremely rare since there are few references in the literature. It is more frequent in younger people, especially children. Histologically it is usually of a lower grade than supratentorial tumours but its inaccessible position more than cancels out this favourable aspect for the tumour is not removable by current methods. The benign piloid cerebellar astrocytoma (which is sometimes cystic) is a tumour restricted to childhood and young teenagers and does not occur in elderly people; however, occasionally a more malignant astrocytic tumour will present in the cerebellar hemisphere. The cerebellar haemangioblastoma is an unusual tumour of the elderly though it formed 12% of Salcman's (1982) series. It may be either solid or cystic and may form part of a von Hippel–Lindau complex, especially if there is a family history. Under such circumstances, however, the tumour is unlikely to present for the first time at an advanced age though recurrence may present at such an age since these can be a significant problem when there is a family history. Acoustic neuromas (schwannoma) may occur in elderly people, the incidence being very variable (low in the series of Friedman and Odom (1972), Twomey (1978), and Pennybacker (1968), and more significant in that of Salcman (1982)). Unfortunately it is likely to be large and to have caused serious brain stem compression before diagnosis since the initial deafness is often attributed to age, and associated vertiginous symptoms ascribed to vertebrobasilar ischaemia.

All infratentorial tumours will tend to produce hydrocephalus due to obstruction of the CSF flow especially in the fourth ventricle and its exit foramina, and sometimes the symptoms of hydrocephalus will be more apparent than the local effects of the tumour.

Clinical Features

There is no certain method by which a benign tumour may be differentiated from a malignant one and differentiation between a primary and metastatic tumour will often depend upon prior identification of a primary. Although a long history might be more suggestive of an underlying benign tumour this is by no means always the case since underlying cerebral atrophy, occurring in an ageing brain, may allow a considerable amount of time to pass, and a large tumour to grow, before there are definite neurological symptoms and signs. Although duration of symptoms has been claimed to be useful in differentiating benign from malignant tumours (Hoessly and Olivecrona, 1955), Twomey (1978) stressed that the discriminant value of this feature was poor.

Supratentorial tumours

The symptoms will depend upon the site of the tumour and the amount of space occupation. The latter will be governed by the size of the tumour, the quantity of surrounding oedema, and any increase in the size of the ventricular system.

Symptoms. Epilepsy is a common symptom and may be obviously focal, of temporal lobe character, or grand mal. Focal and temporal lobe epilepsy may progress to grand mal seizures. Epilepsy was relatively common in the series of Friedman and Odom (1972) (38%) and in the report of Cooney and Solitare (1972) (32%) and rare in Twomey's (1978) series. Certain areas, namely the pre- and post-central regions, are more likely to be epileptogenic than others. Temporal lobe epilepsy may result from a tumour arising in the medial temporal region but review of the literature does not support a clear correlation between this site and the occurrence of temporal lobe epilepsy. Although epilepsy is often associated with meningiomas, it is only slightly more common in such tumours than in gliomas (Cooney and Solitare, 1972).

A frontal tumour may present with general deterioration in intellectual function and ultimately dementia. With involvement of medial frontal regions and midline structures, especially the corpus callosum, sphincter disturbance is common. Almost 50% of the patients of Friedman and Odom (1972) showed personality/mental changes and this was more common than in patients with subdural haematomas. Certainly impairment of mental function is very common in elderly patients with a supratentorial tumour, though this may be overlooked, being attributed either to the ageing process, cerebrovascular disease or cerebral atrophy. While relatively rapid onset may suggest a tumour, slow deterioration due, for example, to a subfrontal meningioma may not suggest this diagnosis until there are more overt focal neurological signs.

Focal symptoms and signs will occur in relation to the appropriate areas: posterior frontal or pre-motor area tumours producing contralateral weakness; parietal or post-central tumours producing contralateral focal sensory epilepsy; occipital tumours producing a contralateral visual field loss. Speech disturbance may occur in dominant hemisphere tumours. Inferior frontal or superior temporal gyrus lesions usually cause expressive symptoms, while posterior temporal or inferior parietal lesions tend to be associated with receptive symptoms. Focal symptoms and signs are reported as being extremely common in brain tumours in elderly patients (Godfrey and Caird, 1984; Twomey, 1978).

Differentiating stroke from intracranial tumour continues to pose a problem, although only 9% of Twomey's (1978) tumour patients were incorrectly diagnosed as having had a stroke. A higher figure was reported by Reichenthal and Shalit (1978) and Sencer (1964) warned of the dangers of assuming that an acute onset always implied a stroke: 33% of his series of tumours presented with an acute stroke-like syndrome.

Raised intracranial pressure symptoms may occur less frequently in the elderly tumour patient because of underlying cerebral atrophy. Moreover, headaches may occur, for example, in cranial arteritis. It may sometimes be unclear whether focal symptoms are transient ischaemic attacks or focal epilepsy. While accompanying amaurosis may help differentiation there is in fact no certain way of knowing whether a focal attack is ischaemic or epileptic. The presence of widespread vascular disease will not always be helpful since this may be co-present in many elderly patients.

Signs. These will of course depend on the site of the tumour, the common signs being hemiparesis and/or hemisensory disturbance. Papilloedema is uncommon (Pennybacker, 1968; Godfrey and Caird, 1984) but visual field defects are common.

Even large tumours occurring in 'silent' areas, such as non-dominant frontal and non-dominant anterior temporal lobes, may not present with focal neurological signs. Some signs may be extremely helpful; for example, unilateral anosmia, which may suggest a sub-frontal olfactory groove meningioma. Lower limb weakness disproportionate to upper limb or facial weakness, or occurring alone, may indicate a contralateral parasagittal/falcine meningioma. Although of course bilateral lower limb weakness is most commonly associated with spinal cord lesions, there are other rare causes of 'cerebral paraplegia', including interhemispheric subdural haematoma and interhemispheric subdural empyema. Sometimes hydrocephalus causes predominantly lower limb signs with a mixture of weakness and ataxia.

At an advanced stage, a large intracranial tumour will produce the features of a transtentorial (uncal) herniation or coning, with increasing drowsiness, pupillary dilatation (usually ipsilateral to the tumour), and hemiparesis (Sharr, 1984). Though it is more commonly contralateral, hemiparesis may sometimes be ipsilateral. This paradox, known as the Kernohan notch effect (Kernohan and Woltman, 1929), is due to the midbrain being shifted away from the side of the tumour, the pyramidal fibres in the opposite cerebral peduncle thereby being indented by the edge of the tentorium. Since these fibres will decussate at medullary level the hemiparesis manifests itself on the same side as the tumour that has produced the initial midbrain displacement.

Pituitary tumour and craniopharyngioma

Both pituitary tumour and craniopharyngioma may cause symptoms and signs of optic nerve and chiasmal compression. Assessment of failing vision in an elderly person may be difficult and awareness of an actual visual field defect may be late. It is all too easy to attribute visual failure to 'the ageing process'. Visual failure, especially if unilateral or very asymmetrical, may occasionally be due to a suprasellar or parasellar meningioma. Such lesions may be difficult to confirm even with sophisticated neuroradiology since a small tumour can nest under one optic nerve very easily. Unfortunately late diagnosis is not infrequent (Garfield and Neil-Dwyer, 1975). As with a younger person, unless failing vision in an elderly patient can easily be explained by a local ocular or ophthalmological disorder, further investigations are mandatory. No patient, whatever the age, should be allowed to go blind without a potentially reversible cause being sought.

Features of hypopituitarism may be missed in an elderly person, especially the typical facial appearance. Loss of secondary sexual characteristics might be difficult to determine in such a patient. Symptoms of pituitary and hypothalamic dysfunction, especially polydipsia and polyuria, may be confused with other disorders including diabetes mellitus. An old person may have very advanced myxoedema before the diagnosis is made and even then an underlying pituitary disorder may be missed. Hypersecreting tumours are comparatively rare in the elderly but do occur (Salcman, 1982).

Acute haemorrhage in relation to supratentorial tumours

Whilst this may occur in any tumour, and suggests an erroneous diagnosis of haemorrhagic stroke, it remains a rare complication. It was recorded in less than 10% of cases of Cooney and Solitare (1972), and all the tumours subsequently proved to be glioblastomas. Nevertheless, malignant melanoma and pituitary tumours have a propensity to bleed. In the latter case, this may occur alone or as a result of a haemorrhagic infarction—so-called pituitary apoplexy, where, with or without symptoms and signs of visual failure, the patient becomes rapidly obtunded with hypotension, acute electrolytic disturbance, and large, poorly reacting or non-reacting pupils.

Infratentorial tumours

Infratentorial tumours are less common in elderly patients than those in the supratentorial compartment (Godfrey and Caird, 1984). As with supratentorial tumours, symptoms and signs depend on the site of the tumour and its space-occupying effect. Because the posterior fossa is more confined, raised intracranial pressure (usually as a consequence of CSF obstruction and hydrocephalus) may be more pronounced than other symptoms. However, as with supratentorial tumours, this may not be as common in elderly patients.

Cerebellar metastases usually have a short history, the commonest symptoms being vertigo and unsteadiness with associated headaches and vomiting. Metastases from breast carcinoma may have an unexpectedly long history. Although raised intracranial pressure may be more common than in a supratentorial tumour, papilloedema is relatively uncommon. Nystagmus and ataxia, affecting the limbs in cerebellar hemisphere lesions and the trunk in vermis lesions, are quite common. Occasionally a cerebellar syndrome may present as a non-metastatic manifestation of an occult neoplasm, when intracranial pressure will not be raised. Since, however, raised intracranial pressure may not occur in elderly patients it may still be difficult to differentiate on clinical grounds alone between a tumour and a non-metastatic syndrome.

Haemangioblastoma is rare in the elderly, only one out of 67 patients being over the age of 70 in Salcman's (1982) series. A family history and the von Hippel–Lindau complex may point to the diagnosis. There may be acute episodes of cerebellar–brain stem dysfunction which may be due to recurrent haemorrhage. There appears to be a relationship between this tumour and polycythaemia, the latter also being associated with a renal neoplasm. It is therefore not without interest that those patients who have the von Hippel–Lindau trait, and who may develop haemangioblastoma, have an increased incidence of renal carcinoma and what may be

initially assumed to be a haemangioblastoma may prove to be a metastasis from a renal carcinoma (Goodbody and Gamlen, 1974).

Acoustic neuroma is comparatively rare in the elderly (Salcman, 1982) and usually presents quite late since deafness is often dismissed as being due to the ageing process. Unilateral deafness should never be disregarded, especially in the absence of an obvious local otological cause. Slow growth of the tumour and a failure to appreciate the significance of deafness will result in a large tumour producing brain stem distortion causing ataxia, and it is this symptom that ultimately leads to a neurological, and eventually neurosurgical, referral. Hydrocephalus may occur and, rarely, it is so marked that CSF rhinorrhoea may result from the enlarged third ventricle eroding through the cribriform plate of the ethmoid. Severe hydrocephalus in this and other slowly growing benign posterior fossa tumours, may lead to dementia which, again, may be attributed to 'old age'. Other cerebellopontine angle tumours, such as mengiomas and trigeminal neuromas, may present in a very similar way to an acoustic neuroma although there may be less pronounced hearing loss and more trigeminal sensory symptoms in a trigeminal neuroma. There is dispute as to whether trigeminal neuralgia resembling the idiopathic variety can result from a cerebellopontine angle trigeminal neuroma (Stookey and Ransohoff, 1959). Very rarely, brain stem glioma (see below) may present as a cerebellopontine angle mass, producing deafness; and indeed neurosurgeons will occasionally carry out posterior fossa exploration and discover that the cerebellopontine angle is occupied by an asymmetrical swelling emanating from the pons. The triad of dementia, ataxia, and incontinence may suggest normal or low pressure hydrocephalus (Hakim and Adams, 1965).

Primary brain stem glioma is a very rare tumour of the elderly and, as in younger patients, symptoms and signs of raised intracranial pressure may be conspicuous by their absence. The usual features are cranial nerve dysfunction (the specific nerves involved depending upon the level in the brain stem at which the tumour is arising) and long tract symptoms and signs. Very occasionally these tumours may extend into the cavity of the fourth ventricle and produce hydrocephalus. Other fourth ventricle tumours include ependymoma and choroid plexus papilloma; both will tend to cause CSF obstruction quite early and hydrocephalus may produce variable symptoms.

Investigations and Treatment

These must be considered together since, if there are clinical grounds for deciding against treatment, investigation will be of academic interest only.

Why investigate?

The fundamental question to be answered is whether or not the patient could benefit from treatment. 'Treatment' usually implies surgery, although conservative treatment of some cerebral tumours using steroids may produce worthwhile results (Graham and Caird, 1978). The ultimate justification for investigation is the hope of finding a neurosurgically remediable lesion, such as a benign tumour, or other non-neoplastic lesion, such as chronic subdural haematoma or cerebral abscess, which may be indistinguishable from an intracranial tumour in their mode of presentation. It is also useful to know if a patient has a malignant tumour. Having said this, the extent to which one would wish to investigate will be influenced by the presence or absence of concurrent medical problems which will greatly influence the outcome of operation.

Investigations

Chest X-ray may reveal a primary tumour or multiple metastases. Past history of a primary neoplasm should not necessarily lead to the assumption that a neurological syndrome is due to metastasis (Raskind *et al.*, 1971). A plain skull X-ray may be useful in that many elderly patients have a calcified pineal gland and displacement may occur in the presence of a supratentorial mass. It must again be stressed that the latter may not necessarily be neoplastic. No pineal shift will of course occur in a patient with an infratentorial tumour. It does not require neuroradiological experience to visualize a calcified pineal gland, although it is surprising how often mistakes can be made. The most useful guide is

a lateral skull X-ray since, if a calcified pineal gland can be seen, visualization should be possible in the Towne's view. In elderly patients there may be other areas of calcification including the falx and lateral ventricle choroid plexus; the former will not be displaced even in the absence of a large supratentorial mass, whereas some displacement of the latter may occur in the presence of such a mass. If only one lateral ventricle choroid plexus is calcified it is important not to mistake it for a shifted pineal. Such a mistake should not occur since pineal displacement to the point where a choroid plexus is usually postioned would be very unlikely to be compatible with life! Another common plain film abnormality, occurring particularly in women, is hyperostosis frontalis interna. This is usually bilateral, classically sparing the midline, and should not be mistaken for enostotic changes of a meningioma. The appearance of the pituitary fossa should be noted as this may reveal raised intracranial pressure or an intrasellar pituitary tumour. The characteristic rarefaction of the dorsum sella and/or pituitary fossa floor that may occur in raised intracranial pressure is not always easy to recognize in elderly patients since some rarefaction will inevitably occur as part of the ageing process. However, the fossa should not enlarge or balloon with age and such changes should be regarded as suggesting a pituitary tumour or craniopharyngioma, although the latter is less likely to affect the pituitary fossa than the former. The characteristic sellar and suprasellar calcification related to childhood and juvenile craniopharyngioma is much less common in adults and certainly in the elderly.

Isotope brain scanning

This is widely available and its value should not be underestimated. Many supratentorial meningiomas may be visualized as will the majority of gliomas. The torcula (confluence of the sinuses) should not be mistaken for a tumour. There is an approximate 15–25% false negative rate in the diagnosis of chronic subdural haematoma (Burrows, 1972). A sylvian 'flare' in the distribution of the middle cerebral artery is sometimes mistakenly identified as a chronic subdural haematoma when, in fact, it represents underlying infarction. Changes of infarction on an isotope scan usually take 7–14 days to appear and may remain for 4–6 weeks before some resolution takes place, a useful point to note when adopting a 'wait and see' policy in an elderly patient in whom the diagnosis falls between tumour or infarction. The place of isotope scanning in the diagnosis of infratentorial tumours is limited, although this investigation will commonly reveal an acoustic neuroma and some infratentorial meningiomas. It will, however, frequently fail to demonstrate most other infratentorial tumours.

Computed tomography (CT)

If available, this investigation will provide the most information about intracranial lesions. Although it may be frequently possible to identify the pathological nature of the lesion on the basis of CT scan appearances, it is often not possible to distinguish between a cystic primary tumour, necrotic metastasis, and cerebral abscess. CT scanning may reveal multiple lesions (usually metastases) and it will also delineate ventricular size. The significance of ventricular enlargement in the elderly may be difficult to evaluate because cortical atrophy is quite common. The size of the cortical sulci may help to distinguish ventricular enlargement associated with this from that due to raised intracranial pressure.

Angiography

This procedure is performed much less often now that CT scanning is available and its use in patients with suspected tumours is largely restricted to meningiomas and some rare posterior fossa tumours. Since the risks of angiography undoubtedly increase with age, this investigation should be employed sparingly in elderly patients. Vertebral angiography may be particularly hazardous in the elderly.

Magnetic resonance imaging

This is available only in a few centres and its clinical application to patients with intracranial and spinal disorders is still in its infancy. While it may become the definitive investigation of choice in the future, at present scanning time remains relatively long and costs are high.

Treatment

The major differences between the method of treatment of younger patients compared with older patients relate to emphasis (Bartlett, 1985). Once as precise a diagnosis as possible has been made from the history, examination, and investigations, the decision to treat will depend as much upon the patient's general condition as upon the neurological diagnosis.

Glioma

Radical surgery is rarely justified in the elderly since they anyway have a poorer prognosis than younger patients. Moreover, the Karnofsky index (a clinical grading on the basis of symptoms and signs), is likely to be lower in the elderly patient with a glioma, due to diminished cerebral reserve. The lower the Karnofsky index the worse the prognosis. The main objective of management is to exclude an underlying benign lesion and prove beyond all doubt with histological confirmation that the tumour is malignant. This can be achieved by means of a burr hole biopsy, a simple surgical procedure that can, if necessary, be performed under local anaesthetic. The simplicity of the procedure, however, should not divert attention from the possible sequelae such as swelling and haemorrhage, which may lead to worsening of a neurological deficit or even death. It should not be forgotten that the procedure is diagnostic and not therapeutic.

Can craniotomy be justified in an elderly patient with a presumed malignant glioma? By and large the answer to this is 'no', but in rare situations, where the patient remains comparatively well and with minimal deficit, but with symptoms of raised intracranial pressure (e.g. headaches, vomiting) that are not effectively controlled by steroids, a craniotomy and decompression might be justified. This is especially applicable to tumours in the non-dominant frontal or temporal lobes. Since headaches and vomiting are uncommon in the elderly, however, this is unlikely to occur very often.

There is considerable controversy surrounding the use of chemotherapy in patients with gliomas. So long as the place of chemotherapy remains uncertain, it is unlikely to be frequently justified in elderly patients with malignant gliomas.

Metastasis

The approach here is very similar to that for a malignant glioma. Occasionally, removal of what appears to be a solitary metastasis can produce surprisingly good results. The discovery of other metastases and the potential curability of a primary tumour if known, as well as the efficacy of any treatment of a previous primary tumour, would all be factors in assessing the value of a craniotomy (Sharr, 1983). Failure to isolate and identify the primary tumour may not necessarily be considered an adverse factor since sometimes a tumour remains occult, and it is well known, for example, that a small breast tumour in an elderly female remains occult or, if palpable, indolent for many years. A more conservative approach using steroids and, where appropriate, radiotherapy may also produce worthwhile benefits (Cairncross et al., 1980).

In summary, anything more than a biopsy should be the exception in an elderly patient with a suspected malignant brain tumour. Nevertheless, each patient should be assessed individually and a decision made as to whether steroids, radiotherapy, or attempted removal of the tumour is the preferred course of action. The available evidence from the literature does not, however, support major surgery as a routine method of treatment.

Meningioma, pituitary tumour, craniopharyngioma

These tumours are discussed together because in all three attempted removal may be worth considering. Both pituitary tumour and craniopharyngioma may undergo sufficient suprasellar extension to cause hydrocephalus. In this situation, insertion of a ventriculo-atrial or ventriculo-peritoneal shunt may be all that is needed to improve the patient's condition. Unfortunately, as with burr hole biopsy, this relatively easy technical procedure may lead to serious sequelae in the elderly. The ensuing relief of hydrocephalus in the atrophic brain leads to an acute subdural haematoma because the brain collapses like a pricked balloon and cortical veins bridging the subdural space may be torn.

When there are severe local visual symptoms and signs it is clearly difficult to withhold surgery. Even though the elderly and infirm person may fare better without surgery, blindness is a symptom which cannot be ignored, especially as the tumour is indolent and benign (even accepting that in reality both pituitary tumours and craniopharyngiomas are difficult to eradicate totally). The symptoms and signs produced by a cystic craniopharyngioma may be relieved by tapping the fluid through a burr hole with, on occasions, quite dramatic improvement. Refilling of a cyst is very likely but in a very elderly patient this may not be such a problem in view of the likely life expectancy.

Meningioma presents a problem intermediate between pituitary tumour and craniopharyngioma on one hand and malignant brain tumours on the other. Meningiomas are more common than is usually supposed (Wood et al., 1957) and with the advent of CT scanning more elderly people are found to have such tumours (Papo, 1983). Clinicians are consequently being increasingly forced to make decisions as to whether surgery should be considered. It must not be forgotten that even a benign tumour may be difficult, indeed hazardous, to remove: a parasagittal meningioma may be close to the superior sagittal sinus; whilst a sphenoid wing meningioma may have an intimate relationship to the middle cerebral and/or carotid artery. Moreover, the tumour may recur, although this may not be such a great problem in an elderly patient whose life expectancy may be limited. Prolonged frontal lobe retraction during removal of a sub-frontal (olfactory groove) meningioma may lead to postoperative cerebral oedema which may in turn result in a serious postoperative deficit or even death. Moreover, preoperative dementia may not be reversed. Even a convexity meningioma, although technically totally removable, may be best treated conservatively if the only symptoms are focal epilepsy, since there is no guarantee that surgery would prevent further fits. However, an otherwise healthy elderly person who is developing a significant focal deficit, or is suffering from symptoms of raised intracranial pressure, may be considered for surgery. Atrophic brain does not always respond favourably to the removal of a long-standing tumour. The postoperative complication rate increases with age and meningioma surgery on patients over the age of 65 still remains a challenge (Papo, 1983).

Infratentorial tumours

Biopsy of a posterior fossa tumour is technically much more difficult and potentially more dangerous than that of a supratentorial tumour. The surgeon is faced with a stark choice between no surgical procedure and a potentially major posterior fossa exploration. In the presence of hydrocephalus, insertion of a shunt may produce impressive improvement with resolution of headache, drowsiness, and confusion. Ataxia, however, responds poorly to shunting, presumably because this symptom is largely due to brain stem distortion. Moreover, shunt insertion in the presence of a large posterior fossa tumour may lead to an upward cone where the higher posterior fossa pressure causes the posterior fossa structures to be displaced in a rostral direction through the tentorial hiatus. Admittedly this complication is rare and where attempts to remove a tumour from within the fourth ventricle (e.g. ependymoma) are unlikely to benefit an elderly patient, a shunt may be all that is required. Excision of a cerebellar hemisphere tumour may be worthwhile in a patient where ataxia is the main problem. Although the surgeon may be tempted to 'back off' if the CT scan suggests a malignant posterior fossa tumour, it is well to remember that a patient with a benign cerebellar tumour (e.g. haemangioblastoma) may have become anorexic due to vomiting and headache and develop a cachectic appearance suggesting underlying malignant disease. The CT scan cannot differentiate with certainty between a malignant metastatic cerebellar tumour and a benign haemangioblastoma. Many of the fourth ventricle tumours, whatever their histological nature, will not be totally removable. If the surgeon does remove a metastatic tumour from the cerebellar hemisphere, search for an asymptomatic primary is not likely to be justified, in contrast with the appropriateness of a more aggressive approach in a younger patient.

The elderly patient with an acoustic neuroma or cerebellopontine angle meningioma should be assessed carefully since surgery is likely to be difficult and dangerous. Since, however, shunting is of limited benefit in ataxia, more radical surgery may be justified, except in very elderly and frail patients. The most important hazard is related to brain stem dysfunction. There may also be damage to the facial nerve. The former is not necessarily due to direct injury, but results from pressure changes and distortion consequent upon manipulation and removal of the tumour. This may be lessened by carrying out an intracapsular removal of the tumour, leaving the capsule attached to the surrounding structure. Unfortunately, there may be heavy bleeding from a meningioma so that partial removal may be less easily achieved than initially expected.

Summary of Treatment

The likely nature of the tumour will influence management although on the whole a conservative approach should be considered, at least initially. Nevertheless, because an infratentorial tumour may cause more physical than mental disability (rather than the opposite which tends to be produced by supratentorial tumours) and because mental function is not likely to be impaired as a result of surgery, operative treatment has its place. Improving the quality of life must always be a priority in an elderly person. As with all surgery in the elderly, deep vein thrombosis and pulmonary embolism pose a significant threat and may adversely affect the outcome of a technically successful operation.

SPINAL TUMOURS (see also Chapter 17)

Classification and Pathology

For practical purposes Table 16.2, although not exhaustive, lists the important varieties of spinal tumour. The commonest tumour causing spinal compression is an extradural metastasis, usually originating from lung, breast, or prostate. Lymphoma may also occur and this may have a better prognosis than other tumours (Sharr, 1982). The two important intradural, extramedullary tumours

TABLE 16.2 SPINAL TUMOURS OF THE ELDERLY

Extradural (metastatic)

Intradural
    Extramedullary (meningioma, neurofibroma)
    Intramedullary (astrocytoma, ependymoma)

are meningioma and neurofibroma, the former being more common than the latter. Intramedullary tumours are usually astrocytomas or ependymomas; these are usually of a lower grade and thus less malignant than their cerebral counterparts.

Symptoms and Signs

Symptoms

Whilst there may be differences in the mode of presentation of intracranial tumours in the elderly as compared with younger patients, these differences are less evident in the case of tumours compressing the spinal cord and cauda equina. This may reflect the fact that spinal function declines less with age than cerebral function and spinal atrophy occurs at a much slower rate. Nevertheless, it is a regrettable fact that if an older person shows a deterioration of lower limb function this is often at first ascribed to advancing years. Delay in diagnosing extradural metastatic compression remains a persistent problem (Shaw *et al.*, 1980; Richardson and Maurice-Williams, 1982).

The hallmark of extradural spinal cord metastatic compression is pain, either midline spinal, or radicular, or both. The pain is severe and unremitting and typically made worse by straining, coughing and sneezing. Although similar symptoms may arise from a neurofibroma, the radicular pain due to that tumour is usually worse than the spinal pain. Of greater significance is the duration of this symptom prior to the appearance of other neurological symptoms, this usually being a matter of weeks or months in extradural metastatic compression whereas it is almost always longer, sometimes years, in a patient with a neurofibroma. Spinal cord compression due

to meningioma is often painless; hence the need to suspect this tumour in any elderly female who gradually 'goes off her legs'.

Other neurological deficits usually become apparent sometime after the onset of the pain, though they may occasionally antedate it. Lower limb weakness and/or sensory dysfunction are common although both upper and lower limbs will obviously be affected in cervical cord lesions. An elderly patient might be somewhat vague about what appear on examination to be significant neurological signs. Descriptions such as 'my legs feel funny' or 'my legs won't do what they should' are relatively common (Sharr, 1985). Sensory symptoms may be even more difficult than motor symptoms to define precisely, although when the patient is aware of them the description is not infrequently one of sensory impairment ascending from the distal part of the lower limbs through the groins and then into the trunk. An elderly patient may be confused and state that the limbs are weak when in practice they are malfunctioning due to sensory ataxia arising out of impaired or absent joint position sense.

A tumour in the region of the lumbar vertebrae may give rise to a cauda equina syndrome. The patient will still describe the legs as being weak, though of course he will not be able to distinguish between lower and upper motor neurone symptoms. If, however, there is a clear description of sensory loss above the groin (i.e. above the L1 dermatome) then the lesion causing lower limb symptoms must be at the level of the cord rather than the cauda equina. It does not follow from this, however, that sensory symptoms confined to below the groin necessarily indicate cauda equina compression since an ascending sensory loss due to spinal cord compression may have been 'caught' early in its evolution. The slow and insidious decline that may occur as a result of a benign spinal tumour may make early diagnosis even more difficult and common misdiagnoses include subacute combined degeneration of the cord, peripheral neuropathy, and motor neurone disease. The radicular pain of a metastatic deposit or of a neurofibroma may sometimes be mistaken for cardiac or abdominal disease, especially in an elderly patient.

Sphincter dysfunction tends to be a late manifestation of spinal cord compression, although its presence usually heralds the beginning of decompensation of spinal cord function and represents a neurosurgical emergency. It may occur early when compression is in the region of the conus medullaris or cauda equina. Although the bladder is more usually affected than the bowel, the presence of sphincter dysfunction is much more important than the question of which sphincter is affected (Sharr, 1985) and in most cases, especially where the cause is extradural spinal cord compression, it usually gets inexorably worse. Its significance may not be appreciated and a diagnosis of 'prostatism' is often made in the male and gynaecological disorders invoked in the female. This underlines the importance of a neurological examination of the lower limbs in an elderly patient with sphincter dysfunction.

Signs

The signs of spinal cord dysfunction include increased tone, hyperreflexia, and a pyramidal distribution of weakness, these being the features of an upper motor neurone lesion. Whilst hypotonia and hyporeflexia may indicate a lower motor neurone lesion, due for example to a cauda equina disturbance, it should be remembered that in some patients with extradural spinal cord lesions, a rapid rate of compression, together with the accompanying vascular problems of ischaemia and venous obstruction that may lead to infarction, may produce a clinical picture akin to 'spinal shock'; hence the apparent lower motor neurone signs of flaccidity, hypotonia and areflexia. True spontaneous spinal vascular incidents are rare, but like their cerebral counterparts have an acute onset and there really should be no excuse for confusing a spinal cord tumour with a spinal cord stroke. Another feature of an extradural metastatic deposit is spinal tenderness due to the destructive effect of the tumour on the bone, in particular the vertebral body. Such tenderness is very rare in a benign spinal tumour and in the common degenerative bony disorders of the spine. Thoracic midline pain and tenderness must therefore never be attributed to degenerative spondylosis since even in the elderly thoracic spinal spondylosis is

rarely severe enough to cause spinal cord compression. Likewise, osteoporosis rarely produces such a degree of vertebral body collapse as to cause spinal cord compression. Exquisite spinal tenderness may be related to underlying bone infection and the extremely uncommon, but lethal in terms of morbidity, spinal extradural abscess.

The signs in a patient with a thoracic benign spinal tumour, more often a meningioma than a neurofibroma in the elderly, are usually those of a spastic paraparesis, a distinct sensory level being less common. If the patient reports a definite deterioration in lower limb function and there is little evidence of any pyramidal disturbance, careful search for posterior column dysfunction should be made. Whilst some impairment of vibration may occur with ageing, joint position function should be retained even into advanced age and any impairment should be assumed to be abnormal. Extensor plantar responses may be seen in the elderly due to cervical myelopathy associated with cervical spondylosis and by themselves are not necessarily of any significance. It has to be conceded that it may often be impossible to differentiate cervical spondylotic myelopathy from a myelopathy due to a benign cervical tumour on clinical grounds alone. Pain in the second and third cervical dermatomes can be common in cervical spondylosis but any other sensory symptoms, and certainly any sensory impairment, should arouse the suspicion of a tumour. Even so, high cervical or foramen magnum benign tumours may be very variable in their presentation and diagnosis extremely difficult. Cauda equina compression due to degenerative spondylotic narrowing, however, will not be confused with thoracic cord compression if the signs are carefully analysed.

In summary, degenerative disease of the cervical and lumbar spine is common in elderly people and may be difficult to differentiate from myelopathy or radiculopathy due to an underlying tumour. However, thoracic myelopathy is almost always due to a tumour and this fact alone should be sufficient to discourage a diagnosis of degenerative disease where the signs are compatible with a tumour. Any patient with midline thoracic pain should be assumed to have a tumour until otherwise proved. Similarly, a developing paraparesis, no matter how slowly progressive, should arouse suspicion of a spinal cord tumour, especially if accompanied by a thoracic sensory level.

Intramedullary tumours

These are very rare indeed in elderly patients, and there is no definite method of differentiating between them and benign extramedullary tumours. Contrary to popular belief, pain is not uncommon whereas early sphincter symptoms are rare (Sloof *et al.*, 1964). It is much less important to fail to differentiate between an intramedullary spinal tumour and a benign extramedullary tumour than to fail to diagnose a spinal tumour at all. Indeed, since treating an intramedullary spinal tumour in an elderly patient is unlikely to be worthwhile, failure to diagnose such a tumour is rarely of any great consequence. However, failure to diagnose a benign extramedullary tumour may be a neurological tragedy.

Investigation and Treatment (see also Chapter 17)

If it is decided that the patient's general medical condition or neurological state does not justify active treatment, then invasive investigations are obviously not warranted. However, it must be stressed that a very advanced neurological deficit due to a benign intradural extramedullary spinal tumour may reverse after surgery even in an elderly patient. For this reason, if there is any suspicion that such a lesion could be present full investigation is mandatory. Equally, of course, a patient with a spinal syndrome, but who also has evidence of a disseminated tumour, will be inappropriate for extensive investigation of this nature. Not all patients with extradural metastatic cord compression would benefit from active treatment. A significant number of patients may indeed be made worse by a conventional decompressive laminectomy (Findlay, 1984). It must not be forgotten, however, that a bony metastasis may be effectively controlled by chemotherapy (e.g. hormone therapy in breast or prostatic carcinoma) and for this reason dissemination of malignant disease is not necessarily a contraindication to further investigation. The history will often suggest the type of tumour: a short history accompanied by spinal or radicular pain is likely to be due to an extradural metastasis; whereas a long history unaccompanied by pain is quite likely to be due to a benign tumour.

Plain X-rays

In extradural metastatic disease it is common to see vertebral body collapse, and/or pedicular destruction. The latter must not be confused with an increase in the interpedicular distance due to a longstanding intramedullary lesion where the pedicles are narrowed but not actually destroyed. Vertebral collapse must be distinguished from the effects of infection where the disc space is altered by the collapsed vertebral body—in contrast to non-involvement in malignant infiltration. Soft tissue shadowing may be seen in malignant disease as well as chronic infection. It may also be rarely seen in Paget's disease, the latter being an important, albeit rare, cause of spinal compression in the elderly. Unless there is clear evidence of plain X-ray changes compatible with a metastatic deposit, it is unwise to assume the diagnosis unless a primary tumour is obviously present. Plain X-ray changes in conjunction with a benign tumour are uncommon, although sometimes an enlarged intervertebral foramen may be seen with a neurofibroma and rarely calcification with a meningioma.

Bone scanning

This is probably most useful where plain X-rays in a patient with suspected malignant disease show only one vertebra to be abnormal. The scan may then reveal multiple lesions. Gallium scanning may help to resolve the question of malignant disease versus infection. Multiple metastases may have a less serious prognosis in a patient with breast or prostatic carcinoma than one with bronchial carcinoma. For this reason, determining the nature of the primary tumour may be very useful in planning treatment.

Myelography

This should be restricted to those patients who are candidates for further treatment, either surgery or radiotherapy. Because the precise level of the myelo-graphic abnormality is crucial to the surgeon, it is almost mandatory for the procedure to be performed if surgery is anticipated. Myelography is usually carried out via the lumbar route, although occasionally the cervical route is used.

Lumbar puncture should not be carried out except as part of a myelographic procedure; otherwise it might make myelography difficult to perform. Moreover, it is associated with the risk of converting a partial lesion of the cord to a complete one.

The value of a myelogram is as follows:

1. It will identify the site of a compressive lesion.
2. It will often differentiate between an extradural and intradural tumour and may differentiate between an extramedullary and intramedullary intradural tumour.
3. It may demonstrate the position of a tumour in relation to the spinal cord, in particular whether the tumour is anterior or posterior to the theca. This is important because anteriorly placed lesions respond less favourably to conventional decompressive laminectomy than posteriorly placed ones. Indeed, the position of the tumour may act as a 'casting vote' either for or against surgical treatment. Similar considerations apply to a benign intradural spinal tumour, since anteriorly placed lesions in the mid-thoracic region (where the blood supply is at its most precarious) still carry a higher risk to cord function than lateral or posterior tumours.

Computed tomography

This may show abnormalities provided the correct level can be ascertained. While details of bony destruction may be obtained, maximum information may require injection of contrast media intrathecally as for conventional myelography. This investigation is still not universally available and its place in the management of the elderly patient with spinal cord compression remains uncertain at present.

Treatment

Surgery in the elderly patient is largely restricted to those in whom there is the possibility of a benign spinal tumour or an extradural metastasis which, for various reasons, may not be suitable for other forms of treatment.

Removal of a benign tumour involves laminectomy followed by opening the dura. This requires patience and a meticulous technique, preferably with the aid of an operating microscope. The tumour must be manoeuvred away from the spinal cord with no or minimal disturbance to the latter. The preservation of segmental vessels is crucial; they tend to be closely related to the nerve roots and any displacement of these roots must not cause damage to the vessels. Spinal cord retraction may be needed in order to remove anteriorly placed tumours; hence the higher risk of morbidity with such tumours as compared with those that are posterior to the cord. Inevitably the spinal cord will be less resilient in older patients and sometimes the surgeon, despite meticulous operative technique, has to face the disappointment of a patient who has been made worse by surgery. Contrariwise, recovery may sometimes exceed initial expectations and a chair- or even bed-bound old person eventually walks and regains independence and normal sphincter function.

The technical problems encountered in removing an intradural meningioma or a neurofibroma are very similar. Because, however, the neurofibroma may have an extradural component, and even an extraspinal component protruding through an enlarged intervertebral foramen (dumb-bell tumour), there may be additional technical problems. Thoracic neurofibromata may have a very large mediastinal component and be relatively asymptomatic until the intraspinal component causes cord compression. On the whole, the removal of the extraspinal component of a neurofibroma is rarely justified in an elderly patient since it may necessitate an additional operation or, in the case of cervical tumours, could cause serious haemorrhage from the vertebral artery. Moreover the slow growth of a residual extraspinal component means that the recurrence of neurological symptoms in an elderly patient's lifetime is relatively uncommon.

The management of extradural metastatic spinal cord compression is influenced by several considerations. There is now good evidence that the traditional laminectomy may well fail and is probably no better than radiotherapy (Findlay, 1984). If the tumour appears to be posterior to the theca then decompressive laminectomy may be successful, although complete tumour removal is the exception rather than the rule. Attempts to remove tumour lateral to, or in front of, the theca are undesirable since this would necessitate retraction on the theca of an already jeopardized cord. There are other technical problems relating to decompressive laminectomy, including those of stripping the muscles from tumour-infiltrated bone and heavy bleeding. Moreover, cardiovascular disturbances may result from an elderly patient being placed in the prone position and this may threaten an already malfunctioning spinal cord.

Because of the unsatisfactory results of conventional decompressive laminectomy, some surgeons have adopted an anterior approach to remove the diseased vertebral body, some form of fusion then being performed (Siegal and Siegal, 1985). This, however, is a major undertaking and requires a thoracotomy. This will be rarely justified in an elderly patient, especially where there is evidence of disseminated disease.

Chemotherapy may be as useful as radiotherapy both as a form of primary treatment and as an adjuvant if surgery, by whatever route, is carried out. Carcinoma of the breast and prostate, lymphomas and myeloma may all respond well both to radiotherapy and chemotherapy. The question sometimes arises as to whether or not such treatment should be instituted in the absence of definite histological confirmation of a tumour of a particular cell type. If, however, it is accepted that there is little evidence of a beneficial effect of laminectomy, then precise histological diagnosis is of academic interest only. Moreover, if the tumour is not radio- or chemosensitive, the prognosis will be poor anyway. If it is possible to obtain a histological diagnosis by closed biopsy (e.g. with a needle), this may be useful and a quick smear technique has been reported (Sandeman and Findlay, 1985). A small number of patients may require urgent decompression because the rate of deterioration allows insufficient time for response to radiotherapy. If surgery is to be worthwhile, the limbs should still have more than a flicker

of movement and sensation and sphincter function should be at least in part preserved.

Decisions in this area tend to be marginal and it could be argued that such patients would still be better treated with radiotherapy and/or chemotherapy. As always, each patient would have to be individually assessed. The final decision will be influenced by ethical and social considerations as well as purely medical ones.

PERIPHERAL TUMOURS

For practical purposes these encompass the so-called neurofibromas. (Other terms such as schwannomas, neurilemmomas, neurinomas, etc., whilst having pathological connotations, are not of real clinical importance.) Irrespective of whether the tumour arises in a single nerve or from a plexus, it will usually present as a mass in the appropriate area and may cause the expected neurological dysfunction. The main indications for removal are either pain or progressive neurological deficit. Compression of part of the brachial plexus may occur in the absence of a palpable mass and the dilemma arises as to whether exploration should be performed. This would depend on whether a deficit is present and how much incapacity is produced by it.

Patients with von Recklinghausen's disease may develop a plexiform neurofibroma and these may grow to quite a large size. They may occur in the eyelid as well as more typically in the limbs and visual impairment may result from the tumour hanging over the eye. Sometimes malignant change takes place. The development of a neurofibrosarcoma may be heralded by a rapid increase in size of the lesion and/or pain in what was previously a painless mass.

Treatment

If symptoms or progressive neurological damage warrant removal of the tumour, this should be performed microsurgically. Preservation of neural fascicles is very important in order to reduce the chances of neurological disability. Even so, damage may occur, possibly because of injury to small vessels.

Whenever a lesion arises on a cutaneous nerve, sacrifice of the latter may be justified since overlap will allow sensory impairment to be reduced to a minimum. Whilst surgery in an elderly patient is best avoided, a patient with a serious deficit, especially if there are other handicapping disorders such as arthritis, may require surgery.

ACKNOWLEDGEMENT

I am grateful to Mrs Jessie Kent for her invaluable secretarial help.

REFERENCES

Bartlett, J. (1971). Craniopharyngiomas. An analysis of some aspects of symptomatology, radiology and histology. *Brain*, **94**, 725–32.

Bartlett, J. (1985). Neurosurgical decisions in the elderly. In: Hildick-Smith, M. (ed.) *Neurological Problems in the Elderly*, Baillière Tindall, London, pp. 239–51.

Burrows, E.H. (1972). The clinical utility of brain scanning in nuclear medicine. In: Potchen, E.J., and McCready, V.R. (eds.) *Progress in Nuclear Medicine*, Karger, Basel, pp. 287–335.

Cairncross, J.G., Kim, J.H., and Posner, J.B. (1980). Radiation therapy for brain metastases. *Ann. Neurol.*, **7**, 529–41.

Cooney, L.M., and Solitare, G.B. (1972). Primary intracranial tumours in the elderly. *Geriatrics*, **27**, 94–104.

Cushing, H. (1932). *Intracranial Tumours*, Thomas, Springfield, Illinois.

Findlay, G.F. (1984). Adverse effects of management of malignant spinal cord compression. *J. Neurol. Neurosurg. Psychiatry*, **47**, 761–8.

Friedman, H., and Odom, G.L. (1972). Expanding intracranial lesions in geriatric patients. *Geriatrics*, **27**, 105–15.

Garfield, J.S., and Neil-Dwyer, G. (1975). Delay in diagnosis of optic nerve and chiasmal compression presenting with unilateral failing vision. *Br. Med. J.*, **1**, 22–5.

Godfrey, J.B., and Caird, F.I. (1984). Intracranial tumours in the elderly; diagnosis and treatment. *Age Ageing*, **13**, 152–8.

Goodbody, R.A., and Gamlen, T.R. (1974). Cerebellar haemangioblastoma and genito urinary tumours. *J. Neurol. Neurosurg. Psychiatry*, **37**, 606–9.

Graham, K., and Caird, F.I. (1978). High dose steroid therapy of intracranial tumour in the elderly. *Age Ageing*, **7**, 146–50.

Hakim, S., and Adams, R.D. (1965). The special clinical problems of symptomatic hydrocephalus with normal cerebrospinal fluid pressure. *J. Neurol. Sci.*, **2**, 307–27.

Hoessly, G.F., and Olivecrona, H. (1955). Report of 280 cases of verified parasagittal meningioma. *J. Neurosurg.*, **12**, 614–26.

Kernohan, J.W., and Woltman, H.W. (1929). Incisura of the crus due to contralateral brain tumour. *Arch. Neurol. Psychiatry*, **21**, 274–87.

Papo, I. (1983). Intracranial meningiomas in the elderly in the CT scan era. *Acta Neurochirurg.*, **67**, 195–204.

Pennybacker, J. (1968). The neurosurgery of old age. *Ceskoslov. Neurol.*, **31**, 73–9.

Raskind, R., Weiss, S.R., Manning, J.J., and Wermuth, R.E. (1971). Survival after surgical excision of a single metastatic brain tumour. *Am. J. Roentgenol. Rad. Ther. Nucl. Med.*, **111**, 323–8.

Reichenthal, E., and Shalit, M.N. (1978). Neurosurgical management of the elderly patient. *Surg. Neurol.*, **10**, 153–6.

Richardson, P., and Maurice-Williams, R. (1982). Auditing the process of referral of a common neurosurgical emergency. *J. Neurol. Neurosurg. Psychiatry*, **45**, 281.

Salcman, M. (1982). Brain tumours and the geriatric patient. *J. Am. Geriatr. Soc.*, **30**, 501–8.

Sandeman, D.R., and Findlay, G.F. (1985). Needle biopsy and quick smear reporting. Paper presented at National Instructional Course "The Spine". Royal Liverpool Hospital, 23–25 October 1985.

Sencer, W. (1964). Problems in diagnosis of intracranial disease among the aged. *Mount Sinai J. Med.*, **31**, 17–29.

Sharr, M.M. (1979). The surgical management of intracranial metastases. In: Whitehouse, J.M.A., and Kay, H.E.M. (eds.) *Central Nervous System Complications of Malignant Disease*, Macmillan, London, pp. 361–9.

Sharr, M.M. (1982). Surgical management of brain and spinal metastases. In Hildebrand, J., and Gangji, D. (eds.) *Treatment of Neoplastic Lesions of the Nervous System*, Pergamon, Oxford, pp. 117–24.

Sharr, M.M. (1983). Intracranial metastases management and the place of the CT scan in patients who are treated with surgery only. *J. Neuro-Oncol.*, **1**, 307–12.

Sharr, M.M. (1984). Mechanics of raised intracranial pressure. *Surgery*, **1**, 187–90.

Sharr, M.M. (1985). Diagnosis of spinal cord and cauda equina metastases. In: Rose, F.C., and Fields, W.S. (eds.) *Neuro-Oncology*, Karger, Basel, pp. 93–104.

Shaw, M.D.M., Rose, J.E., and Paterson, A. (1980). Metastatic extradural malignancy of the spine. *Acta Neurochirurg.*, **52**, 113–20.

Siegal, T., and Siegal, T. (1985). Treatment of malignant epidural and cauda equina compression. In: Rose, F.C., and Fields, W.S. (eds.) *Neuro-Oncology*, Karger, Basel, pp. 225–31.

Sloof, J.L., Kernohan, J.W., and MacCarthy, J.S. (1964). *Primary Intramedullary Tumours of the Spinal Cord and Filum Terminale*, Saunders, Philadelphia.

Stookey, B., and Ransohoff, J. (1959). *Trigeminal Neuralgia. Its History and Treatment*, Thomas, Springfield, Illinois.

Twomey, C. (1978). Brain tumours in the elderly. *Age Ageing*, **7,** 138–45.

Wood, M.W., White, R.J., and Kernohan, J.W. (1957). One hundred intracranial meningiomas found incidentally at necropsy. *J. Neuropathol. Exp. Neurol.*, **16,** 337–40.

The Clinical Neurology of Old Age
Edited by R. Tallis
© 1989 John Wiley & Sons Ltd

Chapter 17

Spinal Cord and Spinal Root Disease, Secondary to Diseases of the Spine

Pauline Monro

Consultant Neurologist, Atkinson Morley's Hospital, London, UK

David Uttley

Consultant Neurosurgeon, Atkinson Morley's Hospital, London, UK

INTRODUCTION

'My walking is not as good as it was', 'I'm falling over more often', 'I can't control my water' or 'I'm losing the use of my hands'.

These are common complaints from elderly patients. They may result from the cumulative effect of a number of minor impairments occurring in an ageing body, but disorders of spinal cord or nerve roots secondary to disease of the spine column also commonly play a part. Assessment of the relative importance of this latter contribution is an essential first step in deciding how best to help the patient and this is not always easy.

In assessing such patients it is important to remember the following points.

1. Patients in the geriatric age group are susceptible to a similar range of pathologies as those below the age of 65. Although degenerative disease of the spine can be shown on X-ray in the vast majority of elderly patients this does not necessarily mean that it is the cause of their symptoms, even if these can be shown to be due to neurological dysfunction (Figures 17.1a and 17.1b).
2. There are many causes of loss of dexterity and disordered gait in the elderly. Arthritis in hips,

knees and hands causes not only loss of mobility and 'stiffness', but also associated muscle wasting. Cerebral ischaemia may contribute to spasticity and weakness, Parkinson's disease to a slow shuffling gait and vestibular dysfunction, postural hypotension or brain stem ischaemia to unsteadiness of gait.

Important factors to be borne in mind in deciding when to investigate and how to manage a geriatric patient in whom it is thought that spinal column disease is contributing to neurological dysfunction are:

1. Elderly patients who have learnt to adapt to inefficiencies in bodily function which have developed gradually over the years may not tolerate interference well, whether this be with drugs (e.g. aimed to relieve spasticity), with mechanical aids, such as corset or collar, or with surgical treatment. However, in recent years technological advances, improved surgical techniques and increasing sophistication in anaesthesia have decreased the risks of surgery. If the patient's general health is good, age alone is no bar to surgery, though surgery should be considered *only* when there is good evidence to suggest that it will

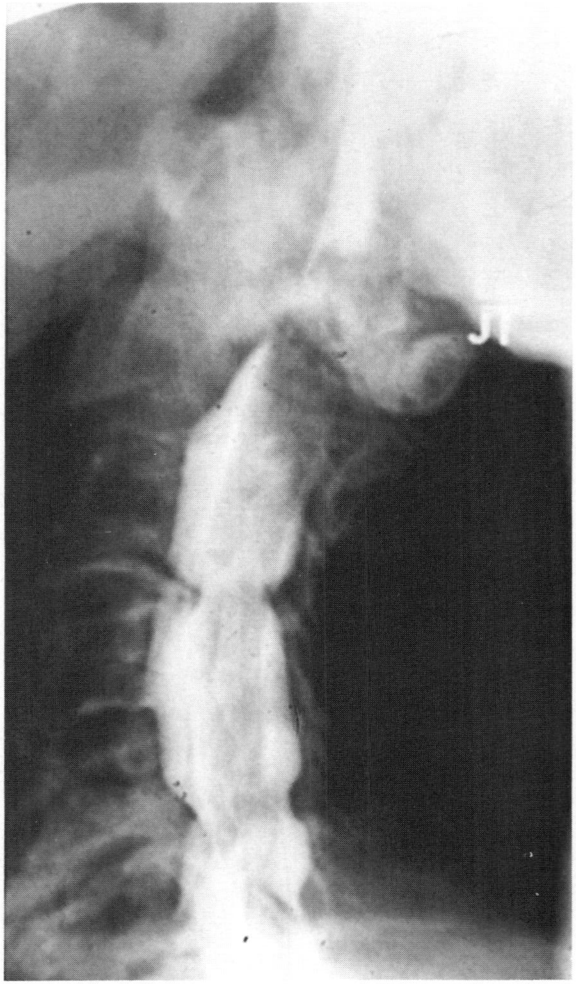

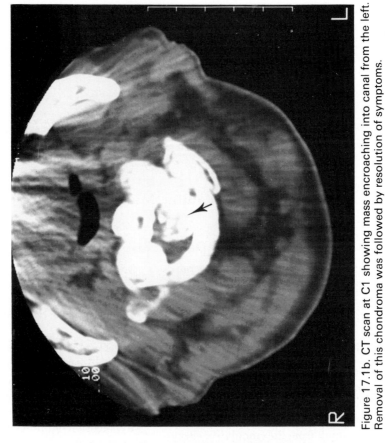

Figure 17.1b. CT scan at C1 showing mass encroaching into canal from the left. Removal of this chondroma was followed by resolution of symptoms.

Figure 17.1a. Myelogram of 82 year old woman with 5 year history of disability due to upper motor neurone disorder and posterior column loss in arms and legs. Temporary improvement for 2 years followed immobilization of the neck in a collar. Distortion of subarachnoid space anteriorly and posteriorly at C3/4 and C5/6 due to spondylotic changes. Failure of contrast flow posteriorly at C1.

be helpful in either halting the progression of the patient's symptoms or allowing improvement.

2. No patient should be subjected to any invasive, uncomfortable or expensive investigation such as myelography, computed tomographic (CT) scanning or magnetic resonance imaging (MRI) unless the decision has first been made that the results will influence the management; this usually implies that the patient would tolerate an operation should a surgically remediable lesion be found.

PATHOLOGY

Dysfunction of the spinal cord and nerve roots may occur when any disorder of the spinal column causes mechanical distortion or compression of the enclosed delicate neural tissues or their blood supply. Cord and nerve roots can adapt to slow progressive distortion. Symptoms arise either when compression with associated ischaemia occurs, or when there is repeated trauma due to intermittent distortion produced by movement. The clinical features at presentation depend on the site of the distorted tissue and the speed with which distortion develops rather than the pathology. Involvement of peripheral nerve tissue by direct spread from the spine either of infection or neoplasia occurs infrequently because of the protection afforded by the ensheathing dura mater.

ANATOMY

In order to understand the pathology, clinical features and principles of management of cord and root disorders due to spinal disease, it is essential to have a clear idea of the normal relationship of the neural tissue to the vertebrae and of the effects ageing has on these.

Spinal Cord

The cord lies within the spinal canal and follows its contours from the foramen magnum to the lower border of the second lumbar vertebra (Figure 17.2). The cord is surrounded and cushioned by cerebrospinal fluid within the subarachnoid space which is

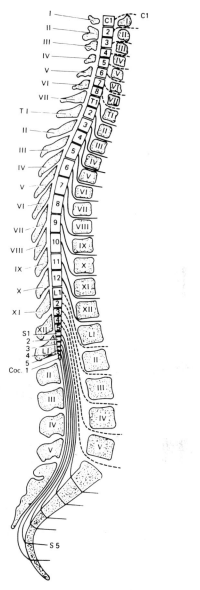

Figure 17.2. Diagram of lateral view of vertebral column illustrating the relationship of spinal cord segments and nerve roots to vertebrae. The cord ends at L2. Note increasing obliquity of descent of nerve roots to reach exit at segmental level from cervical to sacral region. (From *The Neuroanatomic Basis for Clinical Neurology* by T.L. Peele. *Reproduced by permission of McGraw Hill Inc.*)

most capacious in the lower cervical region and narrowest in the thoracic canal. The cord thus lies freely within, but totally enclosed by, the unyielding walls of the canal formed by the vertebrae, the firm ligaments covering the intervertebral joints anteriorly, the apophyseal joints laterally and the lamina joints posteriorly. The movement which occurs at these joints is least in the thoracic region and greatest in the lower cervical and lumbar spine, where lordosis is most marked and through which the line of the centre of gravity and therefore of weight transmission passes (Figure 17.3). It is as a result of this that with advancing years these two sites are most commonly and most severely affected by degenerative disease.

Roots

Nerve roots pass laterally from the spinal cord in the upper cervical segment to pass under their segmental pedicles and into the intervertebral foramina bounded laterally by the apophyseal joints, medially by the intervertebral disc and the opposing lateral borders of the vertebral bodies, and superiorly and inferiorly by the pedicles (Figure 17.4). The emergent roots slope progressively more obliquely and caudally to reach their segmental foramina until, below the conus at the second lumbar vertebra, the lower sacral roots pass almost vertically downwards (see Figures 17.2 and 17.6).

Anatomical factors of importance in determining the pathology and therefore the clinical presentation are described below.

The Separation of Motor and Sensory Nerve Roots at the Exit Foramina

At the entrance of the intervertebral foramen the sensory dorsal root ganglia lie superiorly and may therefore be affected by degenerative changes or other disease occurring in the adjacent apophyseal joints or in the uncinate region of the intervertebral disc (Figure 17.4). The motor root, bounded by its own dural sheath, lies more inferiorly in the exit foramen and may be either spared or differentially affected. Patients may therefore present with radicular sensory or motor symptoms independently. Since

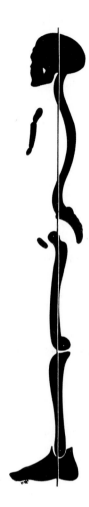

Figure 17.3. Outline of lateral view of skeleton showing line of centre of gravity passing through vertebral column at sites of greatest curvature—lower cervical and lower lumbar regions. These are also sites of greatest mobility and commonest sites of degenerative joint changes. (From *Clinical Neuroanatomy for Medical Students* (1981) by Richard S. Snell. *Reproduced by permission of Little, Brown and Company, Boston.*)

pain may occur as a result of motor root involvement alone (Frykholm, 1951), radicular pain and profound motor loss are not necessarily accompanied by any demonstrable sensory deficit.

Descending Path of Nerve Roots from Cord to Exit Foramina

The obliquity of descent of the nerve roots in the lower cervical region and below is such that disorder at the level of one exit foramen may involve not only that nerve root but also the next adjacent nerve root as it descends (Figure 17.5). A complete obstructing lesion at L3 may catch all the descending nerve roots of the cauda equina, whereas a central lesion, such as a prolapsed intervertebral disc, may catch the lower sacral roots only, producing loss of sacral sensation and sphincter control with no motor or sensory deficit distally in the limb as the laterally situated L3 to S1 roots may be untouched (Figure 17.6).

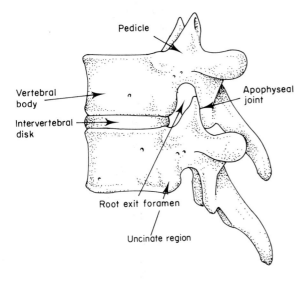

Figure 17.4. Diagram of boundaries of nerve root exit canal.

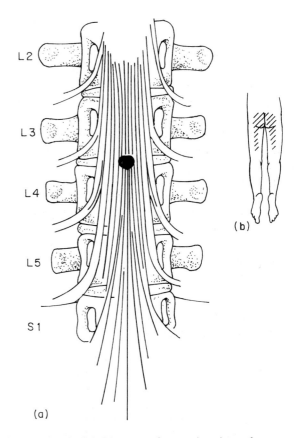

(b)

(a)

Figure 17.6. (a) Diagram of posterior view of conus and cauda equina. A central disc protrusion at L3/4 can impinge on descending sacral roots while more laterally placed lumbar roots may be untouched. (b) Diagram of resultant sacral sensory loss.

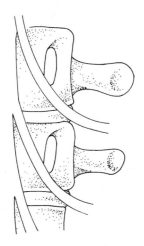

Figure 17.5. Diagram of nerve root descending from cord to exit canal illustrating how a nerve root may be affected by degenerative changes at two intervertebral levels.

Blood Supply

Radicular arteries of varying size and importance in the maintenance of the integrity of the spinal cord also enter through the intervertebral foramen to anastomose with the anterior and posterior spinal arteries. Although the role of these arteries in contributing to pathology in spondylotic disease is not established, involvement with granulation tissue as in tuberculosis, or occlusion following severe subluxation in the cervical region in rheumatoid arthritis, may produce ischaemic changes in the cord.

In cervical rheumatoid disease this is thought to account for the cord atrophy which is sometimes seen below the site of subluxation (Hughes, 1977). Involvement of a radicular artery due to a lumbar disc protrusion may account for the occasional finding of associated cord sensory loss.

Enclosure and Movement

Since the cord and nerve roots lie within unyielding canals, they are susceptible not only to distortion but also to compression by any mass lesion within the canal, whether this be bony or ligamentous hypertrophy, infection or neoplasia. The movement of neural tissue and its blood supply which occurs relative to the vertebral column exacerbates the effect of any distortion. Changes in shape and contour of the canal with movement are most marked in the neck on flexion and extension. The cord normally accommodates by moving upwards (rostrally) and posteriorly on neck flexion, and downwards (caudally) and anteriorly on extension (Reid, 1960; Breig *et al.*, 1966; Adams and Logue, 1971b). Movement of the cord is cushioned by the surrounding cerebrospinal fluid and meninges and limited by the anteriorly emerging spinal nerve roots and, possibly by the dentate ligaments laterally (Kahn, 1947; Stoltman and Blackwood, 1966), so that although the cord does not impinge on the smooth contours of the normal canal, it may be repeatedly deformed by any distorting mass lesion. Alteration of the normal alignment, movement and contours of the canal with secondary root and cord disturbance may thus result from any disease,

whether this be trauma, infection or neoplasia causing collapse of the vertebrae, from any disorder of the apophyseal or intervertebral joints, or from rupture or laxity of the intervertebral ligaments with subsequent prolapse of disc material or subluxation of the vertebrae.

Since movement is greatest in the cervical spine, symptomatic myelopathy may arise here in the absence of compression, whereas in the relatively immobile thoracic spine the onset of symptoms from a slowly progressive lesion usually heralds compression.

SYMPTOMS AND SIGNS

Whether spinal cord compression or root damage develops from disease in the vertebral bodies, disc prolapse or degenerative conditions, its impact on the neural elements is usually stereotyped. There is a loss of function distal to the level of the injury, but the rate of evolution may vary enormously from hours to years. Recognition of impending problems at an early stage is essential to forestall irreversible damage. This is the role of the physician—to identify which patients with cord or root dysfunction require investigation and referral to a neurosurgeon for definitive treatment, and which should be treated symptomatically.

Although the functional neuroanatomy of the spinal cord and roots is generally well understood, the presenting symptoms may be less well apprehended and cause delay in referral.

Pain

The conditions dealt with in this chapter frequently have their real nature obscured by the depressing and seemingly ubiquitous symptom of neck or back pain as a presenting feature. In the UK 2% of the population each year consult a doctor with low back pain, usually arising out of structures external to the neural tissues. A lifetime of intermittent episodes of neck or low back pain may herald major degenerative problems. Back pain appearing for the first time in the elderly should always be considered seriously, especially outside the lumbar region, as it may indicate malignant deposits. Disease of the vertebral bodies is accompanied by a progressively severe deep-seated aching pain, localized to the segments involved and responding badly to analgesics. Frequently worse at night, it disturbs sleep and causes the victim to sit upright or pace about. Sudden intense pain at the thoracolumbar junction should raise the spectre of an extradural abscess.

With root pain the patient complains of severe sharp lancinating pains, along the distribution of the root. The pain is often compared to 'electric shocks', 'knives' or 'burning', raised to new heights of torture with any manoeuvre such as coughing, straining and movement, which momentarily increases intrathecal pressure. Such pains are usually found in compression of the intervertebral foramen by prolapsed disc, malignant involvement of the neural arch and neurofibromas. The intensity of the pain leads the patient to shun movement. When radiating along a limb, the pain is not hard to identify, but confusion may arise with girdle pain around the trunk which may be mistaken for pleurisy, cardiac or renal pain.

Slow compression of the sensory pathways in the spinal cord may produce dysaesthesiae below the level of the lesion often described as burning, tingling or painful numbness. This is best exemplified in the fingers of patients suffering from chronic cervical spondylotic myelopathy whose manual dexterity is also severely constrained by symptoms of posterior column deficit to the point where simple daily tasks such as fastening buttons become impossible.

Vertebral Column

Inspection of the spine may reveal scoliosis due to unilateral muscle spasm or an unnatural rigidity and loss of movement due to bilateral protective spasm of the paraspinal muscles. The presence of angulation when the spine is viewed in profile indicates a kyphos due to collapse of the relevant vertebral body. Pressure or percussion over the spinous processes may elicit pain due to underlying vertebral disease before deformity develops.

Motor

Description of the earliest motor and sensory manifestations may be misleading due to vernacular and local usage. For instance, 'deadness' can be used to indicate either weakness or sensory loss. The greatest care is therefore necessary in interpretation. Power can be gauged objectively by means of the Medical Research Council (MRC) grading, and this should be used during every examination to stand as a baseline for subsequent reference. It is quicker and more accurate to use this system than to employ descriptive terms.

Compression of the spinal cord produces two sets of motor signs. Firstly there is local damage to the anterior horn cells and ventral roots at the level of the compression leading to segmental lower motor neurone signs of wasting, weakness, loss of tone, fasciculation and reduced or absent reflexes. These changes are best seen in the arms and legs, but may be elusive in thoracic lesions and in the obese. Signs of this type can be expressed in root values which will pinpoint the actual level of the lesion. The second set of signs originate from disturbance of the pyramidal tracts so that below the level of compression there are the upper motor neurone signs of weakness again, but this time in a generalized manner, with an associated increase in tone leading to spasticity, pathologically exaggerated reflexes and extensor plantar responses.

The first symptoms of a pyramidal lesion may be a heaviness in the anterior compartment of the thighs, followed by increasing clumsiness, a shorter step, slowing of gait, an inability to hurry, and dragging of the feet leading to falls. Flexor spasms, when present, are a useful indication that the upper motor neurone disorder is due to a lesion within the cord.

It is not unknown for patients to deteriorate in hospital. Serial assessments of power are required to avoid delays in management.

Sensory Symptoms

The complexity and subtlety of sensory change can often exhaust the patient's descriptive powers and lead the examiner into a mire of misunderstanding. All sensory modalities are usually affected in cord lesion, but the degree of involvement may vary considerably.

Lesions of the spinothalamic tract cause an impaired appreciation of pain and temperature on the opposite side of the body, one or two segments below the level of the pathology. This is due to the spread of incoming impulses over several segments in the dorsal horns before crossing the cord to join the contralateral tract. Spinothalamic lesions often result in 'sacral sparing' leaving this area less affected than the trunk or legs. The converse, 'saddle anaesthesiae', occurs when the sacral nerve roots are damaged (Figure 17.6b).

The dorsal columns are the other afferent systems of major clinical significance. These subserve ipsilateral appreciation of light touch, joint position sense and the sense of passive movement crucial to the maintenance of posture and ability to carry out fine hand movements. Defects are described as though the patient were 'walking on cotton wool' or 'sponges', and a sensation of wearing tight garments. The gait becomes clumsy, particularly in the dark. The loss is often asymmetrical and greater on the side of the weaker limb. In most cases of cord compression, sensory changes develop after the onset of motor loss, though with some slowly evolving benign intradural tumours, subtle sensory symptoms may antedate more readily comprehended weakness.

Reflexes

An accurate assessment of the deep tendon reflexes may be invaluable in determining the type and level of spinal lesions. Root damage results in diminished or absent reflexes. Compression of the pyramidal tract in cord lesions will lead to pathologically exaggerated responses which are associated with an increase in tone. Although reflex abnormalities are most valuable in cervical or lumbar lesions, the loss of the segmental abdominal reflexes, provided the abdomen is not too lax, or of the cremasteric reflexes will be evident in upper motor neurone lesions above their level of innervation. Lesions at any point in the cord will result in extensor plantar responses, even in the conus where the deep tendon reflexes are absent.

Sphincters

The neural control of the sphincteric mechanisms is usually affected late in the sequence of cord compression, but the interval between the initial symptoms and complete disruption of sphincter control may be very short, so no time should be lost in referral once

these have been noted. Retention of urine is the end result of cord or root damage, but prior to this there may be complaints of urgency, frequency or hesitancy of micturition with no dysuria. When cord lesions produce these symptoms, since the mechanism of voiding remains intact there is no disturbance of flow or after dribbling unless prostatic obstruction is also present. In defects of the anal sphincter, involuntary soiling against a background of constipation is the common mode of presentation. Non-neurogenic constipation should always be excluded as a contributory cause of urinary retention.

Autonomic

Symptoms of this type are uncommon, but may take the form of abnormal perspiration in dependent regions, or postural hypotension.

Sexual

Perineal sensory loss interferes with sexual function in both sexes. Impotence is the commonest symptom in the male. Reflex erections can occur in cord lesions though the ability to ejaculate is lost. Seminal incontinence without erection may occur in cauda equina lesions.

Mode of Onset

This varies enormously, and the rate at which disability progresses is unpredictable. At one extreme lesions may take years to evolve or may stabilize as in spondylosis, while at the other acute lesions may be complete in hours. In untreated cases of *progressive* cord compression there comes a point where the rate of deterioration increases alarmingly: in pathological terms mechanical compression has reached a degree which causes vascular occlusion. At this critical juncture there is irreversible infarction of the spinal cord with complete loss of all dependent function. Surgery has nothing to offer in this situation. It is imperative to refer for urgent treatment as events gather momentum if any neurological function is to be preserved.

INVESTIGATIONS

Very often accurate diagnosis of cord or root problems can be achieved only by radiological means. Other laboratory facilities such as haematology, bacteriology, biochemistry and serology may play a role in confirming a diagnosis or reflect the patient's general condition and fitness for intervention.

Lumbar Puncture

While this may be valuable in the laboratory investigation of the CSF, it should be avoided in the preliminary investigation of cord compression. The reasons for this are twofold. Firstly, CSF will continue to escape from the subarachnoid space for several days after puncture, creating pools of CSF in the subdural and extradural spaces; this encourages the radiologist at subsequent myelography to believe erroneously that the subarachnoid space has been entered, and to inject the contrast medium into a false space, thus spoiling the investigation. This can be partially mitigated by performing the test under screen control or by introducing the contrast

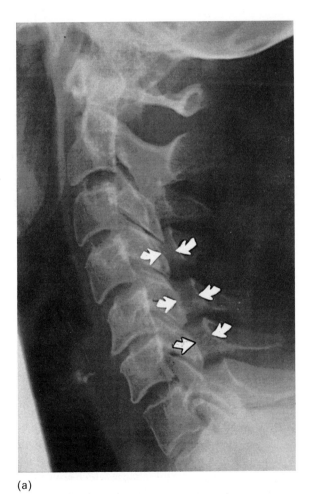

(a)

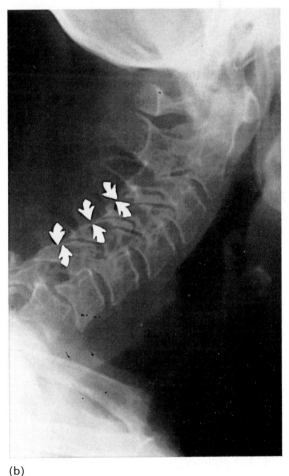

(b)

Figure 17.7. X-ray of cervical spine—lateral views. Arrows indicate posterior surfaces of lateral masses and base of spine. (a) Normal canal. (b) Congenitally narrow canal.

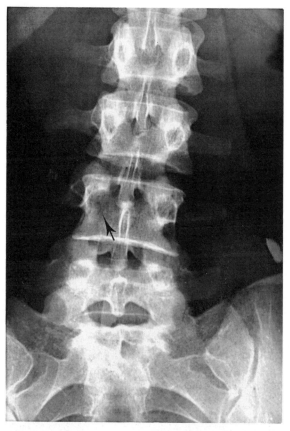

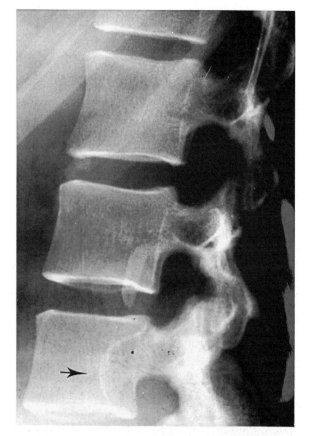

Figure 17.8. X-ray of lumbosacral spine, AP view. Note crescentic shape of right pedicle at L4 with increased interpedicular distance indicative of intradural tumour at this level.

Figure 17.9. X-ray of lumbosacral spine, lateral view. Note scalloping of posterior margin of L4 indicative of intradural tumour at this level.

medium by the more hazardous cervical route. Secondly, the aspiration of CSF together with further leakage may alter the hydrodynamic system within the theca, causing minor displacements of the lesion and a calamitous deterioration in neurological status.

Less common hazards exist with pathology in the lumbar region, namely that the needle may directly enter the lesion and no CSF can be withdrawn, or, in cases of extradural abscess, contamination of the CSF may occur.

CSF can be withdrawn appropriately by the radiologist at myelography. For other than routine studies, arrangements should be made at this time (virology, cytology, serology, immunology) to preclude the necessity for a further lumbar puncture. The technique and hazards of lumbar puncture are described comprehensively by Simpson (1984).

Radio-isotope Studies

Radio-isotope studies may be of considerable value in detecting metastatic vertebral disease before plain X-ray changes are visible. They may indicate also areas of acute degenerative change which have to be distinguished from more sinister pathology. The appearances may help to dictate the most appropriate line of management.

Plain Radiography

Plain X-rays of the spine can be of great value in both the localization and identification of spinal pathology. These changes, however, may take several weeks to appear, and there is thus no likelihood that bone changes will be visible in cases where the interval from the initial pathology to investigation is only a matter of days, such as may occur with an extradural abscess.

Measurement of spinal canal dimensions will reveal canal stenosis. A good indication that the cervical spinal canal is congenitally narrow is given by the distance between the posterior surface of the lateral mass and the base of the spinous process which is reduced to only a millimetre or so (Figure 17.7). The first sign of metastatic disease in the anteroposterior (AP) view is a missing pedicle. The transformation of the pedicles from oval to crescentic structures with an increase in the interpedicular distance is typical of intradural tumour (Figure 17.8).

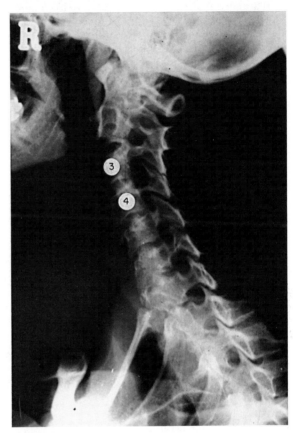

Figure 17.11. X-ray of cervical spine, oblique view to show exit foramina. Enlargement of C3/4 with narrowing of pedicle at C4 due to neurofibroma.

Lateral views may show scalloping of the posterior margins of the vertebral bodies (intramedullary tumour Figure 17.9), collapse of a vertebral body (metastatic disease Figure 17.10), narrowing of a disc space and changes in adjacent bone surfaces (tuberculous disease). Views in an oblique plane may show an enlarged intervertebral foramen indicating the presence of a neurofibroma (Figure 17.11), or an irregular narrowed one typical of degeneration (Figure 17.12). An increase in the

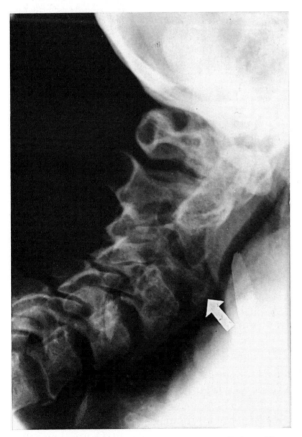

Figure 17.10. X-ray of cervical spine, lateral view. Note collapse of vertebral body at C3 due to metastatic disease.

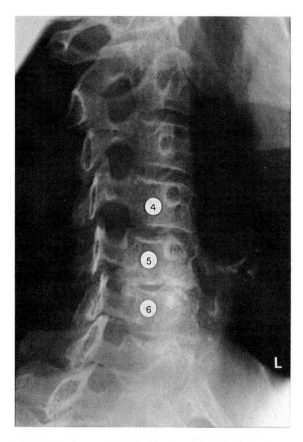

Figure 17.12. X-ray of cervical spine. Oblique view to show exit foramina. Osteophytic encroachment on exit foramen at C5/6 from degenerative disease at intervertebral joint.

paravertebral soft tissue shadows suggests a collection of neoplastic or inflammatory material. Alterations in bone density and texture may be diagnostic. Calcification is occasionally seen in intradural meningiomas, often in thoracic discs.

Myelography

Despite modern developments, this investigation remains the most useful diagnostic tool in the study of spinal compressive conditions, and the examination is usually definitive.

Water-soluble compounds have supplanted the older oil-based contrast media. They give excellent resolution, particularly of nerve root sleeves, and

disappear from the CSF pathways within 24 hours. Adverse reactions are very uncommon, and they do not produce long-term complications such as arachnoiditis.

The contrast medium is injected into the lumbar subarachnoid space and the patient is screened on a tilting table so that the whole extent of the spinal sac can be seen up to the craniovertebral junction. Films taken in the AP and lateral projections will demonstrate the level of the lesion(s), and whether it is extradural or intradural, and, in the latter, whether or not it is intramedullary. In complete obstruction the contrast outlines the lower margin of the lesion. The clinical findings suggest its upper limit, though with an extensive lesion this level can be located more precisely by introducing contrast medium from above via a lateral cervical puncture.

To ensure that the maximal amount of surgical anatomy is displayed, close cooperation between the radiologist and the surgeon is essential; thus the examination is best undertaken in a neurosurgical centre where surgery can quickly follow in case of deterioration. The level of the lesion should be marked on the patient's back, avoiding distortion, as a guide to the surgeon. The films taken during this investigation should have readily identifiable bony landmarks visible to enable subsequent examiners to count both up and down the spine to the appropriate level.

CT Scanning

Increasing sophistication in the latest generation of CT scanners has opened up new approaches to the diagnosis of spinal problems. Because of its frequency the problems of lumbar degenerative disease have attracted most attention, though the rest of the spine is also under scrutiny. The non-invasive nature of the examination has much appeal. Essential prerequisites are a high resolution scanner (HRCT) equipped with a digital scout radiology system for slice selection. The value of the images depends upon careful conduct of the examination. Attention to details such as positioning and reassuring the patient are important to avoid movement. Continuous 5 mm slices of the affected region are obtained for examination and to do this without waste requires close collaboration between radiologist and clinician. The time taken to set up the examination, perform it and reformat the images takes approximately 45 minutes for a three segment scan.

The images generated can provide unparalleled information on the structure of vertebral bodies, discs, nerve root canals, nerve roots, ligaments and the spinal canal itself, together with its contents, and offer a unique opportunity to differentiate between the elements causing the 'failed back surgery syndrome' (Heithoff, 1983). Pitfalls, largely methodological, are encountered (Braun *et al.*, 1984) and can be readily overcome.

The same techniques are being applied to the cervical region for both brachalgia and spondylosis and the results compare favourably with myelographic examination (Daniels *et al.*, 1984). Postmyelographic examination of patients with spinal tumours enables the relationship of the lesion to the cord to be delineated accurately, thus guiding the surgical approach.

Magnetic Resonance Imaging (MRI)

This revolutionary new imaging method can produce anatomical and biochemical information of high quality without ionizing irradiation or invasive procedures. Thus it can be employed on an outpatient basis. Using the appropriate imaging parameters derived from plots of signal intensity versus time, it is possible to produce both sagittal and axial images of high definition. In the latter dimension HRCT images are superior, particularly in the study of the lateral recesses and foramina. In the sagittal plane, however, the MRI images are superior to CT reformats. By varying the time scale of MRI it is possible to study the spinal components individually, thus helping to differentiate the contributory elements of the degenerative processes (Modic *et al.*, 1984).

With advancing technology, improvements in section thickness, spatial resolution, examination time and a better signal-to-noise ratio will enhance image quality. The major clinical drawback lies in the examination of the scoliotic patient where spinal curvature interferes with the production of adequate sagittal images. Despite these limitations MRI will have an increasingly important role to play in the diagnosis of pathology in the spinal column, where it already competes on advantageous terms with HRCT and myelography.

Despite the obvious advantages of the new technology of HRCT and MRI, the expense of these machines and the high running costs mean that they will remain very much the exclusive tool of specialized centres, so that only a handful of the growing elderly population will actually benefit from the ease, convenience and excellence of these methods in the near future.

Electromyographic (EMG) Studies

Studies of nerve conduction often help the interpretation of lower motor neurone lesions. The site of the lesion (e.g. anterior horn, root, plexus or nerve) can be determined. This may indicate the duration of the disease process. Serial examinations may quantify its progress for good or ill. In certain cases the changes are sufficiently distinctive to be diagnostic, e.g. peripheral neuropathy, motor neurone disease. The efficacy of medication or surgery can be monitored by outpatient study at intervals.

CERVICAL SPONDYLOSIS

Pathology

Spinal column

As a result of a lifetime of continual movement of the vertebral column, together with inevitable minor traumas following falls and jolts, degenerative disc disease will develop in both the lumbar and cervical spine in the majority of elderly patients. Pallis *et al.* (1954) showed radiological evidence of cervical spondylosis in 75% of patients over the age of 50, and Holt and Yates (1966) found post-mortem changes in 110 of 120 elderly patients. The intervertebral disc is a hydrostatic load bearing device with two main components: a peripheral fibrous layered structure known as the annulus fibrosus with 80% water content, surrounding and containing the inner semifluid nucleus pulposus which consists of 85–90% water. The reduction of fluid content of these two components to 70% which occurs with age (Lipson and Muir, 1981), results in almost universal loss of disc height throughout the spine. This is frequently associated with herniation of disc material either through the ligaments or into the vertebral bodies, particularly in the lower cervical spine where movement is greatest, and in the lower lumbar spine which bears most weight. The resultant loss of disc volume allows circumferential bulging of the annulus which is then followed by outgrowth of bone at the disc margins. The osteophytic ridges so formed distort the spinal canal anteriorly and laterally protrude into the root exit canals (Figure 17.12). All these degenerative changes which are exacerbated by movement are maximal in the lower cervical and lumbar regions, but also develop, as a result of the stresses thrown on intervertebral joints, above and below fused vertebrae, whether the fusion be congenital, degenerative or secondary to surgery. Compensatory subluxation at such sites may then occur. Loss of disc height and disordered movements between the bodies of vertebrae must inevitably be accompanied by abnormal stresses on the apophyseal joints. The ligamentous and bony hypertrophy which accompanies degeneration of these joints encroaches on the spinal canal laterally and on the nerve root exit canal which the joints bound (see Figure 17.4).

Posteriorly the spinal canal may be narrowed by the ligamentum flavum which may lose its elasticity, becoming markedly hypertrophied and buckled as a result of increased intervertebral movement. Indentation and corrugation of the canal, particularly on neck extension, may be seen (see Figure 17.13). This effect may be exaggerated by 'shingling' or overlap of the laminae on neck extension.

Spinal cord

Pallis showed that three-quarters of patients over the age of 65 with radiological evidence of cervical spondylosis had some signs of a cord disorder, a figure which increases with advancing years. Symptomatic myelopathy, even in the presence of the marked spondylotic distortion of the canal so often seen in the elderly, is less common. The factors which have been shown to determine the development of

clinically significant myelopathy are described below.

1. The degree of narrowing of the spinal canal and deformity of the cord. In most people the cervical canal is so capacious in relation to the size of the cord that even marked encroachment by bone or soft tissue distorts only the subarachnoid space, leaving the cord untouched. The development of cord dysfunction has been shown to be correlated with the acquired width of the canal (Nurick, 1972a). It is likely to occur if the width is less than 15 mm and is almost inevitable if the width is less than 13 mm (the usual cord diameter is approximately 11 mm). Using CT scanning with myelography to outline the contour of the canal Yu *et al.* (1986) concluded that the severity of the clinical features of the myelopathy could be correlated with the degree of deformation of the cord. However, canal width and cord deformity are clearly not the only factor since in disabled patients severe narrowing is not always found, and surgical relief of compression is not always followed by improvement of symptoms. The degree of narrowing and distortion appears to be related to the development of cord symptoms but not to progression of the disease (Nurick, 1972b).

2. The degree of mobility. A close correlation has been shown between the degree of mobility of the cervical spine and the progression of clinical deterioration, both before (Barnes and Saunders, 1984) and after surgery (Adams and Logue, 1971b). It appears therefore that a cord subject to static distortion may continue to function at a reduced capacity, whereas if the cord and its vessels are subject to intermittent distortion and compression further deterioration in function is likely to occur. A canal which may show only minimal distortion in the neutral position may, on movement, show marked distortion of contour and narrowing, either due to buckling of the ligamentum flavum (Figure 17.13) or movement of vertebrae (Figure 17.14 a, b and c).

3. Trauma. Sudden trauma, either relatively minor from a jolt or more severe from a fall, may either precipitate or exacerbate pre-existing cord dysfunc-

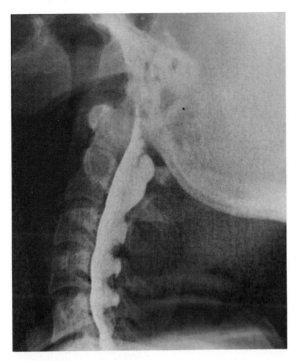

Figure 17.13. Myelogram of cervical spine in extension. Lateral view showing posterior indentation of subarachnoid space due to hypertrophy of ligamentum flavum at level of intervertebral movement.

tion. Although this may be due to vertebral subluxation or, even in the elderly, to prolapse of an intervertebral disc (Young *et al.*, 1986), in some cases spontaneous recovery may occur without surgical intervention, and it seems likely that the symptoms have arisen from contusion produced by rapid movement of the narrowly confined, possibly ischaemic cord over the distorting surfaces.

4. Atherosclerosis. Although Nurick (1972a) showed that progression in cervical spondylotic myelopathy is more likely to occur with advancing years, he showed that there was no association with evidence of atherosclerosis elsewhere and it is unlikely that atherosclerotic ischaemia plays any major part in myelopathy. The rarity of anterior spinal artery thrombosis in cervical spondylosis (Hughes and Brownell, 1964) supports this suggestion. Although the pathological changes seen in the spinal cord resemble those seen in ischaemia (Mair and Druckman, 1953), they are in the boundary zones between the major arteries of supply, i.e. the anterior and posterior spinal arteries (Hawkins *et al.*, 1975), and are more likely to result from distortion and attenuation of small vessels occurring with movement and compression of the cord rather than from major vessel disease.

5. Venous stasis. It has been suggested that venous stasis may contribute to the development of myelopathy in cervical spondylosis since venous distension is often noted at operations. However, there is no pathological support for this; it is possible that the appearances are an artefact of the conditions of surgery.

Nerve roots

The emergent nerve roots occupy less than a quarter of the intervertebral foramina, but either the sensory or motor components may be distorted, compressed or trapped by osteophytic outgrowth from the uncinate region of the intervertebral disc (Figure 17.12) or by distortion of the apophyseal joint. As with the cord, any dysfunction will be exacerbated by movement.

Clinical Features

Disorders of root and cord due to spondylosis can occur independently (Mayfield, 1965). Although in the younger population, radiculopathy is more common than myelopathy, the series of Lees and Turner (1963) and a review of the many reports of patients receiving surgery (Monro, 1984) support a clinical impression that in the geriatric population symptomatic myelopathy is a much more common problem than pure radiculopathy.

Radiculopathy

Radiculopathy may be asymptomatic and shown merely by loss of the triceps or biceps reflexes or may

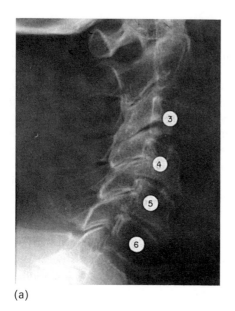

(a)

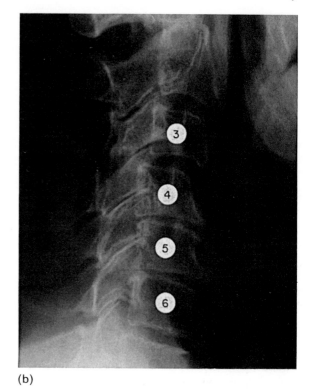

(b)

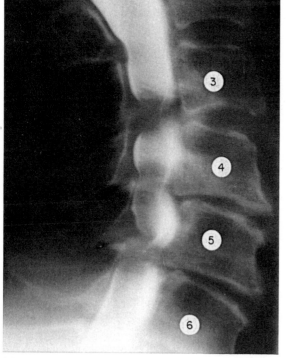

(c)

Figure 17.14. Lateral cervical spine X-rays of 68 year old patient presenting with cervical myelopathy.
(a) Extension. Note congenitally narrow canal. Loss of disc height at C4/5 and C5/6 and increased disc height anteriorly at C3/4.
(b) Flexion. Note forward subluxation of C3 on C4 with loss of alignment of posterior surface of vertebral bodies.
(c) Myelogram. Note indentation of subarachnoid space with distortion of cord outline posteriorly and anteriorly at C3/4, C4/5 and C5/6.
Marked clinical improvement followed anterior discectomy with fusion at C3/4.

present as slowly progressive weakness and wasting, particularly of the small muscles of the hand. In the elderly it less commonly presents acutely or sub-acutely with root pain and sensory deficit.

Myelopathy

The commonest clinical presentation of spondylotic myelopathy is with a combination of multiple root disorders at different levels with sensory root symptoms (usually tingling and numbness of the fingers) more common than motor, and 'upper motor neurone' disorders of the legs, spasticity being more marked than weakness (Clarke and Robinson, 1956; Bradshaw, 1957; Crandell and Batzdorf, 1966). Since myelopathy frequently extends above C5/6 it is common to have mixed upper and lower motor neurone signs in the arms. There may be some wasting and the reflexes may be either brisk or absent, depending on the level of involvement. In addition to spasticity and weakness of the legs, posterior column dysfunction may contribute to ataxia. Spinothalamic loss, either uni- or bilateral, indicating the cervical site of the lesion, occurs less frequently.

The length of history is very variable (Lees and Turner, 1963; Campbell and Phillips, 1960; Lunsford *et al.*, 1980a). A very gradual onset of dysfunction is indicated by the frequent findings of neurological signs in patients with no symptoms. Most commonly the story is of a very gradual onset of spasticity in the legs over many years and, as Lees and Turner showed, there is frequently a fluctuating course with episodes of deterioration followed by long intervals during which there may be no progression or even improvement. Trauma may precede by very varying periods the onset of symptoms. The patient may present with a short history of acute onset and rapid deterioration over days or weeks, not necessarily following a fall.

Radiology

If the clinical features are compatible with myelopathy secondary to spondylosis, X-rays of the cervical spine should be taken with views in flexion and extension. These are highly likely to show spondylo-

sis but myelopathy is unlikely to be secondary to this unless either a significant degree of narrowing of the AP diameter of the canal is shown in at least one position at one level, or a significant degree of hypermobility is shown, i.e. an increased range of movement on flexion or extension, usually with subluxation of one vertebra on another and subsequent loss of the normal smooth canal contours (Figure 17.14). It should, however, be remembered that narrowing of the canal can be produced not only by osteophytes but also by soft tissues not visible on X-rays. Hypertrophy of ligaments, particularly the ligamentum flavum posteriorly, is likely to occur whenever there is hypermobility (Figure 17.13). A canal which is congenitally wide may show extensive degenerative changes at many levels, without any significant impingement on the spinal cord (Figure 17.1a), whereas a patient with a congenitally narrow canal may have significant narrowing and therefore symptomatic myelopathy with only minor degenerative changes.

Oblique views of the cervical spine to show the exit foramina are useful in the presence of radiculopathy since such views clearly demonstrate osteophytic encroachment (Figure 17.12), whereas if tumour or infection are responsible for the symptoms, enlargement or erosion of the foramina may be found (Figure 17.11).

Further Investigation

The diagnosis of spondylotic myelopathy and the exclusion of some other structural cause for cord or root dysfunction requires the demonstration of soft tissues. As previously indicated this can be done by MRI, which is not yet universally available, by CT scanning and by myelography, either alone or in combination. These investigations are expensive, time consuming, tedious and uncomfortable for the patient. Moreover, myelography is not without hazard. Further investigation to define any structural distorting lesion should be undertaken only when other likely medical explanations for the clinical presentation have been excluded, and after it has been ascertained that the patient's clinical condition is such that surgery would be undertaken if a surgically remediable lesion were found.

Differential Diagnosis of Cervical Spondylotic Myelopathy and Radiculopathy

1. Motor neurone disease. This occurs in the elderly and may be responsible for a combination of 'upper' and 'lower' motor neurone signs in arms and legs and quite frequently for weakness and wasting in the arms, associated with brisk reflexes and spasticity and weakness in the legs. When lumbar spondylosis produces lower motor neurone signs in the legs, or cerebrovascular disease produces dysarthria, the differential diagnosis may not be easy, particularly since, as spondylosis is so common in the elderly, motor neurone disease and spondylosis not infrequently coexist. Widespread fasciculation, not only in the arms but also in the trunk, legs and tongue is pathognomonic of motor neurone disease. Marked sensory symptoms cannot be attributed to the disorder. The diagnosis may be confirmed by electromyography and this may also be helpful in establishing the presence of radiculopathy.

2. Subacute combined degeneration of the cord. Vitamin B12 deficiency due to pernicious anaemia or following gastrectomy results in myelopathy with evidence of upper motor neurone and dorsal column dysfunction in the cord, together with peripheral neuropathy producing absent ankle jerks and diminished reflexes in the arms with peripheral sensory deficit. Although macrocytosis and anaemia are commonly present they are not invariably found. The diagnosis can be established by serum B12 estimation, although a recent report suggests levels are not always significantly reduced (Lindenbaum *et al.*, 1988; Beck, 1988).

3. Cord compression due to a mass lesion. Compression due to acute or chronic infection in the vertebrae or to neoplasia, either primary or secondary, will produce cord disorder with evidence of a lesion at a single level. This will frequently but not invariable be accompanied by osteolytic changes on X-ray (see section below on spinal extradural malignancy).

4. Non-metastatic complication of neoplasia. A combination of peripheral neuropathy and upper motor neurone disorder can occur as a remote effect of neoplasia, and electromyography may help clarify this.

5. Syphilis. Although rare, syphilitic hypertrophy in the cervical region may produce a combination of cord and root dysfunction as in cervical spondylosis. Serological tests for treponemal infection should always be made. Interpretation in patients of West Indian extraction is complicated by the possibility of a past history of yaws.

Management of Cervical Spondylotic Myelopathy and Radiculopathy

If on clinical grounds and as a result of the non-invasive investigations outlined above, it seems likely that neurological symptoms and signs are secondary to cervical spondylosis, the logical treatment should be to remove the distorting and compressing tissues and to prevent the mobility thought to be responsible. However, the results of surgery are not always good. Management is dependent on the clinical presentation and in particular whether there is pure radiculopathy or whether myelopathy is present as well.

Patients presenting with myelopathy

Although there is very little recorded evidence of the natural history of spondylotic myelopathy, the few reports there are indicate clearly that once symptoms develop the disorder is by no means always steadily progressive. Analysis of the very few published series of patients not treated surgically and followed for periods between 2 and 40 years (Monro, 1984) revealed that 43% of patients improved over this period, 34% were unchanged and only 23% had deteriorated. However, it should be noted that, although in the series of Lees and Turner (1963) only 4 of 28 patients followed for up to 40 years were worse, the majority of their patients were severely disabled and that deterioration is more likely to occur in the elderly (Nurick, 1972b).

Surgical attempts to improve on this outcome have included removal of the distorting tissues, either posteriorly by laminectomy or anteriorly through the disc space with fusion. While some patients are reported as showing stabilization or even dramatic improvement in their myelopathy, these are counterbalanced by others who deteriorate or die. Lunsford *et al.* (1980a) in a recent well-documented report claimed 50% improvement and 50% deterioration postoperatively. There have been no controlled trials to show whether surgery affects the outcome and the differences in selection of patients, in their assessment, and in the operative techniques and period of follow-up are such that interpretation of published data is difficult. Survey of the literature gives no clear answer (Monro, 1984). However, there are indications that age does not necessarily affect the outcome, that those patients with the most severe disability have the best chance of improvement if they are operated on early, and that those patients with focal disease limited to one or two levels who have an anterior discectomy are those most likely to improve, especially if soft tissue only is removed and if adequate immobilization is achieved postoperatively. Until further evidence is obtained, the pragmatic approach is to select for further investigation with a view to surgery those patients with myelopathy who would be able to withstand surgery, whose symptoms are of sufficient severity to interfere with their mobility and who have a short history or a progressive one with evidence of recent deterioration. It must be borne in mind that the patients who are most likely to proceed to surgery and to benefit from it are those with radiological evidence of narrowing of the canal to a width of less than 15 mm, those with evidence of significant instability of the spine and with disease limited to one or two levels only.

Soft disc protrusion

It should be noted that even elderly patients may develop soft disc protrusion on a background of spondylosis (Young *et al.*, 1986). The characteristic presentation is with a short history of loss of use of the hands due to impairment of joint position sense, often with only a mild spastic paraparesis and only rarely with any preceding history of trauma. Most commonly the disc is at C3/4, above the site of maximum degenerative changes which have rendered the lower intervertebral joints immobile. Such patients respond well to surgery.

Falls in patients with spondylosis

Acute deterioration following a fall does not necessarily indicate fresh pathology, particularly if the spondylotic changes are diffuse with no focal narrowing and no instability. In such cases, if the paresis is incomplete, then an initial trial of conservative management with cervical immobilization provided by a firm collar, possibly aided by bed rest, for a period of up to 48 hours is frequently rewarded by spontaneous improvement. A short course of steroids (dexamethasone 4 mg four times daily) for a period of 10 days is sometimes given with the aim of reducing cord swelling. Since, however, there is good evidence that steroids do not affect cerebral swelling following head injuries nor improve the outcome, there is no reason to suppose that steroids are effective following injury to the spinal cord. Since, in the doses used, steroids have a number of side-effects, they should be given for a limited period only. If improvement does not occur within 48 hours or if paresis is complete or progressive then further investigations should be carried out to see if there is any extrinsic compression of the cord requiring surgery. Management of cord lesions following trauma in elderly patients is discussed later.

Surgery

The anterior cervical approach carries a number of advantages. Stabilization, which has been shown to be of crucial importance in determining the improvement (Adams and Logue 1971b), is more readily achieved and often follows removal of the disc but is usually aided by the insertion of intervertebral bone graft or prosthesis. Soft tissue can readily be removed through the disc space and, following fusion of vertebrae, bony osteophytes have been shown to resorb. Improvement may therefore follow anterior fusion even when the hard distorting tissue is posteriorly situated and is left untouched. A posterior approach necessarily involves the risk of disturbing the cord in order to remove anterior compressive tissue which can be readily reached via an anterior approach, and it is not surprising, therefore, that laminectomy carries an increased morbidity.

Conservative management

Those patients with a myelopathy which is not causing significant difficulty in walking or use of the hands, or in whom there has been no evidence of deterioration in recent months, and those in whom radiology shows diffuse disease with no instability and a capacious canal are unlikely to benefit from surgery. In such patients, therefore, there is no indication for myelography. It should, however, be stressed that patients with a significant degree of difficulty in walking who have insignificant spondylotic changes on X-ray should be investigated to ascertain the cause of their myelopathy (see Figure 17.1). Any patient with myelopathy and radiological evidence of spondylotic change which could be responsible, i.e. with narrowing of the canal and instability, but who is unfit for surgery should be given a cervical collar. A collar is usually provided even in the abence of demonstrable instability, the rationale being that reduction of even normal movement may produce some improvement or prevent further deterioration. Although there is no evidence to indicate that the collar is responsible, improvement undoubtedly occurs in some patients while they are wearing it (Roberts, 1966). It is important to ensure that any collar does adequately immobilize the neck in the neutral or slightly flexed position, since this position not only ensures that the patients can see what they are doing with their hands and can carry on with their normal activities, but it is also the position in which the cervical canal is most capacious. It is also important to check that the patient or somebody who lives with him, knows how to put the collar on and can do so, and that the collar is sufficiently comfortable to be worn continuously during the day. A soft collar should be provided for night wear.

If the patient is liable to falls, or there is instability of the cervical spine, the collar should be worn for as long as the patient is mobile. If no cervical instability has been demonstrated then it seems logical to wear the collar until at least 3 months after the clinical condition has stabilized, resuming it should neurological deterioration occur.

The patient who has been given a collar should be followed at regular intervals, monthly in the first instance and then 3 monthly, in order to detect any deterioration which should prompt further investigation.

Patients presenting with radiculopathy

The majority of patients who present with pain in the neck radiating to the arm attributable to spondylosis improve within 4 weeks with conservative management, whether this be with traction or a collar, with no long-term sequelae (British Association of Physical Medicine, 1966; Lees and Turner, 1963). Patients presenting in this way should have X-rays of the exit foramina to ensure that there is no enlargement or erosion which would indicate other pathology (see Figures 17.11 and 17.12), and should then be treated symptomatically with adequate analgesics and a cervical collar provided in the manner previously described. Although traction may relieve muscle spasm it is unlikely to benefit any spondylotic change and a collar appears to provide comfort and relieve symptoms particularly in the elderly. Manipulation of an unstable spondylotic spine carries the risk of precipitating a myelopathy and should be avoided.

If pain is persistent, severe and unresponsive, electromyography may help localize the site of the root lesion as a preliminary to further investigation with a view to surgical decompression. If pain is accompanied by sensory symptoms or motor weakness then, although there is no evidence to indicate that delay in surgery worsens the prognosis, it is sensible to time intervention depending on the severity of the patient's symptoms and, if disabling weakness is present, to operate before atrophy occurs. If a geriatric patient is found to have motor wasting and weakness attributable to spondylotic radiculopathy it is sensible to proceed to further investigations with a view to intervention only if the patient is significantly disabled by the weakness and if the symptoms are of recent onset or are progressive.

The reported results of surgery for pure radiculopathy are good with a high chance of significant improvement or complete cure with insignificant morbidity, negligible mortality and no long-term sequelae. These good results are obtained whether the approach is posterior by laminectomy and foramenotomy, or by partial removal of adjacent laminae, or anterior through the disc space followed by intervertebral fusion. The anterior approach is now usually adopted as it carries a lower morbidity (Lunsford *et al.*, 1980b).

LUMBAR DEGENERATIVE DISEASE

Accumulated stress, strains and injury to the lumbar spine inexorably lead to degenerative changes seen in 60% of plain radiographs in patients aged 50 years and over, and the incidence increases with advancing years. Between 85 and 95% of people by 50 years have autopsy evidence of lumbar degeneration (Quinet and Hadler, 1979). The majority of this group have only mild occasional attacks of back pain if they are troubled at all. Small wonder though that a small number complain bitterly of persisting symptoms which can lead to limitation of mobility and permanent disability. Acute disc prolapse is rare in the elderly whose symptoms are often less well defined, but no less debilitating for being chronic and unspectacular.

Aetiology

The underlying mechanisms of degenerative change are common to all the various syndromes. Preceding serious back injury or acute disc prolapse in earlier years are obvious predisposing causes to the development of long-term complications, but most patients progress by insidious changes of a less striking nature. The age-related degeneration of intervertebral and apophyseal joints, dehydration and the cumulative trauma of repeated movements have been described in the development of cervical spondylosis. The same pathological mechanisms apply in the lumbar spine, but here the role of the spine in weight transmission is of greater importance. The apophyseal joints in the lumbar region share in this role, they are larger and are recognized as playing an important part in the production of the clinical picture of lumbar spondylosis. The effect of loss of disc height in the lumbar region is shown in Figure 17.15. The superior articular facet of the lower vertebra is allowed to move slightly upwards. The altered disposition of the facets in the synovial joint causes cartilaginous

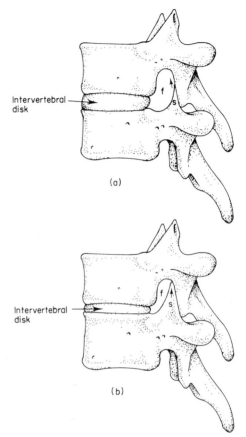

Figure 17.15. (a) Normal appearances. (b) With narrowing of the disc space note the slight upward migration of the superior articular facet(s), the backward displacement of the upper vertebra, and the narrowed intervertebral foramen (f).

damage and bony hypertrophy. The initial symptoms will arise from the facet joint itself, but, later, entrapment of the nerve root together with the entering spinal arteries in the intervertebral foramen may occur. Medial expansion of the superior articular facet may lead to narrowing of the lateral (subarticular) recess causing compression of the root leaving the spinal canal below the level (Figure 17.16).

Pathological disruption of a facet joint cannot

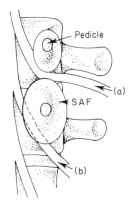

Figure 17.16. Coronal view right half of spinal canal showing effect of an enlarged superior articular facet (SAF) leading to (a) foraminal obstruction, (b) lateral recess stenosis (broken line).

occur in isolation. There will have been preliminary changes in the disc joint; and it is axiomatic that changes will occur in the adjacent paired facet joints. Hence the 'three joint' concept of spinal degeneration suggested by Farfan (1973), in which the disc joint and the two posterolateral facet joints are intimately dependent upon one another at each vertebral level.

As the cycle of degeneration progresses, concentric but asymmetrical encroachment on the circumference of the spinal canal occurs. The shape of the canal slowly changes from roughly oval to a trefoil appearance.

In addition to the bone deformities, changes in the soft tissues also appear: hypertrophy of the ligamentum flavum results in posterior constriction of the canal which, as in the cervical region, is exaggerated by extension. The composite picture in a fully developed case will consist of narrowing of the canal anteriorly by the backwardly bulging annulus, disc prolapse and associated osteophytic excrescences. Posterolaterally, the canal will be encroached upon by the forward and medially projecting hypertrophied facet joints and ligaments. These changes will be exacerbated by extension of the spine, as in standing, causing changes in symptomatology which will be dealt with later. Both intervertebral disc

degeneration and articular facet disease lengthen and narrow the nerve root canal.

After this brief consideration of lumbar degeneration, it is possible to discuss separately the different syndromes, but it should be noted that a continuum of pathology is present and that one symptom complex may coexist with others, compounding the problems of analysis.

Facet Joint Disease

This is one of the early and milder manifestations of degenerative disease. Osteoarthritic changes are present in these small synovial joints and there is a laxity in the joint capsules. The latter have a nerve supply originating in the root leaving at that level. Back ache is the common complaint, with transient exacerbations of a sharper pain on initiation of movement. The pain is usually situated over the joint, i.e. to one or other side of the midline, and may be referred to the buttock, hip or upper posterior thigh. Stiffness is usually present after periods of immobility, e.g. sleeping or sitting, tending to wear off with activity. Sitting itself may be uncomfortable and the patient often complains of being unable to settle for any length of time.

There are no abnormal neurological findings; any that are discovered are likely to be due to antecedent disc prolapse. Pressure over the appropriate joint frequently reproduces the pain and this is perhaps the best diagnostic pointer. Plain X-rays will demonstrate degenerative changes at the appropriate level, but may not be gross. Special investigations are not required.

Treatment consists of general back care and exercises to restrict progression. Non-steroidal anti-inflammatory agents may be of value and in view of the relapsing nature of the problem, repeated courses of treatment may be required. If these measures fail, it is worthwhile injecting the offending joint with local anaesthetic to see if this brings about a short period of relief. If it does, more permanent relief can be obtained by mixing the local anaesthetic with a depot steroid preparation. Recurrent pain may require stronger measures such as an injection of phenol in an aqueous solution. Equally definitive lesions can be made with cryoprobes or radiofre-

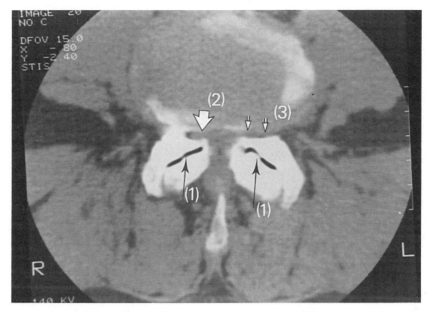

Figure 17.17. HRCl scan at L4/5 interspace shows facetal hypertrophy (1) leading to canal stenosis, lateral recess stenosis (2) and obliteration of root canal (3).

quency generators, but even these may need to be repeated at intervals.

Lateral Recess Stenosis

This uncommon condition afflicting the elderly is caused, as its name implies, by root compression in the lateral (subarticular) recess (Figure 17.16b). Although a variable degree of back discomfort is usually present, the principal clinical feature is one of severe unilateral (or bilateral) leg pain induced by standing or walking for short periods, which is quickly relieved by squatting or sitting (Ciric *et al.*, 1980). No definite signs of root compression may be present, but EMG studies may indicate an abnormality referable to the appropriate root. Myelography may not be diagnostic as partial filling of the root cuff may be present. HRCT is to be preferred as this will demonstrate the anatomy of the subarticular recesses and the root canals throughout their length (Figure 17.17).

Operative intervention is required for relief. Fenestration under screen control to identify the correct level is followed by foramenotomy and removal of the medial third of the facet joint together with any associated disc prolapse. Great care must be exercised during the operation to avoid damage to the nerve and for that reason the operating microscope should be employed. A satisfactory outcome is likely if the nerve is fully mobile throughout its length at the conclusion of the dissection.

Neurogenic Claudication

This term refers to intermittent disturbance of neurological function produced by walking a fixed distance, and relieved by rest, in a person who in a non-active state has no persisting symptoms and usually little in the way of signs. The anatomical background is one of severe canal stenosis due to the degenerative processes previously described, and often superimposed on lumbar canals which are congenitally narrow in the sagittal plane. The lumbosacral junction is usually spared, but the maximal changes are at the L4/5 intervertebral level and may extend upwards over multiple consecutive levels with diminishing severity to the thoracolumbar junction. Pioneering work by Verbiest in the mid 1950s led to increasing awareness of the narrow lumbar canal and its significance for patients with cauda equina compression (Verbiest, 1954 and 1955), but it was Blau and Logue (1978) who observed that patients with severe lumbar canal stenosis developed symptoms on walking that were in some ways akin to the claudication of peripheral arterial insufficiency. The disordered physiology responsible for the symptoms is less easily understood: its basis is customarily held to be vascular, but whether the ischaemic changes occur in the lumbar canal or in the nerve root foramina is not clear. A recent suggestion based on a post-mortem study is that a combination of thickened arachnoid around the roots, disturbing perfusion into the CSF, and very local vascular changes lead to ectopic nerve impulse discharges which produce the symptom complex (Watanable and Parke, 1986).

Clinical features

As the relevant pathological anatomy increases with age so these symptoms usually develop in an elderly population. Males are affected three times more often than females. There is frequently a history of back injury in earlier years.

The symptoms develop after walking a fairly predictable distance, though this can vary: shorter distances can produce symptoms if the patient is walking slowly, or downhill, when extension of the spine occurs sooner. The symptoms consist of spreading pain, paraesthesiae, numbness or clumsiness, which ascend or descend, ultimately involving the whole leg as far as the groin and sometimes up to the waist. These sensations, either individually or in combination, suffice to bring the patient to a halt, until with either sitting or leaning forwards respite occurs. The patient is then able to proceed, only to run up against recurrence after a similar distance. Prolonged standing can also produce these symptoms and may constitute a source of embarrassment to elderly patients attending functions. Other static conditions such as sciatica may be present and obscure presentation (Verbiest, 1980).

On examination there is often nothing to find

beyond the occasionally absent ankle reflex. The symptoms are reliably and conveniently reproduced by asking the patient to stand and then hyperextending the spine. The characteristic symptoms develop usually within 60 seconds. Flexion at this point leads to relief in about half this time. The differential diagnosis is from intermittent claudication of peripheral vascular disease. A careful history and examination is therefore essential.

Investigations

1. Plain X-rays. These may show a lumbar canal which is narrow in the sagittal plane due to congenital factors. Superimposed upon these there may be evidence of previous injury and progressive degener-

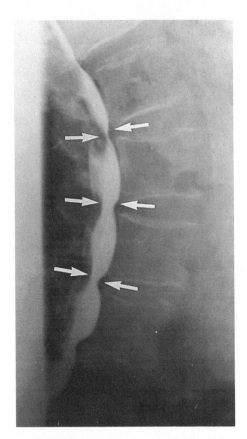

Figure 17.18. Lateral myelogram in lumbar canal stenosis where arrows demonstrate the segmental narrowing of the contrast column adjacent to the disc spaces.

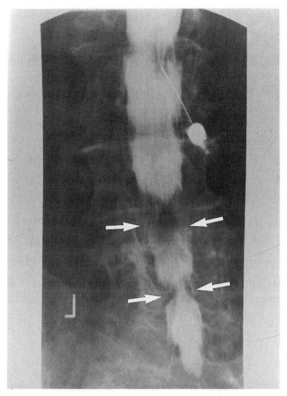

Figure 17.19. AP myelogram in lumbar canal stenosis where the arrows show constriction of the contrast column at multiple levels.

ative changes. Since the latter are a universal feature of the ageing spine, the value of plain films may be questioned. Various studies have been undertaken to measure the dimensions of the spinal canal. Hawkes and Roberts (1980) have summarized the evidence that the sagittal diameter and pedicular length are particularly valuable predictors of overall stenosis. of overall stenosis.

2. Myelography. Water soluble contrast medium is used to outline the subarachnoid space. This should be introduced at a high level under screen control in view of the underlying pathology, which is reflected in waist-like constructions (obstruction) at each interspace in both the AP and lateral views (Figures 17.18 and 17.19).

3. High resolution CT scanning. This has become an extremely useful examination as it reveals the transverse dimensions of the spinal canal in a unique manner. All the contributing elements to the stenotic picture can be seen and identified. The method is non-invasive as contrast medium is not required. Reformating will also demonstrate the canal in the sagittal and coronal planes.

4. Magnetic resonance imaging. This is of growing importance in the investigation of this condition because of its ability to demonstrate the spinal canal in the sagittal plane throughout its length.

Treatment

The mechanical nature of the condition means that conservative treatment is unlikely to be of value, though a carefully structured lumbar sacral support may help those whose poor general medical condition precludes surgery. Operative decompression is usually the obligatory approach. Not only has an adequate posterolateral decompression to be achieved, but the folded and buckled ligamentum flavum has to be excised, and the medial portions of the superior articular facets have to be curetted away to free the theca and the nerve roots. Decompression has to be extensive enough for all affected levels to be encompassed: Omissions are a common cause of unsuccessful surgery. The surgery is tedious, time consuming and should be performed meticulously with an operating microscope to avoid damage to neural elements already compromised and not able to tolerate further abuse.

Prognosis

The outcome of major surgery in the elderly is adversely affected by medical problems and difficulties of mobilization following extensive lumbar operations. These indirect factors play a deleterious role in outcome; if they are not present, however, about two-thirds of patients have lasting benefit, and many more are improved within the limits of their overall exercise tolerance (Verbiest, 1976; Blau and Logue, 1978).

THORACIC DISC PROLAPSE

This is a rare condition constituting only approximately 0.5% of all prolapsed discs. The peak incidence is in the fourth decade, but 15% are over the age of 60 and males predominate. The majority occur below the level of T6 (90%) and the commonest site is at T12 (25%). Most of the discs are centrally placed—an important consideration in planning the optimal surgical approach. The length of history varies from months to years, an acute onset being a rarity. The commonest initial symptom is midline back pain (50%), with girdle pains uncommon (10%), and at the time of diagnosis 70% have evidence of cord compression (Arce and Dohrmann, 1985).

Plain X-rays of the region often demonstrate calcification in the offending disc, but a more reliable investigation is a water soluble myelogram with tomography in the lateral views to see if the disc bulge lies more to one side of the midline. This may dictate the surgical route of access. High resolution CT scanning with or without contrast defines these parameters with ease, and MRI study will also be valuable in determining the number of discs involved.

The treatment of these discs is surgical but laminectomy has been deservedly abandoned as causing an excessive morbidity. Either a lateral costotransversectomy or an anterior transthoracic approach is indicated with a high success rate for cure or improvement.

SPINAL EPIDURAL INFECTION

This is fortunately a rare problem affecting males more than females, and subdividing into roughly equal numbers of acute and chronic cases (Baker *et al.*, 1975). In the acute variety infection arises in distant sites and is often modest in degree: furuncles and dental infections are relatively frequent causes of haematogenous spread; whereas the chronic type usually spreads directly from local osteomyelitis or discitis. By far the commonest infecting organism is *Staphylococcus aureus*. The usual location in acute cases is the thoracolumbar junction where frank pus collects in the epidural space leading to a rapid onset of symptoms comprising intense local pain, worse on palpation or percussion of a rigid spine, together with ingravescent root and cord signs.

Plain spinal X-rays are unlikely to be helpful as the history is likely to be of the order of a few days, but myelography will show the presence of an extradural block. Laminectomy and drainage is the traditional treatment of choice, but if a sample of pus can be obtained via a needle, vigorous treatment with the appropriate antibiotics may be effective and spare surgical intervention.

Chronic cases arising from neighbouring sepsis take longer to evolve before the onset of epidural infection, which again is characterized by local back pain and signs of cord or root compression of slower onset than the acute type.

In these cases bone scans are very often positive, plain X-rays frequently so. Myelography will demonstrate the level of the block caused by a mass of granulation tissue for which surgical decompression allied to prolonged antibiotic treatment is desirable. The prognosis for functional recovery is better in this group.

SPINAL EXTRADURAL MALIGNANCY
(see also Chapter 16)

About 5% of patients suffering from malignant disease will develop spinal deposits at some stage in their illness. The average age at onset is 60. The most common primary sites are lung, breast and prostate, but some malignancies such as lymphoma arise in the vertebral column. Most deposits (70%) occur in the thoracic spine with the rest shared equally between the cervical and lumbar regions.

The presenting symptom is usually that of pain. Due attention has to be paid to complaints of back pain in the elderly patient with no previous history of such trouble if early diagnosis is to be made. Unfortunately at diagnosis the situation is usually more complex and less favourable since in addition to pain, which is a feature in 95%, there are motor signs in 75%, autonomic disturbances in 60% and sensory deficits in 50%. In 80% of cases the disease begins in the vertebral body or pedicle; spinal deformity and instability therefore starts anteriorly. Vertebral collapse and increasing tumour volume

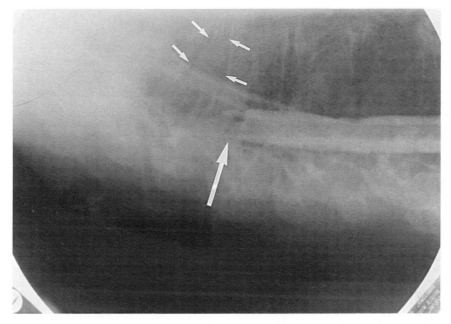

Figure 17.20. Lateral myelogram of spinal metastasis. Note the wedge-shaped collapsed vertebra between the small arrows, and the block in the contrast column.

first compress the theca and its contents leading to a gradual loss of cord functions, which ultimately accelerates alarmingly as vascular insufficiency leads to infarction of the cord and a complete paraplegia.

A radioactive bone scan may be positive before plain X-ray changes occur and may indicate widespread disease in other bone structures. Water soluble myelography should demonstrate the lower end of the lesion and possibly the relationship of the mass to the cord (Figures 17.20 and 17.21). CT scanning with intrathecal contrast is also valuable (Figure 17.22), especially with reformats of the image in other projections. Non-invasive MRI, when available, is the investigation of choice to delineate the contours of the lesion through its sagittal extent.

Treatment should be undertaken with realistic expectations. Palliation rather than cure is the aim. Since laminectomy with radiotherapy appears to produce much the same results as radiotherapy alone (Dunn *et al.*, 1980; Young *et al.*, 1980), the latter, with or without appropriate chemotherapy has become the first line of treatment. But surgery has a

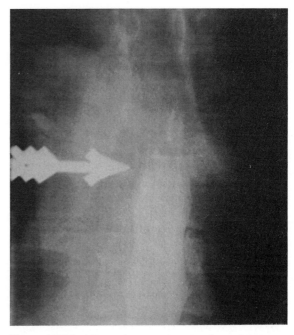

Figure 17.21. AP myelogram showing irregular upper margin of contrast at level of block.

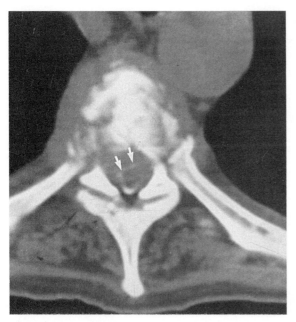

Figure 17.22. HRCT of thoracic vertebra after myelography showing the destruction of the vertebral body and pedicle and the deformity of the cord (arrow) by malignant tissue.

place in management provided the indications are clearly defined. Ideally it should be employed in patients whose disease is under control elsewhere and who are suffering progressive neurological deterioration and/or intractable pain from a single segment lesion. In practice, surgery is employed to establish a histological diagnosis and decompress the cord if a primary diagnosis is not available. It is also used when local relapse occurs after a full course of radiotherapy, or when there is inexorable local deterioration during radiotherapy. There is no place for surgery in fulminating widespread disease.

Until recently, laminectomy has been used widely and uncritically as the decompressive operation of choice. To endanger posterior stability while the disease process is active anteriorly is illogical and the generally poor results of laminectomy have led to a rapid decline in its popularity. The operation should be directed where the disease is producing its maximal impact and recently attention has been focused upon anterior decompression, with some

form of stabilization where necessary. The emphasis is on techniques which eliminate pain and disability, but at the same time promote early mobilization of patients who have a limited life expectancy. Some encouraging results are appearing (Harrington, 1984). For one of us (D.U.) this approach is bringing rewards in selected cases.

SPINAL TRAUMA

Major spinal trauma is fortunately uncommon in the elderly, but the cumulative effects of age, infirmity, systemic illness and advancing degenerative disease may mean that a relatively minor trauma may have a major adverse effect. The neck is the most vulnerable site; even quite trivial low velocity hyper-extension injuries can produce a quadriplegia under predisposing circumstances. Plain X-rays may not reveal evidence of overt bone damage or subluxation, if the pathogenesis is contusion or ischaemia, but CT scanning will show severe canal stenosis. Temporary external immobilization in a collar is indicated. The use of steroids is discretionary; they are of little value if the condition has been present for some days at the time of detection. Fortunately improvement often occurs if the deficit is incomplete (Firooznia *et al.*, 1985). Victims of advanced rheumatoid arthritis are at risk of a dislocation or fracture of the dens after mild injury, and signs of myelopathy should prompt transoral odontoidectomy (Stevens *et al.*, 1986) rather than external fixation or posterior fusion, though in non-rheumatoid patients sustaining fracture of the dens, success has been claimed for early posterior fusion with wire and acrylic (Wisoff, 1984). Paradoxically, radical surgery may have to be undertaken in the frail, elderly patient to achieve the early mobilization so essential to ward off the evils of immobilization in this group. Close collaboration is necessary between the referring physician, anaesthetist and surgeon to evaluate the various risk factors in coming to a decision on management. It is the authors' view that one should err on the active side to avoid the medical and psychological dangers of incapacity. This view also applies to those rare cases of major trauma in this age group, where, again, there is a powerful argument in favour of internal spinal stabilization in selected cases.

RHEUMATOID ARTHRITIS

The geriatric patient with rheumatoid arthritis is at increased risk of developing disorganization of the cervical spine with secondary involvement of the nervous system. Superimposed on the usual spondylotic degeneration found in this age group, rheumatoid destruction of bone and ligaments characteristically results in intervertebral subluxation, often at several levels (Figure 17.23). This is particularly likely to occur in the upper cervical spine where destruction of ligaments holding the odontoid peg in place may result in atlanto-axial dislocation, and rheumatoid changes in the dens may predispose to fracture with dislocation which is sometimes vertical. Not every geriatric patient with rheumatoid arthritis will show such changes; the reported incidence varies between 15% of 962 patients (Smith *et al.*, 1972) and 36% of 100 patients (Stevens *et al.*, 1971). Moreover, although subluxation and formation of rheumatoid pannus within the canal may result in compression of medulla and cord and their blood supply, this is not an invariable sequel. Myelopathy was found in only 12% of 150 patients with rheumatoid subluxation by Stevens *et al.*, (1971) and developed in only 3% of the remaining 130 patients who were followed over the next 9 years. Nahano (1975) similarly estimated that only 2.5% of patients with cervical rheumatoid subluxation developed myelopathy over a 6 year period. It is, however, in the geriatric age group that myelopathy is likely to develop (Marks and Sharp, 1981) and since in some cases rapid deterioration and even death may follow, the possibility of rheumatoid cervical subluxation as a cause of neurological symptoms must be borne in mind.

Clinical Picture

The commonest presentation of myelopathy secondary to rheumatoid disease of the spine is with sensory symptoms, paraesthesiae or numbness in all four limbs. These may mimic a peripheral neuropathy and are usually associated with spastic weakness

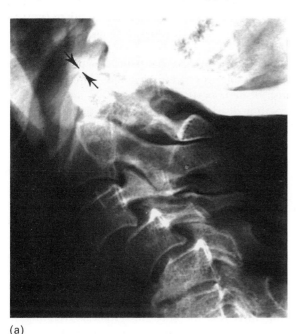
(a)

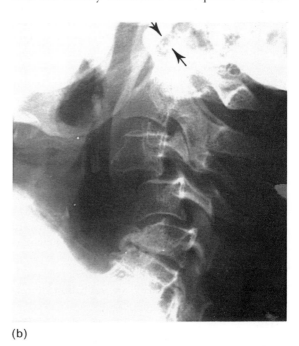
(b)

Figure 17.23. Lateral cervical spine X-ray of patient with rheumatoid arthritis.
(a) Extension. Note disorganization of spinal canal due to subaxial dislocation at C3/4 and C4/5 and degenerative loss of disc height at C4/5. Odontoid peg opposed to arch of atlas (arrowed).
(b) Flexion. Note separation of odontoid peg from arch of atlas (arrowed).

which, as might be expected from a disorder commonly affecting the upper cervical spine, is a quadriparesis rather than a paraparesis (Marks and Sharp, 1981; Stevens *et al.*, 1986). The myelopathy is frequently associated with loss of bladder control. Posterior column sensation is often spared but a sensory level may be found, particularly in patients with rapidly developing symptoms. When myelopathy develops slowly its onset may pass undetected in patients whose rheumatoid arthropathy renders their hands useless and walking impossible. Moreover, in these patients assessment is not easy since the arthritis interferes both with motor testing and the ability to elicit reflexes.

The most dramatic presentation of atlanto-axial subluxation (AAS) results from sudden dislocation of the odontoid peg posteriorly and sometimes vertically, with subsequent pressure on the cord, medulla or vertebral vessels. Acute tetraparesis may result which may be transient or, fortunately less commonly, permanent. Pressure on the vertebral artery as it crosses the axis may cause ischaemia in the brain stem with vertigo, dysarthria and ataxia and this may be associated with symptoms of ischaemia in the distribution of the posterior cerebral artery, teichopsia or visual loss. Although these symptoms are often transient and related to neck movements, in the geriatric population in whom atheromatous narrowing of potential collateral vessels is very likely, permanent infarction may occur and even sudden death (Davis and Markhey, 1951; Jones and Kaufmann, 1976).

Pain, although common, is not an invariable accompaniment of rheumatoid disease of the spine (seven of 31 in the series of Marks and Sharp (1981); nineteen of 31 in the series of Stevens *et al.* (1986)). Its severity is not related to the severity of the changes likely to be shown on X-ray. Pain commonly arises from the disordered joint and, even when referred to the arms, is not necessarily an indication of root compression.

Management

If a geriatric patient has rheumatoid arthritis but none of the neurological features just described, there is little benefit in X-raying the cervical spine simply in order to ascertain whether there is any rheumatoid change unless the patient is to be subjected to anaesthesia. Manipulation of an unstable spine during intubation may have a disastrous effect on the cord or medulla and the anaesthetist should be forewarned of this. However, if the patient is symptom free then even if subluxation is demonstrated, neurological involvement does not necessarily follow (see above) and, as Smith *et al.* (1972) showed, progression of radiological changes is not inevitable. It develops in only 25% of patients over a 9 year period, while 75% remained unchanged or became more stable, irrespective of whether or not a cervical collar was worn. However, if the patient develops any of the symptoms or signs of neurological involvement just described, since these could result from rheumatoid disease of the spine, X-rays of the neck should be taken with views in flexion and extension to detect the mobility likely to be present, either at the atlanto-axial joint or subaxially. The presence of AAS will be shown by a gap of more than 3 mm between the anterior surface of the odontoid peg and the posterior surface of the anterior arch of the axis (Figure 17.23).

Although it is clear that patients with myelopathy attributable to cervical rheumatoid disease are at risk of deterioration which may be rapid or even result in death, the size of this risk is not clear. In the series of Marks and Sharp (1981) nineteen out of 31 patients died within 6 months, although in only four of these was this due to neurological disorders. Other estimates vary between 60% deterioration over 7 years (Winfield *et al.*, 1981) and 25% over 14 years (Nahano, 1975). Those at highest risk on clinical grounds appear to be patients with recent onset of transient symptoms and those with progressive deterioration of myelopathy, especially if this is rapid. Radiological pointers to likely deterioration are, as with cervical spondylosis, a combination of narrowing of the available space for cord or medulla and increased mobility of vertebrae resulting in intermittent distortion of neural tissue. At the craniovertebral junction, narrowing of the residual canal to less than 15 mm and an increase in the dens/axis gap to more than 10 mm is likely to be accompanied by rapid deterioration. However, as

Stevens *et al.* (1986) have shown, the degree of distortion of cord and medulla cannot be determined by plain X-rays alone, or even myelography unaided, but is most clearly demonstrated using a combination of CT scanning with myelography. Using this technique Stevens *et al.* suggest that the severity of clinical features and their rate of deterioration are related to the degree of narrowing of the canal and distortion of soft tissues plus the extent of mobility. Intermittent distortion of the cord anteriorly by the odontoid peg on neck movement is most dangerous and symptoms are more likely to occur if there is also narrowing of the subarachnoid space posteriorly, thus contributing to compression and limiting the possibility of adaptive movement.

Surgical Treatment

If on the clinical or radiological grounds outlined above deterioration seems likely, treatment, as with cervical spondylosis, is aimed at removing distorting tissue and decreasing mobility. However, immobilization is more difficult to achieve in rheumatoid cervical disease than in spondylosis. Neither the clinical nor the radiological findings appear to be affected by wearing a collar. Deterioration, often rapid, may occur with traction (Rona *et al.*, 1973) and, unlike spondylotic disease, surgical attempts at immobilization are often unsuccessful, particularly in patients with AAS. In a review of the literature, Stevens *et al.* (1986) estimated that operative treatment, usually by posterior fusion after attempted reduction of dislocation, sometimes with laminectomy and almost always followed by a period of up to 12 weeks' traction, carried an operative mortality which varied between 10 and 70%, and resulted in improvement in between 0 and 60%. Better results with 86% sustained improvement and no perioperative deaths were reported by this group following transoral removal of the odontoid peg and subsequent posterior fusion. Even in those patients in whom stabilization was not achieved, deterioration was much less likely to occur if the dens had been removed. This approach has the additional advantage of allowing removal of any anteriorly situated rheumatoid pannus which may be preventing reduction of the dislocation of the dens (Chun *et al.*, 1974).

This operation can, however, be offered only to patients who are both fit enough to withstand surgery and who have temporomandibular joints which, although they may be affected by rheumatoid disease, are sufficiently mobile to allow access through the mouth.

Treatment of subaxial rheumatoid subluxation, which is usually combined with spondylotic degeneration, follows the same general principles outlined in the management of cervical spondylosis. Surgery is determined on clinical grounds of progressive myelopathy when combined with radiological evidence of sufficient narrowing of the canal and mobility to account for this.

ACKNOWLEDGEMENTS

We are grateful to Mr Tom Robb for drawing Figures 17.15 and 17.16, to Dr J. Ambrose and Dr G. Hart of the Department of Radiology of Atkinson Morley's Hospital for their kind help with the X-ray plates, and for the unstinting enthusiasm, patience and skill of our secretaries, Miss A. Pollock and Miss S. Rostrom.

REFERENCES

Adams, C.B.T., and Logue, V. (1971a). Studies in cervical myelopathy. I Movement of the cervical roots, dura and cord and their relation to the course of extra-thecal roots. *Brain*, **94**, 557–60.

Adams, C.B.T., and Logue, V. (1971b). Studies in cervical myelopathy. III Some functional effects of operations for cervical spondylotic myelopathy. *Brain*, **94**, 587–95.

Arce, C.A., and Dohrmann, G.J. (1985). Thoracic disc herniation. Improved diagnosis with computed tomographic scanning and a review of the literature. *Surg. Neurol.*, **23**, 356–61.

Baker, A.S., Ojemann, R.G., Swartz, M.N., and Richardson, E.P. Jr. (1975). Spinal epidural abscess. *N. Engl. J. Med.*, **293**, 463–8.

Barnes, M.P., and Saunders, M. (1984). The effect of cervical mobility on the natural history of cervical spondylotic myelopathy. *J. Neurol. Neurosurg. Psychiatry*, **47**, 13–20.

Beck, W.S. (1988) *N. Engl. J. Med.*, **318**, 1752–4.

Blau, J.N., and Logue, V. (1978). The natural history of intermittent claudication of the cauda equina. *Brain*, **101**, 211–22.

Bradshaw, P. (1957). Some aspects of cervical spondylosis. *Q. J. Med.* **46**, 177–208.

Braun, I.F., Lin, J.F., George, A.E., Kricheff, I.I., and

Hoffman, J.C. Jr. (1984). Pitfalls in the computed tomographic evaluation of the lumbar spine in disc disease. *Neuroradiology*, **26**, 15–26.

Breig, A., Turnbull, I., and Hassler, O. (1966). Effects of mechanical stresses on the spinal cord in cervical spondylosis. A study of fresh cadaver material. *J. Neurosurg.*, **25**, 45–56.

British Association of Physical Medicine (1966). Pain in the neck and arm: a multicentre trial of the effects of physiotherapy. *Br. Med. J.*, **1**, 253–8.

Campbell, A.M.G., and Phillips, D.G. (1960). Cervical disc lesions with neurological disorder. *Br. J. Med.*, **ii**, 5197–201.

Chun, C., Messert, B., Winkler, S.S., and Turner, J.H. (1974). Rheumatoid C1–C2 dislocation: pathogenesis and treatment reconsidered. *J. Neurol. Neurosurg. Psychiatry*, **37**, 1069–73.

Ciric, I., Mikhael, M.A., Tarkington, J.A., and Vick, N.A. (1980) The lateral recess syndrome. A variant of spinal stenosis. *J. Neurosurg.*, **53**, 433–44.

Clarke, E., and Robinson, P.K. (1956). Cervical myelopathy, a complication of cervical spondylosis. *Brain*, **79**, 483–510.

Crandell, P.H., and Batzdorf, U. (1966). Cervical spondylotic myelopathy. *J. Neurosurg.*, **25**, 57–66.

Daniels, D.L., Grogan, J.P., Johansen, J.G., Meyer, G.A., Williams, A.L., and Haughton, V.M. (1984). Cervical radiculopathy: computed tomography and myelography compared. *Radiology*, **151**, 109–13.

Davis, F.W., and Markhey, H.E. (1951). Rheumatoid arthritis with death from medullary compression. *Ann. Intern. Med.*, **35**, 451–4.

Dunn, R.C., Kelly, W.A., Wohns, R.N.W., and Howe, J.F. (1980). Spinal epidural neoplasia. A 15 year review of the results of surgical therapy. *J. Neurosurg.*, **52**, 47–51.

Farfan, H.F. (1973). *Mechanical Disorders of the Low Back*, Lee & Febiger, Philadelphia.

Firooznia, H., Ahn, J.H., Rafii, M., and Ragnarsson, K. (1985). Sudden quadriplegia after a minor trauma. The role of pre-existing spinal stenosis. *Surg. Neurol.*, **23**, 165–8.

Frykholm, R. (1951). Cervical nerve root compression resulting from disc degeneration and nerve root fibrosis. A clinical investigation. *Acta Chirurg. Scand. (Suppl.)*, **160**, 1–149.

Harrington, K.D. (1984). Anterior cord decompression and spinal stabilisation for patients with metastatic lesions of the spine. *J. Neurosurg.*, **61**, 107–17.

Hawkes, C.H., and Roberts, G.M. (1980) Lumbar canal stenosis. *Br. J. Hosp. Med.*, **23**, 498–505.

Hawkins, J.C., Yaghmal, F., and Gindin, R.A. (1975). Cervical myelopathy due to spondylosis (Case report). *J. Neurosurg.*, **48**, 297–301.

Heithoff, K.B. (1983). In: Cauthen, J.C. (ed.) *Lumbar Spine Surgery*, Williams & Wilkins, Baltimore, London.

Holt, S., and Yates, P.O. (1966). Cervical spondylosis and nerve root lesions. Incidence at routine necropsy. *J. Bone Joint Surg.*, **48B**, 407–23.

Hughes, J.T. (1977). Spinal cord involvement by C4–C5 vertebral subluxation in rheumatoid arthritis—A description of 2 cases examined at necropsy. *Ann. Neurol.*, **1**, 575–82.

Hughes, J.T., and Brownell, B. (1964). Cervical spondylosis complicated by anterior spinal artery thrombosis. *Neurology*, **14**, 1073–7.

Jones, M.W., and Kaufmann, J.C.E. (1976). Vertebrobasilar artery insufficiency in rheumatoid atlanto-axial subluxation. *J. Neurol. Neurosurg. Psychiatry*, **39**, 122–8.

Kahn, C.A. (1947). The role of the dentate ligaments in spinal cord compression and in the syndrome of lateral sclerosis. *J. Neurosurg.*, **4**, 191–9.

Lees, F., and Turner, J.W.A. (1963). Natural history and prognosis of cervical spondylosis. *Br. Med. J.*, **ii**, 1609–10.

Lindenbaum, J., Healton, E.B., Savage, D.G., Brust, J.C.M., Garrett, T.J., Podell, E.R., Marcell, P.D., Stabler, S.P., and Allen, R.H. (1988) *N. Engl. J. Med.*, **318**, 1720–28.

Lipson, S.J., and Muir, H. (1981). 1981 Volvo Award of Basic Science: Proteoglycans in experimental intervertebral disc degeneration. *Spine*, **6**, 194–210.

Lunsford, L.D., Bissonette, D.J., and Zorub, D.S. (1980a). Anterior surgery for cervical disc disease, Part 2. Treatment of spondylotic myelopathy in 32 cases. *J. Neurosurg.*, **53**, 12–19.

Lunsford, L.D., Bissonette, D.J., Janette, P.J., Scheptak, P.E., and Zorub, D.S. (1980b). Anterior surgery for cervical disc disease, Part 1. Treatment of lateral cervical disc herniation in 253 cases. *J. Neurosurg.*, **53**, 1–11.

Mair, W.G.P., and Druckman, R. (1953). The pathology of spinal cord lesions and their relation to the clinical features on protrusion of cervical intervertebral discs. *Brain*, **76**, 70–91.

Marks, J.S., and Sharp, J. (1981). Rheumatoid cervical myelopathy. *Q. J. Med.*, **50**, 307–19.

Mayfield, G.H. (1965). Cervical spondylosis, observations based on surgical treatment of 400 patients. *Postgrad. Med.* **38**, 345–57.

Modic, M.T., Pavlicek, W., Weinstein, M.A., Boumphrey, F., Ngo, F., Hardy, R., and Duchesneau, P.M. (1984). Magnetic resonance imaging of intervertebral disc disease. *Radiology*, **152**, 103–11.

Monro, P. (1984). What has surgery to offer in cervical spondylosis? In: Warlow, C., and Garfield, J. (eds) *Dilemmas in the Management of the Neurological Patient*, Churchill Livingstone, Edinburgh, pp. 168–87.

Nahano, K.K. (1975). Neurological complications of rheumatoid arthritis. *Ortho. Clin. North Am.*, **6**, 861–79.

Nurick, S. (1972a). The pathogenesis of the spinal cord disorder associated with cervical spondylosis. *Brain*, **95**, 87–100.

Nurick, S. (1972b). The natural history and the results of

surgical treatment of the spinal cord disorder associated with cervical spondylosis. *Brain*, **95**, 101–8.

Pallis, C., Jones, M.A., and Spillane, J.D. (1954). Cervical spondylosis. *Brain*, **77**, 274–89.

Quinet, R.J., and Hadler, N.M. (1979). Diagnosis and treatment of back ache. *Semin. Arthritis Rheum.*, **8**, 261–87.

Reid, J.D. (1960). Effects of flexion-extension movements of the head and spine upon spinal cord and nerve roots. *J. Neurol. Neurosurg. Psychiatry*, **23**, 214–21.

Roberts, A.H. (1966). Myelopathy due to cervical spondylosis treated by collar immobilisation. *Neurology*, **16**, 951–4.

Rona, N.A., Hancock, D.O., Taylor, A.R., and Hill, A.G.S. (1973). Altanto-axial subluxation in rheumatoid arthritis. *J. Bone Joint Surg.*, **55(B)**, 458–70.

Simpson, J.A. (1984). *Contemporary Neurology*, Butterworths, London.

Smith, P.H., Benn, R.T., and Sharp, J. (1972). Natural history of rheumatoid cervical subluxations. *Ann. Rheum. Dis.*, **31**, 431–9.

Stevens, J.C., Cartlidge, N.E.F., Saunders, M., Appleby, A., Hall, M., and Shaw, D.A. (1971). Atlanto-axial subluxation and cervical myelopathy in rheumatoid arthritis. *Q. J. Med.*, **40**, 391–408.

Stevens, J.M., Kendall, B.E., and Crockard, H.A. (1986). The spinal cord in rheumatoid arthritis with clinical myelopathy: a computed myelographic study. *J. Neurol, Neurosurg. Psychiatry*, **49**, 140–51.

Stoltman, H.F., and Blackwood, W. (1966). The role of the dentate ligament in the pathogenesis of myelopathy in cervical spondylosis. *Brain*, **87**, 45–50.

Verbiest, H. (1954). A radicular syndrome from developmental narrowing of the lumbar vertebral canal. *J. Bone Joint Surg.*, **36B**, 236–7.

Verbiest, H. (1955). Further experiences on the pathological influence of a developmental narrowness of the bony lumbar vertebral canal. *J. Bone Joint Surg.*, **37b**, 576.

Verbiest, H. (1976). *Neurogenic Intermittent Claudication*, North Holland Publishing, Amsterdam.

Verbiest, H. (1980). Stenosis of the lumbar vertebral canal and sciatica. *Neurosurg. Rev.* **3**, 75–89.

Watanable, R., and Parke, W.W. (1986). Vascular and neural pathology of lumbosacral spinal stenosis. *J. Neurosurg.*, **64**, 64–7.

Winfield, J., Cooke, D., Brook, A.S., and Corbett, M. (1981). A prospective study of the radiological changes in the cervical spine in early rheumatoid disease. *Ann. Rheum. Dis.*, **40**, 109–14.

Wisoff, H.S. (1984). Fracture of the dens in the aged. *Surg. Neurol.*, **22**, 547–55.

Young, R.F., Post, E.M., and King, G.A. (1980). Treatment of spinal epidural metastases. Randomised prospective comparison of laminectomy and radiotherapy. *J. Neurosurg.*, **53**, 741–8.

Young, S., Tamas, L., and O'Laoire, S.A. (1986). Cervical disc prolapse in elderly patients with cervical spondylosis: an easily overlooked reversible cause of spinal cord compression. *Br. Med. J.*, **293**, 749–50.

Yu, Y.L., Du Boulay, G.H., Stevens, J.M., and Kendall, B.E. (1986). Computer assisted myelography in cervical spondylotic myelopathy and radiculopathy. Clinical correlation and pathogenetic mechanisms. *Brain*, **109**, 259–78.

Chapter 18

Cranio-cerebral Trauma

P. O'Neill

Consultant Neurosurgeon, The National Neurosurgery Centre, Beaumont Hospital, Dublin, Eire

EPIDEMIOLOGY

Head injuries constitute a major health problem in all developed countries. A survey of Scottish hospitals for sample periods during 1974 led to an estimate that approximately one million new cases of head injury present to accident and emergency departments in Britain each year (Lancet, 1977). Six per cent of all attenders are aged 65 years or over. Of those attending accident and emergency departments with head injuries 23% are admitted to hospital (Strang *et al.*, 1978).

Throughout most of Britain only patients with the more severe injuries are transferred to regional neurosurgical units, the remainder who require hospital admission going to primary surgical or orthopaedic wards. There is, however, a surprising range in the proportion transferred, reflecting differences between regions in the neurosurgical facilities available (e.g. number of beds per million population served) and in the policy of individual neurosurgeons. In England and Wales as a whole, 5% of all patients admitted with a head injury go to neurosurgical units according to the published 10% sample of discharges (Office of Population Censuses and Surveys, 1974). In the Mersey Region, however, only 1.2% of admitted head injuries go to the neurosurgical unit, while in Edinburgh the proportion is 35% (Jeffreys and Azzam, 1979; Jennett, 1980). Overall, of those patients who are admitted with head injury to either primary surgical wards or to neurosurgical units, 9% are in the geriatric age group (> 65 years)

(Lancet, 1977). More recently Galbraith reported that head injuries in those over 65 years old accounted for 14% of admissions to a head and spinal injuries unit of a teaching hospital (Galbraith, 1987).

The causes of head injury in the elderly have been documented (Strang *et al.*, 1978). Domestic accidents accounted for 29%, falls for another 28% and road accidents for 24%. Two per cent were due to accidents at work and 1% to assault. Social class has been shown to have a significant effect on the occurrence of head injury but the data pertaining to the geriatric age group are thought to be unreliable (Field, 1976).

PATHOLOGY

The most important factor governing the early clinical picture and ultimate outcome from a non-missile injury is the damage sustained by the brain (Adams *et al.*, 1977). A fundamental principle in any concept of head injury is that part of this damage results from forces engendered at the moment of impact (immediate or primary impact damage) whilst further damage can result from subsequent secondary events, e.g. expanding intracranial haematoma; hypotension or hypoxia; infection; and seizures. Immediate impact damage is caused by linear and rotational shear strains resulting from acceleration and deceleration forces and distortion of the skull (Adams, 1975).

Immediate Impact Damage

Skull fractures

If the force at impact has been of sufficient severity a skull fracture will result. Such fractures were found in 80% of fatal head injuries admitted to a neuro-surgical unit (Jennett, 1980). Most patients with an intracranial haematoma have a skull fracture. This is the case in 85–90% of those with extradural haematomas and in about 70% of those with intradural haematomas. The exceptions for those with an intradural haematoma are predominantly patients over 60 years old. Compound fractures have additional significance due to the increased risk of intracranial infection. It must be remembered that base of skull fractures frequently transgress air sinuses or the middle ear and must then be regarded as compound. Rhinorrhoea or otorrhoea are unequivocal signs of a compound skull fracture as is the presence of intracranial air.

The absence of a skull fracture does not, however, necessarily mean that no significant brain damage has occurred.

Diffuse axonal injury

That nerve axons may be damaged directly by shear strains engendered at the moment of impact was postulated by Strich (1956) when she reported extensive degeneration in the white matter of brains from patients who had survived for months in the vegetative state following head injury. Subsequent studies by Adams *et al.* (1977) have demonstrated easily identifiable lesions in the corpus callosum and in the dorsolateral quadrant of the rostral brain stem in the region of the superior cerebellar peduncles. These show histological evidence of diffuse damage to axons as evidenced by axonal retraction balls, microglial stars and degeneration of specific fibre tracts—these being sequential stages in a continuous pathological process (Adams, 1975).

Patients who have suffered a diffuse axonal injury present characteristic clinical features. All are in coma from the time of impact and frequently have bilateral extensor rigidity of limbs with some autonomic dysfunction. This was previously termed primary brain stem injury. Mitchell and Adams

(1973), however, have clearly shown that brain stem lesions do not occur in the absence of more diffuse axonal injury. There is also a much lower incidence of skull fracture in these patients (32%) compared to that in other fatally head injured patients (88%).

Cerebral contusions

Cerebral contusions are frequently found after head injury and are usually multiple and bilateral but asymmetrical in distribution. They are most common on the undersurface of the temporal and frontal lobes and on the anterior poles of the temporal lobes regardless of the site of impact (Adams, 1975). Recent contusions are haemorrhagic and when superficial are characteristically restricted to the crests of gyri but they often extend through the cortex into the white matter. Severe contusions in the frontal and temporal lobes are often associated with acute subdural and intracerebral blood when the term 'burst lobe' is commonly applied.

There is now abundant evidence, both experimental and clinical, that cerebral contusion can be extensive without there being prolonged (or any) loss of consciousness. The chief significance of contusions lies in the processes that they may initiate (i.e. oedema, hyperaemia and haemorrhage) and the consequences of these secondary events (see below).

Secondary Brain Damage

Raised intracranial pressure

Following head injury several different processes can occur, each of which has the common result of producing an expanding intracranial lesion. As these lesions increase in size there is initially only a slight increase in intracranial pressure (ICP) but there is subsequently a rapid increase (Figure 18.1). This concept of progression from a phase of 'compensation' for the presence of a mass lesion to one of 'decompensation' has been recognized for many years. Four stages of evolution were described by Duret in 1878 and more recently Langfitt (1969, 1978) made an experimental analogue of these. During the first stage, spatial compensation, there is only a minimal increase in intracranial pressure.

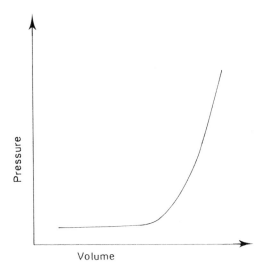

Figure 18.1. Changes in intracranial pressure with an intracranial expanding lesion. The initial phase of compensation is followed by a rapid rise in pressure even in response to small increments of volume.

Decompensation occurs in three successive phases. Initially ICP rises, even in response to small additions to the expanding lesion. Subsequently spontaneous waves of raised ICP occur, cerebral function becomes impaired and the cerebral circulation is unresponsive to physiological stimuli. In the final phase these changes become irreversible. In general the effects of raised ICP on brain function are mediated by changes in cerebral blood flow and by the interplay between ICP and brain shift with herniation. Brain herniations conform to a number of fairly predictable patterns, each associated with characteristic pathological findings and clinical syndromes (Adams, 1975; Plum and Posner, 1972).

Acute Traumatic Intracranial Haematomas

Traumatic intracranial haematomas developed in only approximately 1% of patients with head injury who were admitted to a Glasgow hospital (Galbraith, 1976). They are, however, the most important mechanism by which an initial apparently trivial injury can become life-threatening. Delay in diagnosis or treatment of an intracranial haematoma was the commonest 'preventable' factor in a series of patients with head injury who talked and yet subsequently died (Rose *et al.*, 1977).

Intracranial haematomas are usually classified as extradural, subdural or intracerebral although a clear distinction between wholly subdural and various forms of intracerebral haematomas with swelling, including 'burst lobes', can be difficult. Intradural haematomas are more common in the elderly.

Extradural haematoma

In the Western Infirmary, Glasgow an extradural haematoma (EDH) developed in only 0.2% of patients admited with head injury but was found in from 5 to 10% of fatal blunt head injuries (Adams, 1975; Maloney and Whatmore, 1969). Haemorrhage takes place from meningeal vessels and as the haematoma develops it gradually strips the dura from the skull to form an ovoid mass that progressively indents the adjacent brain. Overall a skull fracture is present in 85% of patients who develop an EDH (Jamieson and Yelland, 1968) and of those who do not have a skull fracture over 90% are under 30 years of age (Galbraith, 1973). In Galbraith's series all cases over 50 years of age had a skull fracture. The commonest site for an EDH is the temporal region but they also occur in the frontal, parietal and occipital regions and within the posterior fossa. Occasionally they can be bilateral.

Acute subdural haematoma (SDH)

Acute subdural haematomas are usually attributed to the rupture of small vessels which bridge the subdural space. Other sources are ruptured vessels at the site of contusions or tears in small branches of the cerebral arteries, particularly the middle cerebral artery. In contrast to the localized nature of EDH, haemorrhage into the subdural space tends to spread diffusely over the hemispheres and is more frequently bilateral. Large acute subdural haematomas are usually associated with severe contusions of the underlying brain, and it is this association with severe underlying primary brain damage which is the reason for the relatively poor prognosis for those with acute subdural haematoma.

Chronic subdural haematoma

In contrast to the acute haematoma, when the effects of secondary brain compression are usually inextricably mixed with the effects of primary brain damage, chronic subdural haematoma represents almost pure brain compression and distortion. The primary subdural bleeding usually occurs following trivial head injury but may also be due to so-called spontaneous bleeding. In this latter case it is thought to be due largely to vascular anomalies, vascular diseases or coagulation disturbances (Loew and Kivelitz, 1976).

As the fluid haematoma becomes larger it is bounded by a membrane which attaches to the dura and arachnoid and which gradually thickens. The gradual expansion of the haematoma is thought to be due to either repeated small haemorrhages or to osmotic changes within the haematoma fluid.

It should be noted that in adults the occurrence of chronic SDH is limited almost exclusively to geriatric patients or alcoholics with brain atrophy. The presence of cerebral atrophy is thought to explain the apparently paradoxical phenomenon of relatively low ICP with severe brain shift frequently found in patients with chronic SDH (Bucy and Oberhill, 1968; Munro, 1942). Because of the absence of significant underlying brain damage the prognosis for chronic SDH is significantly better than for those with acute haematomas.

Acute intracerebral haematoma (ICH)

Intracerebral haematomas may be single or multiple and act as rapidly expanding lesions. They are found in approximately 40% of fatal head injuries. Occasionally the development of an ICH appears to be delayed for several days but it is not clear to what extent this is due to a slowly expanding haematoma or to an actual delay in the occurrence of the haemorrhage. Most ICHs are related to contusions of the brain and occur principally therefore in the subfrontal or temporal regions. They also occur, however, deep within the hemispheres where they are presumably due to shearing strains affecting small blood vessels at the time of impact (Adams, 1975).

Ischaemic Brain Damage

It has long been recognized that focal ischaemic brain damage, ranging from small foci of ischaemic necrosis to frank infarction, is not uncommon in patients dying as a result of blunt head injury. Jellinger and Seitelberger (1970) have emphasized the occurrence of brain ischaemia in those patients who remain severely disabled or vegetative for long periods after head injury, and subsequently Graham and Adams placed the incidence of post-traumatic brain ischaemia in better perspective by their detailed study of more than 150 consecutive fatal head injuries (Graham and Adams, 1971; Graham *et al.*, 1978). Even after diffuse neocortical necrosis resulting from known episodes of cardiac arrest or status epilepticus, infarctions associated with contusion, infarction in the cortex supplied by the posterior cerebral artery in patients with raised ICP, and necrosis attributable to fat embolism has been excluded, the incidence of ischaemic brain damage was still found to be unexpectedly high. Ischaemic foci were seen in the cerebral cortex in 46% of cases. In more than half of these the ischaemic lesions were found in arterial boundary zones but in the remainder the cortical ischaemia lay squarely in the territory of supply of a major intracranial artery. Ischaemic foci were even more common in the basal ganglia and in the hippocampus (80%). After an extensive search for causal factors these authors were unable to incriminate any specific factor which had special significance in the aetiology of these ischaemic lesions. The correlation between angiographic findings and post-traumatic ischaemia has been reported (Macpherson and Graham, 1978).

Systemic Insults to the Injured Brain

Miller *et al.* (1978) reported that of 100 consecutive patients with severe head injury who arrived at a major trauma centre in the USA, 44% had potentially serious systemic disorders. The particular abnormalities included arterial hypotension (13%), anaemia (12%) and hypocarbia (4%), which were almost exclusively associated with multiple injuries, and hypoxia (30%) including several patients with brain injury alone. These systemic insults to an already damaged brain were associated with an increase in mortality and morbidity. Gentleman and Jennett (1981) reported similar findings in a recent British survey.

Infection

Meningitis is a well-recognized complication of head injury and is usually due to the spread of micro-organisms through an open fracture of the calvarium or a fracture of the base of the skull into the air sinuses or middle ear/mastoid. It may also occur following penetrating injury and following craniotomy or ventricular puncture for ICP monitoring or CSF drainage.

Meningitis is one of the most devastating secondary insults that can affect the patient with a severe head injury (Miller, 1976). In unconscious patients the diagnosis is often not made until the patient is already moribund, so the mortality rate continues to be high, despite the use of antibiotics. The later complications of meningitis include an increased risk of epilepsy and impairment of CSF absorption resulting in post-traumatic hydrocephalus.

Seizures

Poorly controlled epilepsy was the second most common avoidable factor contributing to death after head injury found by Rose *et al.* (1977). Secondary hypoxic and ischaemic damage was found at necropsy. Epilepsy also contributed to delay in treating intracranial haematomas because deterioration was sometimes attributed to the post-ictal state.

CLINICAL ASSESSMENT OF HEAD INJURED PATIENT

History

It behoves the doctor to seek as much information as possible concerning the precise time and mechanism of injury. A history of the patient's vital signs and neurological deficits obtained at the scene of the accident and during transport to hospital should always be sought. This information has proved to be practically obtainable (Teasdale and Jennett, 1976).

Clinical Examination

Despite its limitations, the neurological examination remains the single most comprehensive process in the diagnostic evaluation of the patient with head injury, providing a rapidly available index of generalized and focal dysfunction of the nervous system. The depth of the neurological examination will vary according to the type and degree of brain injury. In patients who are alert the initial examination is as thorough as possible, while the scope of the first examination in patients with impaired consciousness is limited. Therefore in patients with altered consciousness, emphasis is given to certain critical aspects of the examination while subsequent examinations are appropriately expanded. The importance of serial examinations cannot be over-emphasized. In the initial examination Teasdale stresses that it is more important to determine if brain damage is lateralized to one or other cerebral hemisphere and whether signs of brain stem dysfunction are present, than to debate the direction of the plantar responses (Teasdale, 1978).

Assessment of impaired consciousness

A continuum of altered consciousness is recognized between the fully alert and the deeply comatose patient (Plum and Posner, 1972). An objective measure of this continuum is a major difficulty in the evaluation of patients with head injury. Recently the need for widely applicable, clearly defined terminology and methods to describe the neurological state of the patient was appreciated. In response to this, Teasdale and Jennett described the Glasgow Coma Scale (GCS) in 1974 (Teasdale and Jennett, 1974). This method of grading the level of consciousness has proved particularly useful and has achieved widespread acceptance. The original authors have confirmed that the simplicity of the chosen terms affords a consistent and accurate assessment when performed by nurses and junior doctors. Langfitt (1978) suggested that the GCS be used in all evaluations of coma in head injured patients.

The GCS incorporates three features which are independently observed: eye opening; best motor response and verbal response. The Glasgow Coma Score is derived by giving the response on each component of the scale a number higher by one than the less responsive grade below it. This allows a minimum score of 3 and a maximum score of 15. Coma is defined as a score of 8 or less.

Other neurological observations

The initial neurological assessment must not be limited to the parameters of unconsciousness in the GCS. Of equal importance is the assessment of vital signs, pupillary response, eye movements and ocular reflexes. Furthermore the pattern of response in all four limbs is of diagnostic and prognostic significance and should be recorded separately from the assessment of the responsiveness of the brain as a whole. When these features are coupled with the GCS a dependable and rapid clinical assessment of the patient's overall neurological status is obtained.

General examination

It must be realized that one-third of head injuries admitted to hospital have another significant injury. This is particularly common in road accidents, both to vehicle occupants and to pedestrians. A careful search must therefore be made for possible associated injuries and these must be treated and any resultant systemic complications corrected.

INITIAL MANAGEMENT AND TREATMENT

It is not within the remit of this chapter to describe in any detail the medical or surgical treatment of the various lesions which can result from cranio-cerebral trauma. Rather its aim is to present a rational approach to head injuries in the elderly.

The initial management of the head injured patient is largely dictated by the condition when first seen. At times immediate resuscitation may have to take precedence over formal assessment, e.g. clearing the airway, ensuring adequate ventilation or restoring an adequate circulating blood volume. Following this, an appropriate clinical neurological assessment, as outlined above, is made. Consideration must also be given to the possible influence of alcohol or other drugs on the patient's condition but one must guard against overestimating their ability to produce a low level of responsiveness.

Following this initial assessment and resuscitation, three questions commonly require to be answered:

(1) Which patient should have a skull X-ray performed?
(2) Which patient should be admitted for observation?
(3) Which patient requires neurosurgical consultation?

No specific guidelines for geriatric patients are available. Guidelines have, however, recently been proposed for the adult population in general (Table 18.1) (*British Medical Journal*, 1984) and are appropriate, with the proviso that in the elderly the indications for transfer for active neurosurgical management are inextricably linked to the effect of age on the ultimate outcome following head injury and the therefore expected prognosis in any particular case. This will be discussed in more detail in a later section.

INVESTIGATIONS

The advent of computed tomography in 1972 revolutionized the optimum investigation of head injured patients and presently the role of magnetic resonance imaging in the assessment of brain damage is being assessed. These facilities, however, will for the foreseeable future be available only in regional neurosurgical units, teaching hospitals and a small number of district general hospitals. Therefore, as trauma is no respecter of geography, many head injuries will continue to be managed, for a time at least, outside centres where these facilities are not available. Less sophisticated but more generally available radiological techniques therefore still retain their importance.

Skull X-ray

Three views are taken routinely: posteroanterior (PA), Towne's or half axial PA view, and lateral. Sometimes additional views are helpful, e.g. tangential views to assess the degree of depression of a fracture or submento-vertical views which show the base of the skull when a basal fracture is suspected. If the pineal gland is visible on the lateral view, it

TABLE 18.1   MANAGEMENT OF RECENT HEAD INJURY

A. Indications for skull X-ray examination
(1) Loss of consciousness or amnesia at any time
(2) Neurological symptoms or signs
(3) Cerebrospinal fluid or blood from nose or ear
(4) Suspected penetrating injury
(5) Scalp bruising or swelling

B. Indications for admission to a general hospital
(1) Confusion or any other depression of the level of consciousness at the time of examination
(2) Skull fracture
(3) Neurological symptoms or signs
(4) Difficulty in assessing the patient, e.g. alcohol, epilepsy or other medical condition
(5) Lack of responsible adult to supervise the patient; other social problems

C. Indications for consultation with a neurosurgeon
(1) Fractured skull with any of the following: confusion or worse impairment of consciousness; one or more epileptic fits or any other neurological symptoms or signs
(2) Coma continuing after resuscitation—even if no skull fracture
(3) Deterioration in level of consciousness
(4) Confusion or other neurological disturbances persisting for more than 8 hours, even if there is no skull fracture
(5) Depressed fracture of the skull vault
(6) Suspected fracture of base of skull (cerebrospinal fluid rhinorrhoea or otorrhoea, bilateral orbital haematoma, mastoid haematoma or evidence of penetrating type of injury such as spike or gunshot)

Reproduced from *British Medical Journal* (1984), with permission.

should be sought in both PA and Towne's views because displacement from its normal midline position may be a vital clue to the presence of a mass lesion. However, a centrally placed pineal gland does not exclude a sizeable subfrontal or subtemporal clot. Fractures running into the basal air sinuses can sometimes be seen on the three views routinely obtained but they can also be suspected from the presence of fluid in an air sinus or intracranial air seen on the brow up lateral view.

Significance of a Skull Fracture

A number of patients who are fully alert, some of whom have never been unconscious, have a fracture of the skull vault. In these, the presence of a skull fracture significantly increases the risk of intracranial haematoma to about one in thirty. The risk of an intracranial haematoma in patients with a skull fracture who are not fully orientated is one in four. Focal signs or an epileptic fit in a patient with skull fracture also indicate a high risk. Patients in coma have a one in four risk of developing an intracranial haematoma even if they do not have a skull fracture.

In contrast, a patient without a skull fracture who is fully orientated has a less than one in a thousand risk of developing an intracranial haematoma. A patient who is confused but without a skull fracture has a one in a hundred risk.

The above statistics are derived from data obtained from an entire adult population. The author is unaware of any equivalent data which pertain only to geriatric patients although it seems probable that the trends are similar in this age group.

Radio-isotope Imaging

Isotope scanning is seldom used in the acute phase of head injury because any associated skull or scalp lesion will also show as an area of high activity at this stage. The greatest use of isotope scanning following head injury is in the detection of chronic subdural haematomas which are most common in the elderly. It is the capsule of the haematoma which is probably responsible for the area of high activity seen on the scan and therefore false negative scans are common only in patients studied within 10 days of injury. After this period 91% of scans are positive.

Although computed tomography is superior in detecting an acute intracranial haematoma when the suspicion is of a chronic subdural haematoma, the two techniques are comparable in their detection rate (Cornell *et al.*, 1978). It is a rapid non-invasive technique without associated morbidity or mortality.

X-Rays of Cervical Spine

The occurrence of cervical spine injury in patients who have suffered a significant head injury is relatively common (Davis *et al.*, 1971) and it has been suggested that in older age groups less severe injuries to the cervical spine may produce spinal cord damage because of pre-existing arthritic changes (Kalsbeek *et al.*, 1980). An anteroposterior and lateral X-ray of the cervical spine is therefore mandatory in all cases of significant head injury. Care must be taken to ensure that all seven cervical vertebrae and the first thoracic vertebra are visualized.

SPECIALIZED NEURORADIOLOGICAL STUDIES (see also Chapter 6)

CT Scanning

Introduced by Hounsfield and Ambrose in 1972, computed tomography (CT) revolutionized the diagnostic evaluation of traumatic intracranial lesions (Ambrose, 1973; Hounsfield, 1973). The general principles of this technique have been discussed elsewhere (Ter-Pogassian, 1977).

The value of CT in the management of head injuries was reported by French and Dublin (1977). CT scanning revealed all cases of extradural haematoma as well as subdural lesions of greater or lesser density than brain tissue. Isodense subdural haematomas were more difficult to diagnose, especially when these were bilateral. Ipsilateral ventricular compression with contralateral ventricular dilatation should always raise the suspicion of an isodense extracerebral mass. It was possible to assess readily what proportion of a parenchymal lesion was intracerebral haematoma, contusion or oedema thereby allowing precise surgical decisions. Overall 51% of patients scanned had abnormal findings and the incidence of demonstrated pathological lesions increased with deteriorating neurological state. Serial scanning was found to be extremely useful in defining the development of new lesions or deterioration in known lesions. With greater experience of this investigative technique it has been possible to correlate CT scan appearances with intracranial pressure, clinical state and prognosis (Lipper *et al.*, 1985; Teasdale *et al.*, 1984).

Others

Since the advent of CT scanning, cerebral angiography and ventriculography are rarely used in the assessment of the head injured patient. Magnetic resonance imaging is presently being evaluated and is likely to prove a significant advance even on CT scanning. However, for the foreseeable future, its availability will be restricted to relatively few regional units.

FACTORS AFFECTING PROGNOSIS

Age

Elderly patients have reduced cerebral reserve and so are less able to withstand even a minor injury. When the effect of such an injury is added to pre-existing impairments, the resulting cognitive impairment may be severe enough to preclude discharge or independent living (Roy *et al.*, 1986).

Teasdale *et al.* (1979) reported a series of patients who had been in coma for a period of at least 6 hours following head injury. Coma was defined as 'not opening eyes, not uttering any recognisable words and not obeying commands'. Mortality was found to increase exponentially with increasing age (Figure 18.2). In a similar series reported by Jennett and colleagues (1976) 88% of those over 60 years of age either died or remained in a persistent vegetative state. Only 5% made a good recovery or were left with a moderate residual disability. This profound effect of age on outcome is independent of state of responsiveness, eye movement and pupil reactions.

For patients with an intracranial haematoma the worse outcome of older patients is more noticeable in cases of extradural haematoma (Jamieson and Yelland, 1968). Age had little effect on outcome from intradural haematoma below the age of 60 years (<60 years, mortality 38%; >60 years, mortality 65%) (Jamieson and Yelland, 1972a, 1972b; Teasdale and Galbraith, 1981), but above 60 years the mortality continues to rise with age. Klun and Fettich (1979) reported a mortality of 71% for patients with acute subdural haematoma who were in their seventh decade. This had risen to 81% for those in their eighth decade (Klun and Fettich, 1979).

Level of Responsiveness

It is now accepted that the most important factor in determining prognosis following head injury is the

n = 44 46 94 63 57 46 39 49 43 43 38 39 32 16 19

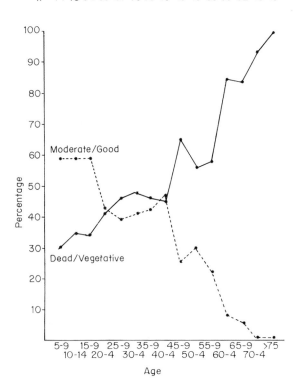

Figure 18.2. Effect of age on outcome following severe head injury in adults. (*Reproduced from Jennett and Teasdale (1981) with permission.*)

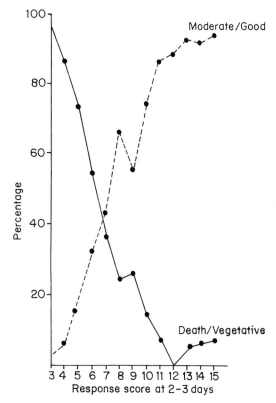

Figure 18.3. Outcome at 6 months for patients with different Glasgow Coma Scores—best in 2-3 day epoch. (*Reproduced from Jennett and Teasdale (1981) with permission.*)

degree of brain damage, which is reflected in the level of impaired responsiveness (Jennett *et al.*, 1979b). This is graphically represented in Figure 18.3. These data were obtained from adults of all age groups (Jennett and Teasdale, 1981).

Other Factors

Other factors found to be strongly related to outcome include pupil reaction, eye movements and motor response pattern (Jennett *et al.*, 1979b). Outcome is better in relation to a given level of brain dysfunction when this was the patient's worst state during a given time epoch, than if it were the best level of responsiveness. All of these factors interact adversely with increasing age in determining the final outcome.

'AVOIDABLE FACTORS' CONTRIBUTING TO DEATH AFTER HEAD INJURY

Rose *et al.* (1977) reviewed 116 patients known to have talked before dying after head injury to discover factors which had contributed to death but which might have been avoided. All patients had been admitted to a neurosurgical unit and had a neuropathological examination. One or more avoidable factors were identified in 74% of patients and were judged to have certainly contributed to death in 54%. The most common avoidable factor was delay in the treatment of an intracranial haematoma; others included poorly controlled epilepsy, meningitis, hypoxia and hypotension.

Galbraith (1976) made a detailed analysis of the causes of misdiagnosis and delayed diagnosis in traumatic intracranial haematoma. He points out that the classically described course of a patient developing a traumatic intracranial haematoma (i.e. an initial period of altered consciousness, followed by a lucid interval, after which the conscious level again begins to deteriorate, the ipsilateral pupil becomes fixed and dilated and a contralateral hemiparesis develops) occurs in only a small minority of patients. More commonly there is an altered level of responsiveness present from the time of injury with progressive deterioration. Failure to appreciate this is one reason why there is sometimes a delay in recognizing intracranial haematoma.

In two-thirds of cases the delay was due to an erroneous diagnosis, either of cerebrovascular accident or of alcohol intoxication. In the patient suspected of having a cerebrovascular accident the detection of a skull fracture is the best clue to management. All but four of 33 patients with traumatic haematomas whose condition was incorrectly diagnosed as a vascular accident had a skull fracture. In contrast, in a retrospective study of 1000 consecutive cases with a cerebrovascular accident, 132 had skull X-rays performed and not one had a skull fracture. Therefore if a patient suspected of having had a cerebrovascular accident has a skull fracture his condition is more likely to be due to a traumatic intracranial haematoma (Galbraith, 1976). In a separate publication Galbraith points out that if the blood alcohol level is less than 200 $\mu g/$ 100 ml then any alteration in consciousness is unlikely to be due to alcohol alone (Galbraith *et al.*, 1976).

REHABILITATION

Doctors dealing with head injured patients are frequently apt to underestimate the extent of the difficulties encountered by patients after they are discharged from the surgical ward. The rehabilitation needs of the head injured patient have been discussed by Lewin (1970). Because rehabilitation is an integral part of geriatric medicine it is not surprising that rehabilitation facilities in many areas are better for the elderly than for younger patients.

In the early post-injury period the main objective is to prevent complications and to give a realistic opinion as to prognosis so that both the patient and

his family can be prepared for the likely time course and degree of recovery. Later every effort should be made to promote recovery by specific graded activities. After approximately a 6 month interval when neurological recovery has largely been completed, an overall assessment of the patient's disabilities and capabilities should be performed and reasonable efforts made to help with the ultimate physical, mental and social adjustments which may be necessary.

CONCLUSIONS

The presently outlined management of the elderly head injured patient should be seen in the light of present day knowledge, facilities and experience. As the number of elderly patients in the population increases and our knowledge and expertise improve these guidelines will require modification and it is inevitable that more elderly head injured patients will be accepted for active neurosurgical management. One must caution, however, against unrealistic expectations of dramatic changes in the near future.

REFERENCES

Adams, J.H. (1975). The neuropathology of head injuries. In: Vinken, P.J., and Bruyn, C.W. (eds) *Handbook of Clinical Neurology*, Vol. 23, pp. 35–65.

Adams, J.H., Mitchell, D.E., Graham, D.I., and Doyle, D. (1977). Diffuse brain damage of immediate impact type. *Brain*, **100**, 489–502.

Ambrose, J. (1973). Computerised transverse axial scanning (tomography) Part 2. Clinical approach. *Br. J. Radiol.*, **46**, 1023–46.

British Medical Journal (1984). Guidelines for initial management after head injury in adults: Suggestions from a group of neurosurgeons. *Br. Med. J.*, **i**, 983–5.

Bucy, P.C., and Oberhill, H.R. (1968). Subdural haematoma in adults. *Arizona Med.*, **25**, 186–9.

Cornell, S.H., Chiu, L.C., and Christie, J.H. (1978). Diagnosis of extracerebral fluid collections by computed tomography. *Am. J. Roentgenol.*, **131**, 107–10.

Davis, D., Bohlman, H., Walker, A.E., Russell, F., and Robinson, R. (1971). The pathological findings in fatal cranio-spinal injuries. *J. Neurosurg.*, **34**, 603–13.

Duret, H. (1878). Études expérimentales et clinique sur les traumatismes cérébaux. 86ffi 6 8(76ffi (1920), Traumatismes Cranio-cérébaux, 2 Alcan, Paris.

Field, J.H. (1976). *Epidemiology of Head Injuries in England & Wales*, H.M.S.O., London.

French, B.N., and Dublin, A.B. (1977). The value of computerised tomography in the management of 1000 consecutive head injuries. *Surg. Neurol.*, **7**, 171–83.

Galbraith, S. (1973). Age distribution of extradural haemorrhage without skull fracture. *Lancet*, **i**, 1217–18.

Galbraith, S. (1976). Misdiagnosis and delayed diagnosis in traumatic intracranial haematoma. *Br. Med. J.*, **i**, 1438–9.

Galbraith, S. (1978). Traumatic intracranial haematoma. *Scott. Med. J.*, **23**(1), 95.

Galbraith, S. (1987). Head injuries in the elderly. Leading article. *Br. Med. J.*, **294**, 325.

Galbraith, S., Murray, W.R., Patel, A.R., and Kwill-Jones, R. (1976). The relationship between alcohol and head injury and its effect on the conscious level. *Br. J. Surg.*, **63**, 128–30.

Gentleman, D., and Jennett, B. (1981). Hazards of inter-hospital transfer of comatose head injured patients. *Lancet*, **ii**, 853–5.

Graham, D.I., and Adams, J.H. (1971). Ischaemic brain damage in fatal head injuries. *Lancet*, **i**, 265–6.

Graham, D.I., Adams, J.H., and Doyle, D. (1978). Ischaemic brain damage in fatal non-missile head injuries. *J. Neurol. Sci.*, **39**, 213–34.

Hounsfield, G.N. (1973). Computerised transverse axial scanning (tomography): Part I. Description of system. *Br. J. Radiol.*, **46**, 1016–22.

Jamieson, K.G., and Yelland, J.D.N. (1968). Extradural haematoma. Report of 167 cases. *J. Neurosurg.*, **29**, 13–23.

Jamieson, K.G., and Yelland, J.D.N. (1972a). Surgically treated traumatic subdural haematomas. *J. Neurosurg.*, **37**, 137–49.

Jamieson, K.G., and Yelland, J.D.N. (1972b). Traumatic haematoma. Report of 63 surgically treated cases. *J. Neurosurg.*, **37**, 528–32.

Jeffreys, R.V., and Azzam, N.I. (1979). Experiences with head injuries in a Regional Neurosurgical Unit. *Br. J. Surg.*, **66**, 562–4.

Jellinger, K., and Seitelberger, G. (1970). Protracted post-traumatic encephalopathy: pathology, pathogenesis and clinical implications. *J. Neurol. Sci.*, **10**, 51–94.

Jennett, B. (1980). Skull X-rays after recent head injury. *Clin. Radiol.*, **31**, 463–9.

Jennett, B., and Teasdale, G. (1981). *Management of Head Injuries*, F.A. Davis, Philadelphia.

Jennett, B., Teasdale, G., Braakman, R. et al. (1976). Predicting outcome in individual patients after severe head injury. *Lancet*, **i**, 1031–4.

Jennett, B., Murray, A., Carlin, J. et al. (1979a). Head injuries in three Scottish neurosurgical units. *Br. Med. J.*, **ii**, 955–8.

Jennett, B., Teasdale, G., Braakman, R. et al. (1979b). Prognosis of patients with severe head injury. *Neurosurgery*, **4**, 283–9.

Kalsbeek, W.D., McLaurin, R.L., Harris, B.S.H., and

Miller, J.D. (1980). The national head and spinal cord injury survey—Major findings. *J. Neurosurg.*, **53**, 519–31.

Klun, B., and Fettich, M. (1979). Factors determining prognosis in acute subdural haematoma. *Acta Neurochir.*, Suppl. 28, 134–6.

Lancet (1977). Head injuries in Scottish hospitals: Scottish head injury management study. *Lancet*, **ii**, 696–8.

Langfitt, T.W. (1969). Increased intracranial pressure. *Clin. Neurosurg.*, **16**, 436.

Langfitt, T.W. (1978). Measuring the outcome from head injuries. *J. Neurosurg.*, **48**, 673–8.

Lewin, W. (1970). Rehabilitation needs of the brain injured patient. *Proc. Roy. Soc. Med.*, **63**, 28–32.

Lipper, M.H., Kishore, P.R.S., Enas, G.G. et al. (1985). Computed tomography in the prediction of outcome in head injury. *A.J.N.R.*, **6**, 7–10.

Loew, F., and Kivelitz, R. (1976). Chronic subdural haematomas. In: Vinken, P.J., and Bruyn, G.W. (eds.) *Handbook of Clinical Neurology*, Vol. 24, pp. 297–327.

Macpherson, P., and Graham, D.I. (1978). Correlation between angiographic findings and the ischemia of head injury. *J. Neurol. Neurosurg Psychiatry*, **41**, 122–7.

Maloney, S.F.J., and Whatmore, W.J. (1969). Clinical and pathological observations in fatal head injuries: five year survey of 173 cases. *Br. J. Surg.*, **56**, 23–31.

Miller, J.D. (1976). Infection after head injury. In: Vinken, P.J., and Bruyn, G.W. (eds.) *Handbook of Clinical Neurology*, Vol. 24, pp. 215–30.

Miller, J.D., Sweet, R.C., Narayan, R., and Becker, D.P. (1978). Early insults to the injured brain. *J.A.M.A.*, **240**, 439–42.

Mitchell, D.E., and Adams, J.H. (1973). Primary focal impact damage to the brain stem in blunt head injuries: does it exist? *Lancet*, **ii**, 215–18.

Munro, D. (1942). Cerebral subdural haematomas. A study of 310 verified cases. *N. Engl. J. Med.*, **227**, 87–95.

Office of Population Censuses and Surveys (1974). *Hospital Inpatient Enquiry for England and Wales*, H.M.S.O., London.

Plum, F., and Posner, J.B. (1972). *Diagnosis of Stupor and Coma*, Davis, Philadelphia.

Rose, J., Valtonen, S., and Jennett, B. (1977). Avoidable factors contributing to death after head injury. *Br. Med. J.*, **ii**, 615–18.

Roy, C.W., Pentland, B., and Miller, J.D. (1986). The causes and consequences of minor head injury in the elderly. *Injury*, **17**, 220–3.

Strang, I., MacMillan, R., and Jennett, B. (1978). Head injuries in accident and emergency departments at Scottish hospitals. *Injury*, **10**, 154–9.

Strich, S.J. (1956). Diffuse degeneration of the cerebral white matter in severe dementia following head injury. *J. Neurol. Neurosurg. Psychiatry*, **19**, 163–85.

Teasdale, G. (1978). Assessment of head injuries. *Scott. Med. J.*, **23**(1), 97.

Teasdale, G., and Galbraith, S. (1981). Acute traumatic intracranial haematomas. *Prog. Neurol. Surg.*, **10**, 252–90.

Teasdale, G., and Jennett, B. (1974). Assessment of coma and impaired consciousness. *Lancet*, **ii**, 81–4.

Teasdale, G., and Jennett, B. (1976). Assessment and prognosis of coma after head injury. *Acta. Neurochir. (Wien.)*, **34**, 45–55.

Teasdale, G., Skene, A., Parker, L., and Jennett, B. (1979).

Age and outcome of severe head injury. *Acta Neurochir.* Suppl. 28, 140–3.

Teasdale, E., Cardoso, E., Galbraith, S., and Teasdale, G. (1984). CT scan in severe diffuse head injury: Physiological and clinical correlations. *J. Neurol. Neurosurg. Psychiatry*, **47**, 600–3.

Ter-Pogassian, M.M. (1977). Computerised cranial tomography: Equipment and physics. *Semin. Roentgenol.*, **12**, 13–25.

The Clinical Neurology of Old Age
Edited by R. Tallis
© 1989 John Wiley & Sons Ltd

Chapter 19

Infectious Diseases of the Nervous System

Rachel Angus

Senior Registrar, Department of Geriatric Medicine, Northwick Park Hospital, Harrow, Middlesex, UK

BACTERIAL MENINGITIS

Bacterial meningitis is a rare disease in old age and is, even now, associated with a high mortality. In the pre-antibiotic era the mortality rate for all ages exceeded 90% and most survivors were neurologically devastated. Effective antibiotic treatment has reduced the overall mortality to about 10 to 20% but it remains between 44 and 77% for the elderly (Newton and Wilczynski, 1979; Finland and Barnes, 1977; Gorse *et al.*, 1984).

Factors contributing to increased mortality and morbidity in pneumococcal meningitis have been analysed (Ispahani, 1983; Bohr *et al.*, 1984). Co-existing illness was found to be the most important factor; but coma, confusion, fits, a CSF protein of more than 2.8 g/l and a CSF sugar of less than 0.8 mmol/l were also bad prognostic signs. In a recent British study (Davey *et al.*, 1982), 55% of the patients with pneumococcal meningitis had a significant history of conditions associated with impaired resistance to infection such as diabetes mellitus.

Delay in making the diagnosis in an elderly patient is probably the most important factor contributing to a poor prognosis.

Incidence

Data from the Communicable Diseases Surveillance Centre show that of a total number of 1447 cases of meningitis in England and Wales in 1975 4.5% were patients over 65 years (Newton and Wilczynski,

1979). Between 1975 and 1978 the number of cases of meningitis in the elderly has more than doubled. A similar increase has been noted in the USA (Fraser *et al.*, 1973). This rise is far more than can be accounted for by the increase in population of this age group and can therefore be explained by either a true rise in incidence or greater interest in diagnosis in elderly patients, or both.

Predisposing Factors and Bacteriology

The most common route of meningeal infection in the elderly is blood-borne from an extracranial source. Meningitis can also follow from bacterial seeding of the meninges by contagious spread from a pericranial focus of infection or direct inoculation of bacteria as a result of head trauma or neurosurgery. In some cases it is impossible to demonstrate a predisposing cause. The site of primary infection may sometimes be useful in indicating the causative organism (Table 19.1). Over half the cases of meningitis in the elderly are due to *Streptococcus pneumoniae*. *Neisseria meningitidis* and *Listeria monocytogenes* are less common but each occur in about 10% of cases (Newton and Wilczynski, 1979). Other pathogens including Gram-negative organisms, *Staphylococcus aureus* and *Mycobacterium tuberculosis* account for about 25% of cases. The distribution of organisms appears constant from year to year in most studies when hospital acquired infections, particularly immune suppressed patients, are included (Massanari, 1977).

TABLE 19.1   FACTORS PREDISPOSING TO MEN-
INGITIS IN THE ELDERLY RELATED TO ORGANISM
COMMONLY FOUND

Pneumonia Skull trauma Ear and sinus infection	*Streptococcus pneumoniae*
Neurosurgery Osteomyelitis Cellulitis	*Staphylococcus aureus*

Abdominal surgery
Urinary tract
    infection
Urinary tract
    instrumentation
Pressure ulcers
Neurosurgery
Osteomyelitis
Cellulitis
	Gram-negative organisms
	Anaerobes

Impaired immunity
    (malignant disease,
    steroid treatment,
    alcoholism,
    diabetes mellitus,
    etc.)
	Gram-negative organisms
	Listeria monocytogenes

Listeria monocytogenes infection typically occurs in the immunosuppressed patient with lymphoprolifer-ative disease and those on steroids. Epidemiological data suggest that age per se predisposes to *Listeria* infection in otherwise healthy elderly people. The source of infection in *Listeria* meningitis can often not be identified.

Meningitis caused by *Haemophilus influenzae* is extremely rare in the elderly (Eykyn *et al.*, 1974) and like *Neisseria meningitidis* it may present in an atypical manner.

Clinical Features

There is little difficulty in making the diagnosis when there is a short history of headache and fever with neck stiffness. The history may be as short as 1 to 3 days in pneumococcal meningitis with rapid deterio-ration. A longer history of up to 2 weeks would suggest infection with one of the less common organisms or *Listeria monocytogenes* or the progression of pneumococcal pneumonia to meningitis (Ander-

son, 1984). Presentation in the elderly patient is often non-specific with malaise and confusion. Many other common conditions such as cerebrovascular disease, toxic confusional states, or intoxication of drugs may be considered the cause of the illness.

Focal signs in the CNS are more common in elderly patients with meningitis than in younger patients (Lambert, 1983a). Patients with diabetes are particularly at risk from misdiagnosis because meningitis may induce diabetic ketoacidosis and diabetic ketoacidosis may mimic meningitis. The mortality of diabetics with meningitis is high (Anderson, 1974). Fever, although often absent in infective diseases of the elderly (Anderson, 1985), is almost always present in meningitis. Neck stiffness is an unreliable sign and may be attributed to cervical spondylosis (Puxty, 1983). However, it should be possible to flex the head at the atlanto-occipital joint in patients with cervical spondylosis and therefore complete rigidity should suggest meningitis or a subarachnoid haemorrhage (Coakley, 1981). The presence of focal neurological signs and cognitive defects may be misleading and be attributed to pre-existing disease such as cerebrovascular disease or to a fresh stroke. Progression of symptoms beyond 12 hours should make the clinician suspicious of a non-vascular disease including meningitis (Editorial, 1978a).

The optic fundi should be examined for evidence of raised intracranial pressure, choroidal tubercles or haemorrhages associated with bacterial endo-carditis. In suspected meningitis accompanied by focal neurological signs or coma, computed tomography (CT) should be considered before lumbar puncture. The presence of papilloedema makes CT mandatory and lumbar puncture contraindicated. The systemic features of meningococcal septicaemia may result in the clinical features of pericarditis, arrhythmias, ST depression on ECG and arthralgia. These may be mistaken for more common ischaemic heart disease or degenerative joint disease. Rashes, especially those due to antibiotics, are common in the elderly and should be differentiated from the petechial or maculopapular rash of meningococcal infection. A purpuric rash occasionally occurs in pneumococcal infection, and a diffuse pink macular rash can occur on the trunk in *Listeria* infection.

The key to early diagnosis of meningitis is a high index of suspicion in an ill patient with signs of infection and neurological deficit.

Investigation of Bacterial Meningitis

The principal investigations are lumbar puncture, blood culture and blood glucose estimation.

Lumbar puncture

There is no evidence to suggest that there are any CSF findings peculiar to the elderly either in normal circumstances or in meningitis. The combination of turbidity, pleocytosis, a raised protein and a low glucose is diagnostic. *Listeria monocytogenes* infection may give a lymphocytic predominance. The Gram-stained smear of centrifuged CSF deposit is vitally important since it may be the only indication of the infecting organism. *Listeria monocytogenes* is a small Gram-positive rod and has been mistaken for Gram-positive cocci. *Haemophilus influenzae* is sometimes difficult to identify due to Gram variability and pleomorphism (Eykyn *et al.*, 1974). Countercurrent immunoelectrophoresis sometimes indicates a bacterial antigen in the CSF when other tests are negative.

There is no evidence that incidental antibiotic therapy prior to admission to hospital affects prognosis although some laboratory findings may be altered (Ispahani, 1983).

Other bacteriological investigations

Blood culture may help in identifying a causal organism which may fail to grow in the CSF, particularly *Listeria monocytogenes*. Sputum and swabs from obvious sites of infection, e.g. ulcers or wounds, may be helpful.

Blood glucose

This should be estimated at the same time as CSF glucose, since diabetes precipitated by meningitis can cause the CSF glucose to be raised or apparently normal. If the cell count and protein level in the CSF are raised but the glucose concentration is normal, herpes simplex encephalitis should also be suspected.

Treatment of Pyogenic Meningitis— Antibiotics

Meningitis in the elderly is a medical emergency. Urgent, aggressive treatment should be started as soon as the basic investigations have been performed.

Since the most likely organisms in the elderly are *Streptococcus pneumoniae*, *Neisseria meningitidis* and *Listeria monocytogenes*, high dose intravenous benzylpenicillin 1.2–2.4 g (2–4 MU) 4 hourly should be given. Postoperative neurosurgical patients or those in whom Gram-negative meningitis is suspected should be given chloramphenicol 25 mg/kg 6 hourly intravenously. Later definitive treatment will be guided by the bacteriological results. Intrathecal antibiotic treatment is unnecessary and potentially dangerous in the common forms of meningitis.

Pneumococcal meningitis

Most pneumococci are still sensitive to penicillin and high dose intravenous benzylpenicillin should be continued for 7–10 days. Pneumococcal susceptibility to penicillin varies from area to area within Britain and minimal inhibiting concentrations should be determined for all CSF isolates of pneumococci. This is particularly important to patients who do not respond to penicillin treatment. Several of the third generation cephalosporins, including cefotaxime, have excellent in vitro activity against the pneumococcus and have good CSF penetration. However, benzylpenicillin remains the drug of choice for pneumococcal meningitis.

Patients allergic to penicillin can be treated effectively with chloramphenicol. Combinations of drugs are no longer used routinely.

Meningococcal meningitis

Sulphonamides are no longer used for initial treatment due to the increasing resistance of *Neisseria meningitidis*. The treatment of choice is intravenous benzylpenicillin 1.2–2.4 g (2–4 MU) 4 hourly. However, a long course of intravenous therapy can sometimes be abbreviated by using oral sulphadiazine, sulphadimidine, or sulphafurazole if the organism is sensitive.

Listeria monocytogenes meningitis

Treatment of *Listeria* meningitis with either penicillin or ampicillin is effective.

Gram-negative meningitis

Chloramphenicol is the initial treatment choice for *Haemophilus influenzae* meningitis since about 10% of isolates produce beta lactamase which inactivates ampicillin. Gram-negative meningitis due to organisms other than *Haemophilus influenzae* presents a difficult antibiotic choice. Ampicillin, chloramphenicol and gentamicin were the mainstays of treatment. However, the CSF penetration of aminoglycosides does not allow CSF concentrations adequate to kill bacteria if gentamicin is given systemically. Even lumbar intrathecal administration is unreliable in achieving effective levels. The third generation cephalosporins show promise in the treatment of Gram-negative meningitis. Moxalactam and cefotaxime both have excellent activity against many Gram-negative organisms and penetrate the CSF in bactericidal concentrations when given systemically (Lambert, 1983b; Beam, 1984).

Treatment of Pyogenic Meningitis—Other Aspects

Steroids have limited value since they are ineffective in reducing cerebral oedema secondary to infection and may render the blood–brain barrier less permeable to antimicrobial agents (Editorial, 1982).

Fits should be controlled with short-term anticonvulsants such as phenytoin. Phenobarbitone should be avoided because it may cloud the evaluation of the mental state.

Repeating lumbar puncture routinely to assess progress is not recommended since it may be harmful in generating further symptoms and encourages unnecessary changes in treatment (Lambert, 1983a). It should only be repeated if persistent infection is suspected.

CEREBRAL ABSCESS

The incidence of cerebral abscess is bimodally distributed. One peak occurs in the first two decades and the second in the two decades between 50 and 70 years (Brewer *et al.*, 1975). In 1981, for example, the Office of Population Censuses and Surveys for England and Wales recorded 43 deaths due to intracranial abscess (23 male, 20 female). This is probably an underestimate of the true incidence. In a group of 24 patients whose abscesses were diagnosed only at post-mortem examination, one-third were over 60 years and the ratio of men to women was 2:1.

Early diagnosis and treatment is extremely important because antibiotic response is more effective before capsule formation occurs round the abscess thus reducing the need for neurosurgery.

Predisposing Factors

Cerebral abscesses arise from blood-borne infection or local spread from infections arising from either outside the body, as in penetrating injuries or neurosurgery, or from inside such as dental or paranasal sinus infections. In 25% of cases the site of the original infection remains unknown. Nearly one-quarter of fatal cases of cerebral abscess have bacterial endocarditis (Brewer *et al.*, 1975).

Diagnosis of Cerebral Abscess

The predominant presenting features are those of an expanding intracerebral lesion with headache and focal signs rather than an infectious process (Brewer *et al.*, 1975). In the elderly the symptoms and signs may be attributed to other more common conditions and pre-existing diseases may cause further difficulty in diagnosis. Fever is frequently absent and the peripheral leucocyte count is frequently lower than 10 000 per mm^3. Many patients present with a major central nervous system deficit including hemiparesis, visual field defect, cerebellar syndrome or fits. The signs develop subacutely over 1 or 2 weeks but still may be mistaken for a cerebrovascular incident particularly when there is rapid development of oedema surrounding the abscess. Neck stiffness is present in about 50% of cases, due either to raised intracranial pressure or associated meningitis.

Lumbar puncture

Lumbar puncture should be avoided in patients with the features of cerebral abscess because of the risk of tentorial herniation. However, when CSF is examined it may be normal, show a leucocytosis or frank meningitis, but culture is rarely rewarding.

Computed Tomography

CT is helpful in diagnosis and assessment of response to treatment. An unenhanced scan shows only an area of hypoattenuation and the mass effect of the abscess. Contrast enhancement shows a ring around the abscess due to release of contrast into areas of increased vascular permeability surrounding the focus (Garvey, 1983). Instillation of radio-opaque material into the abscess cavity is obsolete because it interferes with subsequent CT scanning.

Management of Cerebral Abscess

Antibiotics and neurosurgery form the basis of management of cerebral abscess although the timing of neurosurgery is debated.

Antibiotic treatment

The microbiology of intracranial abscesses is complex and facultative anaerobes, obligate anaerobes and carbon dioxide dependent bacteria may be present. Multiple organisms are recovered from up to 60% of cases (Brewer *et al.*, 1975) and consequently combination antibiotic therapy will often be needed. The commonest organisms are streptococci; since most of these are penicillin sensitive, intravenous benzylpenicillin 1.2–2.4 g (2–4 MU) should be given 4 hourly. This is combined with systemic metronidazole to cover obligate anaerobes and chloramphenicol. Gram-negative organisms are often found in mixed cultures of post-traumatic or post-neurosurgical abscesses. In these cases gentamicin should be added or one of the third generation cephalosporins. If trauma or osteomyelitis is thought to be the cause of the abscess, the treatment should include an anti-staphylococcal drug. Treatment should continue for at least 6 weeks.

Neurosurgery

Some neurosurgeons recommend primary excision of the abscess followed by antibiotics (Garvey, 1983). Others favour simple aspiration and antibiotics except in cerebellar abscesses (Editorial, 1978b). Once abscess formation has occurred, surgical intervention is the only definitive method for eradicating infection inaccessible to antibiotics and for preventing the pressure-related complications of brain abscess.

Anticonvulsants

Anticonvulsants are prescribed routinely because the risk of fits is high not only during the illness, but also as a later complication. They should be continued for at least 5 years.

Steroids

Dexamethasone may be used to control cerebral oedema but the use of steroids remains controversial because of their adverse effect on the access of antibiotics to the site of infection.

TUBERCULOUS MENINGITIS (TBM)

Formerly a complication of primary tuberculosis in infancy and childhood, TBM is now seen in adults as a result of reactivated infection. It is less often a part of miliary disease and more commonly a reactivation and rupture of a caseous focus in the meninges, cerebral or spinal tissue. The subsequent features depend on the inflammatory reaction and arteritis resulting in ischaemia and infarction.

Incidence and Mortality

The overall incidence of TBM in England and Wales is 30 cases per year, but less than 10% of these are elderly (Kennedy and Fallon, 1979). The mortality rate is high and is at least partly due to delay in diagnosis and presence of underlying disease (Fallon and Kennedy, 1981). TBM is more common in Asians and language difficulties may add to the diagnostic problem. It also occurs in Caucasians especially where there is a history of tuberculosis contact (Traub et al., 1984). A Scottish study found over half of the cases had close contact with tuberculosis (Kennedy and Fallon, 1979). The contacts in 21% of these were receiving or had recently received treatment and 25% were regarded as cured.

Clinical Features

The clinical presentation is of a subacute meningitis with symptoms of tuberculous toxaemia. Initially the symptoms are non-specific with general malaise, low grade fever, anorexia, vague headaches and muscle pains. The elderly patient may have exhibited a toxic confusional state with fluctuating confusion, personality change and drowsiness. After a few weeks, definite neurological features develop, including persistent headache, neck stiffness, oculomotor palsies, hemiparesis and sometimes tremor and involuntary movements. Choroidal tubercles are seen only as part of miliary disease. Progressive coma, multiple cranial nerve palsies and hemiplegia are associated with a poor prognosis.

Investigation

Lumbar puncture

Absolute confirmation of TBM depends on the identification of *Mycobacterium tuberculosis* in the CSF, although this is achieved only in under 40% of initial specimens (Fallon and Kennedy, 1981). The cell count rises to $400/mm^3$, mainly lymphocytes, and the protein concentration rises to 0.8–4.0 g/l. The glucose level falls, sometimes to zero. Proven cases of TBM with tubercle bacilli in the CSF have, however, been associated with normal CSF findings, especially in patients who are severely ill, on steroids or those with impaired immunological function. The CSF 48 hours later has shown the usual abnormalities. Consequently, when clinical suspicion is high, lumbar puncture should be repeated 24 hours after a normal result.

Other investigations

A chest X-ray may give useful information, though miliary changes are found in only about 40% of cases

(Kennedy and Fallon, 1979). The peripheral leucocyte count and ESR may be normal in elderly patients. The tuberculin reaction may be negative. A history of past immunization with BCG vaccine does not preclude the diagnosis of TBM.

Treatment of TBM

Chemotherapy

Four antituberculous drugs should be given initially until sensitivities are available. Only isoniazid, ethionamide and pyrazinamide penetrate non-inflamed meninges effectively. Rifampicin, ethambutol and systemically administered streptomycin penetrate only if the meninges are inflamed in the first 4 to 6 weeks of illness. Intramuscular streptomycin 1 g daily is given with oral isoniazid 300–600 mg daily, rifampicin 600 mg daily and pyrazinamide 40 mg/kg daily. Intrathecal use of streptomycin is nowadays normally omitted. Chemotherapy is continued for 18–24 months since there is no evidence that shorter courses are both safe and effective for TBM in the elderly.

If a positive bacteriological diagnosis of TBM cannot be made and the possibility of pyogenic meningitis remains, a severely ill patient should be treated with penicillin in addition to the full antituberculous regimen until the diagnosis is clarified.

The problem of drug compliance in the elderly is well known and close supervision is required to prevent development of resistant organisms. Toxic effects are also more common in the elderly, particularly liver toxicity with rifampicin and isoniazid (Kennedy and Fallon, 1979). Renal insufficiency may result in higher than expected levels of ethambutol, thus potentiating the development of optic neuritis. Ototoxicity is more likely to occur with streptomycin in renal failure. Isoniazid interferes with the metabolism of other drugs such as phenytoin which may be needed to control fits. Serum levels of phenytoin should be monitored regularly.

Steroids

There have been no properly controlled trials of steroids in TBM (Gordon and Parsons, 1972).

Dexamethasone is probably justified in very ill patients, those with cerebral oedema, adrenal failure or severe drug reactions and in those suspected of developing hydrocephalus or spinal block. Steroids complicate management by increasing the risk of secondary infection and electrolyte disturbance and diminishing drug penetration through the blood–brain barrier.

Neurosurgery

This can be life-saving in patients who have pronounced cerebral oedema (Fallon and Kennedy, 1981).

INTRACRANIAL TUBERCULOMA

Tuberculomas are usually single and behave as space-occupying lesions. A minority develop in the course of TBM even during antituberculous treatment (Lees *et al.*, 1980). A high proportion of patients are Asian (Loizou and Anderson, 1982). Diagnosis may be difficult in the absence of fever and malaise, but a past history of tuberculosis, contact with it or evidence of tuberculosis outside the CNS is helpful. Nearly 70% of cases, however, have a normal chest X-ray. Computed tomography has been a major advance in the diagnosis and management of intracranial tuberculoma (Loizou and Anderson, 1982). Treatment is similar to that of tuberculous meningitis. A trial of antituberculous therapy should be given without biopsy confirmation of the diagnosis in those patients where there is very high clinical suspicion. Improvement in clinical and CT features can be monitored and avoids the need for surgery, which is then reserved for patients who do not respond to medical treatment.

HERPES SIMPLEX VIRUS (HSV) ENCEPHALITIS

Herpes simplex virus is the one most commonly isolated from cases of sporadic severe encephalitis. It is important to diagnose HSV encephalitis not only because a non-toxic and effective treatment is available but also because treatment of the conditions it may mimic (cerebral tumour, cerebral abscess, tuberculous meningitis) is different.

TABLE 19.2 CLINICAL FINDINGS IN 112 BRAIN BIOPSY OR AUTOPSY POSITIVE PATIENTS WITH HSV ENCEPHALITIS

	Percentage
CSF pleocytosis	97
Fever	97
Alteration of consciousness	90
Focal neurological signs	90
Headache	81
Dysphasia	76
Personality change	71
Seizures	38
Memory loss	24

From Whitely *et al.* (1982).

HSV encephalitis has an incidence of one case per million per year and occurs at all ages (Kennedy, 1984). The mortality rate of HSV encephalitis treated with acyclovir is about 19% (Skoldenberg *et al.*, 1984).

Clinical Features

HSV encephalitis is almost always localized to the orbitofrontal and temporal lobes which show haemorrhagic necrosis, often unilateral. As a result of this, focal neurological signs and fits are common (Table 19.2). The patient may present with a short history of psychological symptoms of personality change, a speech disturbance or loss of memory, suggesting a psychiatric illness. Focal neurological signs, headache or signs of raised intracranial pressure may mimic a cerebral tumour or abscess or tuberculous meningitis (Whitely *et al.*, 1982). The illness is usually severe and brain oedema is the most common cause of death. Coma and focal signs are associated with a poor prognosis.

Concomitant or preceding herpetic skin lesions are found with only the same frequency in patients with HSV encephalitis as in the general population (Whitely *et al.*, 1982).

Investigation

Lumbar CSF

Examination of the CSF is more important to

exclude other conditions in the differential diagnosis than to make a definitive diagnosis of HSV encephalitis. There is a variable lymphocytosis and there may be a large number of red cells. The CSF may be normal.

A specific radioimmunoassay for serum and CSF HSV antibodies has been described (Klapper *et al.*, 1981) but information from such tests would provide only a retrospective diagnosis after antiviral treatment had been started.

Electroencephalography (EEG)

This may be very useful by showing characteristic abnormalities at an early stage in the illness when CT may be normal (Illis and Taylor, 1972; Dutt and Johnston, 1982).

Computed tomography

The predominant CT finding in HSV encephalitis is an area of attenuation in one or both temporal lobes, sometimes accompanied by evidence of haemorrhage into those areas. Antiviral treatment is most effective before necrosis has occurred and thus CT is less useful than EEG in the earliest stages of the disease. Over-dependence on CT may delay diagnosis and institution of therapy. It is hoped that nuclear magnetic resonance scanning may contribute to the early assessment of HSV encephalitis.

Brain biopsy

Examination of brain tissue is still the most certain method of achieving an early diagnosis (Skoldenberg *et al.*, 1984). It must be performed as early as possible in the course of the illness to give the patient the chance of a good recovery. Some physicians treat presumed HSV encephalitis without craniotomy, in view of the safety of acyclovir, and use antibody tests to make a retrospective diagnosis (Longson *et al.*, 1983). However, complications of brain biopsy are extremely uncommon (Whitely *et al.*, 1981). There are several treatable illnesses which mimic HSV encephalitis and early use of antiviral drugs can be fatal if they give a false sense of security. In a recent series of 132 cases of suspected HSV encephalitis 23% had other diseases requiring other forms of treatment (Whitely *et al.*, 1981).

Treatment of HSV encephalitis

HSV encephalitis is best treated by an experienced physician in a specialist unit.

Antiviral drugs

Acyclovir is the present drug of choice for HSV encephalitis. It is activated specifically in HSV-infected cells by virus thymidine kinase. It has the great advantage of being non-toxic to normal human cells but of selectively inhibiting the HSV-specific DNA polymerase (Timbury, 1982). Treatment should be started as soon as possible in the illness to prevent viral replication and cell damage. Acyclovir is given intravenously 10 mg/kg 8 hourly, each injection being infused over at least 1 hour. Treatment should last 10 days (Skoldenberg *et al.*, 1984). Trials are in progress to establish whether oral acyclovir should be used after an initial period of intravenous drug. Acyclovir is excreted by the kidneys and the dose should be reduced in patients with impaired renal function.

Brain oedema

Early measures to control cerebral oedema before the antiviral drug has had an effect may be life-saving. Hypertonic solutions and dexamethasone may be effective and surgical decompression may be necessary.

Anticonvulsant drugs

These are normally necessary in view of the high incidence of fits.

VARICELLA ZOSTER (SHINGLES)

Varicella zoster is the most important herpesvirus in the elderly because of the often devastating pain shingles causes. Chickenpox can be caught from zoster vesicles but shingles patients are less infectious than chickenpox patients. The incidence in healthy people is 4/1000/year at 55 years and 10/1000/year at 90 years. A second attack is unusual (5%) (Juel-Jensen and MacCallum, 1972). Few patients remember having had chickenpox.

Clinical Features

Zoster or 'shingles' is a vesicular eruption usually localized to a single dermatome frequently in the distribution of the trigeminal nerve or spinal segments T3 to L2. There is often intense paraesthesia, burning or tenderness. Pain is common, starting as long as 3 weeks before the rash and persisting for 2 weeks or longer. The initial pain is due to inflammation of the skin as a result of histamine release and is distinct from the pain of post-herpetic neuralgia which is due to post-inflammatory fibrosis and is perpetuated by central mechanisms. The skin eruption progresses from macules to vesicles then crusts. Fresh vesicles may appear over a few days. The lesions can be superinfected with *Staphylococcus aureus*. Scarring and pigmentation may occur, particularly if there has been superinfection. Systemic illness with mild fever and malaise accompanies the rash and there may be mild thrombocytopenia but no change in white cell count or ESR. Up to 50% of patients with uncomplicated zoster have mild CSF abnormalities. In about a third of cases satellite lesions are found, probably due to temporary viraemia. In some cases there is no rash (zoster sine herpete) (Lewis, 1958) and the symptoms may be confused with cord lesions, renal colic, appendicitis, myocardial pain or Bornholm disease.

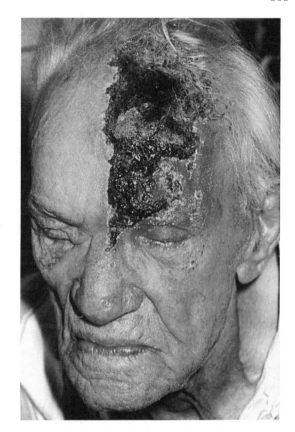

Figure 19.1. Ophthalmic zoster.

Complications of Varicella Zoster Infection

Ophthalmic zoster (Figure 19.1) occurs when the first division of the trigeminal nerve is affected. This is most serious when the nasociliary branch is involved and the eye may be damaged in 70% of cases (Womack and Liesegang, 1983). Examination of the eye with a slit lamp is required. Failure to treat ocular zoster may result in keratitis (55%), uveitis (43%) or secondary glaucoma (9%), all of which have the potential for major visual impairment.

Post-herpetic neuralgia occurs in 30–40% of untreated patients over the age of 60 years. Of these, 45% have pain for less than 8 weeks but 22% have pain for more than one year, the highest incidence being in the elderly and following ophthalmic zoster.

Generalized zoster may occur in immunosuppressed patients.

Zoster encephalitis carries an untreated mortality of 30% and is associated with cranial nerve palsies.

Bladder involvement may result from bilateral or unilateral zoster of the sacral segments below S2 and often results in paralysis of the bladder.

Treatment of Varicella Zoster

Antiviral agents

The key to successful treatment of zoster is specific chemotherapy as early as possible after development of the rash. Acyclovir acts through virus coded enzymes and affects only the development of early lesions or the spread of viruses from cell to cell. It cannot be expected to benefit lesions or complications when already fully developed (Balfour, 1984).

Initial acute pain is diminished by oral acyclovir (McKendrick et al., 1984; Peterslund et al., 1984). Post-herpetic neuralgia is probably also reduced (Balfour et al., 1983) by early acyclovir treatment but further studies are required to establish statistical significance of this effect. It would be expected, however, that if damage to nerve endings could be prevented by acyclovir then post-herpetic neuralgia would be less likely to occur.

Oral acyclovir 200–400/mg five times daily for 5 days is given, preferably within 24 hours of the appearance of the rash (Finn and Smith, 1984; McKendrick et al., 1984; Peterslund et al., 1984). Other authorities use topical idoxuridine 5–35% in dimethyl sulphoxide (DMSO) for 5 days (Juel-Jensen and McCallum, 1974; Dawber, 1974). When further trials of oral acyclovir are published it is possible that topical treatment will be obsolete.

Successful use of acyclovir in the treatment of herpes zoster in immunocompromised patients is well described (Balfour et al., 1983). The question remains which immunologically competent patient with herpes zoster should receive acyclovir in view of the possibility of development of resistant strains. Viral resistance can be developed in the laboratory and although it is not yet a clinical reality, widespread use of oral acyclovir may select resistant strains. Some physicians would reserve acyclovir for only the most severe cases of zoster infection (Jeffries, 1985).

Complicated zoster (ocular, visceral, encephalitis or generalized zoster) should be treated with high dose intravenous acyclovir 10 mg/kg 8 hourly, each dose given over at least one hour. A lower dose is given if the creatinine clearance is impaired. Intravenous treatment should be continued for 5 days (Bean et al., 1983; Nicholson, 1984).

General measures

Zoster patients should be nursed away from immunosuppressed patients because of the risk of chickenpox. Simple analgesics should be used to control pain and calamine lotion applied to relieve itching.

Antibiotics

Severe secondary infection of the lesions can be treated with oral flucloxacillin and topical fucidin.

Steroids

In healthy elderly patients who develop trigeminal zoster, a moderate dose of prednisolone, 40 mg daily for 10 days, which is gradually tailed off over the following 3 weeks may be effective in reducing the occurrence of post-herpetic neuralgia (Keczkes and Basheer, 1980). The treatment is effective only if started within 7 days of the onset but may not be necessary if acyclovir is also used.

Post-herpetic neuralgia (see also Chapter 22)

This is notoriously difficult to treat. Some benefit has been described with early treatment with prednisolone (Keczkes and Basheer, 1980). The rationale of steroids is to try to inhibit the inflammatory process in the acute phase. The early use of acyclovir has been shown to reduce the incidence of post-herpetic neuralgia but this requires further study.

Amitriptyline, phenytoin, and carbamazepine are of limited value. Amantidine (100 mg twice a day for 28 days) is occasionally successful (Galbraith, 1983). Thalidomide has also been used in desperate cases under hospital supervison (Peto and Juel-Jensen, 1986).

Nerve blockade, temporary or permanent, is sometimes required if analgesic drugs fail.

NEUROSYPHILIS

The clinical features of neurosyphilis may be modified by inadequate chance treatment with broad spectrum antibiotics and clinical and laboratory features may become more subtle and difficult to recognize (Alani and Millac, 1982; Hooshmand et al., 1972). Neurosyphilis has become a rare disease. The incidence is estimated at 0.18–10.30 per 100 000 per year (Alani and Millac, 1982; Nordenbo and Sorensen, 1981). The treatment is usually a total of 7.2 MU of benzathine penicillin (2.4 MU weekly) or a total of 9 MU of procaine penicillin (600 000 units daily).

REFERENCES

Alani, I., and Millac, P. (1982). Neurosyphilis in the Leicester area. *Postgrad. Med. J.*, **58**, 685.

Anderson, F. (1985). An historical overview of geriatric medicine: definition and aims. In: Pathy, M.S.J. (ed.) *Principles and Practice of Geriatric Medicine*, John Wiley & Sons, Chichester, p. 11

Anderson, J.M. (1974). Diabetic ketoacidosis presenting as neurosurgical emergencies. *Br. Med. J.*, **iii**, 22.

Anderson, J.M. (1984). Bacterial meningitis. In: Matthews, W.B., and Glaser, G.H. (eds.) *Recent Advances in Clinical Neurology*, Churchill Livingstone, Edinburgh Vol. 4, p. 90.

Balfour, H.H. (1984). Acyclovir and other chemotherapy for Herpes group viral infections. *Ann. Rev. Med.*, **35**, 279–91.

Balfour, H.H., Bean, B., Laskin, O.L., Ambinder, R.F., Myers, J.D., Wade J.C., Zaia, J.A., Aeppli, D., Kirk, L.E., Segreti, A.C., and Keeney, R.E. (1983). Acyclovir halts progression of Herpes Zoster in immunocompromised patients. *N. Engl. J. Med.*, **308**, 1448–53.

Beam, T.R. (1984). Cephalosporins in adult meningitis. *Bull. N.Y. Acad. Med.*, **60**, 380.

Bean, B., Aeppli, D., and Balfour, H. (1983). Acyclovir in shingles. *J. Antimicrob. Chemother.* **12** (Suppl. B), 123.

Bohr, V., Paulson, O.B., and Rasmussen, N. (1984). Pneumococcal meningitis. Late neurologic sequelae and features of prognostic impact. *Arch. Neurol.*, **41**, 1045.

Brewer, N.S., MacCarty, C.S., and Wellman, W.E. (1975). Brain abscess: A review of recent experience. *Ann. Intern. Med.*, **82**, 571.

Coakley, D. (1981). *Acute Geriatric Medicine*, Croom-Helm, London, p. 74.

Davey, P.G., Cruikshank, J.K., McManus, J.C., Mahood, B., Snow, M.H., and Gedes, A.M. (1982). Bacterial meningitis—ten years' experience. *J. Hyg. Camb.*, **88**, 383.

Dawber, R. (1974). Idoxuridine in herpes zoster—further evaluation of intermittent topical therapy. *Br. Med. J.*, **ii**, 526.

Dutt, M.K., and Johnston, I.D.A. (1982). Computer tomography and EEG in herpes simplex encephalitis. *Arch. Neurol.*, **39**, 99.

Editorial (1978a). Investigating stroke. *Br. Med. J.*, **i**, 1503.

Editorial (1978b). Chemotherapy of brain abscess. *Lancet*, **ii**, 1081.

Editorial (1982). Steroids in bacterial meningitis—helpful or harmful? *Lancet*, **i**, 1164.

Eykyn, S.J., Thomas, R.D., and Phillips, I. (1974). Haemophilus influenzae meningitis in adults. *Br. Med. J.*, **ii**, 463.

Fallon, R.J., and Kennedy, D.H. (1981). Treatment and prognosis in tuberculous meningitis. *J. Infect.*, 3 (Suppl. 1), 39.

Finland, M., and Barnes, M.W. (1977). Acute bacterial meningitis at Boston City Hospital during 12 selected years 1935–1972. *J. Infect. Dis.*, **13**, 400–15.

Finn, R., and Smith, M.A. (1984). Oral acyclovir for herpes zoster. *Lancet*, **ii**, 575.

Fraser, D.W., Henke, C.E., and Feldman, R.A. (1973). Changing patterns of bacterial meningitis in Olmstead County, Minesota 1935–1970. *J. Infect. Dis.*, **128**, 300.

Galbraith, A.W. (1983). Prevention of post-herpetic neuralgia by amantidine. *Br. J. Clin. Pract.*, **37**, 304–6.

Garvey, G. (1983). Current concepts of bacterial infections of the central nervous system. *J. Neurosurg.*, **59**, 735.

Gordon, A., and Parsons, M. (1972). The place of corticosteroids in the management of tuberculous meningitis. *Br. J. Hosp. Med.*, **7**, 651.

Gorse, G.J., Thrupp, L.D., Nudleman, K.L., Wyle, F.A., Hawkins, B., and Cesario, T.C. (1984). Bacterial meningitis in the elderly. *Arch. Intern. Med.*, **144**, 1603.

Hooshmand, H., Escobar, M.R., and Kopf, S.W. (1972). Neurosyphilis, a study of 241 patients. *J.A.M.A.*, **219**, 726.

Illis, L.S., and Taylor, F.M. (1972). The electroencephalogram in herpes simplex encephalitis. *Lancet*, **i**, 718.

Ispahani, P. (1983). Bacterial meningitis in Nottingham. *J. Hyg., Camb.*, **91**, 189.

Jeffries, D.J. (1985). Clinical use of acyclovir. *Br. Med. J.*, **290**, 177–8.

Juel-Jensen, B., and MacCallum, F.O. (1972). *Herpes Simplex, Varicella and Zoster, Clinical Manifestations and Treatment*, Heinemann, London.

Juel-Jensen, B., and MacCallum, F.O. (1974). Idoxuridine in herpes zoster. *Br. Med. J.*, **iii**, 41.

Keczkes, K., and Basheer, A.M. (1980). Do corticosteroids prevent post-herpetic neuralgia? *Br. J. Dermatol.*, **102**, 551.

Kennedy, D.H., and Fallon, R.J. (1979). Tuberculous meningitis. *J.A.M.A.*, **241**, 264.

Kennedy, P.G.E. (1984). Herpes simplex virus and the nervous system. *Postgrad. Med. J.*, **60**, 253.

Klapper, P.E., Laing, I., and Longson, M. (1981). Rapid non-invasive diagnosis of herpes encephalitis. *Lancet*, **ii**, 607.

Lambert, H.P. (1983a). Management problems in meningitis. *Br. J. Hosp. Med.*, 128.

Lambert, H.P. (1983b). Treatment of bacterial meningitis. *Br. Med. J.*, **286**, 741.

Lees, A.J., MacLeod, A.F., and Marshall, J. (1980). Cerebral tuberculomas developing during treatment of tuberculous meningitis. *Lancet*, **i**, 1208.

Lewis, G.W. (1958). Zoster Sine Herpete. *Br. Med. J.*, **ii**, 418.

Loizou, L.A., and Anderson, M. (1982). Intracranial tuberculomas: correlation of computerised tomography with clinico-pathological findings. *Q. J. Med.*, **201**, 104.

Longson, M., Klapper, P.E., and Cleator, G.M. (1983). The treatment of herpes encephalitis. *J. Infect.* **6**, 15.

Massanari, R.M. (1977). Purulent meningitis in the elderly: when to suspect an unusual pathogen. *Geriatrics*, **32**, 55.

McKendrick, M.W., Care, C., Burke, C., Hickmott, E., and McKendrick, G.D.W. (1984). Oral acyclovir in herpes zoster. *J. Antimicrob. Chemother.*, **14**, 661.

Newton, J.E., and Wilczynski, P.J.G. (1979). Meningitis in the elderly. *Lancet*, **ii**, 157.

Nicholson, K.G. (1984). Antiviral therapy. Varicella-zoster virus infections, herpes labialis and mucocutaneous herpes and cytomegalovirus infections. *Lancet*, **ii**, 677.

Nordenbo, A.M., and Sorensen, P.S. (1981). The incidence and clinical presentation of neurosyphilis in Greater Copenhagen 1974 through 1978. *Acta Neurol. Scand.*, **63**, 237–46.

Peterslund, N.A., Esmann, J., Ipsen, K., Christensen, D., and Petersen, C.M. (1984). Oral and intravenous acyclovir are equally effective in herpes zoster. *J. Antimicrob. Chemother.*, **14**, 185–9.

Peto, T.E.A., and Juel-Jensen, B.E. (1986). Herpes simplex and varicella zoster virus infection in the elderly. In: Denham, M.J. (ed.) *Infections in the Elderly*, MTP Press, Lancaster, p. 184.

Puxty, J.A.H. (1983). The frequency of physical signs usually attributed to meningeal irritation in elderly patients. *J. Am. Geriatr. Soc.*, **31**, 590.

Skoldenberg, B., Alestig, K., Burman, L., Forkman, A., Lovgren, K., Norrby, R., Stiernstedt, G., Forsgren, M., Bergstrom, T., Dahlqvist, E., Fryden, A., Norlin, K., Olding-Stenkvist, E., Uhnoo, I., and Devahl, K. (1984). Acyclovir versus vidarabine in herpes simplex encephalitis. *Lancet*, **ii**, 707.

Timbury, M. (1982). Acyclovir. *Br. Med. J.*, **285**, 1223.

Traub, M., Colchester, A.C.F., Kingsley, D.P.E., and Swash, M. (1984). Tuberculosis of the central nervous system. *Q. J. Med.*, **209**, 81.

Whitely, R.J., Soon, S.-J., Hirsch, M.S., Karchmar, A.W., Dohn, R., Galasso, G., Dunnick, J.K., and Alford, C.A. (1981). Herpes simplex encephalitis. Vidarabine therapy and diagnostic problems. *N. Engl. J. Med.*, **304**, 313.

Whitely, R.J., Soong, S.-J., Linneman, C., Lin, C., Pazin, G., and Alford, C.A. (1982). Herpes simplex encephalitis, clinical assessment. *J.A.M.A.*, **247**, 317.

Womack, L.W., and Liesegang, T.J. (1983). Complications of herpes zoster Ophthalmicus. *Arch. Ophthalmol.* **101**, 42.

Chapter 20

The Neurological Complications of Metabolic, Nutritional and Endocrine Disorders

John Puxty

Associate Professor, Geriatric Assessment Unit, Ottawa General Hospital, Ottawa, Ontario, Canada

Neurological interrelationships between metabolic, endocrine and nutritional disorders are common but rarely as obvious as for instance the local compressive manifestations of pituitary tumours. An awareness of their existence is helpful in the evaluation of encephalopathies, neuropathies, spinal cord syndromes and myopathies.

COMMON PRESENTATIONS

Neurobehavioural Disturbances

A variety of endocrine and metabolic disorders may produce similar behavioural disturbances. They can be roughly classified into four different types of reactions:

1. The release of specific substances such as adrenaline as a primary or secondary effect may produce a panic attack with anxiety, sweating, hyperventilation and somatic symptoms.
2. Modification of the individual's normal 'setting' for energy, mood, level of arousal, activity and appetite. These symptoms imply an alteration of central regulatory mechanisms concerned with homeostasis. The clinical picture will depend upon the rate of onset of the imbalance.
3. Classical functional psychoses with hallucinations, delusions and paranoia. Endocrine or metabolic changes may lower the threshold for depressive or schizophrenic psychoses.
4. Confusional states, characterized by clouding of consciousness, disorientation, fragmentation of speech and illusions, appear in severe endocrine or metabolic disturbances.

Intellectual functions are probably the most complex and demanding activities performed by the brain and are especially vulnerable to disruption. Prolonged or recurrent interruption of the availability of metabolites will eventually compromise integrated cellular function and produce an impairment of intellectual abilities. If the metabolic disturbance is acute and overwhelming an acute confusional state results and the major behavioural defect is a deficit in attention. This is often accompanied by slowness of response, disorientation in time and space, fluctuating arousal, changes in mood, and hallucinations. If the metabolic disturbance occurs slowly the clinical picture is often more like that of a slowly progressive dementia. The features are usually more that of a subcortical dementia with psychomotor retardation, impairment of memory and cognition, and mood changes. Disturbances of motor function such as tremor, myoclonus, choreoathetosis, asterixis, tone changes and bradykinesia may be present. Table 20.1 summarizes the principal metabolic conditions associated with a gradual and chronic disturbance of cognition.

TABLE 20.1 PRINCIPAL METABOLIC CONDITIONS ASSOCIATED WITH 'DEMENTIA SYNDROMES'

Conditions associated with anoxia:
  Anoxic anoxia
    Pulmonary insufficiency
  Stagnant anoxia
    Cardiac disease
    Hyperviscosity states
  Anaemic anoxia
  Postanoxic
    Cardiorespiratory arrest

Chronic renal failure:
  Uraemic encephalopathy
  Dialysis encephalopathy

Pancreatic disorders:
  Hypoglycaemia
  Pancreatic encephalopathy

Hepatic disorders:
  Portosystemic encephalopathy

Electrolyte abnormalities
  Hyponatraemia
  Hypernatraemia

Vitamin deficiency states:
  Thiamine
  B12
  Folate
  Niacin

Endocrine disorders:
  Hypothyroidism
  Parathyroid abnormalities

Adrenal disease:
  Panhypopituitarism

Disorders of Consciousness

Faints, fits or coma may be seen in many of the conditions under consideration in this chapter.

Faints of syncope arise from vasomotor disturbances and are therefore especially likely to be seen in the presence of the peripheral neuropathies associated with diabetes and uraemia. Hyponatraemia will predispose to postural hypotension and therefore syncope.

Changes in the distribution and amounts of body fluids, with or without disturbances in levels of ions important in nerve function, will predispose to seizures (see also Chapter 15). Adrenal and parathyroid disorders and the inappropriate antidiuretic

hormone (ADH) syndrome are likely to present with epilepsy. Thyroid disease, particularly hypothyroidism, may also present with seizures. Hypoglycaemia may produce convulsions.

Diabetics may present with more profound disturbances of consciousness because of hyper- or hypoglycaemia. In parathyroid and adrenal disorders, prolonged disturbances of consciousness tend to be associated with raised intracranial pressure. In thyroid disease, coma may occur with both hypo- and hyperthyroidism.

Paraesthesiae and Limb Pain

These subjects are discussed in detail in other chapters (e.g. Chapter 22) but there is a considerable overlap in the aetiologies of these presentations. They include the peripheral neuropathies of diabetes, thyroid disease, uraemia, and avitaminosis, and the myopathies of osteomalacia and thyroid and adrenal disease (Chapter 12).

SPECIFIC CONDITIONS

Anoxia

Chronic cerebral anoxia may produce a picture similar to that of a dementia syndrome. It may be divided into anoxic anoxia arising from inadequate blood oxygenation; ischaemic anoxia secondary to impaired cerebral perfusion; and anaemic anoxia caused by poor oxygen-carrying capacity of the blood.

Chronic pulmonary insufficiency and anoxic anoxia

Occasionally chronic impairment of cognition is the presenting feature of pulmonary disease (Cummings *et al.*, 1980). Neuropsychological studies of individuals with chronic pulmonary insufficiency reveal that reversible intellectual deficits are common (Krop *et al.*, 1973). Tremulousness and asterixis are frequently also present. When hypoxia and hypercapnoea are severe, a more extensive syndrome of headache, papilloedema, tremor and twitching of the extremities is seen along with signs of cardiopulmonary decompensation. Mental changes include inattention, drowsiness, lethargy and forgetfulness.

Chronic cardiac disease and stagnant anoxia

Although the brain represents only 2% of the total body weight, it accounts for nearly 20% of the total oxygen consumption (Hall, 1981). Any interruption of flow of oxygenated blood to the brain will have deleterious effects on mental function. The principal clinical features are irritability, disorientation, impaired memory and somnolence.

Reversible cognitive changes may be associated with chronic stagnant anoxia syndromes produced by hyperviscosity syndromes such as Waldenström's macroglobulinaemia and polycythaemia rubra vera.

If oxygen deprivation has been acute and severe, injury or death to cerebral neurones may occur. Three degrees of postanoxic encephalopathy may be seen. The most severe is brain death, where anoxia is so severe as effectively to destroy all neuronal activity. Bodily functions will continue only if artificially maintained. The second category is characterized by maintenance of brain stem functions governing autonomous respiration and circulation, without evidence of higher cortical activity. This persistent vegetative state is to be distinguished from akinetic mutism, where arousal is present but volitional activity absent, and from the locked-in syndrome, in which the patient is cognitively intact but paralysed and anarthric. The third category is that of a dementia syndrome, where partial cortical function is preserved. The severity of the dementia and the extent to which recovery may occur vary greatly. Aphasia, visuo-spatial disorientation, constructional disturbances, memory disorders, acalculia and impaired abstraction may be combined with degrees of spasticity, paresis, ataxia, and pseudobulbar palsy.

Anaemic anoxia

Low haemoglobin concentration with impaired oxygen-carrying capacity and cerebral anoxia produces intellectual impairment, poor attention, emotional lability, restlessness and, occasionally, myoclonus.

Chronic Renal Failure

Many conditions associated with chronic renal failure produce disturbance of cognition (Table 20.2).

TABLE 20.2　CAUSES OF MENTAL STATUS CHANGES IN CHRONIC RENAL FAILURE

Uraemic encephalopathy
Electrolyte imbalance
Anaemia
Hypertensive encephalopathy
Hypertensive cerebrovascular disease
Hypertensive cardiovascular disease
Altered drug metabolism
Dialysis
　　Dialysis encephalopathy
　　Subdural haematoma
　　Emboli
　　Disequilibrium syndrome
Immunosuppression
　　Steroid psychosis
　　Viral encephalitis

Some clinical disorders are a direct consequence of the renal failure and others of the treatment such as dialysis, transplantation or immunosuppression.

Disruption of renal function results in a number of metabolic effects. These include elevations of blood urea, creatinine, potassium and urate, and depression of blood calcium, bicarbonate and sodium. There may be a metabolic acidosis. The overall effects of these metabolic disturbances on mental status include fatigue, drowsiness, poor concentration, erratic memory, irritability, hallucinations and paranoia. In one study of elderly patients, uraemia was thought to account for 10% of all cases of delirium (Flint and Richards, 1956).

Disturbances of motor function are common and include increased muscle tone, asterixis, myoclonus and tremor. Convulsions may occur late in the clinical course (Raskin and Fishman, 1976).

Peripheral neuropathy (see also Chapter 13) may occur early in the disease and worsens as renal function deteriorates (Avran *et al.*, 1978). The neuropathy is distal, symmetrical and sensorimotor and characterized by axonal degeneration of the large diameter fibres. Pain may be a prominent feature. Many patients also complain of the restless legs syndrome. An autonomic neuropathy may be present but is usually mild.

Uraemic polyneuropathy is one of the few metabolic neuropathies which regularly improves with treatment of the underlying disease. Severe established polyneuropathy may, however, respond poorly and, on occasion, rapid deterioration occurs within the first few weeks of dialysis (Jebsen *et al.*, 1967).

The EEG is abnormal in uraemia. The most frequently observed changes are disorganization and slowing of the background rhythm. Bursts of paroxysmal, bilaterally synchronous slow waves are also seen (Jacobs *et al.*, 1965).

Hepatic Disease

Portosystemic encephalopathy (hepatic coma, hepatic encephalopathy) is a neuropsychiatric disorder associated with severe impairment of hepatic function and shunting of portal venous blood through collateral vessels into the peripheral circulation. The main clinical manifestations are an altered mental state, asterixis, increased muscle tone, hyperreflexia, gait ataxia and a typical fetor. Neurobehavioural disturbances include changes in mood, with euphoria or depression, impaired concentration and attention, poor memory, fluctuating arousal and often bizarre behaviour (Hoffman, 1981; Sherlock *et al.*, 1954). Constructional disturbances and motor impersistence are common. Asterixis is present in most patients. It usually manifests as intermittent lapse in posture (flap) of hands when the arms are held outstretched with the hands dorsiflexed at the wrist. Occasionally the same phenomenon is present in the arms, neck, jaws, with a protruded tongue, retracted mouth or tightly closed eyelids (Leavitt and Tyler, 1964; Sherlock *et al.*, 1954). Asterixis is usually accompanied by an irregular postural tremor.

The pathogenesis of portosystemic encephalopathy is not fully understood. Several compounds, including ammonia, short chain fatty-acids, mercaptens and false neurotransmitter amines, have been proposed as solely or partly responsible (Conn, 1969; Hoffman, 1981; Soeters and Fischer, 1976). Abnormalities of ammonia metabolism appear to show the closest correlation with the severity of encephalopathy.

In addition to abnormalities of serum ammonia and CSF glutamate, there are characteristic changes in the EEG. Disorganization and slowing of the background alpha activity and generalized slow waves in the theta and delta range occur with bursts of 2 Hz bilaterally, and synchronous triphasic waves with frontal predominance (Kiloh *et al.*, 1972; Silverman, 1962).

Treatment of portosystemic encephalopathy is aimed at minimizing gut protein, modifying intestinal bacterial activity and limiting protein absorption. Strict control of dietary protein and oral lactulose or neomycin are the mainstays of treatment (Hoffman, 1981). Improvement in mental status commonly follows. Some patients have shown additional improvement in intellectual function from treatment with levodopa or bromocriptine (Lunzer *et al.*, 1974; Morgan *et al.*, 1977).

Hypoglycaemia

Chronic or recurrent hypoglycaemia results in mental status impairment with personality alterations, aggressive behaviour, apathy and emotional lability (Lishman, 1978; Markowitz *et al.*, 1961; Tom and Richardson, 1951). Memory disturbance is often severe and at times may be the major behavioural disturbance. Peripheral neuropathy can occur and transient focal neurological deficits may be observed during a hypoglycaemic episode. The causes of recurrent hypoglycaemia include over-administration of hypoglycaemic agents, insulinoma, postgastrectomy hypoglycaemia, liver necrosis and retroperitoneal tumours.

Pancreatic Encephalopathy

Acute pancreatitis is sometimes associated with a subacute encephalopathy manifesting as confusion, agitation, hallucination, paranoia, lack of insight and incoherent speech (Pallis and Lewis, 1974). It is associated with dysarthria and extrapyramidal rigidity and seizures may occur. Pathological findings include focal loss of neurones and areas of demyelination. The CNS changes are thought to be produced by the released lipases and proteolytic enzymes (Pallis and Lewis, 1974).

Electrolyte Abnormalities

Hyponatraemia

Chronic or recurrent hyponatraemia can occur in a variety of situations: inappropriate secretion of anti-diuretic hormone (ISAH), Addison's disease, chronic renal failure, congestive cardiac failure, cirrhosis of the liver, inappropriate water consumption, and idiopathic sodium depletion. The ISAH syndrome can be associated with bronchial carcinoma, cerebral infections, and injuries such as subdural haematomas, and tuberculosis. ISAH can also be stimulated by sulphonylureas, cytotoxic drugs such as vincristine and cyclophosphamide, tricyclic compounds such as amitriptyline, diuretics and major tranquillizers.

The symptoms of hyponatraemia depend upon the cause, the level of serum sodium and the speed of onset. Where the prime lesion is sodium depletion, neurological symptoms dominate; whereas with water overload, gastrointestinal symptoms occur (Kennedy and Early, 1970; Arieff *et al.*, 1976). Once the serum sodium drops below 125 mEq/l neurological symptoms and signs are usually present.

Neuropsychiatric manifestations of hyponatraemia include weakness, anorexia, lethargy, disorientation, psychosis and seizures (Arieff *et al.*, 1976; Dubovsky *et al.*, 1973). Seizures may occur when the serum sodium gets as low as 110 to 112 mEq/l, but cerebral oedema may occur with any value below 125 mEq/l.

Treatment will depend upon the underlying mechanism of the hyponatraemia. Where there is excess sodium loss, from the renal or gastrointestinal tract, replacement of sodium and water is required. The administration of hypertonic saline solution is rarely required and potentially dangerous.

In some situations, hyponatraemia is in fact associated with an *increased* total body sodium, as may be seen in chronic cardiac failure, cirrhosis or nephrotic syndrome. Such patients are suffering from secondary hyperaldosteronism. Treatment of the underlying condition with fluid and salt restriction is the mainstay of therapy. The angiotensin-converting enzyme (ACE) inhibitors are useful in this situation.

Most cases of IADH syndrome are self-limiting since the commonest cause in the elderly is respiratory infection. If drugs are implicated, they should be stopped. IADH syndrome in association with malignancy may be more serious, especially if the patient consumes excess hypotonic fluids, such as beer, thereby precipitating a further and dangerous drop in serum sodium. In such cases, it may on occasions be necessary to resort to hypertonic saline.

Hypernatraemia

Hypernatraemia is usually due to decreased fluid intake. The elderly appear to be particularly prone to dehydration partly because of an age-related diminution of the thirst threshold (Miller *et al.*, 1982).

The brain is generally able to tolerate dehydration, hypernatraemia and hyperosmolarity. The elderly, however, appear to be more sensitive to fluctuations in serum sodium, and intellectual impairment may be seen with relatively mild degrees of hypernatraemia. Hypernatraemia usually occurs when there is decreased or absent fluid intake; increased fluid loss; or disorders of fluid and electrolyte regulation. The principal neurobehavioural abnormalities are confusion, disorientation and restlessness. Severe hypernatraemia may be associated with drowsiness, coma, muscular rigidity and fits.

Deficiency States

Thiamine: classical thiamine deficiency syndromes

1. Wernicke–Korsakoff syndrome. Wernicke's encephalopathy is characterized by a sudden onset of confusion associated with paralysis of eye movements and an ataxic gait. Peripheral nerves are also commonly involved: Victor *et al.* (1971) found peripheral neuropathies in more than 80% of the patients studied. Postural hypotension and disturbances of vestibular function are often seen (Birchfield, 1964; Ghez, 1969). It is usually associated with alcoholism but even Wernicke's original three cases included a non-alcoholic with pyloric stenosis.

The pathological alterations that affect the cerebrum and brain stem are remarkably constant. They are usually bilaterally symmetrical. Lesions are invariably seen in the mamillary bodies and the terminal fornices. Lesions in the periaqueductal region of the midbrain, in the floor of the fourth ventricle, in the vicinity of the dorsal motor nucleus of the vagus and the anterior superior parts of the cerebellar vermices probably account for the paralysis of gaze, nystagmus and ataxia.

The earliest abnormality is glial oedema but later there is necrosis of nerve cells and myelinated structures. A marked glial reaction characterizes the centre of the lesion. Endothelial proliferation and haemorrhages are found. In the vermis of the cerebellum the principal change consists of a loss of Purkinje cells and gliosis of the molecular layer of the cortex.

A post-mortem study of 2891 cadavers over a 4 year period revealed that 51 cases (1.7%), 45 of whom were alcoholics, had evidence of Wernicke's encephalopathy (Harper, 1979). Only seven had been diagnosed during life. This suggests that it is commonly undiagnosed.

It is probable that Wernicke's encephalopathy and Korsakoff's psychosis are manifestations of the same pathological process, albeit at successive stages. Of 186 patients with Wernicke's encephalopathy 84% had evidence of Korsakoff's psychosis (Victor *et al.*, 1971). It is essentially a disorder in which the disturbance in memory is out of proportion to that of other cognitive functions. Loss of recent memory (retrograde amnesia) and impaired ability to form new memories (anterograde amnesia) are common. Confabulation is seen in many patients.

Early treatment with thiamine may result in rapid reversal of the ophthalmoplegia and the other abnormalities improve gradually over a period of several days. Amnesia may become apparent as the confusion lifts (Cravioto *et al.*, 1961; Malamud and Skillicorn, 1956; Victor *et al.*, 1971). Some degree of spontaneous recovery does appear to occur. Claims for improved performance on memory tests have been claimed following administration of clonidine or vasopressin (McEntee and Mair, 1980; Oliveros *et al.*, 1978).

2. Peripheral neuropathy. The peripheral neuropathy of thiamine deficiency involves both sensory and motor nerves and is symmetrical in distribution. Axonal degeneration with destruction of both the axon and myelin sheath is seen pathologically. The most pronounced changes occur in the longest and largest myelinated fibres. The vagus and the paravertebral sympathetic chains may be involved in advanced cases. In very advanced cases the anterior and dorsal root ganglia show chromatolysis.

The legs are typically involved earlier and more severely than the arms. Motor disability usually predominates with only a quarter of patients having pain or paraesthesia as their main complaint (Victor and Adams, 1971). Tenderness of the muscles on pressure is common. The depression of deep tendon reflexes in the legs is often out of proportion to the degree of weakness.

Brin (1962) has proposed that in addition to the well-recognized syndromes of thiamine deficiency, there is a poorly defined cluster of non-specific symptoms such as anorexia, insomnia, irritability and difficulty in concentrating, due to milder degrees of thiamine deficiency.

The observations of de Wardner and Lennox (1947) on 32 000 British troops following the surrender of Singapore in 1942 support Brin's concept of progression from non-specific symptoms to the more classical manifestations of thiamine deficiency. The abrupt change from normal British army rations to a diet of polished rice was followed in about 6 weeks by an eruption of numerous symptoms. Of the 52 cases chosen for study the symptoms observed included anorexia (88%), nausea and vomiting (57%), nystagmus (100%), mental changes (78%), and other central nervous symptoms (11%). The mental changes started with anxiety, followed by progressive memory loss for recent events over a period of 2 to 3 weeks, followed by disorientation for time and then place. Once parenteral thiamine was administered, recovery occurred in the reverse order as the signs had developed. A number improved dramatically within 2 days and memory for recent events returned in 2 to 7 days.

Lonsdale and Shamberger (1980) reported an apparent association of functional neurotic symptoms with abnormality of red cell transketolase activity. Common symptoms were abdominal or chest pain, sleep disturbances, personality changes, fatigue, fluctuating bowel habit, anorexia and nausea and headaches. All of the subjects claimed symptomatic improvement after thiamine supplementation. A double-blind study by Wood *et al.* (1980), however, failed to show significant difference between controls and subjects with respect to symptoms, findings on examination, the results of psychological testing, nerve conduction studies or work performance. There was some suggestion, however, that fatigue, irritability and hyperaesthesia occurred more commonly in the thiamine restricted group.

Delirium is a common presentation of disease in the elderly, especially in the presence of infection (Hodkinson, 1973). Older and Dickerson (1982) made the interesting observation that confusion following surgery for a fractured neck of femur was more common in patients with an initially abnormal thiamine status. Changes in pyruvate metabolism have also been described, both in confusional states of the elderly (Mitra, 1971) and in febrile infected patients (Gilbert, 1968). Gilbert *et al.* (1969) reported changes in thiamine status in 23 out of 48 febrile patients with an age range of 22–56 years. A longitudinal study of biochemical measures of thiamine status in elderly inpatients demonstrated significant changes at the time of onset of delirium associated with infection (Puxty, 1985). It is possible, therefore, that changes in thiamine status with infection might play some part in the development of delirium.

Vitamin B12 deficiency

Neurological manifestations of vitamin B12 deficiency include peripheral neuropathy, myelopathy, optic neuropathy and encephalopathy.

The cerebral and spinal lesions of vitamin B12 deficiency are similar. There is a diffuse though uneven degeneration of the white matter with little proliferation of the fibrous glia. Within the foci of demyelination, histological changes include fusiform swelling of myelin sheaths, followed by destruction of myelin and axons and the appearance of lipid-laden macrophages (Smith, 1976). In the spinal cord, the white matter changes begin in the posterior columns at the thoracic level. Demyelination then extends up

and down the cord and anteriorly to the lateral columns (Pant *et al.*, 1968; Victor and Lear, 1956).

The main features of the encephalopathy include slowness of mental reactions, confusion, memory defects and depression. Agitation, delusions, paranoid behaviour and hallucinations also occur. The encephalopathy may have a fluctuating course and can precede any haematological or marrow changes (Pallis and Lewis, 1974; Strachan and Henderson, 1965). The typical neuropathy in vitamin B12 deficiency includes superficial sensory impairment with burning paraesthesia, tender peripheral nerves, early loss of ankle jerks and distal weakness (Abransky, 1972; Pallis and Lewis, 1974; Victor and Lear, 1956). The myelopathy involves the posterior and lateral columns of the spinal cord and produces impairment of vibration sense, limb weakness, spasticity, exaggerated tendon reflexes and extensor plantar responses.

Folate deficiency

Although folate deficiency is very common it rarely has neurological consequences. On occasions it may mimic vitamin B12 deficiency, with neuropathy, myelopathy and encephalopathy (Fehling *et al.*, 1974; Pincus *et al.*, 1972; Strachan and Henderson, 1967).

Nicotinic acid deficiency

Nicotinic acid deficiency results in cutaneous lesions, lesions of the gastrointestinal tract and nervous system abnormalities (pellagra).

The most striking histological lesion of niacin deficiency is central chromatolysis of neurones. The changes are most prominent in Betz cells and in brain stem nuclei. Neurones are rounded with peripheral displacement of the Nissl substance and nuclei. Electron microscopy reveals that RNA granules and lipofuscin pigment deposits are pushed to the periphery of the cytoplasm, whereas the central portion of the cytoplasm is occupied by mitochondria, lysosomes, and dilated vesicles (Nobuyoshi and Nishihara, 1981; Smith *et al.*, 1976).

The neurological abnormalities include peripheral neuropathy, myelopathy and neurobehavioural disturbances. A pellagrous dementia and an acute niacin-deficiency encephalopathy (Jolliffe syndrome) have been reported. The dementia syndrome includes lassitude, depression, irritability, apprehension, memory impairment, confabulation and psychomotor retardation (Spillane, 1947; Sydenstricker, 1943). Acute symptoms from niacin deficiency include clouding of consciousness, cogwheel rigidity, and marked sucking and grasping responses (Jolliffe *et al.*, 1940).

Niacin deficiency results from chronic dietary neglect such as may occur in alcoholics or in the presence of a variety of systemic disorders including cirrhosis, inflammatory bowel disease, diabetes mellitus, neoplasms and hyperthyroidism.

Endocrine Disturbances

Hyperthyroidism

Neurological manifestations of excessive thyroid hormone production include myopathy, peripheral neuropathy, corticospinal tract disease, chorea, seizures, neurobehavioural disturbances, optic neuropathy, retinopathy and exophthalmic ophthalmoplegia (see also Chapter 12).

The encephalopathy associated with hyperthyroidism is typically characterized by subjective feelings of anxiety, restlessness, irritability and emotional lability. Distractability leads to poor attention, impaired memory and difficulty with calculation (Lishman, 1978; Logothetis, 1961; Whybrow *et al.*, 1969). Depression, euphoria, and schizophrenia-like psychoses may also manifest in the hyperthyroid state (Lishman, 1978). If hyperthyroidism progresses, intellectual function is increasingly compromised, apathy and somnolence progress and coma supervenes (Weaver *et al.*, 1956; Waldenström, 1945). The encephalopathy is associated with evidence of cardiovascular strain and pyrexia. Myeloencephalopathy, paralysis of cranial nerves and choreiform movements have also been reported (Sutherland, 1903).

In the elderly, hyperthyroidism may present in an atypical or masked form that obscures the diagnosis. Anxiety, tremor, tachycardia and restlessness may be completely lacking and the only manifestation may be lethargy, apathy and psychomotor retardation (Arnold *et al.*, 1974; Gordon and Gryfe, 1981).

The EEG is abnormal in most patients with hyperthyroid encephalopathy. Slow-wave activity is present and approximately half the patients have diffuse, paroxysmal sharp waves and spikes occurring with slow waves (Condon *et al.*, 1954; Olsen *et al.*, 1972). Large-amplitude fast-wave activity may be present and a few patients have triphasic delta activity (Scherokman, 1980). Cerebral blood flow is increased in hyperthyroidism (Sensenbach *et al.*, 1954).

Generalized convulsive seizures in hyperthyroidism may not be as uncommon as previously thought. It was found that 9% of admissions to a general hospital presented with seizures (Jabbari and Huott, 1980) while hyperthyroidism was the apparent cause of the first fit in 1.2% of seizure cases.

Patients with hyperthyroidism commonly complain of weakness and fatiguability but a minority present with a proximal myopathy (see Chapter 12). In the older patient, severe proximal myopathy may be the dominant clinical presentation of hyperthyroidism.

An important association between thyroid dysfunction and myasthenia gravis is well reported (Drachman, 1962). In a study using phrenic nerve preparations from hyperthyroid animals (Hoffmann and Denys, 1972), a significant reduction in the amplitude of miniature end plates was found. It was speculated that hyperthyroidism could predispose to the development of disorders of neuromuscular transmission, because of an effect on the amount of acetylcholine release.

Hypothyroidism

Diminished thyroid activity has profound effects on the nervous system and may cause myopathy, peripheral neuropathy, cranial nerve abnormalities, ataxia and other cerebellar signs, psychosis and dementia, coma and seizures (Nickel and Frame, 1958; Sanders, 1962; Swanson *et al.*, 1981). The psychosis of hypothyroidism has no pathognomonic features but inattention, disorientation, paranoia and hallucinations are common (Asher 1949; Logothetis 1963). Neuropsychiatric problems occur in approximately 5% of hypothyroid individuals and are manifested by psychic retardation, memory impairment, poor attention and impaired abstraction (Swanson *et al.*, 1981; Whybrow *et al.*, 1969). If hypothyroidism progresses untreated, the patient becomes obtunded and eventually comatose and may die. EEG studies demonstrate slowing of background rhythms with diminished wave amplitude (Olivarius and Roder, 1970), and cerebral flow studies show increased cerebral vascular resistance and reduced blood flow (Sensenbach *et al.*, 1954?).

Varying degrees of deafness occur in hypothyroidism due to a direct involvement of the eighth cranial nerve in about 15% of patients (Deol, 1973). It is usually sensorineural and may improve with thyroxine replacement therapy.

The cerebellar disorder associated with hypothyroidism is largely reversible and usually seen in long-standing cases although cases with symptoms of hypothyroidism as short as one month have been reported (Cremer *et al.*, 1969). The most severely affected cases are so ataxic they cannot stand or walk. The midline cerebellar structures controlling stance are mainly affected. Myxoedematous deposits and 'round bodies' containing glycogen have been found at autopsy in the cerebellum of a patient with long-standing hypothyroidism and ataxia (Price and Netsky, 1966).

The early descriptions of hypothyroidism mentioned the symptoms of peripheral nerve dysfunction (Ord, 1878). (See also Chapter 13.) Not infrequently these are due to an entrapment neuropathy, with, most commonly, compression of the median nerve at the wrist producing a carpal tunnel syndrome. The more diffuse polyneuritis of hypothyroidism is probably related to the metabolic disorder rather than myxoedematous material deposition.

The myopathy of hypothyroidism is characterized by weakness, slowing of muscle contraction and relaxation ('pseudomyotonia'), muscle stiffness and in severe cases increased muscle mass (Hoffmann's syndrome). In such cases, an elevated creatinine phosphokinase is found. Electromyographic and biopsy findings are inconsistent and non-specific.

Muscle cramps may be a feature of hypothyroidism and less commonly of hyperthyroidism (Hurwitz *et al.*, 1970). They are thought to be due to the myopathic processes producing hyperexcitable foci, especially at distal portions of the nerves. 'Myokymic' muscular twitches caused by the spontaneous repetitive discharges of single motor fibres have been reported in both hypo- and hyperthyroidism. This phenomenon usually disappears with correction of the thyroid dysfunction (Harman and Richardson, 1954).

Hyperparathyroidism

The most prominent manifestations of hyperparathyroidism are weakness, fatiguability, renal colic, weight loss, mental disturbances, constipation, abdominal pain, anorexia, arthralgia and bone pain (Mallette *et al.*, 1974). Mental changes are seen in approximately half of patients who are apathetic and depressed. This may progress to disorientation with impaired memory, impaired concentration and calculation ability, paranoia and hallucinations (Fitz and Hallman, 1952; Gatewood *et al.*, 1975; Henson, 1968). Catatonia may occur (Gelenberg, 1976). In the advanced stages of the disease, obtundation and coma are seen. The changes in mental state correlate with the raised serum calcium and are not unique to hyperparathyroidism. Similar neurobehavioural disturbances are seen with other causes of hypercalcaemia (Lehrer and Levitt, 1960).

The EEG in hypercalcaemic patients may be normal or may show slowing of the posterior background rhythms, excess theta and delta activity, and high-voltage bilaterally synchronous frontal delta activity (Cohn and Sode, 1971).

Hypoparathyroidism

Hypoparathyroidism affects many different organ systems. Typical manifestations include chronic tetany, seizures, dementia, cataracts, coarseness of skin and trophic nail changes (Robinson *et al.*, 1954). Hyperactivity of tendon reflexes is the basis of the Chvostek sign. Calcification of the basal ganglia and an extrapyramidal motor syndrome with parkinsonism or choreoathetosis are distinctive features of this metabolic disturbance (Hossain, 1970; Muenter and Whisnant, 1968). The dementia syndrome is characterized by poor concentration, impaired memory, disorientation, apathy and hallucinations (Eraut, 1974; Slyter, 1979). In some cases the extrapyramidal and dementia syndromes respond to normalization of the serum calcium (Berger and Ross, 1981; Slyter, 1979).

Hypocalcaemia in pseudohyperparathyroidism is thought to be due to an end-organ failure to respond to parathyroid hormone. In some a dementia syndrome, seizures, tics and athetoid movements occur as well. The basal ganglia may also be calcified (Ettigi and Brown, 1978).

Adrenal Disorders

Cushing's disease

The clinical manifestations of Cushing's disease include obesity, rounding of the face, thickening of the supraclavicular fat pads and abdominal panniculus, thinning of the skin, with an increased tendency to bruising, striae formation, hirsutism, acne, oligomenorrhoea, limb weakness, osteoporosis, hypertension, diabetes and neurobehavioural disturbances (Liddle, 1971). The latter include depression, psychomotor retardation, irritability, poor concentration and memory, disturbed sleep pattern and psychosis (Glaser, 1953; Starkman and Schteingart, 1981; Trethowan and Cobb, 1952). The severity of the neurobehavioural disturbance is claimed by some authors to correlate with the degree of cortisol elevation (Starkman and Schteingart, 1981). It usually reverses with normalization of cortisol status.

A review of 29 cases by Cohen *et al.* (1980) suggested that 25 had depressive symptoms. In those patients who had tumours, depression improved following surgery. Kelly *et al.* (1980) have investigated the possibility that the increased cortisol level in Cushing's syndrome increases the activity of the enzyme tryptophanase. This would tend to lower levels of brain 5-HT. They found that although there were lower levels of tryptophan than in controls the differences were not significant.

The commonest muscle disorder in Cushing's disease is a proximal muscle weakness particularly affecting the pelvic girdle and, to a lesser extent, the shoulder girdle. The muscle weakness is usually associated with wasting (see Chapter 12).

Addison's disease

The patient in Addison's disease feels languid, weak and apathetic. There is associated anorexia, weight loss and hypotension. The mental changes include apathy, irritability, depression, suspiciousness, agitation and memory impairment (Lishman, 1978). They are present in half to two-thirds of cases (Meyer, 1982). Treatment of the adrenal insufficiency normalizes mental state in most cases.

Pituitary Disorders

Panhypopituitarism

Combined hypothyroidism and adrenal insufficiency associated with panhypopituitarism can produce neurobehavioural disturbances with apathy, lethargy, depression, impaired concentration and memory, delusions and hallucinations (Cleghorn, 1951; Hanna, 1970). Endocrine replacement reverses these disturbances.

The empty sella syndrome

The empty sella syndrome is a diagnosis made after radiographic or surgical exploration when the sella is found to contain cerebrospinal fluid from the basal cisterns. It is not a primary diagnosis and therefore published series tend to be highly selective. Neelon *et al.* (1973) published a series of 31 patients, five of whom had major endocrine abnormalities. Despite the almost complete absence of macroscopic pituitary tissue, routine pituitary function tests were normal.

Metabolic Bone Disease

The finding of proximal muscle weakness and muscle fatiguability in osteomalacia has been taken to indicate the presence of a myopathy. There is no association between these symptoms and the biochemical abnormality. The lack of any characteristic abnormality on muscle biopsy or of an elevation of creatinine phosphokinase throws some doubt on whether this is a genuine myopathy.

REFERENCES

Abramsky, O. (1972). Common and uncommon neurological manifestations as presenting symptoms of vitamin B12 deficiency. *J. Am. Geriatr. Soc.*, **20**, 93–6.

Arieff, A.I., Llach, F., and Massry, S.G. (1976). Neurological manifestations and study of hyponatraemia. Correlation with brain water and electrolytes. *Medicine (Baltimore)*, **55**, 121–9.

Arnold, B.M., Casal, G., and Higgins, H.P. (1974). Apathetic thyrotoxicosis. *Can. Med. Assoc. J.*, **3**, 957–8.

Asher, R. (1949). Myxoedematous madness. *Br. Med. J.*, **ii**: 555–62.

Avran, M.M., Feinfeld, D.A., and Huatuco, A.H. (1978). Search for the uremic toxin. *N. Engl. J. Med.*, **298**, 1000–3.

Berger, J.R., and Ross, D.B. (1981). Reversible Parkinson syndrome complicating postoperative hypoparathyroidism. *Neurology*, **31**, 881–2.

Birchfield, R.I. (1964). Postural hypotension in Wernicke's disease, a manifestation of autonomic nervous system involvement. *Am. J. Med.*, **36**, 404–14.

Brin, M. (1962). Erythrocyte transketolase in early thiamin deficiency. *Ann. N.Y. Acad. Sci.*, **98**, 528.

Cleghorn, R.A. (1951). Adrenal cortical insufficiency: psychological and neurological observations. *Can. Med. Assoc. J.*, **65**, 449–54.

Cohen, C.R., Duchesneau, P.M., and Weinstein, M.A. (1980). Calcification of the basal ganglia as visualised by computed tomography. *Radiology*, **134**, 97–9.

Cohn, R., and Sode, J. (1971). The EEG in hypercalcemia. *Neurology*, **21**, 154–61.

Condon, J.V., Backa, D.R., and Gibbs, F.A. (1954). Electroencephalographic abnormalities in hyperthyroidism. *J. Clin. Endocrinol. Metabol.*, **14**, 1511–18.

Conn, H.O. (1969). A rational programme for the management of hepatic coma. *Gastroenterology*, **57**, 715–23.

Cravioto, H., Korein, J., and Silberman, J. (1961). Wernicke's encephalopathy. *Arch. Neurol.*, **4**, 510–19.

Cremer, G.M., Goldstein, N.P., and Paris, J. (1969). Myxoedema and ataxia. *Neurology*, **19**, 37–46.

Cummings, J.L., Benson, D.E., and LoVerme, S. Jr (1980). Reversible dementia. *J.A.M.A.*, **243**, 2434–9.

Deol, M.S. (1973). An experimental approach to the understanding and treatment of hereditary syndromes with congenital deafness and hypothyroidism. *J. Med. Genet.*, **10**, 235–42.

De Wardener, H.E., and Lennox, B. (1947). Cerebral beri beri (Wernicke's encephalopathy). *Lancet*, **1**, 11–17.

Drachman, D.B. (1962). Myasthenia gravis and the thyroid gland. *N. Engl. J. Med.*, **266**, 330–3.

Dubovsky, S.L., Grabon, S., Bert, T., and Schrier, R.W. (1973). Syndrome of inappropriate secretion of antidiuretic hormone with exacerbated psychosis. *Ann. Intern. Med.*, **79**, 552–4.

Eraut, D. (1974). Idiopathic hypoparathyroidism presenting as dementia. *Br. Med. J.*, **i**, 429–30.

Ettigi, P.G., and Brown, G.M. (1978). Brain disorders associated with endocrine dysfunction. *Psychiatr. Clin. North Am.*, **1**, 117–36.

Fehling, C., Jagerstad, M., Linstrand, K., and Elmqvist, D. (1974). Folate deficiency and neurological disease. *Arch. Neurol.*, **30**, 263–5.

Fitz, T.E., and Hallman, B.L. (1952). Mental changes associated with hyperparathyroidism. *Arch. Intern. Med.*, **89**, 547–51.

Flint, F.J., and Richards, S.M. (1956). Organic basis of confusional states in the elderly. *Br. Med. J.*, **ii**, 1537–9.

Gatewood, J.W., Organ, C.H.Jr., and Mead, B.T. (1975). Mental changes associated with hyperparathyroidism. *Am. J. Psychiatry*, **132**, 129–32.

Gelenberg, A. (1976). The catatonic syndrome. *Lancet*, **i**, 1339–41.

Ghez, C. (1969). Vestibular paresis: a clinical feature of Wernicke's disease. *J. Neurol. Neurosurg. Psychiatry*, **32**, 134–9.

Gilbert, V.E. (1968). Blood pyruvate and lactate during febrile human infections. *Metabolism*, **17**, 943.

Gilbert, V.E., Susser, M.C., and Nolte, A. (1969). Deficient thiamin pyrophosphate and blood alpha-ketoglutarate-pyruvate relationships during febrile human infections. *Metabolism*, **18**(9), 789.

Glaser, G.H. (1953). Psychotic reactions induced by corticotropin (ACTH) and cortisone. *Psychosomat. Med.*, **15**, 280–91.

Gordon, M., and Gryfe, C.I. (1981). Hyperthyroidism with painless subacute thyroiditis in the elderly. *J.A.M.A.*, **246**, 2354–5.

Hall, W.J. (1981). Psychiatric problems in the elderly related to organic pulmonary disease. In: Levenson, A.J., and Hall, R.C.W. (eds.) *Neuropsychiatric Manifestations of Physical Disease in the Elderly*, Raven Press, New York, pp. 41–8.

Hanna, S.M. (1970). Hypopituitarism (Sheehan's syndrome) presenting with organic psychosis. *J. Neurol. Neurosurg. Psychiatry*, **33**, 192–3.

Harman, J.B., and Richardson, J.T. (1954). Generalised myokymia in thyrotoxicosis. *Lancet*, **ii**, 473–4.

Harper, C. (1979). Wernicke's Encephalopathy: a more common disease than realised. A neuropathological study of 51 cases. *J. Neurol. Neurosurg. Psychiatry*, **42**, 226.

Henson, R.A. (1968). The neurological aspects of hypercalcemia: with special reference to primary hyperparathyroidism. *J. Roy. Coll. Physicians Lond.*, **1**, 41–50.

Hoch, F.L. (1970). Thyrotoxicosis as a disease of mitochondria. *N. Engl. J. Med.*, **266**, 446–55, 488, 505.

Hodkinson, H.M. (1973). Mental impairment in the elderly. *J. Roy. Coll. Physicians Lond.*, **7**, 305.

Hoffman, N.E. (1981). Gastrointestinal disease presenting as psychiatric symptoms. In: Levenson, A.J., and Hall, R.C.W. (eds.) *Neuropsychiatric Manifestations of Physical Disease in the Elderly*, Raven Press, New York, pp. 49–57.

Hoffmann, W.W., and Denys, E.H. (1972). Effect of the

thyroid hormone at the neuromuscular junction. *Am. J. Physiol.*, **223**, 283–7.

Hossain, M. (1970). Neurological and psychiatric manifestations in idiopathic hypoparathyroidism: response to treatment. *J. Neurol. Neurosurg. Psychiatry*, **33**, 153–6.

Hurwitz, L.J., McCormick, D., and Allen, I.V. (1970). Reduced muscle-glucosidase (acid-maltase) activity in hypothyroid myopathy. *Lancet*, **i**, 67–9.

Jabbari, B., and Huott, A.D. (1980). Seizures in thyrotoxicosis. *Epilepsia*, **21**, 91–6.

Jacobs, J.C., Gloor, P., Elwan, O.H., Dossetor, J.B., and Pateras, V.R. (1965). Electroencephalographic changes in chronic renal failure. *Neurology*, **15**, 419–29.

Jebsen, R.H., Tenckhoff, H., and Honet, J.C. (1967). Natural history of uraemic polyneuropathy and the effects of dialysis. *N. Engl. J. Med.*, **308**, 119–25.

Jolliffe, N., Bowman, K.M., Rosenblum, L.A., and Fein, H.D. (1940). Nicotinic acid deficiency encephalopathy. *J.A.M.A.*, **114**, 307–12.

Kelly, M.P., Garron, D.C., and Javid, H. (1980). Carotid artery disease, carotid endarterectomy, and behaviour. *Arch. Neurol.*, **37**, 178–80.

Kennedy, R.M., and Early, L.E. (1970). Profound hyponatraemia resulting from a thiazide-induced decrease in urinary diluting capacity in a patient with primary polydipsia. *N. Engl. J. Med.*, **202**, 1185–6.

Kiloh, L.G., McComas, A.J., and Osselton, J.W. (1972). *Clinical Electroencephalography*, third edition, Butterworths, London.

Krop, H.D., Block, A.J., and Cohen, E. (1973). Neuropsychiatric effects of continuous oxygen therapy in chronic obstructive pulmonary disease. *Chest*, **64**, 317–22.

Leavitt, S., and Tyler, H.R. (1964). Studies in asterixis. *Arch. Neurol.*, **10**, 360–8.

Lehrer, G.M., and Levitt, M.F. (1960). Neuropsychiatric presentation of hypercalcemia. *J. Mount Sinai Hosp.*, **27**, 10–18.

Liddle, G.W. (1971). Adrenal cortex. In: Beeson, P.B., and McDermott, W. (eds.) *Cecil and Loeb: Textbook of Medicine*, 13th edition, W.B. Saunders, Philadelphia, pp. 1780–99.

Lishman, W.A. (1978). *Organic Psychiatry*. Blackwell Scientific Publications, Oxford.

Logothetis, J. (1961). Neurologic and muscular manifestations of hyperthyroidism. *Arch. Neurol.*, **5**, 533–44.

Logothetis, J. (1963). Psychotic behaviour as the initial indicator of adult myxedema. *J. Nerv. Ment. Dis.*, **136**, 561–8.

Lonsdale, D., and Shamberger, R.J. (1980). Red cell transketolase as an indicator of nutritional deficiency. *Am. J. Clin. Nutr.*, **33**, 205.

Lunzer, M., James, I.M., Weinman, J., and Sherlock, S. (1974). Treatment of chronic hepatic encephalopathy with levadopa. *Gut*, **15**, 555–61.

McEntee, W.J., and Mair, R.G. (1980). Memory enhancement in Korsakoff's psychosis by clonidine:

further evidence for a noradrenergic deficit. *Ann. Neurol.*, **7**, 466–70.

Malamud, N., and Skillicorn, S.A. (1956). Relationship between the Wernicke and Korsakoff syndromes. *Arch. Neurol. Psychiatry*, **76**, 585–96.

Mallette, L.E., Bilezikian, J.P., Heath, D.A., and Auerbach, G.D. (1974). Primary hyperthyroidism: clinical and biochemical features. *Medicine*, **53**, 127–46.

Markowitz, A.M., Slanetz, C.A. Jr, and Frantz, V.K. (1961). Functioning islet cell tumours of the pancreas. *Ann. Surg.*, **154**, 877–84.

Meyer, A. (1982). The psychiatry of Addison's disease. *Schweiz. Arch. Neurol. Psychiat.*, **70**, 58–68.

Miller, P.D., Krebs, K.A., Neal, B.J., and McIntyre, D.O. (1982). Hypodipsia in geriatric patients. *Am. J. Med.*, **73**, 354–6.

Mitra, M.L. (1971). Confusional states in relation to vitamin deficiencies in the elderly. *J. Am. Geriatr. Soc.*, **19**(6), 536.

Morgan, M.Y., Jakobivits, A., Elithorn, A., James, I.M., and Sherlock, S. (1977). Successful use of bromocriptine in the treatment of patients with chronic protasystemic encephalopathy. *N. Engl. J. Med.*, **296**, 793–4.

Muenter, M.D., and Whisnant, J.P. (1968). Basal ganglia calcification, hypoparathyroidism, and extrapyramidal motor manifestations. *Neurology*, **18**, 1075–83.

Neelon, F.A., Goree, J., and Lebovitz, H. (1973). The primary empty sella: endocrine function. *Medicine*, **52**, 73–92.

Nickel, S.N., and Frame, B. (1958). Neurologic manifestations of myxedema. *Neurology*, **8**, 511–17.

Nobuyoshi, I., and Nishihara, Y. (1981). Pellagra among chronic alcoholics: clinical and pathological study of 20 necropsy cases. *J. Neurol. Neurosurg. Psychiatry*, **44**, 209–15.

Older, M.J.W., and Dickerson, J.W.T. (1982). Thiamin and the elderly orthopaedic patient. *Age Ageing*, **11**, 101.

Olivarius, B. de F., and Roder, E. (1970). Reversible psychosis and dementia in myxedema. *Acta Psychiatr. Scand.*, **46**, 1–13.

Oliveros, J.C., Jandali, M.K., Timsit-Berthier, M. *et al.* (1978). Vasopressin in amnesia. *Lancet*, **1**, 42.

Olsen, P.Z., Stoier, M., Sierksbaek-Nielson, K., Hansen, J.M., Shioler, M., and Kristensen, M. (1972). Electroencephalographic findings in hyperthyroidism. *Electroencephalogr. Clin. Neurophysiol.* **32**, 171–7.

Ord, W.M. (1878). On myxoedema, a term to be applied to an essential condition in the "cretinoid", affecting occasionally middle-aged women. *Medico-Surgical Transactions*, **61**, 57–78.

Pallis, C.A., and Lewis, P.D. (1974). *The Neurology of Gastrointestinal Disease*, W.B. Saunders, Philadelphia.

Pant, S.S., Asbury, A.K., and Richardson, E.P. Jr. (1968). The myelopathy of pernicious anaemia. *Acta Neurol. Scand.* **44** (Suppl. 35), 8–36.

Pincus, J.H., Respiolds, E.H., and Glaser, G.H. (1972).

Subacute combined system degeneration with folate deficiency. *J.A.M.A.*, **221**, 496–7.

Price, T.R., and Netsky, M.G. (1966). Myxedema and ataxia: cerebellar alterations and "neural myxedema bodies". *Neurology*, **16**, 957–62.

Puxty, J.A.H. (1985). Infections, vitamins and confusion in the elderly. In: Kemm, J.R. (ed.) *Vitamin Deficiency in the Elderly*, Blackwell Scientific Publications, Oxford, pp. 103–16.

Raskin, N.H., and Fishman, R.A. (1976). Neurologic disorders in renal failure. *N. Engl. J. Med.*, **294**, 143–8, 204–10.

Robinson, K.C., Kallbery, M.H., and Crowley, M.F. (1954). Idiopathic hypoparathyroidism presenting as dementia. *Br. Med. J.*, **ii**, 1203–6.

Sanders, V. (1962). Neurologic manifestations of myxedema. *N. Engl. J. Med.*, **266**, 547–52.

Scherokman, B.J. (1980). Triphasic delta waves in a patient with acute hyperthyroidism. *Arch. Neurol.*, **37**, 731.

Sensenbach, W., Madison, L., Iesenberg, S., and Ochs, L. (1954). The cerebral circulation and metabolism in hyperthyroidism and myxoedema. *J. Clin.*, **33**, 1434–40.

Sherlock, S., Summerskill, W.H.J., White, L.P., and Phear, E.A. (1954). Portasystemic encephalopathy. *Lancet*, **ii**, 453–7.

Silverman, D. (1962). Some observations on the EEG in hepatic coma. *Electroencephalogr. Clin. Neurophysiol.*, **14**, 53–9.

Slyter, H. (1979). Idiopathic hypoparathyroidism presenting as dementia. *Neurology*, **29**, 393–4.

Smith, J.S., Kiloh, L.G., Ratnavale, G.S., and Grant, D.A. (1976). The investigation of dementia. *Med. J. Aust.*, **2**, 403–5.

Smith, W.T. (1960). Nutritional deficiencies and disorders. In: Blackwood, W., and Corsellis, J.A.N. (eds.) *Greenfield's Neuropathology*, Year Book Medical Publishers, Chicago, pp. 148–93.

Soeters, P.B., and Fischer, J.E. (1976). Insulin, glucagon, amino acid imbalance, and hepatic encephalopathy. *Lancet*, **ii**, 880–2.

Spillane, J.D. (1947). *Nutritional Disorders of the Nervous System*, Williams and Wilkins, Philadelphia.

Starkman, M.N., and Schteingart, D.E. (1981). Neuropsychiatric manifestations of patients with Cushing's syndrome. *Arch. Intern. Med.*, **142**, 215–19.

Strachan, R.W., and Henderson, J.G. (1965). Psychiatric syndromes due to avitaminosis B12 with normal blood and marrow. *Q. J. Med.*, **34**, 303–17.

Strachan, R.W., and Henderson, J.G. (1967). Dementia and folate deficiency. *Q. J. Med.*, **36**, 189–204.

Sutherland, G.A. (1903). Chorea and Graves disease. *Brain*, **26**, 210–14.

Swanson, J.W., Kelly, J.J. Jr, and McConahey, W.M. (1981). Neurologic aspects of thyroid dysfunction. *Mayo Clin. Proc.*, **56**, 504–12.

Sydenstricker, V.P. (1943). The neurological complications of malnutrition. Psychic manifestations of nicotinic acid deficiency. *Proc. Roy. Soc. Med.*, **36**, 169–71.

Thompson, R.H.S., and Johnson, R.E. (1935). Blood pyruvate in vitamin B-1 deficiency. *Biochem. J.*, **29**, 694.

Tom, M.I., and Richardson, J.C. (1951). Hypoglycaemia from islet cell tumour of pancreas with amyotrophy and cerebrospinal nerve cell changes. *J. Neuropathol. Exp. Neurol.*, **10**, 57–66.

Trethowan, W.H., and Cobb, S. (1952). Neuropsychiatric aspects of Cushing's syndrome. *Arch. Neurol. Psychiatry*, **67**, 283–309.

Victor, M., and Adams, R.D. (1971). On the aetiology of the alcoholic neurologic diseases: with special reference to the role of nutrition. *Am. J. Clin. Nutr.*, **9**, 379–97.

Victor, M., Adams, R.D., and Collins, G.H. (1971). *The Wernicke–Korsakoff Syndrome*, F.A. Davis, Philadelphia.

Victor, M., and Lear, A.A. (1956). Subacute combined degeneration of the spinal cord. *Am. J. Med.*, **20**, 896.

Waldenström, J. (1945). Acute thyrotoxic encephalomyelopathy, its cause and treatment. *Acta Med. Scand.*, **121**, 251–94.

Weaver, J.A., Jones, A., and Smith, R.A. (1942). Cerebello-olivary degeneration: an example of heredo-familial incidence. *Brain*, **65**, 220–31.

Whybrow, P.C., Prange, A.J. Jr, and Treadway, C.R. (1969). Mental changes accompanying thyroid gland dysfunction. *Arch. Gen. Psychiatry*, **20**, 48–63.

Wood, B., Gijsbers, A., Goode, A., Davis, S., Mulholland, J., and Breen, K. (1980). A study of partial thiamine restriction in human volunteers. *Am. J. Clin. Nutr.*, **33**, 848–61.

Chapter 21

Paraneoplastic Neurological Syndromes

H. M. Warenius

Professor of Radiation Oncology, the Department of Radiation Oncology, Clatterbridge Hospital, Bebington, Wirral, Merseyside, UK

To the practising caring physician whose major concern is with the extent and quality of life of the patient suffering from malignancy, the neurological paraneoplastic syndromes may often seem to be of more academic than practical interest. This may particularly be the case in the elderly. Although the incidence of malignancy increases with age, the expected concomitant increased incidence of paraneoplastic syndromes may not be detected. One clinicopathological analysis (Zuffa *et al.*, 1984) of 1694 medical oncology patients has been reported in which 127 patients developed paraneoplastic syndromes. The age range was from 19 to 85 years, with a mean of 62.7 years. Apart from this series, few recent reports discuss patients over the age of 65 years.

It would thus appear that paraneoplastic syndromes may not be sought so avidly in the elderly. The reasons for this are:

1. These syndromes are relatively rare and the diagnosis is one of exclusion.
2. In the elderly a multiplicity of diseases may often coexist. The diagnosis of paraneoplastic syndrome in this situation is thus more difficult. To be certain that dementia in the elderly patient is a result of paraneoplastic encephalomyelitis and not vascular disease is not always possible and the answer may become apparent only at autopsy.
3. Whilst paraneoplastic neurological syndromes may herald a primary tumour, their course does

not necessarily parallel that of the malignancy. Thus treatment of the primary tumour may not necessarily cause a remission in the paraneoplastic syndrome. Moreover, in the elderly patient normal tissue tolerance may limit doses of radiotherapy and chemotherapy and the general condition of the patient may cancel the beneficial effect of surgical approach. The diagnosis of a neurological syndrome as paraneoplastic and the subsequent hunt for a primary tumour may therefore not appear justified.

Nevertheless, many elderly patients may be extremely fit and well prior to presenting with a paraneoplastic neurological syndrome. The improvements in radiotherapy and chemotherapy which can both control the primary tumour and frequently palliate disease effectively for acceptable periods of time, even when cure is not possible, should not be dismissed. Skilful use of radiotherapy using properly protracted fractionation regimens may often prove as well tolerated in the elderly patient as in the younger. Research in chemotherapy continues to yield new, less toxic agents and regimens, as well as producing new agents which are more effective against specific tumours. Examples of less toxic agents are mitozantrone, which produces less alopecia and cardiotoxicity than Adriamycin, and the recently available carboplatin, which has less renal toxicity than cisplatin. Thus, both the relative fitness of many elderly patients and improvements in our therapeutic modalities make us less reluctant to attempt good palliation and possibly cure in the elderly patient. An awareness of the neurological paraneoplastic syndromes that may occur in the elderly is thus important.

In a number of patients a paraneoplastic syndrome may itself be the first presentation of malignancy. Patients with no known cancer who develop certain neurological syndromes should be considered as having a high suspicion of occult cancer requiring full investigation. The syndromes which excite a high suspicion of cancer include: subacute cerebellar degeneration, encephalitis, subacute motor neurone disease, sensory motor peripheral neuropathy, Eaton–Lambert syndrome and dermatomyositis. Other syndromes such as amyotropic lateral sclerosis, sensory neuropathy and ascending acute polyneuropathy have a less definite association with malignancy and should not prompt energetic attempts to discover an underlying primary tumour. Syndromes such as subacute cerebellar degeneration may be associated with a number of solid tumours where local control of the primary is possible by surgery or radiotherapy, e.g. prostate, colorectal, cervix. Where the paraneoplastic syndrome is the first clinical evidence of such solid tumours the possibility of local control and even cure may exist and in addition there are reports of improvements of the syndrome accompanying removal of the primary tumour.

It should be remembered that sooner or later the majority of primary tumours do produce symptoms which are distressing and inconvenient to the patient. These, however, may initially be overshadowed by the presentation of the paraneoplastic syndrome. The neurological symptoms of the latter may mislead the physician to whom they present, either by focusing attention upon the neurological problem itself, thus leading to a delay in diagnosis of the underlying malignancy, or by suggesting that the patient is suffering from metastatic disease. Whilst it is true that neurological signs and symptoms are most frequently the result of metastatic disease, failure to identify a paraneoplastic neurological syndrome may wrongly result in the assumption that the patient does have metastases and thus the possibility of effective local treatment to the primary

may erroneously be dismissed. Attempts to treat the presumed metastasis in this situation for palliative reasons may also prove unsuccessful. Thus, radiotherapy to the posterior fossa would be an inappropriate treatment for subacute cerebellar degeneration, although it can prove most effective for metastases from a bronchial carcinoma.

INCIDENCE

True paraneoplastic syndromes are relatively rare and form only a small proportion of neurological problems occurring in the older patient with malignancy. Their precise incidence is uncertain because of an absence of control studies, most data having come from uncontrolled series. The incidence also varies from series to series. Croft and Wilkinson (1965) found neuromyopathies in 7% of 1476 cancer patients, of which the majority had lung cancer.

Zuffa *et al.* (1984) found paraneoplastic syndromes as a first manifestation of disease in 7.4% of 127 cases and the syndrome preceded malignancy in 4.6%. Wilner and Brody (1967), by contrast, found no difference in the frequency of neurological syndromes between patients with lung cancer and controls with chronic lung disease. The incidence of paraneoplastic syndrome should be placed in the context of the non-paraneoplastic neurological syndromes occurring in the patient with malignancy; thus 17% of all admissions for cancer to the Memorial Sloan-Kettering Cancer Centre had signs and symptoms requiring neurological consultation (Allen *et al.*, 1979). The majority of these were due to metastatic disease. At autopsy, 24% of all patients were shown to have intracranial metastases (Nugent *et al.*, 1979; Posner and Chernik, 1978).

In certain tumours a higher incidence of neurological paraneoplastic syndromes than that given above may be expected. Small cell bronchial carcinoma and ovarian carcinoma may have an incidence as high as 15% (Spence, 1978). Similarly, approximately 70% of paraneoplastic encephalomyelitis is associated with bronchial carcinomas, mainly of the small cell type, but it may also occur with tumours of the ovary, breast, stomach, uterus and larynx and in Hodgkin's disease (Henson and Urich, 1982). Eaton–Lambert syndrome also has a strong association with small cell bronchial carcinoma. Of 40 cases of Eaton–Lambert syndrome described at the Mayo Clinic 28 had malignant tumours and 20 of these were diagnosed as small cell bronchial carcinoma (Hildebrand, 1982).

CLASSIFICATION

Paraneoplastic neurological syndromes may be a remote manifestation of malignancy, primarily directed at the nervous system (Table 21.1); or they may produce neurological signs and symptoms as a result of more generalized paraneoplastic processes (Table 21.2), such as hypercalcaemia due to ectopic parathormone production or disturbances in sodium and potassium as a result of inappropriate antidiuretic hormone or corticotrophin. Vascular disease as a cause of neurological signs and symptoms is also of importance in the cancer patient. In elderly patients subarachnoid haemorrhage or hemiplegia due to thrombosis or embolism may frequently occur as a parallel event, unrelated to the malignancy from which the patient is suffering. It is of interest, however, that vascular problems in patients with

TABLE 21.1 CLASSIFICATION OF PARANEO-PLASTIC NEUROLOGICAL SYNDROMES: PRIMARY NERVOUS SYSTEM

Intracranial	Subacute cerebellar degeneration
	Progressive multifocal
	leucoencephalopathy
	Encephalomyelitis
	diffuse (dementia)
	limbic
	bulbar
Optic	Neuritis
	Uveomeningitis
	Retinopathy
Spinal	Amyotropic lateral sclerosis
	Subacute necrotizing myelopathy
	Subacute motor neuropathy
Peripheral	Sensorimotor peripheral neuropathy
	Sensory neuropathy
	Ascending acute polyneuropathy
Neuromuscular	Myasthenia gravis
	Eaton–Lambert
	Dermatomyositis
	Polymyositis

TABLE 21.2 CLASSIFICATION OF PARANEO-PLASTIC NEUROLOGICAL SYNDROMES: NEUROLOGICAL MANIFESTATIONS DUE TO GENERALIZED PARANEOPLASTIC PROCESSES

Vascular	Disseminated intravascular coagulation
	Non-bacterial thrombotic endocarditis
	Primary cerebral thrombosis
	(superior sagittal sinus thrombosis)
	Hyperviscosity syndrome
Endocrine	Inappropriate antidiuretic hormone
	Inappropriate corticotrophin
	Hypercalcaemia
	Inappropriate parathormone
	Bone metastases
	Hypoglycaemia (insulinoma)
	Carcinoid syndrome
Metabolic	Hepatic
	Renal

malignancy may show a strikingly dissimilar picture from that in the general population (Minna and Bunn, 1982). Thus, marantic and septic emboli, disseminated intravascular coagulation, tumour related haemorrhage, superior sagittal sinus occlusion and many cases of subarachnoid haemorrhage were noted to be directly tumour related and account for well over 50% of strokes in some series of cancer patients (Rosen and Armstrong, 1973; Collins *et al.*, 1975; Sigsbee *et al.*, 1979).

Risk factors for the general population such as hypertension, arteriosclerotic heart disease and diabetes were noted to be less important in the cancer patient. Marantic emboli following marantic endocarditis (non-bacterial thrombotic endocarditis) occur predominantly in patients with adenocarcinomas, especially of the lung, and may present neurologically as multifocal abnormalities, focal abnormalities or encephalopathy without any focal defects. Haemorrhage occurs most frequently in leukaemia and septic emboli as a result of fungal infection.

A further generalized vascular syndrome which may present neurologically is hyperviscosity syndrome. This may occur in Waldenström's macroglobulinaemia or in some IgA secreting myelomas.

Table 21.1 gives a classification of the majority of the specific neurological syndromes reported to have a neoplastic association. Amongst these, subacute cerebellar degeneration, encephalomyelitis, subacute motor neuropathy, Eaton–Lambert syndrome, sensory motor peripheral neuropathy and dermatomyositis have the strongest associations with malignancy and are the most frequently encountered.

AETIOLOGY

Except for those syndromes where there is an identifiable primary pathophysiology, such as that due to hyperviscosity, carcinoid, ectopic hormone production or a vascular problem such as diffuse intravascular coagulation (DIC), the aetiology of most neurological paraneoplastic syndromes is uncertain. Attempts to explain the aetiology have invoked either infectious or humoral mechanisms. Recent evidence suggests that at least one syndrome has a direct infectious aetiology and should probably not be considered a true paraneoplastic neurological syndrome, whilst an autoimmune mechanism has been suggested for another.

Progressive multifocal leucoencephalopathy associated with dementia, paralysis, aphasia, ataxia, dysarthria and visual field defects, and characterized by pathological demyelination of white matter, was initially thought to be a paraneoplastic syndrome associated with leukaemias, lymphomas and sarcomas. It is now known (Padgett *et al.*, 1971; Weiner *et al.*, 1972) to be due to infection by papovaviruses which may be of two types, an SV40-like virus or one Padgett *et al.* designated as JC virus (Padgett *et al.*, 1971). With regard to other syndromes, there is scant evidence of an infectious aetiology although virus-like particles have been detected in patients suffering from Hodgkin's disease (Walton *et al.*, 1968; Norris *et al.*, 1970) accompanied by subacute motor neuropathy, and in one case (Glaser and Pincus, 1969) of encephalomyelitis intranuclear inclusion bodies suggestive of a viral infection have been detected.

An immunological attack upon specific neurological tissue has been suggested as one humoral pathophysiological mechanism by which some tumours cause a paraneoplastic neurological syndrome. Increasing evidence has now been provided that in some cases of subacute cerebellar degeneration associated with ovarian carcinoma, antibodies directed against cerebellar tissue and in particular Purkinje

cells can be detected. This evidence was based on studies where sera from two ovarian cancer patients with a paraneoplastic cerebellar syndrome confirmed at autopsy gave positive immunofluorescence, with bright cytoplasmic staining of Purkinje cells and neurones within deep cerebellar nuclei (Greenlee and Brashear, 1983).

However, 50% of cases of cerebellar degeneration may occur in the absence of cancer and further studies (Jaeckle *et al.*, 1985) have shown that antibody to Purkinje cells was not detected in 160 patients including neurologically normal cancer patients or 130 ovarian cancer patients. Moreover, this study also showed that the antibodies which reacted with Purkinje cells and which were circulating in the serum of patients with subacute degeneration did not react with the primary tumour. This latter finding was incompatible with an aetiological theory suggesting that the presence of the tumour had invoked an antibody which fortuitously reacted against shared antigenic components on both tumour cells and neurological tissue.

One further piece of evidence for a possible humoral aetiology of a paraneoplastic syndrome is the description (Fukumara *et al.*, 1972) of the effect of an acetone extract of tumour tissue taken from a patient with Eaton–Lambert syndrome. This extract produced an in vitro defect in neuromuscular transmission in frog muscle by reducing acetylcholine release.

DIFFERENTIAL DIAGNOSIS

In the differential diagnosis of all CNS paraneoplastic syndromes, intraparenchymal and leptomeningeal metastatic neoplasms usually head the list when there is a known primary. Vascular disease is the second most likely cause of neurological symptoms and/or signs. Infectious complications associated with depressed immunity from either the underlying malignancy or from chemotherapeutic agents must also be ruled out. There are many such infections associated with depressed immunity; the more common ones include encephalitis due to *Toxoplasma*, aspergillosis or mucormycosis, meningitis from *Cryptococcus* or *Listeria monocytogenes* and herpes zoster encephalitis and/or myelitis.

The differential diagnosis also encompasses a lengthy list of secondary metabolic disorders including hypercalcaemia, disseminated intravascular coagulation (DIC), hyponatraemia secondary to inappropriate antidiuretic hormone secretion, hypoglycaemia, hepatic encephalopathy and deficiency of vitamins B1, B12 or folate. Alcoholic neuropathy with Wernicke's encephalopathy or Korsakoff's psychosis should also be considered and hypothyroidism should be excluded as should the iatrogenic effects of medication.

INTRACRANIAL SYNDROMES

These are less common than paraneoplastic syndromes involving other areas of the neuraxis and in one large series of 1476 cancer patients, only fifteen were noted to have intracranial paraneoplastic lesions (Croft and Wilkinson, 1965). All these cases had subacute cerebellar degeneration.

Subacute Cerebellar Degeneration

Subacute cerebellar degeneration is characterized by cerebellar atrophy with destruction of Purkinje cells, variable loss of granule cells and in some cases loss of basket cells (Spence, 1983).

It has been reported most frequently with carcinoma of the ovary and lung but also occurs with Hodgkin's disease, non-Hodgkin's lymphoma and cancer of the breast, uterus, stomach, colon and larynx (Brain and Wilkinson, 1965). It may occur alone or accompany Eaton–Lambert syndrome, encephalomyelitis or paraneoplastic peripheral neuropathy.

Subacute cerebellar atrophy is characterized clinically by progressive ataxia, vertigo, dysarthria and nystagmus. Pathological changes consistent with the syndrome have, however, been found in the cerebellum in patients undergoing autopsy following death from other neoplastic disorders such as cerebral or spinal encephalomyelitis. It would thus appear that obvious cerebellar damage can occur before the clinical syndrome becomes manifest. The diagnosis of subacute cerebellar atrophy is one of exclusion and in the elderly patient it is particularly difficult to differentiate from vascular disease, but may be distinguished clinically from cerebellar metastases by its symmetry. An absence of raised intracranial pressure should also exclude the diagnosis of cerebellar metastases as should a negative CT scan. The latter, however, can appear normal despite the presence of posterior fossa metastases. Subacute cerebellar atrophy may usually be clinically separated from alcoholic cerebellar degeneration in which dysarthria and upper extremity ataxia are usually mild or absent. In the elderly the insidious onset of myxoedema must also be considered.

Whilst earlier experience suggested that removal of the primary and more recently plasmapheresis (Cocconi *et al.*, 1985) could affect the progress of this syndrome, one of the most recent studies suggests that the disease is in general progressive (Jaeckle *et al.*, 1985). This may be due to the pathological observations recorded above, in which quite severe damage to Purkinje cells may occur before the syndrome becomes clinically manifest. Removing the stimulus to the syndrome, either by treatment of the primary tumour or by lowering circulating immunoglobulin levels by plasmapheresis, may thus be too late in the natural history to effect a clinical recovery. Even in those cases where claims have been made for clinical improvement, this has usually only been partial and transient, although raised circulating IgG levels and low C1q complement levels have been returned to normal by the plasmapheresis.

Future progress may well require detecting the immune response which produces subacute cerebellar degeneration before clinical signs have become manifest. This would, however, require screening immunoglobulin and complement levels in relatively large numbers of patients with ovarian, lung, breast and possibly other cancers. It should also be borne in mind that 50% of cases of subacute cerebellar degeneration occur in the absence of any evidence of cancer and that 50% of cases in patients with cancer may not have detectable antibodies. The aetiology in this latter situation is still uncertain.

PROGRESSIVE MULTIFOCAL LEUCOENCEPHALOPATHY

Progressive multifocal leucoencephalopathy (PML) is a well-defined syndrome in which demyelination of white matter is found throughout the nervous system. It occurs most often in malignancies associated with impaired immunity (leukaemias and lymphomas) but also occurs in benign conditions with altered immunity (sarcoid or steroid therapy). Its viral aetiology was confirmed in 1965 by electron microscopy (Zurhein and Chou, 1965; Silverman and Rubenstein, 1965). Viral particles were seen to be present in the nuclei of oligodendrocytes in PML lesions. The neuropathological changes rather than the clinical features distinguish PML. The lesions occur predominantly in the cerebrum, less often in cerebellum and brain stem, and only rarely in the spinal cord. They are yellow, necrotic and vary in size from millimetres to several centimetres as they become confluent. Oligodendroglial cells and myelin sheaths are completely destroyed in the central regions of advanced lesions. Around the periphery of the lesions, the oligodendrocytes have enlarged nuclei and the chromatin is displaced by large intranuclear inclusion bodies. Neurones and axons tend to be spared but astrocytes assume features of neoplastic change, with pleomorphism and bizarrely shaped hyperchromatic enlarged nuclei. Inflammatory changes are usually lacking. Most cases demonstrate reduction of delayed hypersensitivity responses to skin tests with purified protein derivative, and keyhole-limpet haemocyanin, etc.

The clinical features of PML are protean. With few exceptions, however, this disease is relentlessly progressive to death in 4–6 months. The onset of PML is usually months to years after the primary malignancy has been diagnosed and treated, or after some other chronic wasting disease has been active. PML typically presents as insidious onset of weakness in one limb or one side of the body. Personality changes, gait disturbance and symptoms of dementia, dysarthria or impaired vision are the complaints. Such a presentation may frequently be attributed to vascular problems in the elderly, particularly when occurring a considerable period of time after treatment of the primary disease. CSF analysis is usually normal, although the protein may be slightly elevated.

Certain diagnosis of PML can be made only by brain biopsy, which demonstrates the light and electron microscopic pathological features. Frozen tissue sections can be treated with specific antiviral antibodies, in an indirect immunofluorescence assay, to yield a precise virological diagnosis. Specific serum antibodies against the viral agent can be detected. Their use diagnostically is, however, not helpful because 65% of the population demonstrate positive antibodies by the age of 14 (Walker, 1978).

In the immunocompromised patient other infections in addition to the JC or SV40-like virus should be sought, especially toxoplasmosis and aspergillosis.

Some reports have suggested successful treatment of PML with cytosine arabinoside (Baver *et al.*, 1973; Marriott *et al.*, 1975). Other drugs such as iododeoxyuridine have not been reported as being successful.

ENCEPHALOMYELITIS

Approximately 70% of cases of paraneoplastic encephalomyelitis are associated with bronchial carcinoma, mainly of the small cell type (Henson and Urich, 1982). The other 30% have been reported in association with a wide spectrum of other tumour types which include Hodgkin's disease and cancer of the ovary, breast, stomach, uterus and larynx.

Paraneoplastic encephalomyelitis is distinguished by an inflammatory histological pattern involving the cerebral grey matter diffusely. Though the syndrome may affect multiple sites including the spinal cord, it has usually been classified as (1) diffuse encephalitis, (2) limbic encephalitis or (3) bulbar encephalitis.

It is unusual to see macroscopic changes in the brain, except in limbic encephalitis where the lesions are occasionally extensive enough to be visible grossly as discoloration and thinning of the cortical grey matter band. Characteristically the histological pattern of encephalomyelitis is one of neuronophagia, monocytic infiltration in the meninges and perivascular spaces and microglial infiltration and nodule formation in the parenchyma. Intranuclear inclusions suggestive of a viral aetiology are lacking with only one case report of such an occurrence.

Diffuse encephalitis produces a subacute dementia with or without seizures that are myoclonic or of a generalized grand mal character. Limbic encephalitis is characterized by involvement of the hippocampal formation, amygdaloid nuclei, cingulate gyri, insula and orbital cortex. This produces a clinical syndrome of personality change, anxiety, depression and loss of recent memory. In bulbar encephalitis the medulla and pons are usually the sites of greatest inflammatory reaction. This may result in progressive paralysis of the muscles innervated by cranial nerves V, VII, IX, X and XII. Lesions in the vestibular nuclei, vestibular cerebellar connections and vestibular oculomotor pathways lead to vertigo, nausea, vomiting, nystagmus and ataxia. Other symptoms and signs reported include diffuse muscular rigidity and involuntary movements. Cerebellar signs may also occur due to involvement of cerebellar afferent and efferent pathways.

Cerebral paraneoplastic encephalomyelitis may show abnormal electroencephalographic patterns. Non-specific slowing or irregularities in the background may be detected, or epileptiform discharges which correlate with a clinically evident seizure. Cerebrospinal fluid changes have also been noted, with an increase in the protein level, sometimes as high as hundreds of milligrams per decilitre. A mild monocytic pleocytosis is also often encountered.

In most patients who develop paraneoplastic encephalomyelitis there is a steadily deteriorating clinical course over weeks to months. Attempts to affect the progress of this syndrome with ACTH steroids or vitamins have not been successful.

OPTIC PARANEOPLASTIC SYNDROMES

Ophthalmological signs and symptoms may be the result of primary paraneoplastic problems such as optic neuritis, uveomeningitis or paraneoplastic retinopathy. They may also occur as a result of more generalized paraneoplastic processes. Ophthalmoplegia and nystagmus may thus be secondary to paraneoplastic encephalomyelitis with bulbar involvement (Klingele *et al.*, 1984; Halperin *et al.*, 1981) or ptosis; ophthalmoplegia, nystagmus and facial weakness may be associated with subacute cerebellar degeneration (Brain and Wilkinson, 1965). Opsoclonus (Ellenberger *et al.*, 1968), though a well-recognized paraneoplastic syndrome has not been recorded as occurring in the elderly. The

syndrome is most common between 8 months and 5 years with peak incidence of 2 years. Occasional adult cases have been reported, but not in the elderly (Spence, 1983). Disturbances of ocular movement may be seen as a result of paraneoplastic myasthenia gravis (Rowland *et al.*, 1973) in association with thymoma where ptosis and ophthalmoparesis may be the presenting signs. Other generalized paraneoplastic syndromes which may produce optic signs and symptoms are hyperviscosity syndrome, resulting in chorioretinopathy and optic disc oedema, and nutritional amblyopia resulting in visual field defects.

Primary paraneoplastic retinopathy (Sawyer *et al.*, 1976; Keltner *et al.*, 1983) has been described in association with cancer of the lung, breast, uterus or kidney. Total degeneration of the photoreceptor cell layer, with a marked loss of nuclei from the outer nuclear layer, is noted. This may be accompanied by melanophages in the retina. Clinically it presents with decreased visual acuity, visual field defects, nyctalopia and absent electroretinographic response. Uveomeningitic syndrome (Rudge, 1973) has been described in association with breast cancer where decreased visual acuity, mild anterior uveitis, macular oedema and papillitis may be found.

SPINAL PARANEOPLASTIC NEUROLOGICAL SYNDROMES

Amyotropic Lateral Sclerosis (ALS)

In a series of 130 patients with amyotropic lateral sclerosis (Norris and Engel, 1965) 10% were reported as having an underlying malignancy. When associated with cancer the sex distribution appeared to be predominantly male and the age of onset was older. Also the course of the disease appeared to progress more slowly in cancer patients. These findings have not been confirmed by later reports (Barrow and Rodichok, 1982).

Subacute Motor Neuropathy

Schold *et al.* (1979) assigned ten patients with lymphomas who developed subacute lower motor neurone weakness to the diagnostic category subacute motor neuropathy. Whilst this disease complex may overlap with that of the amyotrophic lateral sclerosis previously described, it does appear to be different from ALS both clinically and pathologically. The weakness may be proximal or distal and often asymmetric. Atrophy, fasciculation and reduced tendon jerks were common but involvement of bulbar respiratory muscles was not prominent. Nerve conduction velocities were unremarkable, but electromyography (EMG) showed denervation potentials. Pathologically there was loss of anterior horn neurones accompanied by inflammatory infiltration in the anterior horns, partial degeneration of the posterior columns, degeneration of ventral spinal groups and denervation changes in muscle. In most patients the motor neurone weakness tended to stabilize or even improve. The pathology resembles that of poliomyelitis so that the possibility of opportunistic viral aetiology cannot be discounted. This syndrome appears to be most common in irradiated patients suffering from lymphoma.

Subacute Necrotic Myelopathy

Subacute necrotic myelopathy (Mancall and Rosales, 1964) is characterized by a rapid motor and sensory paralysis which is most severe in the thoracic region. It usually terminates in death in a matter of days or weeks. There are often degenerative lesions in areas of grey and white matter. The CSF protein level is usually elevated. The syndrome is most often reported in association with lung cancer but may occur with other tumours. It has been reported in association with cerebellar degeneration (Renkawek and Kida, 1983; Greenfield, 1934).

Peripheral Paraneoplastic Neurological Syndromes

The peripheral nerves are the most frequent site in which paraneoplastic syndromes have been observed. The first observations of this association were reported before the beginning of the twentieth century. In 1965 Croft and Wilkinson divided these peripheral neuropathies into asymmetrical sensory peripheral neuropathy and acute or subacute sensory motor neuropathy. This paraneoplastic syndrome has been found to occur most frequently with multiple myeloma or lymphoma rather than with

carcinoma. Even in those cases associated with carcinoma it is possible that the picture was one of acute demyelinating neuropathy rather than subacute sensory motor neuropathy. Presentation may be similar to that of Guillain–Barré syndrome with weakness, clumsiness, numbness and tingling of the lower extremities, elevated CSF protein level and delayed nerve conduction velocity rates (Lisak, 1977). The syndrome has often progressed to paralysis before signs of the primary malignancy have arisen. It may run a progressively fatal course, but there are reports of patients having recovered from the neuropathy. Because the pattern of neuropathy is associated with lymphoproliferative malignancies it has been suggested that pathogenesis involves disordered immune function. Direct evidence to support this speculation, however, is lacking.

Subacute Sensory Neuropathy

Pure sensory neuropathy associated with degeneration of dorsal root ganglia (dorsal root ganglionitis) is strongly associated with malignancy. In the majority of cases the tumour has been reported as localized to the chest (Denny Brown, 1948; Smith and Whitfield, 1953). These reports have included lung cancer, thymoma, lymphomas involving the mediastinum, and laryngeal or oesophageal carcinoma (Horwich and Chol Porro, 1977).

Subacute sensory neuropathy may show considerable overlap with paraneoplastic encephalomyelitis (Henson and Urich, 1982). The syndrome is characterized by subacute development of distal sensory loss, especially proprioception and loss of deep tendon reflexes with normal muscle strength. Motor nerve conduction velocities are normal and CSF proteins often elevated. The patient is usually severely disabled and the syndrome rarely improves.

Ascending Acute Polyneuropathy (Guillain–Barré Syndrome)

Although this syndrome has been reported in some patients with malignancy, particularly Hodgkin's and non-Hodgkin's lymphoma, it is identical to that found clinically in the absence of malignancy. For this reason the association may be coincidental.

Peripheral nerve abnormalities may also be found as a result of other phenomena associated with cancer. Mononeuritis multiplex may develop as a result of tumour related vasculitis limited to the peripheral nervous system (Johnson *et al.*, 1979), or as a result of amyloid deposition. Amyloid deposition occurs most commonly in patients with multiple myeloma (Kelly *et al.*, 1981), where it may be the cause of carpal tunnel syndrome as a result of amyloid deposition in the flexor retinaculum at the wrist.

NEUROMUSCULAR PARANEOPLASTIC NEUROLOGICAL SYNDROMES

Dermatomyositis and Polymyositis

Some reports based on uncontrolled single institution studies suggest that patients with dermatomyositis and polymyositis have five to seven times the incidence of malignancy as the general population (Williams, 1959; Barnes, 1976). This association is most striking in males over 50 years of age, where over 50% have developed cancer. The association between dermatomyositis and occult cancer is stronger than with polymyositis. The clinical features of the syndrome are gradually progressive proximal muscle weakness occurring over weeks to months. Reflexes are usually present but diminished. The rash of dermatomyositis is an erythematous and oedematous eruption involving eyelids, malar areas, anterior chest, extensor surfaces on large joints and knuckles and the periungual skin. The erythrocyte sedimentation rate (ESR) is usually elevated.

The diagnosis of dermatomyositis is based on the presence of the rash plus at least two of the following:

1. Elevated serum levels of muscle associated enzymes such as creatine kinase.
2. A myopathic pattern of EMG.
3. Proximal muscle weakness.
4. The presence of inflammatory changes in a muscle biopsy specimen.

When all the muscle related changes above are present without a rash, polymyositis is the correct diagnosis.

In most instances the myopathy and cancer present within one year of one another. There have been no long-term follow-up studies to determine whether patients with dermatomyositis who do not develop cancer within one year continue to be at a high risk for developing cancer.

Eaton–Lambert Syndrome

Eaton–Lambert syndrome is an uncommon paraneoplastic manifestation of malignancy. It is strongly associated with small cell undifferentiated brochogenic carcinoma and has been reported to occur in 6% of small cell lung cancer patients in one series as compared to 1% of all lung cancer patients (Lambert and Rooke, 1965). Carcinoma of the breast, prostate, stomach, rectum and non-Hodgkin's lymphoma have also been implicated (Rooke *et al.*, 1960; Elmquist and Lambert, 1968). The syndrome has been described rarely in the absence of any evidence of malignancy.

The symptoms frequently develop several months before the underlying carcinoma is detected. The diagnosis of Eaton–Lambert syndrome thus makes a careful search for lung cancer mandatory. Both in the literature and in the author's experience, response of small cell lung cancer to combination chemotherapy has resulted in improvement in the Eaton–Lambert syndrome.

The syndrome is characterized by weakness and easy fatiguability predominantly in the proximal limb muscles. Patients also complain of aching of the thighs and dryness of the mouth. In contrast to myasthenia gravis there is usually little involvement of bulbar or extra-ocular muscles. The tendon reflexes are reduced or absent. In contrast to true myasthenia gravis, muscle strength improves with exercise. EMG confirms the increase in muscle action potential with repeated nerve stimulation at rates greater than 10/sec.

In addition to treatment of the primary tumour with combination chemotherapy, in the majority of cases of Eaton–Lambert syndrome (where small cell bronchial carcinoma is the primary cause) guanidine hydrochloride is an effective agent in providing symptomatic relief by increasing the amount of acetylcholine liberated by nerve terminals. Plasma-pheresis and 4-aminopyridine have proved less useful.

Myasthenia Gravis

Myasthenia gravis is strongly associated with thymoma. A number of other tumours including lymphomas and carcinoma of the pancreas, breast, prostate, ovary, thyroids, cervix, kidney, rectum and palate have been reported in association with myasthenia gravis but uncertainty remains as to whether myasthenia gravis is a true paraneoplastic syndrome accompanying these tumours.

More than 85% of patients with myasthenia gravis have abnormalities of the thymus (Elias and Appel, 1979) and between 9% and 15% have thymomas (Namba et al., 1978). More than 70% have thymic hyperplasia with an increased number of germinal centres (Castleman, 1966). Thymoma occurs with equal frequency in men and women. Approximately 30% of patients with thymoma have myasthenia gravis when the tumour is detected.

The recommended treatment for patients with thymoma with or without myasthenia gravis is complete surgical removal of the tumour. Approximately 70% of thymomas are encapsulated and completely resectable. Where the thymoma cannot be fully resected because of local invasion of pleura, lung or pericardium, radiotherapy should be added since these tumours are relatively radioresponsive. Patients suffering from myasthenia gravis as a result of thymoma are treated with anticholinesterase drugs, glucocorticoids, plasmapheresis and immunosuppressive drugs in an identical manner to patients without a thymoma. The patients with thymoma, however, have a distinctly worse prognosis.

Malignant Cachexia

In addition to the above well-characterized paraneoplastic neuromuscular disorders, it should be noted that many patients with malignancy suffer from cachexia, particularly involving loss of muscle bulk. These may occur more with some tumours such as lung cancer than with others such as breast cancer. Whilst malignant cachexia is at present not classified as a paraneoplastic disorder, it does show many features which suggest that it might be added to the syndromes included under this heading. Its aetiology at present remains obscure.

CONCLUSION

The paraneoplastic neurological syndromes thus show many features which merit careful documentation when they occur in patients, irrespective of age. An increased understanding of the aetiology of at least some of these syndromes and some evidence of responses to treatment, albeit partial, in some situations should encourage the physician to diagnose them accurately where they exist so that he may be in a better position to make relevant decisions about how to manage the elderly patient with malignancy who presents with any of these particular problems.

REFERENCES

Allen, J.C., Deck, M.D.F., Foley, K.M., Galicich, J.H., Holland, J.C.B., Morten, B., Pasternak, J.B., Posner, J.B., Price, R.W., Rottenberg, D.A., Shapiro, W.R., and Young, D.F. (1979). Neuro-oncology II, Dept. of Neurology, Memorial Sloan-Kettering Cancer Centre, N.Y.

Barnes, B.E. (1976). Dermatomyositis and malignancy: A review of the literature. Ann. Intern. Med., 84, 68–76.

Barrow, K.D., and Rodichok, L.D. (1982). Cancer and disorders of motor neurons. In: Rowland, P. (ed.) Human Motor Neuron Disease, Raven Press, New York, pp. 267–72.

Baver, W.R., Turel, A.P., and Johnson, K.P. (1973). Progressive multifocal leucoencephalopathy and cytoarabine. J.A.M.A., 266, 174–5.

Brain, W.R., and Wilkinson, M. (1965). Subacute cerebellar degeneration associated with neoplasms. Brain, 88, 465–78.

Castleman, B. (1966). The pathology of the thymus gland in myasthenia gravis. Ann. N.Y. Acad. Sci., 135, 496–9.

Cocconi, G., Ceci, G., Juvarra, G., Minopoli, M.R., Cocchi, T., Fiaccadori, F., Lechi, A., and Boni, P. (1985). Successful treatment of subacute cerebellar degeneration in ovarian carcinoma with plasmaphoresis. Cancer, 56, 2318–20.

Collins, R.C., Al-Mandhiry, H., Chernik, N.L., and Posner, J.B. (1975). Neurologic manifestations of intravascular coagulation in patients with cancer. A clinico-pathological analysis of 12 cases. *Neurology*, **25**, 795–806.

Croft, P., and Wilkinson, M. (1965). The incidence of carcinomatous neuromyopathy in patients with various types of carcinoma. *Brain*, **88**, 427–34.

Denny Brown, D. (1948). Primary sensory neuropathy with muscular changes associated with carcinoma. *J. Neurol. Neurosurg. Psychiatry*, **11**, 73–80.

Elias, S.B., and Appel, S.H. (1979). Current concepts in the pathogenesis and treatment of myasthenia gravis. *Med. Clin. North Am.*, **63**, 745–56.

Ellenberger, C. Jr, Campa, J.F., and Netsky, M.G. (1968). Opsoclonus and parenchymatous degeneration of the cerebellum. The cerebellar origin of an abnormal ocular movement. *Neurology*, **18**, 1041–6.

Elmquist, D., and Lambert, E.H. (1968). Detailed analysis of neuromuscular transmission in a patient with the myasthenic syndrome sometimes associated with bronchial carcinoma. *Mayo Clin. Proc.*, **43**, 689–95.

Fukumara, N., Takamori, M., Gutmann, L., and Chou, S.M. (1972). Eaton–Lambert syndrome ultrastructural study of the motor end plates. *Arch. Neurol.*, **27**, 67–78.

Glaser, G.H., and Pincus, J.H. (1969). Limbic encephalitis. *J. Nerv. Ment. Dis.*, **149**, 59–65.

Greenfield, J.G. (1934). Subacute spinocerebellar degeneration occurring in elderly patients. *Brain*, **57**, 161–76.

Greenlee, J.E., and Brashear, H.R. (1983). Antibodies to cerebellar purkinje cells in patients with paraneoplastic cerebellar degeneration and ovarian carcinoma. *Ann. Neurol.*, **14**, 609–13.

Halperin, J.J., Richardson, E.P. Jr, Ellis, J., Ross, J.S., and Wray, S.A. (1981). Paraneoplastic encephalomyelitis and neuropathy. *Arch. Neurol.*, **38**, 773–5.

Henson, R.A., and Urich, H. (1982). Cortical cerebellar degeneration. In: *Cancer and the Nervous System. The Neurological Manifestations of Systemic Malignant Disease*, Blackwell, Oxford, pp. 346–57.

Hildebrand, J. (1982). Neurological paraneoplasia. *Eur. J. Cancer Clin. Oncol.*, **17**(9), 985–90.

Horwich, M.S., and Chol Porro, R.S. (1977). Subacute sensory neuropathy a remote effect of carcinoma. *Ann. Neurol.*, **2**, 7–11.

Jaeckle, K.A., Grans, F., Houghton, A., Cardon-Cardo, C., Nielson, S.L., and Posner, J.B. (1985). Autoimmune response of patients with a paraneoplastic cerebellar degeneration to a Purkinje cell cytoplasmic protein antigen. *Ann. Neurol.*, **18**, 592–600.

Johnson, P.C., Polak, L.A., and Hamilton, R.H. (1979). Paraneoplastic vasculitis of nerve. A remote effect of cancer. *Ann. Neurol.*, **5**, 437–42.

Kelly, J.J., Kyle, R.A., and Miles, J.M. (1981). The spectrum of peripheral neuropathy in myeloma. *Neurology*, **31**, 24–34.

Keltmer, J.L., Roth, A.M., and Chang, S. (1983). Photoreceptor degeneration: a possible autoimmune disease. *Arch. Ophthalmol.*, **101**, 564–9.

Klingele, T.G., Burde, R.M., Rapazzo, A.J., Isserman, M.J., Burgess, D., and Kantor, O. (1984). Paraneoplastic retinopathy. *J. Clin. Neuro-Ophthalmol.*, **4**, 239–45.

Lambert, E.H., and Rooke, E.D. (1965). Myasthenic state and lung cancer. In: Brain, W.R., and Norris, F.H. Jr. (eds.) *The Remote Effects of Cancer on the Nervous System*, Grune and Stratton, New York, pp. 67–80.

Lisak, R.P. (1977). Guillain–Barré syndrome and Hodgkin's disease. Three cases with immunological studies. *Ann. Neurol.*, **1**, 72–8.

Mancall, E.L., and Rosales, R.K. (1964). Necrotising myelopathy associated with visceral carcinoma. *Brain*, **87**, 636–41.

Marriott, P.J., O'Brien, M.D., and Mackenzie, I.C.K. (1975). Progressive multifocal leucoencephalopathy; remission with cytoarabine. *J. Neurol. Neurosurg. Psychiatry*, **38**, 205–8.

Minna, J.D., and Bunn, P.A. Jr (1982). Paraneoplastic syndromes. In: Devita, V.T. Jr, Hellindi, S., and Rosenberg, S.A. (eds.) *Cancer. Principles and Practice of Oncology*, J.B. Lippincott, Philadelphia, Toronto, pp. 1476–517.

Namba, T., Brunner, N.G., and Grob, D. (1978). Myasthenia gravis in patients with thymoma with particular reference to onset after thymectomy. *Medicine*, **57**, 411–20.

Norris, F.H., and Engel, W.K. (1965). Carcinomatous amyotrophic lateral sclerosis. In: Brain, L., and Norris, F.H. (eds.) *The Remote Effects of Cancer on the Nervous System*, Grune and Stratton, New York, pp. 24–34.

Norris, F.H. Jr, Mcmenemey, W.H., and Barnard, R.O. (1970). Unusual particles in a case of carcinomatous neuronal disease. *Acta Neuropathol.*, **14**, 350–4.

Nugent, J.L., Bonn, P.A. Jr, Matthews, M.J., Ihde, D.C., Cohen, M.A., Gazdar, A., and Minna, J.D. (1979). Metastases in small cell bronchogenic carcinoma. Increasing frequency and changing pattern with lengthening survival. *Cancer*, **44**, 1855–93.

Padgett, B.L., Walker, D.L., and Zurhein, G.M. (1971). Cultivation of papova-like virus from human brain with progressive multifocal leucoencephalopathy. *Lancet*, **i**, 1257–60.

Posner, J.B., and Chernik, N.L. (1978). Intracranial metastases from systemic cancer. *Adv. Neurol.*, **19**, 575–87.

Renkawek, K., and Kida, E. (1983). Combined acute necrotic myelopathy (ANM) and cerebellar degeneration associated with malignant disease. *Clin. Neuropathol.*, **2**(2), 90–4.

Rooke, E.D., Eaton, L.M., and Lambert, E.H. (1960). Myasthenia and malignant intrathoracic tumour. *Med. Clin. North Am.*, **44**, 977–88.

Rosen, P., and Armstrong, D. (1973). Nonbacterial thrombotic endocarditis in patients with malignant neoplastic disease. *Am. J. Med.*, **54**, 23–9.

Rowland, L.P., Lisak, R.P., Schotland, D.L., De Jesus,

J.V., and Berg, P. (1973). Myasthenic myopathy and thymoma. *Neurology*, **23**, 282–8.

Rudge, P. (1973). Optic neuritis as a complication of carcinoma of the breast. *Proc. Roy. Soc. Med.*, **66**, 1106–7.

Sawyer, R.A., Selhorst, J.B., Zimmerman, L.E., and Hoyt, W.F. (1976). Blindness caused by photoreceptor degeneration as a remote effect of cancer. *Am. J. Ophthalmol.*, **81**, 606–13.

Schold, S.C., Cho, E.S., and Somasundaram, M. (1979). Subacute motor neuropathy: A remote effect of lymphoma. *Ann. Neurol.*, **5**, 271–8.

Sigsbee, B., Deck, M.D.F., and Posner, J.B. (1979). Non-metastatic superior sagittal sinus thrombosis complicating systemic cancer. *Neurology*, **29**, 139–46.

Silverman, L., and Rubenstein, L.J. (1965). Electron microscopic observations on a case of progressive multi-focal leucoencephalopathy. *Acta Neuropathol.*, **5**, 215–18.

Smith, W.T., and Whitfield, A.G.W. (1953). Malignant sensory neuropathy. *Lancet*, **i**, 282–5.

Spence, A.M. (1983). Paraneoplastic syndromes that involve the nervous system. *Current Problems in Cancer*, **8**(3), 4–43.

Walker, D.L. (1978). Professive multifocal leucoencephalopathy. An opportunistic viral infection of the central nervous system. In: Vinker, P.J., and Bruyn, G.W. (eds.) *Handbook of Clinical Neurology*, Vol. 34, North-Holland Publishing, Amsterdam, pp. 307–29.

Walton, J.N., Tomlinson, B.E., and Pearce, G.W. (1968). Subacute "poliomyelitis" and Hodgkin's disease. *J. Neurol. Sci.*, **6**, 435–9.

Weiner, L.P., Herndon, R.M., and Narayan, O. (1972). Isolation of virus related to SV40 from patients with progressive multifocal leucoencephalopathy. *N. Engl. J. Med.*, **286**, 385–7.

Williams, R.C. Jr (1959). Dermatomyositis and malignancy: A review of the literature. *Ann. Intern. Med.*, **501**, 1174–81.

Wilner, E.C., and Brody, J.A. (1967). An evaluation of the remote effects of cancer on the nervous system. *Neurology*, **18**, 1120–4.

Zuffa, M., Kubancok, J., Rusnak, I., Mensatoris, K., and Horvath, A. (1984). Early paraneoplastic syndrome in medical oncology: Clinicopathological analysis of 1,694 patients treated over 20 years. *Neoplasma*, **31**(2), 231–6.

Zurhein, G.M., and Chou, S.M. (1965). Particles resembling papova viruses in human cerebral demyelinating disease. *Science*, **148**, 1477–80.

The Clinical Neurology of Old Age
Edited by R. Tallis
© 1989 John Wiley & Sons Ltd

Chapter 22

Neurological Pain Syndromes

Christopher Wells

Consultant Anaesthetist and Director, Pain Relief Clinic, Walton Hospital, Liverpool, UK

PREVALENCE OF NEUROLOGICAL PROBLEMS IN THE ELDERLY

It has been estimated that 60% of all consultations with doctors occur primarily because of pain. Naturally, as the elderly tend to be more frequently ill and consult more, it might be expected that this would result in a large proportion of elderly patients consulting their doctors about this symptom. Since neurological pain is notoriously difficult to treat successfully, it might also be expected that pain clinics, which take on the management of the more difficult pain syndromes, would be dominated by the elderly. In fact, this is not the case. The mean age of patients attending our pain clinic is about 54, with an even spread across the age groups. Some conditions such as chronic back pain present in younger patients and the mean age for this condition at our unit is 48 years. Other conditions appear more often in the elderly; for instance, the average age of post-herpetic neuralgia sufferers is 70.

This kind of observation has suggested to some that old people do not perceive pain as readily as the young. In fact, what little experimental evidence there is, proves the reverse to be the case. Woodrow *et al.* (1967) looked at over 40 000 patients using a pressure test on the heel and showed clearly that tolerance to pain *decreased* with age. Harkins and Chapman (1976) compared old and young men in their ability to discriminate between painful signals by using dental pain, and showed that the threshold was the same for the two groups. However, older people appear to have greater difficulty judging the differential strength of a pain signal. Harkins and Chapman (1977) also investigated young and elderly normal female volunteers. Again, there was no difference in pain threshold with age.

If older people are either more sensitive to pain or at least as sensitive to pain as the young, why are they not better represented in pain clinics? It may well be that they have come to expect to suffer pain and are prepared to live with it, or, indeed, that their referring doctor believes this and thinks that there is little point in cluttering up such clinics with elderly patients and thus denying younger patients the chance for an expert opinion. Although there are no figures in this country regarding the prevalence of pain in the population, in the USA over 25% of the population is partially or totally disabled by pain for a few days to months every year and this prevalence tends to increase in the elderly (Bonica, 1980).

CHARACTERISTICS OF NEUROLOGICAL PAIN

There are several general features of pain associated with lesions of the nervous system. Such pain is often referred to the skin which may result in false localization. The pain is often prolonged over many years and treatment may be unsatisfactory. Since the nervous system is not intact and conduction is faulty, modulating mechanisms may have become disruptive. Lesions may involve peripheral nerves, the spinal cord or higher centres. Aetiology, pathology and appropriate treatment can be extremely difficult to determine. When a nerve axon is damaged in any way, a whole series of complex and long-lasting effects occurs, and full healing is rare. Axons may demonstrate spontaneous firing, increased mechanical sensitivity and enhanced sensitivity to adrenaline (Wall and Gutnik, 1974). There are also similar changes in the dorsal root ganglia (Wall and Devor, 1981) and further loss of peptides and chemicals by these cells (Barbut *et al.*, 1981). Thus a nerve, once damaged, may continue to act in an abnormal, and thus pain-producing, manner for months or years.

THERAPEUTIC APPROACHES

There are many different therapies to treat chronic pain (Budd, 1982). In older people, however, available treatments may be less well tolerated.

Drug treatment

For neurological pain, standard analgesics are rarely of use. Non-steroidal anti-inflammatory agents have little effect, apart from as a placebo, as there is no inflammation. Opiates too may be ineffective and may only confuse and constipate. The most commonly used drugs are the so-called secondary analgesics, particularly psychoactive drugs. Antidepressants tend to be used for burning neurological pain syndromes. The tricyclics are those most commonly used as the difficulties relating to limitations of diet and drug therapy with monoamine oxidase inhibitors virtually prohibit their use. Tricyclics probably exert their activity by preventing the re-uptake of transmitter amines into presynaptic stores following the release of these substances during neuronal activity. This appears to be a specific analgesic action rather than an antidepressant one, occurring in small doses. Thus, amitriptyline, 10–50 mg at night, is the kind of dose used in many pain clinics for burning dysaesthetic pain. Pain relief may take 2 weeks to become apparent whilst the anticholinergic side-effects of dry mouth and drowsiness appear immediately. Compliance may consequently be poor. Moreover, such drugs may be contraindicated because of cardiovascular disease and may cause

urinary retention, especially in elderly males with prostatic hypertrophy. They may also affect vision and may cause hypotension and confusion in the elderly. Mianserin hydrochloride can be used, in doses of 10–30 mg, but this is sometimes not as effective. It will be noted that these doses are rather lower than conventional antidepressant doses. In fact those whose pain is going to respond to antidepressants usually respond at low doses provided the antidepressants are not being used primarily for an antidepressant effect.

Anticonvulsants have been used as analgesics in neurological pain syndromes since carbamazepine was found to be effective for trigeminal neuralgia (Crill, 1973). The usual initial dose is 100 mg three times a day and this can be increased to a total of 1600 mg a day. Unfortunately, carbamazepine often causes drowsiness and dizziness, thus limiting its usefulness in the elderly. Sodium valproate, starting at 200 mg three times a day and increasing as tolerated, may also be used and it is better tolerated than carbamazepine. Enteric coated tablets reduce the risk of gastric irritation and nausea; however, there may be transient hair loss, oedema and purpura, and it should not be used in the presence of hepatic impairment. Phenytoin is less frequently used because in our experience it appears to have a depressant effect, which may be particularly troublesome in the elderly.

Transcutaneous Nerve Stimulation

Since drugs are poorly tolerated in the elderly, it is reasonable to look towards physical therapies for pain relief. Although apparently a recent invention, electrical stimulation of the nervous system to relieve pain has been used for many centuries. Scribonius Longus employed the electric torpedo fish to treat arthritis and headache and Aristotle used the electric eel to treat gout. Transcutaneous nerve stimulation (TNS) may be useful in certain neurological pain syndromes. The stimulator consists of a device which supplies a small voltage to two or four carbon rubber electrodes placed on the skin. Since Melzack and Wall developed the gate control theory of pain in 1965, it has been recognized that stimulation of large A beta fibres can inhibit pain. The effect usually lasts only while the machine is in place and functioning, but some patients derive relief for some hours after a short period of stimulation. Usually patients are loaned a unit for their own use at home, after receiving instructions in the technique. If the device is found to be useful, patients are encouraged to purchase their own. Some health authorities have a budget set aside for purchase of such devices, but in most cases, stimulators are not provided. Elderly patients may sometimes find it more difficult to understand the concept of stimulation and may experience problems fitting the electrodes and turning the equipment on and off, especially if they have conditions such as rheumatoid arthritis. Moreover, age-related changes in the skin appear to predispose to local adverse reactions.

Acupuncture

This form of treatment also has a long history. It can be safely used in the elderly but, unfortunately, it rarely has a beneficial effect on neurological pain. Some therapists believe that it is less useful in the elderly than the young (J. Kenyon, personal communication).

Psychological Treatments

Psychotherapy is used especially in the USA in pain clinics and is being used increasingly in this country in chronic pain states. Even though it is easy to appreciate the underlying cause of neurological pain syndromes and their unpleasantness, often the only help that can be offered to the patient is an attempt to improve his ability to cope with pain. Many psychological techniques have been developed to this end. They may have a limited efficacy in the elderly who may, after a lifetime of believing that medicine should answer their problems, find it difficult to accept that they should do the job themselves. Interestingly, hypnotizability has been shown to diminish with age (Morgan and Hilgard, 1973). The Pain Management Programme at Walton Hospital is run on psychological lines and it is clear to us that most elderly patients do less well than their younger counterparts in this respect, although there are notable exceptional cases of patients who

have done extremely well in learning how to handle and reduce their pain and diminish its impact on their lives.

Nerve Block

The disadvantage of permanent nerve blocks is that over time there is a tendency to develop uncomfortable dysaesthetic pain. For this reason, permanent lesions are rarely performed on patients with a long life expectancy. They are usually reserved for those patients with terminal cancer and may sometimes be used in the elderly. The procedure is relatively straightforward and may be appropriate even for the very ill. Nevertheless, there may be side-effects and the place of such treatment has to be very carefully calculated in each case.

INDIVIDUAL PAIN SYNDROMES

We shall now consider the different neurological pain syndromes and possible therapies.

Back Pain and Chronic Root Pain

Back pain and chronic root pain are common, especially in middle age. Most back pain patients have musculoskeletal problems and at present it seems that these tend to improve with age in contrast to pain due to degenerative disease. Root pain is especially common because the spinal roots, emerging through the intravertebral foramina, are particularly vulnerable to damage. There may be compression from a disc or irritation from an inflamed facet joint. There are also pain fibres travelling in the sympathetic trunks lying anterolaterally to the vertebral column. These are liable to irritation from instability or injury of the vertebrae or the surrounding muscles and ligaments. Sympathetic pain may radiate down the leg and the affected limb may be colder than the opposite side. Disc or facet pain also radiates down the leg in a dermatomal distribution, although the accuracy of localization in defining the affected root is not now thought to be very good. Last (1978) states that 'dermatome charts of the limb are probably today about as accurate as maps of the world were in the 16th Century'.

Spondylosis, spondylolisthesis and spinal stenosis may all cause radicular pain. If only a single root is affected, corrective surgery may be appropriate. More typically, patients with chronic pain turn out to have more than an isolated root lesion as the cause of their symptoms. Nevertheless, when root damage is thought to be the cause of the pain, it is important to determine if this could explain all of this patient's symptoms and signs. If it does not, the next step is to consider whether more than one root may be involved. If symptoms and signs still do not fit, a different cause for the pain must be sought. Even then, root pain may be a contributory factor, though if attention is focused exclusively on this, other causes such as disuse atrophy, muscle spasm and many psychological factors may be missed.

Arachnoiditis is a popular diagnosis in patients with a vague generalized distribution of pain. Shaw et al. (1978) reported that most cases are lumbosacral and that pain is the presenting symptom. The diagnosis can be made with certainty only on the basis of myelography. Even this may be misleading, as many patients with similar radiographic findings to sufferers, do not appear to suffer pain. The pain of arachnoiditis tends to be continuous and worse with movement, a pattern which is similar to that of chronic psychological pain syndromes, often seen in pain clinics. Treatment is extremely difficult, as surgery to remove arachnoid scarring seems usually only to exacerbate the symptoms. Root pain may also be caused by tabes dorsalis, the symptoms appearing 10–20 years after the disease begins. There is also a diabetic pseudo-tabes described by Gilroy and Meyer (1975).

Treatment of the lesion depends on the diagnosis. Clearly if a specific surgically remediable cause, such as a prolapsed disc, can be identified, then surgery may be justified. In chronic pain states this is rarely the case. Occasionally the pain may originate from facet joints and injection of these joints with local anaesthetic and cortisone under X-ray control (Mehta, 1973) may help. Nerve blocks, which may be diagnostic as well as therapeutic, may produce an improvement for 2 weeks to 3 months. They may be repeated as necessary. Attempts have also been made to denervate facet joints, but this is a difficult procedure and results are often no better than those

obtained with facet joint injections. It should be stressed that facet joint disease as the sole cause of back and root pain is rare and probably over-diagnosed.

Analgesic drugs are not usually especially successful in cases of chronic back and root pain. If there is a shooting element to the pain, anticonvulsants should be used while antidepressants may be helpful where there is burning pain. Antidepressants may also be employed for their specific mood-elevating effect, especially as depression may predate or follow the development of chronic back pain. Transcutaneous nerve stimulators may be used provided the patient is able to deal with the equipment. Acupuncture is rarely effective. Pain from tabes dorsalis is often refractory to all treatments short of high cordotomy (White and Sweet, 1969). It is rarely used now because of the side-effects if the patient lives for more than one year following the procedure.

The treatment of chronic arachnoiditis is especially difficult. Intrathecal steroids have been used, but long-term results are poor, in spite of benefits demonstrated in animal studies (Howland and Curry, 1966). Dorsal rhizotomy, ganglionectomy or dorsal column stimulation have been used with benefit in selected cases (Jain, 1974). Johnston and Matheny (1978) showed that surgery was no better than conservative treatment and myelography demonstrated reaccumulation of arachnoid loculations one year later in all cases examined.

Epidural corticosteroid injections have been widely used for a variety of causes of low back pain. They are often given in association with long-acting drugs such as Depo-Medrone (methylprednisolone). Few randomized controlled trials are available, but Dilke et al. (1973) showed methylprednisolone to be helpful in patients with radicular pain due to lumbar disc disease, as measured both by relief of pain and ability to return to work. Forrest (1980) showed the benefits of extradural steroids in post-traumatic root pain. Diagnostic lumbar sympathetic block with local anaesthetics is sometimes helpful, especially if the pain is burning in character or radiating down the leg and the limb is cold. If a diagnostic procedure demonstrates benefit, a chemical sympathectomy may be performed, using 10% phenol in Myodil at the anterolateral border of the second, third and fourth lumbar vertebrae. The procedure is performed with light sedation and under X-ray control. It is well tolerated by most patients, with very few side-effects. Even chemical sympathectomy tends to last only for about 6 months and it can be repeated with good effect if the pain returns after this time.

Pain following Nerve Injury

There is considerable overlap between this kind of pain and chronic root pain. Peripheral nerves and nerve roots may be damaged by a wide variety of agents. These include nerve section, other forms of direct trauma, mechanical compression due to degenerative disease, entrapment neuropathies such as carpal tunnel syndrome and ulnar nerve compression at the elbow, and transection of nerves during amputation. Nerve injury may also be due to infectious lesions such as herpes zoster or metabolic causes such as diabetes. There is an overlap with peripheral neuropathies. Some neuralgias are of unknown aetiology—for instance, trigeminal neuralgia, which probably has a wide variety of causes (Loeser, 1984).

Nerve injury may lead to a wide variety of pain syndromes. The classical symptom is causalgia, a constant burning pain exacerbated by light touch and many other factors. It is thought to be due to the increased sensitivity of regenerating nerve axons to adrenaline. Stimulation of the sympathetic nervous system releases noradrenaline, increasing activity in sensory afferents. This in turn triggers reflex sympathetic discharges, so there is constant positive feedback (Wall and Gutnik, 1974). The burning pain may be accompanied by coldness of the limb, the skin may appear red and shiny and there may be wasting of the muscles and osteoporosis, as in a classical Sudeck's atrophy.

Once a syndrome has been present for more than a year, it is extremely difficult to treat. Prior to this, sympathetic blockade may produce excellent results. This can be carried out as a diagnostic procedure at the lumbar level, followed if successful by phenol. Alternatively, the guanethidine block technique, as described by Hannington Kiff (1974), may be used. Serial procedures can be carried out at intervals of days to weeks. Guanethidine, a powerful adrenergic

neuronal blocking agent, is instilled intravenously into the affected limb, distal to a tourniquet which has been inflated above systolic pressure after exsanguination of the limb. The drug is selectively taken up by noradrenergic nerve endings and takes up to 21 days to be clear from the tissues. Loh and Nathan (1978) showed that patients with marked hyperpathia are far more likely to respond to this blockade than those without.

Transcutaneous nerve stimulation (TNS) has been used and has been reported as being of great value by Wynn Parry (1984). It is necessary to spend a long period of time with the patients, experimenting with different positions of electrodes, and different values of the parameters of stimulation, such as frequency, amplitude and pulse width. Dorsal column stimulation has also been used, but the long-term results are disappointing and it is a costly and time-consuming therapy. Nashold and Ostdahl (1979) described destruction of the dorsal root entry zone in an attempt to destroy the area of the cord where abnormal central firing is occurring. Again, long-term results have been disappointing. A direct surgical approach on damaged nerves is usually unsuccessful and may make symptoms worse. Wynn Parry (1981) reports that 21 out of 28 patients had worsening pain following a surgical procedure.

Less aggressive treatments include the use of anticonvulsants and antidepressants and some have used L-tryptophan with benefit in certain patients (Budd, 1982). Intravenous lignocaine and chloroprocaine have been used and the response from intravenous lignocaine has been used to predict those patients in whom sodium valproate will be of benefit.

The pain of avulsion injuries of the brachial plexus often has two elements: a severe background burning crushing pain; and periodic spasms of pain lasting for a few seconds. This syndrome typically occurs in the young, especially young men who fall off their motor bikes. The pain may persist for decades and may, in consequence, be seen occasionally in elderly patients. It is often worse in cold weather and when there is intercurrent illness. Once established, it is difficult to treat. TNS and distraction appear to be the most successful forms of therapy.

Intercostal neuralgias may be amenable to nerve blocks, either with local anaesthetic, alcohol or more recently the cryoprobe. The latter technique freezes the cytoplasm of the nerve, in an iceball formed at the tip of the cryoprobe needle, without damaging the nerve membrane. The nerve will then regenerate slowly over a period of months and it is hoped that when this has occurred, it will function normally and neuralgic pain will no longer be present. If an initial response is not sustained, the procedure may sometimes be repeated with good effect. The advantage of a cryoprobe lesion is that it very rarely appears to do any harm, though it is difficult to get good needle placement without direct exposure of the nerve. This will often require multiple small procedures at regular intervals.

Post-herpetic neuralgia is one of the most difficult and distressing syndromes occurring in the elderly. Although only 10% of patients with herpes zoster go on to develop post-herpetic neuralgia (Weiss *et al.*, 1982), the incidence in the elderly may rise to more than 50%. Symptoms usually abate over months, but may persist for up to 15 years. Since herpes occurs more often in the elderly (Harding *et al.*, 1988), it is not surprising that post-herpetic neuralgia is one of the major common pain syndromes presenting at pain clinics and that the average age of patients with this condition in our clinic is over 70. The success rate for treatment is extremely low. In Harding's study, the mean age for those suffering with zoster who developed post-herpetic neuralgia was 70, significantly higher than those who did not (58 years). Thirty per cent of patients over 60 were afflicted with post-herpetic neuralgia and the incidence rose to 70% in those over 80. The pain is classically of two types. There is a constant background aching, gnawing or burning, and a more unpleasant, but transient shooting or stabbing pain.

Numerous types of treatment have been tried with varying degrees of success. In the acute phase, systemic corticosteroids (Keczes and Bashir, 1980), acyclovir (Bean *et al.*, 1982) and sympathetic blockade (Colding, 1969) have all been recommended. Chronically, analgesics (Marsh, 1976) anticonvulsants (Juel-Jenson, 1973) and tricyclic antidepressants and TNS (Hass, 1977) have all been recommended. The variety of methods is perhaps evidence of a lack of satisfactory treatment. A study by Harding *et al.* (1988) showed that although initially

sympathetic blockade relieved the pain of acute zoster, the incidence of post-herpetic neuralgia was not affected. More permanent blockade may result in short-term pain relief, but there are long-term complications and it is therefore contraindicated. Drug treatment is reported to have a success rate in the region of 60% (Milligan and Nash, 1985) and the same authors showed 56% of patients having some improvement with TNS, although the duration of improvement was not reported. It is my own experience that many patients have an initial benefit, but that this wears off rapidly and they return to haunt the pain clinic doctor.

In the present state of knowledge, it would seem reasonable to treat herpes zoster in the acute phase with acyclovir to reduce the incidence of post-herpetic neuralgia and a sympathetic block to control acute pain. TNS in combination with anticonvulsants and antidepressants should be the treatment for post-herpetic pain. Cold (PR Spray or ethyl chloride), subcutaneous lignocaine or intravenous lignocaine and iontophoresis of vincristine, ultrasound, hypnosis and many other treatments have been used. None of these has stood up to critical evaluation.

Phantom Limb Pain

Amputees generally experience phantom limb sensations (Jenson and Rasmussen, 1984). Shukla (1982) reported that 86% of his patients experienced pain and in half of these patients, pain developed within 24 hours. Sherman *et al.* (1980) studied 5000 consecutive cases of amputation in servicemen, of whom 78% had phantom limb pain, even though the interval since amputation was on average 26 years. Half of these patients reported a decrease in pain with time. The patients between them reported over 40 different types of therapy and only 1% indicated any lasting benefit. Many amputations have been related to war injury and these patients are now elderly. In peace time, most amputations in the elderly are due to vascular disease, although trauma is still also a major cause. Several studies (Browder and Gallagher, 1948; Parkes, 1973) have indicated that phantom pain is more frequent in patients who have suffered from severe pre-amputation pain than in those who have not had such pain and this is a major problem in the elderly with ischaemic limbs.

Many patients cope well with their pain. In those who do not, there is, as suggested, a vast range of treatments similar to those used in nerve injuries. Patients may respond to TNS or indeed dorsal column stimulation. Early treatment probably influences the outcome favourably; every effort should be made to alleviate the pain of the damaged or ischaemic limb prior to amputation, for example, by means of an epidural catheter, and instillation of local anaesthetic or morphine. This is reported as lessening the incidence of phantom limb pain (M. Roberts, personal communication). Sympathectomy was found to be useful in some patients by Kallio (1950), and treatments such as acupuncture, relaxation training, biofeedback, ultrasound and hypnosis have been claimed to be useful in certain cases. These have been reviewed by Sherman *et al.* (1980). Medical treatment includes antidepressants and anticonvulsants. Narcotics have also been used, although some patients rapidly become addicted and develop tolerance. They should be used only as a last resort. Marsland *et al.* (1982) has reported beta blockers as being of value.

Tension Headaches

Tension headache is usually generalized and described in terms of tightness or band-like sensations, an aching weight, a pressure or soreness. They may be unilateral or bilateral and may be fleeting or sustained with varying intensity for months or even years. Within the diffusely aching muscles, tender nodules or trigger points can be found.

It has been known for some time that if muscles are exercised in the absence of adequate circulation, this gives rise to discomfort or even severe pain (Lewis *et al.*, 1931). Unaccustomed exercise of any bodily part, especially under conditions of emotion or tension, may give rise to pain. This may be an explanation of some cases of so-called tension headache. That is to say, headaches in which no other cause can be found and in patients in whom there is clear evidence of anxiety. Unfortunately, many

studies have shown that such patients have *less* frontal muscle tension than patients with migraine (Pozniak–Patewicz, 1976; Bakal and Kaganov, 1977). The pain is more clearly related to personality disorder (Harper and Steger, 1978). Although techniques of relaxation, anxiolytics and psychotherapy may help in the short term, there is no convincing beneficial effect in the long term.

Most patients should be reassured as to the benign nature of their pain once investigations have excluded any more serious cause. They should then be encouraged to live with the pain and perhaps non-toxic techniques such as acupuncture, relaxation training, biofeedback, hypnosis and mild analgesics may be used as appropriate. Potent medication, including long-term anxiolytics, and any permanent attack on neural tissue are contraindicated.

Thalamic Pain

The thalamic syndrome was first described by Dejerine and Roussy in 1906. It is usually due to ischaemic vascular lesions, though sometimes haemorrhagic lesions, arteriovenous malformations, tumours or trauma may give rise to the same symptoms. The pain tends to come on sometime after a stroke, typically about 6 months. An intense shooting or burning pain is experienced on the side affected by the stroke and no peripheral lesions can be discovered to account for it. The original description included signs of hemianaesthesia, hemiataxia and choreoathetotic movements. The term thalamic syndrome is now usually confined to pain caused by damage to parts of the thalamus. There has been much debate as to the mechanism of the pain and this has been recently well reviewed by Pagni (1984).

Management is difficult: standard analgesics are notoriously unsuccessful and narcotics generally have no effect. Anticonvulsants have been recommended, but are usually unsuccessful in pure thalamic pain (Gibson and White, 1971). Peripheral nerve blocks are either short-lasting or have no effect and permanent lesions may often make the pain worse. Sympathetic blocks may cause hyperaesthesia in some patients and our success with these is comparable to that of Loh *et al.* (1981). Peripheral and central electrical stimulation has been used by some, usually unsuccessfully (Sedan *et al.*, 1978), although we have noted symptomatic improvement in some patients. Budd (1982) has reported success with intravenous naloxone, but we were able to reproduce these findings in only one of 24 patients. Psychological and psychiatric support may be necessary and may need to be long term.

Trigeminal Neuralgia

Trigeminal neuralgia typically begins in old age. It is usually intermittent and may well be the worst pain anyone may experience. Unlike many chronic pain syndromes, it is easy to diagnose and treatment is usually successful. The pain is sharp and shooting and often occurs in response to specific triggers such as light touch or eating. It is localized in the distribution of the trigeminal nerve and the attack is confined to one side. Pain free intervals occur between attacks and the latter are usually of abrupt onset and abrupt termination. The usually good response to anticonvulsants helps to distinguish it from atypical facial pain. There is minimal sensory loss in the untreated patient. Janetta (1967) and other neurosurgeons believe that the syndrome is caused by compression of the trigeminal root adjacent to the pons, usually by an artery, but possibly by a vein or a neoplasm. The condition may also occur in association with other neurological diseases such as multiple sclerosis. Investigations should be undertaken to exclude a remediable cause. Our own work shows that up to 10% of patients have some treatable dental cause.

Standard analgesics are notoriously unsuccessful and the pain is often resistant to narcotics. These should certainly be avoided during long-term management, although occasionally they can be given short term during a severe crisis of pain. Anticonvulsants are the mainstay of treatment (Crill, 1973). Carbamazepine is the drug of first choice, starting with initial dose 100 mg twice daily and increasing as necessary up to a maximum dose of 400 mg four times a day. Many patients, especially the elderly, may be unable to tolerate these doses. Common side-effects of carbamazepine are nausea, dizziness,

slurred speech, drowsiness and loss of balance. If difficulties are experienced, serum carbamazepine levels should be estimated and should be in the range of 24–43 μmol/l (Tomson *et al.*, 1980). Sodium valproate has also been used and, more recently, baclofen has been reported as having success, although our experience has been disappointing.

Diagnostic blocks of the affected segments may reduce the pain either temporarily or may indeed produce a long remission. Nerve blocks with alcohol last longer, but rarely more than one year, and repeated blocks are associated with an unacceptable level of complications. More recently, the cryoprobe lesion has been used as this produces a reversible numbness to the face, lasting for about 3 months. Unfortunately, our experience with this is that the pain usually recurs when the numbness wears off, or soon afterwards. Radiofrequency lesions appear to be the treatment of choice in the elderly. The technique is a simple percutaneous one performed under local anaesthesia with X-ray control. An insulated needle is placed into the foramen ovale and the appropriate division is precisely and partially damaged. The object is to produce loss of pinprick sensation in the region of the pain and not complete numbness. Many studies have been done and most of these indicate satisfactory pain relief in 80% of patients for more than one year and 50% for more than 5 years, with a complication rate of less than 1% (Loeser, 1977).

Other techniques include injection of glycerol into the arachnoid around the gasserian ganglion, insertion into this area of a balloon catheter which is then inflated, and stimulation of the trigeminal ganglion. All these techniques, although minimizing side-effects, do not have long-lasting results and most of our patients express greater satisfaction after a radiofrequency lesion. Microvascular decompression of the trigeminal nerve has been recommended by Janetta (1976). However, most elderly patients are not keen to have major neurological surgery, especially as it does not guarantee success; the quoted success rate is 85% long term with a 3% morbidity and a 1% mortality. The only advantage of decompression is that there is no sensory loss in the face. Nevertheless, it should usually be regarded as a last resort.

Peripheral Neuropathies

There is clearly an overlap here with peripheral nerve disorders and damage and also with trigeminal neuralgia. The causes of peripheral neuropathy are discussed in Chapter 13. All forms of peripheral neuropathy may produce pain. There may be spontaneous discomfort and hyperaesthesia and, as with the neuralgias, there is often a deep aching as well as a superficial burning and shooting pain. Treatment is directed primarily at the underlying condition if this is treatable. Unfortunately, even where treatment of the underlying condition is successful, the painful neuropathy may not necessarily go away. Nevertheless, this may limit worsening of the pain. Further treatment will then be on a symptomatic basis as previously discussed. Though it is tempting to perform nerve blocks, these usually make the pain worse, implying that whatever the peripheral nature of the damage, major secondary central changes have also occurred. Anticonvulsants and tricyclic antidepressants, electrical stimulation techniques and psychological management may all be tried and have a limited degree of success.

Perineal Pain and Coccydynia

Severe burning pain around the coccyx in the absence of tumour or other disease is termed 'coccydynia' or 'coccygodynia'. The pain is unilateral or bilateral and usually occurs in middle-aged or elderly women. Typically it is produced only on sitting, or is exacerbated by sitting and the patient has to spend much of the time upright or pacing around. Understandably, there is often psychological and psychiatric distress, although in some cases it is thought that psychiatric disturbance may predate the pain. Treatment is notoriously unsuccessful. The fact that a spinal block often does not ablate the pain indicates that there may be a central cause. Some patients have been said to have a psychosexual disorder; however, counselling and therapy often produce no improvement and the patient becomes distressed by suggestions as to the nature of the origin of the pain. The standard treatments for central pain are usually tried and usually found wanting.

CONCLUSION

Neurological pain in the elderly is unfortunately quite common and this precludes referral of all such patients to specialized centres. Many neurological pain syndromes occur more frequently in this age group and their tolerance of this pain is no better than that of any other age. Response to treatment may also be poor and this may lead to considerable frustration on the part of both the patient and the physician. A detailed history, careful examination and full investigations to determine underlying causes are mandatory, as there may be some improvement if these can be treated. Treatment should not be over-aggressive, particularly in view of its limited success. Anticonvulsants and antidepressants are the drugs most likely to help. If these first-line treatments are not effective, then referral to a specialized clinic may be helpful in order that more sophisticated therapeutic modalities may be tried. Unfortunately, transcutaneous nerve stimulation and acupuncture have a limited role. Diagnostic nerve blocks may have a part to play. Permanent nerve blocks and surgical procedures, however, are rarely indicated and usually make matters worse. A considerable amount of psychological support and distraction therapy may be needed. For this reason it is particularly unfortunate that pain clinics are grossly over-subscribed so that they may not be able to maintain the long-term support desirable in many cases. The family should be encouraged to keep the patient mentally active and to maintain interests. Only too often, as old age comes on and interests wane, a neurological pain state may develop. This may be extremely badly tolerated and ruin the remaining years of life. In such situations, good families may have a more important part to play than good physicians.

REFERENCES

Bakal, D.A., and Kaganov, J.A. (1977). Muscle contraction and migraine headache: Psychophysiological comparisons. *Headache*, **17**, 208–15.

Barbut, D., Polak, J.M., and Wall, P.D. (1981). Substance P in spinal cord dorsal horn decreases following peripheral nerve injury. *Brain Res.*,**205**, 289–98.

Bean, B., Braun, C., and Balfour, H.H. (1982). Acyclovir therapy for acute herpes zoster. *Lancet*, **i**, 118–21.

Bonica, J.J. (1980). Pain research therapy: Past and current status and future needs. In: Ng, L.K.V., and Bonica, J.J. (eds.) *Pain Discomfort and Humanitarian Care*, Elsevier/North Holland, pp. 1–46.

Browder, J., and Gallagher, J.P. (1948). Dorsal cordotomy for painful phantom limbs. *Ann. Surg.*, **128**, 456–69.

Budd, K. (1982). *Pain (Update Postgraduate Centre Series)* Update Publications, London.

Colding, A. (1969). The effect of regional sympathetic blocks on the treatment of herpes zoster. *Acta Anaesth. Scand.*, **13**, 133–41.

Crill, W. (1973). Carbamazepine. *Ann. Intern. Med.*, **79**, 79–80.

Dejerine, J., and Roussy, G. (1906). La Syndrome Thalamique. *Rev. Neurol.*,**12**, 521–32.

Dilke, T.F.W., Burry, H.C., and Grahame, R. (1973). Extradural corticosteroid injection in management of lumbar nerve root compression. *Br. Med. J.*, **ii**, 635–7.

Forrest, J.B. (1980). The response to epidural steroid injection in chronic dorsal root pain. *Can. Anaesth. Soc. J.*, **27**, 40–6.

Gibson, J.C., and White, L.E. Jr. (1971). Denervation hyperpathia: A convulsive syndrome of the spinal cord responsive to carbamazepine therapy. *J. Neurosurg.*, **35**, 287–90.

Gilroy, J., and Meyer, J.S. (1975). *Medical Neurology*, Macmillan, New York, pp. 235.

Hannington Kiff, J.G. (1974). Intravenous regional sympathetic block with guanethidine. *Lancet*, **i**, 1019–20.

Harding, S.P., Lipton, J.R., and Wells, J.C.D. (1987). The natural history of herpes zoster ophthalmicus: Predictions of post-herpetic neuralgia and ocular involvement. *Br. J. Ophthalmol.*, **71**, 353–8.

Harkins, S.W., and Chapman, C.R. (1976). Detection and decision factors in pain perception in young and elderly men. *Pain* **2**(3), 253–64.

Harkins, S.W., and Chapman, C.R. (1977). The perception of induced dental pain in young and elderly women. *J. Gerontol.*, **32**(4), 428–35.

Harper, R.C., and Steger, J.C. (1978). Psychological correlations of frontalis EMG and pain in tension headache. *Headache*, **18**, 215–18.

Hass, L.F. (1977). Post herpetic neuralgia: Treatment and prevention. *Trans. Ophthlmol. Soc. N. Z.*, **29**, 133–6.

Howland, W.J., and Curry, J.L. (1966). Pantopaque arachnoiditis: Experimental study of blood as a potentiating agent and corticosteroids as an amelioratory agent. *Acta Radiol.*, **5**, 1032–41.

Jain, K.K. (1974). Nerve root scarring and arachnoiditis as a complication of lumbar intervertebral disc surgery. Surgical treatment. *Neurochirurgica*, **17**, 185–92.

Janetta, P.J. (1967). Arterial compression of the trigeminal nerve at the pons in patients with trigeminal neuralgia. *J. Neurosurg.*, **26**, 159–62.

Janetta, P.J. (1976). Microsurgical approach to the trigeminal nerve for tic doloreux. *Progr. Neurol. Surg.*, **7**, 180–200.

Jenson, T.S., and Rasmussen, P. (1984). Amputation. In:

Wall., P., and Melzack, R. (eds.) Textbook of Pain, Churchill Livingstone, Edinburgh, pp. 402–12.

Johnston, J.D.H., and Matheny, J.B. (1978). Microscopic lysis of lumbar adhesive arachnoiditis. *Spine*, **3**, 36–9.

Juel-Jenson, B.E. (1973). Herpes simplex and zoster. *Br. Med. J.*, **19**, 406.

Kallio, K.E. (1950). Permanence of results obtained by sympathetic surgery in the treatment of phantom pain. *Acta Orthopaed. Scand.*, **19**, 391–7.

Keczes, K., and Bashir, A.M. (1980). Do corticosteroids prevent postherpetic neuralgai? *Br. J. Dermatol.*, **102**, 551–5.

Last, R.J. (1978). *Anatomy, Regional and Applied*, sixth edition, Churchill Livingstone, Edinburgh, p. 22.

Lewis, T., Pickering, G.W., and Rothschild, P. (1931). Observations upon muscular pain in intermittent claudication. *Heart*, **15**, 359–83.

Loeser, J.D. (1977). The management of tic doloreux. *Pain*, **3**, 155–62.

Loeser, J.D. (1984). Tic doloreux and atypical facial pain. In: Wall, P., and Melzack, R. (eds.) Textbook of Pain, Churchill Livingstone, Edinburgh.

Loh, L., and Nathan, P.W. (1978). Painful peripheral states and sympathetic blocks. *J. Neurol. Neurosurg. Psychiatry*, **41**, 664–71.

Loh, L., Nathan, P.W., and Schott, G.D. (1981). Pain due to lesions of central nervous system removed by sympathetic block. *Br. Med. J.*, **282**, 1026–8.

Marsh, R.J. (1976). Current management of ophthalmic herpes zoster. *Trans. Ophthalmol. Soc. U.K.*, **96**, 334.

Marsland, A.R., Weekes, J.W.N., Atkinson, R.L., and Leong, M.G. (1982). Phantom limb pain—A case for beta blockers? *Pain*, **12**, 295–7.

Mehta, M. (1973). *Intractable Pain*, W.B. Saunders, London, pp. 242–5.

Melzack, R., and Wall, P.D. (1965). Pain mechanisms: A new theory. *Science*, **150**, 971–9.

Milligan, N.S., and Nash, T.P. (1985). Treatment of postherpetic neuralgia: A review of 77 consecutive cases. *Pain*, **23**, 381–6.

Morgan, A.H., and Hilgard, E.R. (1973). Age differences in susceptibility to hypnosis. *Int. J. Clin. Exp. Hypnosis*, **21**, 78–85.

Nashold, B.S., and Ostdahl, R.H. (1979). Dorsal root entry zone lesions for pain relief. *J. Neurosurg.*, **54**, 59–69.

Pagni, C.A. (1984). Central pain due to spinal cord and brainstem damage. In: Wall, P., and Melzack, R. (eds.) *Textbook of Pain*, Churchill Livingstone, Edinburgh, pp. 481–95.

Parkes, C.M. (1973). Factors determining the persistence of phantom pain in the amputee. *J. Psychosom. Res.*, **17**, 97–108.

Pozniak-Patewicz, E. (1976). "Cephalgic" spasm of the head and neck muscles. *Headache*, **15**, 261–6.

Sedan, R., Lazorthes, Y., Verdi, J.C., and Peragut, J.C. (1978). La neurostimulation électrique thérapeutique. *Neurochirurgie*, **24** (Suppl. 1), 1–138.

Shaw, M.D.M., Russell, J.A., and Grossart, K.W. (1978).

The changing pattern of Spinal arachnoiditis. *J. Neurol. Neurosurg. Psychiat.*, **41**, 97–107.

Sherman, R.A., Sherman, C.J., and Gall, N.G. (1980). A survey of current phantom limb pain treatments in the United States. *Pain*, **8**, 85–9.

Shukla, G.P., Sahu, S.C., Tripathi, R.P., and Gupta, D.K. (1982). Phantom limb, a phenomenological study. *Br. J. Psychiatry*, **141**, 54–8.

Tomson, T., Tybring, G., Bertilsson, L., Ekbom, K., and Rome, A. (1980). Carbamazepine in trigeminal neuralgia. *Uppsala J. Med. Sci.*, (Suppl. 31), 45–6.

Wall, P.D., and Devor, M. (1981). The effect of peripheral nerve injury on dorsal root potentials and on transmission of afferent signals into the spinal cord. *Brain Res.*, **209**, 95–111.

Wall, P.D., and Gutnick, M. (1974). Ongoing activity in peripheral nerves, 2. The physiology and pharmacology of impulses originating in a neuroma. *Exp. Neurol.*, **43**, 580–93.

Weiss, O., Striwatanakal, K., and Weintraub, M. (1982). Treatment of post-herpetic neuralgia and acute herpetic pain amitriptyline and perphenazine. *S. Afr. Med. J.*, **62**, 274–5.

White, J.C., and Sweet, W.H. (1969). *Pain and the Neurosurgeon*, Charles C. Thomas, Springfield, Illinois.

Woodrow, K.M., Friedman, G.D., Siegelaub, A.B., and Collen, M.F. (1967). *Psychosom. Med.*, **34**, 548–56.

Wynn Parry, C.B., and Withrington, R. (1984). The management of painful peripheral nerve disorders. In: Wall, P., and Melzack, R. (eds.) *Textbook of Pain*, Churchill Livingstone, Edinburgh, pp. 395–401.

Wynn Parry, C.B. (1981). *Rehabilitation of the Hand*, fourth edition, Butterworth, London.

The Clinical Neurology of Old Age
Edited by R. Tallis
© 1989 John Wiley & Sons Ltd

Chapter 23

Visual Failure

Iain Chisholm

Consultant Ophthalmic Surgeon, Southampton Eye Hospital, Southampton, UK

Total loss of sight is fortunately a rare occurrence in both ophthalmic and neurological practice. Visual failure and loss of vision is, however, a constant fear particularly amongst the elderly not only because of the possibility of blindness but also because of the loss of independence and mobility that may result.

Visual failure may arise from damage to any point within the visual system. Some conditions such as cataract are treatable whilst others cause permanent failure and are often associated with the vascular or degenerative effects of ageing. The loss of visual acuity, visual field or eye movement control brings its own problems. False additional information such as distortion, monocular diplopia or hallucination may compound the difficulties experienced by patients.

CAUSES OF VISUAL LOSS IN THE UK

In 1966 Sorsby showed that cataract, senile macular degeneration and glaucoma were the three main causes of blindness in the elderly (Sorsby, 1966). More recently it has been shown that senile macular degeneration accounted for 48.6% of the blind registrations in Scotland amongst those over 65 whilst glaucoma accounted for 16.8%, cataract for 12.5%, diabetic retinopathy for 6.5% and optic atrophy 4.5% (Ghafour *et al.*, 1983). A population study involving subjects over 76 years of age carried out in the Melton Mowbray area showed that senile cataract was present in 46.1% of those examined,

senile macular degeneration in 41.5% and open angle glaucoma in 6.6% (Gibson *et al.*, 1985). These findings were broadly in keeping with the Framingham study (Framingham Eye Study Monograph, 1979). It is estimated that there is a much higher prevalence of visual handicap in the population than the registration figures would suggest. The figures will also have a bias towards those ophthalmic causes which involve a loss of acuity rather than relative or incomplete loss of function.

ASSESSMENT OF VISUAL FUNCTION

Visual Acuity

The usual measurement of acuity is expressed in the Snellen's test, which compares the patient's vision at a standard distance of 6 metres with that of a supposed normal. The lines are such that the 6/6 letters subtend an angle 5 degrees when viewed at 6 metres with each space or line subtending 1 degree. The 6/12 line subtends the same angle when viewed at 12 metres. Thus a patient with 6/12 vision can see at 6 metres what the 'normal' eye can see at 12. Single letter charts are more readily recognized than multiple ones whilst numerical charts or the 'E' test are easier to interpret by those who are illiterate or who have other causes of visual agnosia. At lower levels of acuity the ability to count a number of fingers at a stated distance, to recognize hand movements or simply the presence of a light is

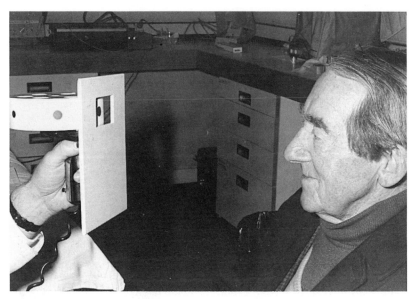

Figure 23.1. The Catford drum. This test, which can be used to assess visual acuity, employs the opticokinetic response to detect a response to different sized spot targets.

recorded as a measure of function. The corrected visual acuity tends to improve up to about the age of 10, only to fall away after the age of 60 (Slataper, 1950).

In recent years the use of contrast sensitivity gratings has given additional information about acuity and function. This is of particular value in patients with early or degenerative disease. In the age range 50–87 a linear decline in contrast sensitivity occurs. This is due to various factors including lenticular yellowing with age, retinal receptor loss and neuronal drop out either in the retina or visual cortex (Ross *et al.*, 1985). Walsh has also shown a diminution of the central processing of images with age (Walsh, 1976).

Near visual acuity is assessed using a standard reading chart held at 30 cm with glasses if needed. Good illumination is important when testing the near acuity in the elderly. The numerical values attached to the N notation of near acuity represent the point size of the typeface. Whilst this measures, to some extent, the visual acuity (N5 is approximately equivalent to 6/18), it is also a test of reading ability, comprehension and integrity of the visual fields and central pathways. The Catford drum employs graded size targets moving to and fro and the opticokinetic response to assess acuity at close range (Figure 23.1). Its use is of value in young children and patients with expressive difficulties. The absence of a response indicates reduced acuity, non-cooperation or a corticopontine lesion.

Visual Fields

Visual fields are assessed using either static or kinetic targets and in both cases it is usual to test from non-seeing to seeing rather than vice versa. The size, intensity and colour of the target can be varied to help in the identification of a relative field defect. Kinetic testing causes difficulty for the elderly who do not find it easy to maintain central fixation, tending to seek out the moving target. Static field testing avoids this disadvantage as the patient is unaware of the direction from which the target is to appear only indicating when he is aware of its presence. The use of a variable number of targets helps to identify a relative field defect. Both eyes should always be examined to avoid missing an homonymous or other diagnostic lesion.

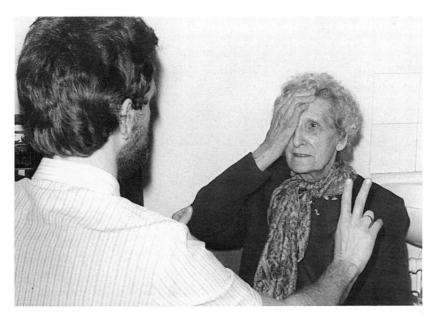

Figure 23.2. Finger counting confrontation fields. These are easy to perform on the elderly and help to detect relative as well as absolute loss.

Field loss confined to one eye indicates a lesion anterior to the optic chiasm although contralateral temporal loss may occur when the lesion is just anterior to the chiasm. Bitemporal loss usually results from a chiasmal lesion although the extent of this loss may differ on the two sides. Loss of one field of vision in a reasonably symmetrical manner is indicative of a contralateral optic tract lesion. This homonymous loss is not, however, truly congruous. A congruous and homonymous loss is due to a lesion occurring behind the lateral geniculate body or in the cortex. Differences in the extreme periphery may modify the loss due to the unilateral ocular representation of this field.

Confrontation fields avoid some of the problems of formal instruments particularly for the elderly. The presentation, for a brief moment, of a variable count of fingers in different quadrants eliminates the tendency to look in that direction. Relative and early defects can be identified and the whole test has the advantage of simplicity (Figure 23.2).

A range of instruments is available for testing central fields or more simply the Bjerrum screen is used. Alternatively the examiner's field and blind spot can be compared with that of the patient. This last method allows the patient's fixation and concentration to be monitored closely. Coloured targets give information about some specific conditions but are also used to reduce the illumination of the target.

The Amsler grid used with reading glasses assesses the central and parafoveal regions within the major vascular arcades. The patient fixates the central spot and notes any distortion of shape, form or size of the grid of squares. Paracentral scotomata are sometimes identified even if due to retrobulbar disease but the main value of this test is in the identification of changes related to macular disease (Figure 23.3). A relative dimming centrally may be due to cataract whilst patchiness of the grid is suggestive of vascular and optic nerve disease.

Ocular Movement

Acquired movement disorders are usually associated with the onset of visual symptoms. Complete horizontal muscle palsies are relatively easy to identify as the patient complains of double vision in the field of action of the muscle concerned. The more peripheral

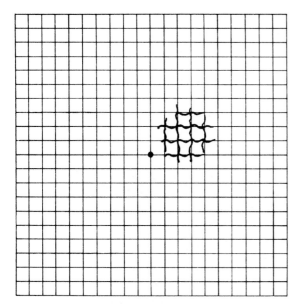

Figure 23.3. The Amsler grid. This aids in the identification of macular and paracentral field disturbance. The distortion of the lines is often the first indication of progressive and possibly treatable macular degeneration (see Figure 23.5(a)).

object seen stems from the affected eye. Vertical, oblique and partial muscle palsies are more difficult to diagnose. The development of an abnormal head posture is suggestive of a weakness of gaze in the direction of the altered posture and a head tilt suggests the involvement of an oblique muscle. The Hess test assists in the identification of the paretic or overacting muscle. The two eyes are dissociated using one to fixate the target while the other projects its position onto a second screen. False localization of the target corresponds to the muscle imbalance.

Central disturbances of eye movement involve more than the weakness of a single muscle. Non-conjugate movement in which the two eyes do not move fully together is seen in internuclear ophthalmoplegia and, in the elderly, is usually the result of brain stem ischaemia. The development of nystagmus in any field of gaze is a pointer to pathology in the cerebellum, brain stem, vestibular apparatus or higher centres.

For the elderly patient the development of a movement disorder is often distressing, particularly if there has previously been good binocular function. A

second, and false, image causes confusion particularly when associated with other symptoms of unsteadiness due to brain stem disease. For the doctor a movement disorder should be a signal to exclude other focal neurological signs such as pupil disorders, long tract signs, or evidence of cortical disease.

Higher Visual Function

The assessment of higher visual function is initially based on the features of acuity, field and movement but to these must be added the patient's interpretation of vision. There may be specific deficits in the form, colour, movement or depth of the perception. Cortical visual loss is sometimes associated with hallucinations in the blind field which can be very distressing. The assessment of disturbances at this level is as much the field of the neurologist as the ophthalmologist. Often a careful history will indicate the area of abnormality in advance of resorting to specific tests of function.

Pupil Responses

A normal response is seen in disease located in front of the retina. Macular disease does not usually produce an afferent defect unless it is particularly extensive. Widespread retinal disturbance, such as that due to retinal vascular obstruction or retinal detachment, gives rise to an afferent defect. To the ophthalmologist the presence of a relative difference between the afferent pathways of the two eyes is often of greater value than a formal assessment of the response to light and accommodation. To the neurologist, however, the reverse may be true as consideration is being given to the different central and peripheral pathways followed. In the elderly many pupils are small due to senile miosis and often react poorly. It is necessary, therefore, to examine them in reduced even illumination and to recognize that an apparent abnormality may be due to local eye disease or treatment.

An afferent pupil defect is elicited by comparing the effect produced by shining a light on one eye with that produced on the other. Relaxation of the pupil tone in the affected eye on transferring the light from the unaffected to the affected eye indicates an afferent defect on that side. Conversely increased constriction of the pupils occurs when the light is transferred back to the unaffected eye. If one pupil is normal the integrity of both afferent pathways can be assessed and pupil signs due to trauma, medication or other eye disease excluded. The suspicion of an afferent defect can be tested by enquiring about the subjective brightness of colour or light as seen by the patient.

A comparison of the afferent arc for light with that for accommodation differentiates lesions behind the lateral geniculate body. The pathway for accommodation relays there and is projected to the cortex by way of the optic radiation whilst that for light passes to the pre-tectal region via the superior quadrigeminate brachium. The Argyll Robertson pupil shows these features and in addition is often irregular and dilates poorly.

The interruption of the sympathetic pathway in Horner's syndrome produces ptosis, miosis and ipsilateral anhydrosis. The instillation of 1% hydroxyamphetamine causes pupillary dilatation in preganglionic lesions but not in complete postganglionic ones (Thompson and Mensher, 1971). Whilst it is unusual for this to produce visual failure its recognition can prove to be a valuable localizing sign. Third nerve lesions have their own localizing value. A pupil-sparing third nerve palsy is more likely to be medical in origin (hypertension or diabetes), whereas a pupil-involving palsy is usually associated with compression of the nerve (tumour or aneurysm). Paresis of the ciliary ganglion (Adie's pupil) is unusual in the elderly. It reacts very poorly, if at all, to light and contracts slowly and in a writhing fashion to accommodation. It dilates in the dark or with homatropine and contracts readily with weak pilocarpine or 2.5% methacholine unlike the normal pupil. Argyll Robertson pupils, which are often irregular, in contrast, do not react to light or dilate with atropine.

SPECIAL INVESTIGATIONS

Fluorescein angiography

When intravenous fluorescein is stimulated by blue light it emits a longer yellow green wavelength.

Suitable filters, inserted into the stimulating and emitting pathways, exclude other wavelengths so that only the fluorescence is seen. Healthy retinal vessels have tight endothelial junctions and the fluorescein remains strictly intravascular. The choriocapillaris lacks such junctions and the dye leaks out readily but is not usually seen due to the masking effect of the pigment epithelium. New vessels, found in many degenerative and ischaemic vascular eye diseases, lack tight junctions and leak dye. In disease, dye leaks into the surrounding tissue or is unmasked due to pigment epithelial defects. This technique is a useful tool for ophthalmic diagnosis.

Ophthalmologists are not infrequently asked to determine the basis for disc swelling by angiography. A swollen disc with normal acuity is suggestive of papilloedema. On angiography there is capillary dilatation and late leakage (Figure 23.4). A similar clinical appearance occurs in pseudo-papilloedema in which there is no evidence of intracranial disease and the disc tends not to leak but other signs of local disc abnormality may be present. Disc swelling with visual failure is indicative of local disc, retinal or nerve disease. Although angiography assists in the

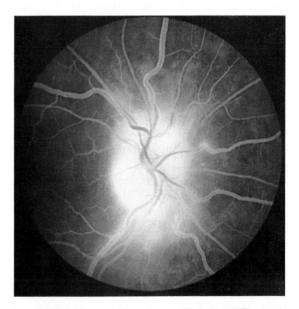

Figure 23.4. Disc oedema in papilloedema. The early fluorescein angiogram shows capillary dilatation and the disc later leaks dye, remaining stained after the background has faded.

diagnosis many of the features can be identified by careful clinical evaluation alone.

Fluorescein angiography is of great value in the diagnosis of macular disease involving sub-retinal neovascularization both to identify its presence and to establish if treatment might be beneficial (Figure 23.5a, b). Similarly it can be of value in determining the extent and severity of retinal vascular disease (Figure 23.6a, b).

Electrophysiology

Embryologically the retina and visual pathways are part of the primitive forebrain. The electroretinogram (ERG) records the electrical activity in the retina in response to light. The electro-oculogram (EOG) reflects the change in standing potential as the eye deviates from side to side and is greater in the light than in the dark. This light rise is reduced or lost in disorders of the pigment epithelium and receptors. These two tests are more strictly of value to the ophthalmologist but help to determine the location of a visual defect within the eye.

Visually evoked responses (VERs) (see also Chapter 7) measure the conduction of visual impulses to the cortex and are used to investigate the higher order neurones. A flash VER represents the simplest stimulus and confirms the integrity of the visual pathway. A reduction in amplitude in the flash VER occurs when there is pathway obstruction, whilst a delay in the conduction suggests optic atrophy or demyelinating disease. In cortical blindness an absent VER is associated with an intact pupil light reflex. More information as to acuity and function may be obtained by a pattern VER which, with varying pattern size, can give an objective assessment of visual acuity. The VER can thus be used to help in the determination of integrity of the visual pathways.

Opticokinetic Nystagmus

This is elicited when a banded drum is rotated in front of the eye. It is this reflex that causes the discomfort experienced on looking out of a moving train at close objects. The eye will follow the rotating stripes in the direction of rotation (slow phase). This smooth pursuit is followed by a rapid re-fixation movement to the primary position (fast phase). The reflex is mediated through the pre-occipital and frontal lobes on the side towards which the drum is rotating. Cortical lesions producing visual and other loss may thus be determined as to side. A normal response together with normal pupils and other findings may point to a functional rather than organic problem.

CONDITIONS THAT CAN MIMIC NEUROLOGICAL CAUSES FOR VISUAL FAILURE

Refractive Error

After the age of 65 glasses tend to need changing only as other problems such as cataract or macular degeneration develop. The addition of a tint to the distance prescription frequently helps considerably. Stronger reading glasses are needed as the acuity falls away and these can incorporate a prism to reduce the need for vergence. Simple magnifiers also help with tasks such as reading telephone directories. Advice about lighting is all important as it is often not realized that the use of an angle poise light close to the written material is much more effective than a remote ceiling light.

Assessment

Formal refraction will show if a change of glasses is needed. The use of a pin hole overcomes any refractive error, reduces the effect of cataract and will show the corrected visual potential of the eye. In macular disease, however, a pin hole often makes the vision worse. The effectiveness of a lens varies with its position relative to the eye so that a hypermetropic correction, which magnifies objects, is more effective and powerful if held away from the eye, while the reverse is true of a myopic lens. It is for this reason many an elderly person wears reading glasses well down the nose. A check on whether altering the lens position improves the vision is always worthwhile.

Cataract

The common presenting features of cataract are visual failure, loss of contrast and acuity, glare and

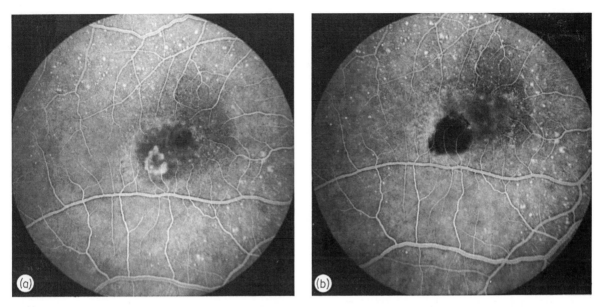

Figure 23.5. Neovascular disciform senile macular degeneration. In a treatable lesion the membrane is seen on angiography to be located just away from fixation. Drusen are also shown as hyperfluorescent spots in the macula (a). After laser photocoagulation the membrane is seen to have been obliterated although the other changes remain (b).

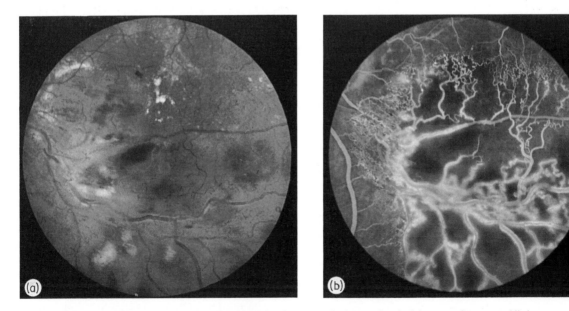

Figure 23.6. Retinal branch vein occlusion. A plain photograph shows the dark haemorrhages and lighter exudates. There is retinal oedema over much of the area below fixation, seen as a greying of the reflex with loss of underlying detail (a). The fluorescein angiogram shows that there is considerable non-perfusion of the affected retina which may later lead to the development of neovascularization in the affected area (b).

monocular diplopia. This double vision is present even when the second eye is covered, being caused by splitting of the image in front of the retina. Not infrequently the history is one of apparent sudden loss of vision which is subsequently shown to be due to cataract. The onset of symptoms was gradual but the recognition sudden.

Assessment

The assessment of cataract warrants ophthalmic referral. The pupil responses should be normal and the Amsler grid should show no distortion. In some cataracts there may be central fading of the grid but the lines are regular whilst in others there is a ghosting of the lines which is sometimes described as diplopia. The confrontation fields are full and the eye movements normal although a secondary divergent squint may develop in a long-standing uniocular cataract.

Management

Cataract surgery with or without an intraocular lens should restore vision. The use of an intraocular lens avoids the image size problems of aphakia produced by glasses or contact lenses.

The Dry Eye Syndrome

This is one of the commonest problems for the elderly and can mimic many ophthalmic and neurological problems. Grittiness and pain around the eyes is a frequent complaint. The pain may radiate back over the scalp or to the temple. There is, however, no local temporal tenderness or other symptoms suggestive of cranial arteritis. The eyes may feel heavy especially in the morning and there may be a mild ptosis. The eyes are often red and infected. The optical properties of the cornea are disturbed, resulting in drying and breaking up of the precorneal tear film. This in turn produces intermittent blurring of the vision which can be mistaken for amaurotic attacks.

Assessment

It is important to consider the possibility of the dry eye syndrome as a cause of visual disturbance. A

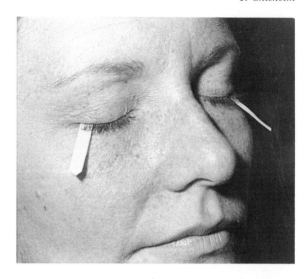

Figure 23.7. The Schirmer's test. Absorbent strips of paper are inserted in the lower fornix of the unanaesthetized eye for 5 minutes. The distance of fluid progression is then measured. In the dry eye this is often only 2–3 mm as opposed to a normal migration of approximately 15 mm.

Schirmer's test is helpful in establishing this diagnosis. The length of capillary migration of the tear film along an absorbent paper in 5 minutes is measured (Figure 23.7). The flow in the unanaesthetized normal eye is about 15 mm but is grossly reduced (often 2–3 mm) in the dry eye. The frequent use of artificial tears helps to confirm or refute the diagnosis once it has been suspected.

Chronic Glaucoma

About 1 in 200 of the population suffers from glaucoma, its prevalence increasing with age. One in ten of first degree relatives will develop the problem in time and should be screened appropriately. The optic disc changes are those of excavation and pallor. The field changes are progressive and characteristic. The intraocular pressure is raised (usually well above 20 mmHg). Glaucoma should be considered as a major differential diagnosis for chronic ischaemic optic neuropathy although in this condition the intraocular pressure is normal.

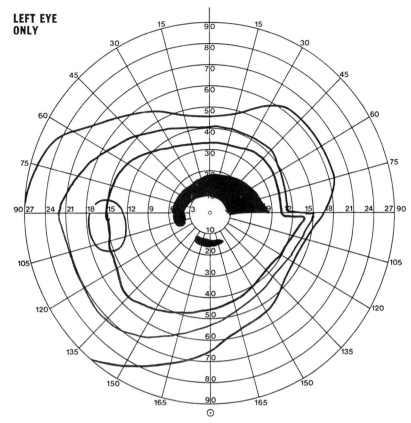

LEFT EYE ONLY

Figure 23.8. Glaucomatous field defect. There is an upper arcuate (Bjerrum) scotoma, a small nasal step to the right and an early inferior defect. Any of these changes, particularly with progression, is indicative of a possible diagnosis of glaucoma which will be supported by the finding of a raised intraocular pressure.

Assessment

This is strictly an ophthalmic diagnosis based on the finding of raised intraocular pressure, disc cupping, pallor and progressive field loss. In the early stages an upper and lower arcuate (Bjerrum) scotoma develops which later extends into a markedly constricted field (Figure 23.8). In contrast the ischaemic disc is often flatter in appearance, has normal intraocular pressure and fields which show generalized constriction, or altitudinal or central loss, normally without progression.

Retinal Irritation

Flashes or patterns of light confined to one eye are evidence of ocular ischaemia, focal macular scarring or peripheral retinal irritation. These conditions may be confused with the symptoms of occipital ischaemic episodes which produce photopsia and a migraine-like aura in one field.

DEGENERATIVE RETINAL DISEASE

Senile Macular Degeneration

Senile macular degeneration is the commonest cause of visual loss in the elderly. Lysosomal breakdown material accumulates within and under the pigment epithelium. Some of this material is visible as yellowish white deposits or drusen. Drusen are probably universal in the elderly and are part of the ageing process. In time, atrophy of the retinal elements causes a fading of the central acuity.

Sub-retinal neovascularization is widespread in the elderly but usually remains under the pigment epithelium. It can cause a more rapid loss of visual acuity if it breaks through the pigment epithelium and proliferates under the retina. Haemorrhage, serous detachment and exudate follow, with ultimate cystic degeneration of the retina. The other eye becomes involved in 50% of patients within 5 years. Photocoagulation can be used to arrest the process if it does not involve fixation. Three studies have shown benefit from treatment but each indicates that to be successful laser photocoagulation should be offered while the visual acuity remains good (6/12 or better) and the symptoms recent (usually less than 1 month) (Grey *et al.*, 1979; Moorfields Macular Study Group, 1982; Coscas and Soubrane, 1982; Macular Photocoagulation Study Group, 1982).

Assessment

Early recognition of developing neovascularization and serous detachment is important if treatment is to be offered. Although sometimes difficult to achieve, referral to an eye department should occur within a day or so of the recognition of the symptoms. Early symptoms are distortion shown on the Amsler grid and the development of central visual loss. The pupil responses are normal. Fundoscopy reveals a loss of choroidal detail and the presence of drusen with central elevation of the retina. An urgent fluorescein angiogram is required to identify the exact location of the neovascular membrane and to determine whether treatment might be beneficial. In advanced, and usually untreatable, cases the vision is poor and the symptoms of much longer duration and there is extensive sub-retinal scarring, exudate and haemorrhage. The angiogram shows widespread sub-retinal neovascular involvement.

Treatment

Laser photocoagulation is beneficial in cases of serous detachment when fixation is not involved and the vision is still good. Even with successful ablation of the neovascular membrane there remains the risk of recurrence of about 12%/year so that continued

ophthalmic surveillance is needed (Figure 23.5b). Low vision aids are of value if the vision deteriorates and treatment is not possible.

Receptor Dystrophies

Retinal dystrophies develop slowly and, whilst usually presenting early in life, can become manifest in the elderly (e.g. the female carrier of the X linked retinitis pigmentosa). They produce visual failure corresponding to the area of involvement. Distortion is not usual although the grid may appear faded, and the pupils are normal until late in the disease. Night vision loss and loss of peripheral field are features of rod dystrophies whilst day blindness, central scotoma, colour vision and acuity loss characterize the cone and macular dystrophies.

Assessment and treatment

Clinical assessment, fluorescein angiography and electrophysiology help to typify the dystrophy. Although considerable progress is now being made in the identification of the underlying pathology, specific treatment is not as yet available. Low vision aids are helpful when loss of central acuity is a problem.

RETINAL VASCULAR DISEASE

Both the arterial and venous retinal circulations are subject to obstruction which may be partial or complete, transient or permanent. The choroidal circulation which supplies the outer retina, is affected much more often than is usually recognized (Gaudric *et al.*, 1982). The arterial supply may be interrupted intermittently in transient ischaemic attacks, or permanently with corresponding, well-defined, visual loss. The venous drainage, when obstructed, has a more variable presentation both as to severity and duration of symptoms. Retinal neovascularization develops in venous obstruction when there is extensive retinal ischaemia. Hypertension is a frequent finding in retinal vascular disease and arterial disease may be an underlying factor in venous occlusion.

Venous Obstruction

Venous obstruction can occur at any age but is rare in patients under 30 and usually occurs in those over 60. It may affect the central, hemisphere or branch retinal vein. Obstruction in a branch vein produces symptoms corresponding to its distribution. These may initially be somewhat variable and intermittent. Visual acuity is affected when fixation is involved either directly or indirectly by haemorrhage, spread of oedema or exudate. Later, if neovascularization develops, vitreous haemorrhage can occur. Similar symptoms develop during the early stages of a central vein occlusion which is more common in the elderly (63% of 232 patients in the group reviewed by Raitta (1965) were over 60). Thrombotic glaucoma, causing a painful and blind eye and vitreous haemorrhage, may complicate ischaemic central vein occlusions.

Assessment

In branch vein occlusion fundus examination shows flame shaped haemorrhages within the superfial retina either localized to a small area or extending out to the retinal periphery. In some areas darker haemorrhages are seen deeper within the retina (Figure 23.6b). The site of the occlusion may be identified at an arteriovenous crossing and the retinal veins are frequently dilated. Localized ring exudate systems are found and there is a loss of background detail suggesting a thickened and oedematous retina. In central vein occlusions the whole retina is involved and the disc itself is often swollen. The pupil responses are normal in branch vein occlusions, when the area of retinal involvement is small, but abnormal with an afferent defect in central vein occlusions.

Apart from the visual effects, the major risk of venous obstruction is development of neovascularization consequent on the ocular ischaemia. This occurs in both forms of venous obstruction and carries with it the risk of vitreous haemorrhage and, in central occlusions, thrombotic glaucoma. A fluorescein angiogram will demonstrate the amount of leakage from the retinal vessels, the extent of ocular ischaemia and the risk of these further complications.

The patient should also be screened for hypertension, diabetes, blood dyscrasia and other causes of hyperviscosity.

Treatment

Hypertension or other systemic disease should be treated but often no ocular treatment is required. There is no evidence that anticoagulants, fibrinolytic agents or steroids favourably influence visual prognosis. Laser photocoagulation can be applied to areas of retinal ischaemia. In branch vein occlusions this is performed when new vessels develop or there is a suggestion of vitreous haemorrhage (Branch Vein Occlusion Study Group, 1986). Focal treatment of an area of exudate or oedema may reduce visual loss. In the early stages of ischaemic central retinal vein occlusion, as identified by fluorescein angiography, pan-retinal photocoagulation reduces the future risk of vitreous haemorrhage and thrombotic glaucoma.

Arterial Occlusion

Arterial occlusion, in contrast to venous obstruction, occurs suddenly causing transient or permanent visual loss. The area of loss corresponds to the end artery occluded. Arterial occlusion is usually embolic. An atheromatous plaque becomes dislodged and impacts in the bifurcation of a retinal artery where it is recognized as a Hollenhorst plaque. Platelet emboli, dislodged from a mural plaque, impact into the retinal circulation where they break up producing only transient symptoms. Sometimes there is a history of intermittent patchiness of the vision in the period immediately prior to the event. In repeated episodes of amaurosis fugax the onset is sudden, almost like a light being extinguished. As recovery occurs, the area of disturbance fades like a mist clearing. Once arterial occlusion is established the visual loss becomes permanent and there is whitening and thickening of the affected retina. 'Cattle trucking' may be seen in the affected vessels and at fixation, where the retina remains relatively thinner than elsewhere, a cherry red spot of underlying choroid is seen (Figure 23.9). Later the retina may return ophthalmoscopically to normal.

Although focal choroidal ischaemia may be commoner than is usually supposed, it is seldom recog-

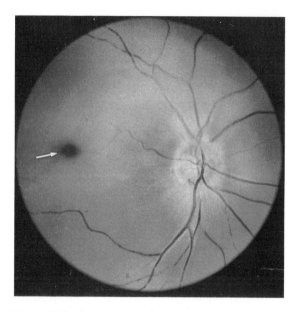

Figure 23.9. Central retinal artery occlusion. There is extensive central retinal oedema but a cherry red spot at fixation where the retina is thinner and the underlying choroid can still be seen.

nized in the acute stage on purely clinical grounds away from the central retinal areas. Local spots, streaks and triangles of atrophy of the pigment epithelium are pointers to previous focal choroidal ischaemia. It is often associated with systemic hypertension.

Assessment

The history is suggestive of a retinal arterial occlusive event. The pupil shows an afferent defect when the central retinal artery is involved. The retinal artery pulsates readily with light pressure on the eye if there is significant ophthalmic or carotid stenosis. Diabetes, hypertension and haematological abnormality must be excluded. An erythrocyte sedimentation rate (ESR) will exclude cranial arteritis. Carotid angiography may be needed to establish if stenosis is the cause. Fluorescein angiography often shows a lengthened arm–eye time, patchy choroidal filling and slow or absent filling of the retinal circulation. After the occlusive event it may return to normal.

Treatment

The treatment of amaurosis fugax is aimed at the underlying cause, be it hypertension, carotid stenosis or cranial arteritis. Simple control of hypertension often resolves the problem. The use of low dose aspirin (perhaps as little as 75–150 mg on alternate days—see Chapter 8) reduces platelet stickiness and the propensity to form emboli.

The treatment of threatened permanent occlusion is aimed at trying to restore flow through the obstructed vessel. It is, however, questionable as to how often it is really effective. Local firm pressure on the eye followed by rapid release can dislodge an embolus. Rebreathing expired air increases the P_{CO_2} causing reflex retinal arteriolar dilatation. The intraocular pressure can be reduced by intravenous acetazolamide 500 mg or surgically by paracentesis. Once the attack has become established it seems that recovery of full vision is rare although there may be some slight return of peripheral vision. Some of this recovery may be due to improvement in the ischaemia on the edge of the infarcted retina rather than true recovery.

VISUAL LOSS DUE TO OPTIC NERVE DISEASE

Disc swelling due to obstruction of the axoplasmic flow may result from a number of causes. Papilloedema does not usually cause visual disturbance beyond that of occasional mild blurring (although visual failure when it comes is usually rapid, severe and often irreversible). Ischaemic anterior optic neuropathy on the other hand is usually associated with marked visual loss. Demyelinating disease produces visual loss and disc swelling although it is not common in the elderly. Herpes zoster and other viral disease can produce an optic neuropathy. When there is visual loss an associated afferent pupil defect is to be expected. In the late stages the disc becomes pale, atrophic and flat.

Anterior Ischaemic Neuropathy

Anterior ischaemic optic neuropathy is a frequent cause of visual loss after the age of 50 and may be arteritic or non-arteritic. In a review of 196 patients

27 patients were found to have giant cell arteritis as the cause for the visual loss but 169 did not (Repka *et al.*, 1983). In this series 25% of those with arteritis suffered involvement of the second eye over a mean follow-up period of 5 years. Younger patients with ischaemic neuropathy have an above normal prevalence of hypertension, diabetes and coronary vascular disease but this does not appear to be so true of older patients.

Premonitory obscurations may precede the onset of visual failure. The loss may fluctuate and be associated with a subjective dimming of both light and colour. The visual field is sometimes described as being patchy. Pain is a variable symptom ranging from a dull local ache, pain with ocular movement to the more widespread symptoms and headache associated with giant cell arteritis. Headache, malaise, temporal tenderness together with insidious onset of vague debility and polymyalgic pain should alert to this diagnosis particularly as blindness can occur within a few hours and with minimal warning (see also Chapters 12 and 29).

Repka found that non-arteritic neuropathy produced a range of visual acuity from 6/6 to non-perception of light. The final visual acuity varied, being either better than 6/9 or worse than 6/36. In giant cell arteritis the final vision tended to be worse than this, being 6/60 or lower in over 50% (26 out of 45 eyes).

The most frequent field loss in Repka's series of ischaemic neuropathy was an inferior altitudinal hemianopia. The defect encroaches on the central 10 degrees giving a horizontal cut to the loss unlike that seen in the arcuate scotoma of chronic glaucoma. Much less frequently, upper altitudinal or central scotomata were recorded although the latter were more commonly found in giant cell arteritis.

Assessment

The diagnosis of ischaemic neuropathy is usually made by the history and clinical findings. Clinically the disc is found to be swollen and either pale or hyperaemic. Involvement may be total, altitudinal or segmental, often with solitary linear haemorrhages on or adjacent to the disc. The visual fields are correspondingly affected (Eagling *et al.*, 1974). The retinal vessels are often arteriosclerotic in appearance and emboli are sometimes seen on the nerve head or at major bifurcations of vessels. In the ensuing months the disc becomes segmentally or diffusely pale and atrophic sometimes with a shallowly cupped appearance which mimics chronic open angle glaucoma. The intraocular pressure will, however, be normal. There is normally an afferent pupil defect.

In giant cell arteritis the ESR is markedly raised, often to levels above 100 mm in the hour. Temporal artery biopsy, when positive, is helpful particularly if the ESR is not grossly elevated. In view of the skip lesions that occur in this disease a negative biopsy does not exclude its possibility. Biopsy shows gross narrowing of the affected vessel with fraying and fragmentation of the internal elastic lamina associated with multinucleated giant cells. All layers, particularly the media, are infiltrated by lymphocytes and plasma cells. Similar lesions can occur in the posterior ciliary, cerebral and vertebral arteries all of which contain an elastic tissue component.

Hypertension, diabetes and other haematological abnormalities such as pernicious anaemia must be excluded. Further investigation is aimed at the exclusion of other disease, especially when the acute episode of disc swelling has not been observed. Fluorescein angiography shows a variety of findings. In the early phase there may be absent or deficient choroidal filling around the disc with dilatation of the disc capillaries. In the late stages the disc leaks dye. As the acute ischaemia subsides, the peripapillary circulation improves and vascular shunts often develop on the surface of the nerve head.

Management

When from the history, ESR and biopsy, giant cell arteritis is suspected as being the basis for the visual loss, treatment with systemic steroids is urgently needed. Patients should be admitted immediately to hospital. Intravenous, intramuscular and oral steroid is given until the ESR falls and the symptoms subside (10 mg of intravenous dexamethasone is followed by 4 mg intramuscularly and up to 100 mg of oral steroid daily). To this may be added acetazolamide (initially 500 mg and then 250 mg four times daily). After the initial treatment the ESR and symptoms must be monitored, varying the steroid dosage accordingly. In the face of an only moderately raised ESR and/or a negative biopsy a trial of treatment with steroids is sometimes justified.

An attack of non-arteritic ischaemic neuropathy will subside and is usually not treated. Systemic steroids may shorten the duration of an attack and prove helpful in some cases. Aspirin reduces platelet stickiness. Diabetes, hypertension and pernicious anaemia need appropriate treatment.

Optic Atrophy

A pale disc with visual loss may follow previous ischaemic optic neuropathy, a more posterior lesion, the late stages of glaucoma or diffuse retinal disease. Fundus examination should exclude the last diagnosis. In glaucoma, the disc tends to be deeply cupped with preferential loss on the upper and lower poles. The field loss in glaucoma is usually characteristic and progressive. The intraocular pressure is found to be raised above the normal range of 10–21 mmHg. In ischaemic neuropathy or atrophy from other causes the disc is flat or shallowly depressed and the intraocular pressure normal. Examination of visual fields of both eyes is vital to exclude a chiasmal or junctional scotoma. Plain skull views and computed tomography (CT) studies may be needed to exclude pathology in the chiasmal region and apex of the orbit. In the absence of definite changes repeated field and contrast studies may be needed.

VISUAL FAILURE DUE TO LESIONS ALONG THE VISUAL PATHWAYS

The majority of such lesions occur in younger patients and relate to demyelination. In the elderly, local ischaemia and neoplasms are likely causes of visual losses.

Optic Nerve and Chiasmal Lesions

Tumours within the orbit displace the eye and compromise ocular movement producing diplopia in the appropriate position of gaze. Secondary deposits and neoplasms in the region of the sphenoidal sinus

and optic canal cause a junctional scotoma when ipsilateral blindness with variable optic atrophy is associated with a contralateral temporal field loss. This loss of field in the second eye stresses the need to examine both visual fields in all cases of neurological visual disturbance.

Investigation of this region involves X-ray, CT scanning and sometimes venography. The extent of the lesion will determine whether the pupil is involved. In optic nerve involvement, the visual evoked response shows an ipsilateral loss of amplitude with variable delay. It is, however, possible to miss small lesions at the apex of the orbit and clinical evaluation remains an all important feature of diagnosis in this region.

Chiasmal lesions in the elderly are more likely to be vascular than due to pituitary compression. The field changes will, in turn, depend on the exact location of the abnormality.

Optic Tract Lesions

Lesions of the optic tract anterior to the lateral geniculate body are similarly difficult to diagnose, with ischaemia being the most common cause. Although homonymous, the visual fields may still be incongruous in shape. The midline of vision is respected save in the most anterior lesions adjacent to the chiasm. A comparison of the VER on the two sides may suggest a lesion of the tract or optic radiation. The pupil responses may be reduced on hemifield testing when the lesion is anterior to the lateral geniculate body.

Optic Radiation Lesions

A lesion in the optic radiation, behind the lateral geniculate body, is more common in the elderly and results from strokes and space-occupying lesions of the parietal, temporal and occipital lobes. The field loss is congruous and is classified according to whether the upper or lower fibres are affected. A superior quadrantanopia is caused by fibres that loop forward into the temporal lobe (Meyer's loop). An inferior quadrantanopia is produced by a parietal lesion which may also cause other forms of visual disorder relating to the preoccipital cortex. The visual evoked responses to that side will be altered but the pupil response to light will be spared.

VISUAL DISTURBANCE DUE TO CORTICAL LESIONS

Transient Visual Loss

Episodes of amaurosis fugax usually affect the ophthalmic circulation but in many elderly patients it is difficult to distinguish between these attacks and those due to disturbances in the basilar supply. The temporal field extends outwards about 100 degrees but the nasal only 60–70 degrees where it is further obscured by the presence of the nose and glasses when worn. The loss of a right hemifield can thus easily be misinterpreted as a loss of vision in the right eye. An association with other sensory or motor disturbances supports a cortical diagnosis. Hypertension, giant cell arteritis or generalized arteriosclerosis are likely to underlie such a disturbance and should be treated accordingly.

Photopsia

A migraine-like aura and visual disturbance may occur in the elderly due to focal ischaemia. The disturbance may consist of a central scotoma or of shifting patterns of light which expand or contract and which are followed at times by a migraine-like headache. Flashes or patterns of light when strictly confined to one eye are evidence of ocular ischaemia, focal macular scarring or peripheral retinal irritation. In macular disease there is usually distortion of the Amsler grid which is not present in the other conditions. Shimmering lights, better seen in reduced illumination such as that on entering a darkened room or building, are suggestive of peripheral vitreo-retinal traction. Flashes associated with the recent onset of floaters may indicate a retinal break and the possibility of a retinal detachment. Ophthalmic review is necessary to identify changes that might predispose to retinal detachment and which might benefit from local treatment.

CORTICAL VISUAL FIELD LOSS

Contralateral congruous visual loss is a feature of lesions located behind the lateral geniculate body. Some incongruity, however, result from the greater temporal field of the eye on the side of the visual loss when compared with the nasal field of the other eye. The calcarine artery supplies the visual cortex above and below the calcarine fissure. Local obstruction or haemorrhage produces appropriate hononymous field loss. Lesions affecting the posterior occipital pole are said to spare the macula. This may be due to the fine saccadic movements that are a feature of fixation resulting in apparent vision on both sides of fixation. The occipital pole lies on the watershed of the posterior and middle cerebral arteries which fact may also account for some sparing in this region.

Occipital stroke is often accompanied by photic symptoms. There may be persistent hallucinations in an area of established field loss. Unformed sensations derive from a posterior occipital lesion whereas hallucinations of real objects stem from a more anterior or temporal lobe lesion. Both can be disturbing for the elderly. Objects also appear in the blind field as if from nowhere thereby increasing the confusion—the so-called Jack in the Box phenomenon.

Cortical blindness due to stroke or other cause produces a total unawareness of loss of vision. Lesser degrees of visual agnosia and disturbance will occur in response to local lesions. Monocular diplopia and polyopia, which are usually ascribed to ocular causes such as cataract, can on rare occasions result from focal posterior cortical lesions although the basis for this is obscure.

Assessment

The pupillary light reflexes are normal in cortical lesions but accommodation reflexes and pursuit movements may be lacking. The opticokinetic nystagmus reflex is interrupted so that the pursuit system follows towards the side of the lesion but the compensatory saccadic refixation in the opposite direction does not occur. The visual evoked responses are also depressed or lacking on the affected side.

VISUAL FAILURE DUE TO MOVEMENT DISORDERS

Disorders of eye movement control do not usually cause visual failure but are often very disturbing to the elderly patient. Acquired central nystagmus, although not necessarily affecting acuity, can give rise to difficulty in maintaining fixation to which may be added difficulties related to oscillopsia, giddiness and double vision.

Diplopia is often minimized in muscle palsy by adopting an altered head posture such that the head rather than the eyes is turned to the affected field. False localization of images occurs and may prove distressing to the elderly who often spontaneously close or cover one eye. Continued lid closure or the effort to overcome the weakness can produce symptoms of ocular pain, aesthenopia, local discomfort and headache. The use of occlusion or temporary prisms on glasses will reduce this problem.

Arteriosclerosis, hypertension and diabetes are the most common causes of brain stem ischaemia in the elderly. Pain is a feature of muscle palsies associated with giant cell arteritis, herpes zoster infection and compressive lesions along the oculomotor pathways. Medical causes of gaze palsy tend to resolve spontaneously over a 3 month period and are usually pupil sparing. Myasthenia gravis should be remembered as a rare cause of intermittent and varying muscle paresis. The basis for the problem should be identified and treated when appropriate. The control of hypertension, arteritis, and diabetes reduces the risk of further problems.

REFERENCES

Branch Vein Occlusion Study Group (1986). Argon laser scatter photocoagulation for prevention of neovascularisation and vitreous haemorrhage in branch vein occlusion. *Arch. Ophthalmol.*, **104**, 34–41.

Coscas, G., and Soubrane, G. (1982). Photocoagulation des néovaisseaux sous rétiniens dans la dégénérescence maculaire sénile par le laser à argon: résultats de l'étude randomisée de 60 cas. *Bull. Soc. Ophthalmol. Fr.*, **94**, 149–54.

Eagling, E.M., Sanders, M.D., and Miller, S.J.H. (1974). Ischaemic papillopathy. Clinical and fluorescein angiographic review of 40 cases. *Br. J. Ophthalmol.*, **58**, 990–1008.

Framingham Eye Study Monograph (1979). National Eye Institute, Bethesda, Maryland.

Gauric, A., Coscas, G., and Bird, A.C. (1982). Choroidal ischaemia. *Am. J. Ophthalmol.*, **94**, 489–98.

Ghafour, I.M., Allen, D., and Foulds, W.S. (1983). Common causes of blindness and visual handicap in the West of Scotland. *Br. J. Ophthalmol.*, **67**, 209–13.

Gibson, J.M., Rossenthal, A.R., and Lavery, J. (1985). A study of the prevalence of eye disease in the elderly in an English community. *Trans. Ophthalmol. Soc. U.K.*, **104**, 196–203.

Grey, R.H.B., Bird, A.C., and Chisholm, I.H. (1979). Senile disciform macular degeneration: features indicating suitability for photocoagulation. *Br. J. Ophthalmol.*, **63**, 85–9.

Macular Photocoagulation Study Group (1982). Argon laser photocoagulation for senile macular degeneration. Results of a randomised clinical trial. *Arch. Ophthalmol.*, **100**, 912–18.

Moorfields Macular Study Group (1982). Treatment of senile disciform macular degeneration: a single blind randomised trial by argon laser photocoagulation. *Br. J. Ophthalmol.*, **66**, 745–53.

Raitta, C. (1965). Der Zentralvenum- und netzhautvenenverschluss. *Acta. Ophthal.*, Suppl. 83, 1–125.

Repka, M.X., Sevino, P.J., Schatz, N.J., and Sergott, R.C. (1983). Clinical profile and long term implications of anterior ischaemic optic neuropathy. *Am. J. Ophthalmol.*, **96**, 478–83.

Ross, J.E., Clarke, D.D., and Bron, A.J. (1985). The effect of age on contrast sensitivity function: uniocular and binocular findings. *Br. J. Ophthalmol.*, **69**, 51–6.

Slataper, F.J. (1950). Age norms of refraction and vision. *Arch. Ophthalmol.*, **43**, 466–81.

Sorsby, A. (1966). The incidence and causes of blindness in England and Wales 1948–1962. Reports on public health and medical subjects. HMSO, London No. 114.

Thompson, H.S., and Mensher, J.H. (1971). Adrenergic mydriasis in Horner's syndrome. Hydroxyamphetamine test for postganglionic defects. *Am. J. Ophthalmol.*, **72**, 472–80.

Walsh, D.A. (1976). Age differences in central perceptual processes. A dichoptic backward masking investigation. *J. Gerontol.*, **31**, 178–85.

Chapter 24

Disturbances of Hearing and Balance

Ian Mackenzie

Consultant Neuro-otologist, Neurosciences Department, Walton Hospital, Liverpool, UK

Loss of hearing or deafness is a common problem and presents throughout life, from birth to old age, in a variety of ways. Hearing loss may be divided into three main categories: sensorineural; conductive; and psychogenic. A patient may suffer from a mixture of sensorineural and conductive deafness.

Sensorineural hearing loss, sometimes referred to as 'perceptive', 'nerve', 'cochlear' or inner ear deafness, results from pathology affecting the cochlear labyrinth, the eighth cranial nerve from the hair cells of the cochlea to the brain stem ganglion, or the central connections ascending from the brain stem. Conductive hearing loss may arise from any physical or pathological obstruction of the sound wave from the point at which it enters the external auditory meatus to the stapes footplate. Psychogenic or non-organic deafness is uncommon. Diagnosis may be extremely difficult, but audiological tests summarized in Table 24.1 will be able to give a true picture of the patient's hearing.

CONDUCTIVE DEAFNESS (see Table 24.2)

Probably the most common cause of this type of deafness is accumulation of wax in the outer ear. Wax normally travels outwards, but in some cases it may collect in the external auditory canal so that the canal becomes occluded. Cotton buds used by patients to remove wax may impact it further into the canal. If it is impacted on to the tympanic

membrane itself, there will also be pain. Wax may be removed with a wax hook under direct vision or with syringeing. Syringeing may require prior softening of the wax. It should not be carried out in the presence of a known perforation.

Foreign bodies in the external canal will also give rise to conductive deafness; cotton wool is the commonest culprit in adults.

In otitis externa the skin of the canal becomes oedematous or infected. In addition to deafness there will be itchiness and discharge. This condition is more common in diabetics. A very serious condition called otitis externa malignans, resulting from a *Pseudomonas* infection, occurs in elderly diabetics and gives rise to an osteitis or osteomyelitis which will spread to the jugular foramen and the petrous apex and subsequently to the sigmoid sinus and may even result in death. Early diagnosis with control of both the ear infection and diabetes will prevent serious sequelae.

Otitis media may be either acute or chronic. Acute otitis media is commoner in children than adults, the main symptoms being pain and conductive deafness. Often the condition resolves spontaneously, the tympanic membrane bursting with a resulting perforation; antibiotics or myringotomy may prevent this. Acute otitis media may give rise to acute mastoiditis. Serous otitis media is also common in children after a cold and is characterized by non-infectious fluid within the middle ear but without the pain of acute

TABLE 24.1 AUDIOLOGICAL TESTS

1. Live voice and whisper tests, single words or short sentences
   Limited value as standardization difficult.
2. Tuning fork tests:
   (a) Rinne test
       Compares air conduction with bone conduction.
       512 Hz most commonly used.
       Air conduction usually better than bone conduction.
       Conductive deafness: bone conduction is better than air conduction.
   (b) Weber test
       Lateralization of sound of tuning fork placed on vertex.
       Conductive deafness: sound lateralized to affected side.
       Sensorineural deafness: sound lateralized to normal side.
   (c) Stenger test
       Using two tuning forks will reveal feigned deafness.

AUDIOMETRY

1. Pure tone audiometry:
   Determines threshold of hearing for pure tones of several seconds' duration delivered through earphones to the ear under test. Frequencies tested from 125 Hz to 8000 Hz and at intensities from 10 to 120 dB.
2. Békésy audiometry:
   Sweep frequency testing and resulting curve indicates pure tone threshold. More objective than pure tone audiometry.
3. Impedance audiometry:
   Shows characteristic changes in middle ear pathology

---

otitis media. It usually resolves spontaneously in adults but in children medical or operative treatment may be necessary.

Suppurative, chronic otitis media is the sequel to incomplete resolution of an acute otitis media. It may be classified as tubo-tympanic or attic. In tubo-tympanic disease the tympanic membrane has a central or marginal perforation and there is a mucoid or mucopurulent discharge which may resolve with antibiotic treatment but commonly recurs after an upper respiratory tract infection. Recurrent infection may give rise to a thickening of the middle ear mucosa which may result in polyp formation but, apart from conductive deafness and a discharging moist ear, many patients are not greatly affected.

Attic disease is much more sinister and is characterized by a posterior or posterosuperior perforation of the tympanic membrane. There may be an ingrowth of squamous epithelium from the ear canal into the middle ear. This collection of squamous cells

may give rise to a cholesteatoma. Cholesteatoma has an erosive potential which can result in the destruction of the boundaries of the attic and mastoid bone and of the osseous labyrinth, and this in turn may lead to intracranial or labyrinthine infection. The ossicles, particularly the incus and stapes, may be destroyed and the integrity of the facial nerve is at risk. Although attic disease may be controlled by frequent removal of the debris in the ear by suction, this is not always possible. In such cases, or where there is evidence of erosion, the mastoid bone must be opened up and all evidence of cholesteatoma removed. It may in addition be necessary to reconstruct the ossicular chain and tympanic membrane to improve the patient's hearing.

In otosclerosis there is new bone formation around the stapes footplate. This stops the movement of the stapes and gives rise to a conductive deafness. In over 90% of cases it affects both ears. It has a strong familial tendency and is more common in women. Tinnitus may be a feature. It may be treated either

TABLE 24.2 CAUSES OF CONDUCTIVE DEAFNESS

1. Congenital:
   Imperforate external auditory meatus
   Ossicular abnormalities

2. Traumatic:
   Perforation of the tympanic membrane

3. Neoplastic:
   Benign
   Bony exostoses in canal (common in swimmers)
   Glomus tumour (chemodectomas)
   Malignant
   Squamous cell carcinoma of nasopharynx
   Squamous cell carcinoma of the external ear

4. Inflammatory:
   Eustachian tube infection
   Otitis media
   Otitis externa

5. Otosclerosis:
   Familial (may be bilateral)

6. Wax:
   Common—may be hard or soft

TABLE 24.3 SENSORINEURAL DEAFNESS

1. Congenital
   Rubella of pregnancy
   Birth trauma
   Rhesus incompatibility
2. Noise-induced deafness
3. Toxic
   Ototoxic drugs, e.g. aminoglycosides
4. Infection
   Meningitis—viral, tuberculosis, bacterial
   Other, e.g., mumps, measles
5. Traumatic
   Especially base of skull fracture
6. Vascular
   Medullary cerebrovascular accident
7. Presbyacusis
8. Menière's disease
9. Neoplastic
   Acoustic neuroma

by fitting a hearing aid or carrying out the operation of stapedectomy, where the stapes bone is replaced by a Teflon piston. In any patient with a normal looking ear drum and conductive deafness, otosclerosis should be considered as a diagnosis. In older patients there is a higher incidence of postoperative dizziness; for this reason, operations are less commonly performed over the age of 60.

Following trauma the ossicles within the middle ear may become dislodged and conductive deafness ensue.

Malignant tumours of the ear are rare and characterized by pain and deafness. Successful treatment is difficult. Glomus tumours and nasopharyngeal carcinoma both may present as conductive deafness.

SENSORINEURAL DEAFNESS
(see Table 24.3)

Sensorineural deafness is more common in adults than a conductive loss. It may present in the young as a result of rubella in pregnancy, rhesus incompatibility, birth trauma, prematurity, congenital syphilis or other congenital causes. This deafness may be severe, sometimes total, and the aim in these high risk groups is to diagnose the hearing loss as early as possible and try and have hearing aids fitted to the baby by the age of 6 months.

In severe trauma to the skull the integrity of the eighth cranial nerve may be damaged or divided resulting in deafness. There may be an associated damage to the vestibular apparatus. Neurosyphilis is a rare cause of deafness.

Certain drugs have ototoxic properties. The best known are the aminoglycoside antibiotics including streptomycin, gentamicin, neomycin and tobramycin, and it is important when using these drugs to keep blood levels within the therapeutic range. Diuretics such as ethacrynic acid and frusemide have also been implicated in deafness but usually after large doses given in life-threatening situations. Chloroquine and quinine are known to cause deafness.

Viral illnesses such as mumps and measles may result in deafness although fortunately often just one ear is affected. Bacterial infections, in particular meningococcal and pneumococcal meningitis, may also cause eighth nerve damage. Any infection which damages the labyrinth will also cause hearing loss because of the continuity of the latter with the cochlea.

Noise induced deafness is a condition which has received a lot of attention in the last few years, although it was noticed in Roman times that blacksmiths were often deaf. It may result either from brief exposure to very loud noise or from prolonged exposure to loud noise at lower levels—especially in association with heavy industry. Noise over the level of 85 dB may damage the hair cells of the cochlea although there is a marked difference in individual susceptibility. The damage to the cochlea is predominantly in the basal rim, the area for detecting frequencies of 4 kHz. The audiogram of affected individuals shows a characteristic dip at this level. Prevention by the wearing of ear plugs or protectors is the best approach, for it is difficult to devise a hearing aid that will increase the hearing level at 4 kHz without increasing the volume at other frequencies to an intolerable level.

Acoustic neuroma (see also Chapter 16) is an uncommon condition but it must always be considered in cases of unilateral sensorineural hearing loss. This is a benign tumour arising usually from the vestibular branch of the eighth nerve but affecting the cochlear branch as well. The commonest site is at the entrance of the internal auditory canal and its initial features are due to local expansion. It will eventually expand to form a true cerebellopontine angle tumour. Unilateral deafness is often the first symptom, followed by vertigo and tinnitus. If the trigeminal nerve is affected, there will be an absent or depressed corneal reflex. If a seventh nerve palsy develops, this usually means that the tumour is large. Audiological tests, tomography of the internal auditory meatus and computed tomography will confirm the diagnosis and if the patient is fit enough excision of the tumour with preservation if possible of the seventh nerve should be carried out.

Acoustic neuroma may need to be differentiated from the much more common Menière's disease. This is characterized by vertigo, tinnitus and fluctuating sensorineural deafness. The aetiology is unknown, but it is thought to be due to an excess of endolymphatic fluid. The diagnosis is arrived at by exclusion of other conditions and the management may be with medication or surgery. Vertigo is an especially distressing feature of the disease.

PRESBYACUSIS

The loss of hearing caused by degenerative changes due to ageing is called presbyacusis and is determined by genetic factors or physical stresses that the ears have been subjected to during life.

Zwardemaker (1899) first described the loss of high tone hearing loss from ageing, and much research has been carried out on the pathology of the condition. The work of Schuknecht (1974) has set out four main types of pathological changes that take place in the process of presbyacusis.

Sensory Presbyacusis

This is associated with high tone hearing loss. Histologically there is atrophy of the organ of Corti in the basal end of the cochlea. The condition usually starts in middle age and progress is very slow.

Neural Presbyacusis

There is a loss of cochlear neurones often involving the whole cochlea and there is a fall in the ganglion cell count from an average 37 000 in the first decade to 20 000 in the ninth decade. In neural presbyacusis the ganglion cell count will fall below this level. Usually there is very poor speech discrimination and speech amplification by hearing aid is often of no help.

Strial Presbyacusis

Histologically there is a patchy atrophy of the stria vascularis in the cochlea which is most marked in the apical half of the cochlea. All three layers of the stria may be affected and cystic changes may be seen with associated basophilic deposits. It is thought that the stria vascularis provides the energy of the scala media. This energy supply is dependent upon the oxidative enzymes of the stria; in consequence, strial degeneration is initially associated with a flat audiometric pattern with good speech discrimination. This discrimination deteriorates rapidly when the hearing loss is greater than 50 dB.

Cochlear Conductive Presbyacusis

This is characterized by descending audiometric patterns. Histological studies show no morphological changes in the cochlear structures to explain the hearing loss and it is postulated that there is a disorder in the motion mechanisms of the basilar membrane.

Schucknecht pointed out that the audiograms showing bilateral sensorineural hearing loss for frequencies over 1–2 kHz also occur in ears with chronic suppurative disease and otosclerosis, diseases which cause an acceleration of the age-related atrophic changes normally occurring in the supporting tissues. Atrophic changes commence in the second decade and continue throughout life. At first there is a loss of fibrocytes in the region of the ligament adjacent to the attachment of the basilar membrane. This is followed by the appearance of a zone of acellularity in the mid-portion of the ligament. Two distinct zones become apparent: a thin external zone consisting of densely packed fibrocytes in a fibrillar stroma; and a larger internal zone, mostly acellular and containing large cystic spaces.

Central Changes

The perception of speech at different stages of life is related to both central and peripheral mechanisms. Efficiency of central processing is critical in speech perception and may be the key to the socially disturbing changes in speech understanding which accompany ageing.

Speech perception is based upon knowledge of the linguistic content and the physical attributes of the message. The latter include its phonological, transmission and environmental acoustics. The auditory, linguistic and psychological abilities of the listener are all important in the reception of the spoken message.

Konigsmark and Murphy (1972), in a study of the ventral cochlear nuclei, found no evidence of age-related degeneration but Kirikae *et al.* (1964) described age-related changes in the cochlear nucleus, the superior olive, the inferior colliculus and medial geniculate body. Hansen and Reske-Neilson (1965) found atrophic changes in parts of the central auditory pathways and their nuclei as well as in the cortical areas.

Dublin (1976) points out that the central auditory pathway may be affected by the arterial insufficiency attendant upon degenerative arterial disease associated with ageing and he reported a correlation between hearing loss and the degree of arteriosclerosis.

These changes may be responsible for impaired auditory discrimination, decreased perceptive judgement, impaired comprehension of moderately distorted speech and decreased ability to recall long sentences.

The term 'phonemic regression' was coined by Gaeth (1948) to describe the abnormal mishearing of the consonants found in older persons. There has been debate as to whether this impairment of word discrimination occurs gradually throughout life or is present significantly only in older persons.

Blumenfeld *et al.* (1969) used the Fairbanks–Rinne test on a sample population drawn entirely from outside clinics and found that performance deteriorated with age. The correlation was stronger for subjects over 60. Feldman and Reger (1967) agreed that the 'phonemic regression' findings of Gaeth and others are more pronounced in ageing adults seen in the audiology clinics than in non-clinic populations.

Clinical Features

Over the years novelists and playwrights have linked ageing with deafness, and any character who has a breakdown in communication because of deafness is naturally assumed to be old.

Hinchcliffe (1962) pointed out that problems in hearing speech are greater than can be accounted for on the basis of a pure tone audiogram. Wood (1975) argued that the best way to measure speech perception disability is by speech discrimination testing. Subjects are presented with a list of 25 words at standard decibel levels and the percentage of words repeated correctly is noted. The graph for the patient with sensory impairment does not reach 100% as ageing causes deterioration of speech reception at higher intensities.

But there is debate as to the validity of this type of testing. Patients do not normally listen to words and sounds in a noise protected box in a clinical situation. Efforts have been made to test speech comprehension under real-life conditions including testing in such places as churches and halls, and over telephones.

Calearo and Lazzaroni (1957) compared the performance of persons over the age of 70 with that of younger adults on the perception of speech produced at various speaking rates in Italy. There was no doubt that there was a significant loss of discrimination in the elderly as speech became faster. Experiments have been carried out by employing talkers of different voices and speech characteristics and this has shown the relative difficulties in speech perception experienced by older listeners.

The elderly often hide their deafness for as long as they can, even though this may result in increasing isolation and loneliness. Kay *et al.* (1964) estimated that 62% of the elderly with organic brain syndromes had impaired hearing while only 31% of the mentally normal had impaired hearing. Gilhome-Herbst and Humphrey (1980) found an apparently closer association between impaired hearing and dementia such that 79% of the demented patients also had a hearing defect.

There is of course a danger of regarding elderly people as demented or confused when they actually have a severe hearing loss.

HEARING AIDS

According to Humphrey *et al.* (1981), less than a quarter of patients in Western countries who have a hearing loss and who might reasonably benefit from help actually possess hearing aids. He also noted that those who develop hearing loss before retirement are more likely to have a hearing aid than those impaired after retirement.

Hearing aids are the mainstay of treatment of presbyacusis. Fitting a hearing aid requires careful assessment of individual requirements. The number and variety of hearing aids available on the market indicates that the perfect aid has yet to be developed. There have been significant improvements over the last few years, but, with further technological advances, further improvements are to be expected in the near future.

Hearing aids are divided into two main groups: aural aids and body worn aids. The aids have two main components, a microphone and an amplifier. The post-aural aids (fitting behind the pinna) usually have an electronic microphone. The ampli-

fier is characterized in terms of degree of amplification in decibels and it is in here that much advance has been made.

Bone conductive aids have vibrators instead of ear phones, and these vibrations act on the mastoid bone and bone conduction is attained. Ear moulds hold the ear phones in place and they also prevent acoustic feedback.

Most people nowadays want a hearing aid that is as unobtrusive as possible. The advantage of aural aids is that they may be fitted post-aurally, intra-aurally or can be attached to spectacles. The main disadvantage is that they are very fiddly and patients with impaired manipulative skills may be unable to use them. Body worn aids have the advantage of a higher gain and amplification and larger controls. They can be used for conductive deafness. The main disadvantage is they are more cumbersome and there is a temptation to cover the box with layers of clothing.

The ear mould itself may present problems. Irrespective of whether it is a solid or vented mould, it may aggravate ear infection, particularly otitis externa. Some may cause local allergic irritation and severe otitis externa relieved only by removing the mould. There are non-toxic, non-allergic moulds but these are often aesthetically less attractive.

Although it is probably ideal to fit a hearing aid in both ears, this is not usually recommended in the elderly—mainly because of cost—and monaural amplification is most commonly used. In right-handed people it is preferable to fit the aid in the right ear, but sometimes better results may be obtained by fitting the aid in the least impaired ear. Audiometricians take impressions for ear moulds and fit the appropriate hearing aid when it has been prepared.

Nowadays hearing therapists are becoming available in centres and they follow up the patients to check that the hearing aid is being worn correctly and the best results are being obtained from the aid that has been issued. Hearing therapists are also available to give general advice on how to cope with deafness and may, for example, suggest readily available aids to amplify the telephone and the sound of the telephone bell.

The NHS provides three principal series of aural

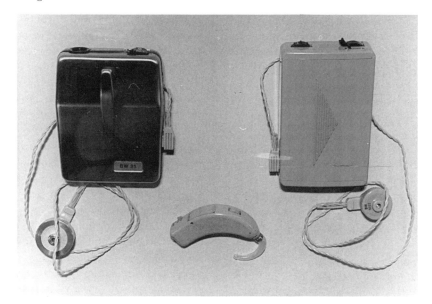

Figure 24.1. Hearing aids available on the National Health Service.
Left: very powerful body worn aid BW81.
Right: easy to control body worn aid BW61.
Centre: behind the ear aid BE11 (small but awkward to control).

aids: BE10, BE30 and BE50. The BE50 series is the most powerful. There are two types of body worn aids (BW81 and BW61) and these are illustrated in Figure 24.1. The batteries are replaced on a one for one basis free of charge on production of a log book and the used batteries. The NHS also provides a repair service and a replacement will normally be supplied while the aid is being fixed.

There are many private companies supplying a variety of aids, sometimes at exorbitant costs. Reputable companies will allow the patient a trial of the aid or even a variety of different aids. The claims of some newspaper adverts for hearing aids tend to be exaggerated and older people are advised either to attend a reputable dealer or to attend the NHS Ear, Nose and Throat Service.

Goldstein and Stephens (1981) felt that three factors should be considered when selecting the correct hearing aid for the patient: auditory sensitivity; the level at which noise becomes uncomfortable; and speech discrimination. Most hearing aids can be adjusted to take account of all three of these factors and if the patient experiences problems, the aid can be adjusted accordingly.

Although regarded by many as belonging to the last century, the ear trumpet is still a very useful instrument and is helpful in those people who cannot manage a hearing aid. It may amplify a voice by as much as 30 dB and is easy to carry around in a handbag or resting by a bed.

Meetings are particularly a problem for those with presbyacusis. Patients should inform others that they have a hearing problem or somehow encourage persons to speak at them. This can be done by placing a body worn hearing aid on to the table in front of them so that the speaker looks towards them as he speaks towards the microphone.

With an increasing number of persons wearing hearing aids it is important that meeting places, theatres and churches take account of this fact. Induction loop systems have been in use for some time working on the principle of an audio frequency amplifier. The amplifier drives an electric current around the loop which generates a magnetic field. This in turn carries the energy generated in this manner to the amplifier of the subject. Hearing aids fitted with a pick up coil have a switch marked 'T' which is sensitive to the varying magnetic field. The listener picks up the voice without outside interference. Although there have been many problems with induction loop systems, they are improving and hopefully they will become more readily available.

TINNITUS (see Table 24.4)

Unfortunately presbyacusis is often accompanied by a ringing or tinkling in the ear. These noises must be distinguished from auditory hallucinations, which take the form of words, music or meaningful sounds, such as occur in neurological or psychiatric conditions. Haggard (1980) reported that about 22% of patients over the age of 60 had experienced either intermittent or permanent tinnitus, but in only 0.5% of patients did the symptom interfere in normal life. The basis of tinnitus is still uncertain and in many cases the underlying cause is unknown.

There is an increased incidence of tinnitus in cases of noice-induced deafness related to previous occupation or to acoustic trauma incurred during the World Wars. As such patients reach older age, tinnitus is going to be encountered more frequently.

Although most tinnitus is subjective, in certain circumstances an 'objective' tinnitus may be present, as where, for example, there is myoclonus of the palate, or a visible lesion such as a vascular malformation (e.g. an aneurysm), a glomus tumour or a cervical arterial abnormality.

There is usually an associated hearing defect. The symptom in most cases seems to be related to one ear. Conditions such as vestibulo-cochlear schwannomas, syphilis and ear infections should all be ruled out as they may give rise to tinnitus and deafness.

TABLE 24.4   FACTORS PREDISPOSING TO TINNITUS

1. Age over 50
2. Exposure to loud noises in the past
3. High frequency hearing loss
4. Exposure to ototoxic drugs including aspirin
5. Otosclerosis
6. Acoustic neuroma
7. Menière's disease
8. Conductive hearing loss

The management of tinnitus is difficult and often reassurance that the patient does not have a tumour helps greatly. The main method of treatment at present is to give a hearing aid which not only improves communication, but also masks tinnitus by amplifying the ambient sounds. In some patients this amplification makes communication more difficult.

Another approach is to present the ear with a sound of sufficient intensity that the tinnitus disappears. Patients seem to prefer external noise produced by the tinnitus masker to their own 'noise'. The apparatus looks and fits just like a hearing aid and has volume and frequency control, so that the masker sounds can be matched for the patient's own noise. Sometimes after wearing the masker for some length of time the patient's noise disappears by a process of residual inhibition even after the masker is removed.

Of the available drugs, only intravenous lignocaine gives relief and the effect is short-lived. There is no convincing evidence of the value of vasodilators that have been used in the hope of increasing blood flow to the inner ear.

Morrison (1975) suggested sectioning the vestibulo-cochlear nerve for those with a severe hearing loss and tinnitus but the results were very disappointing. Tinnitus tends to be severest in those patients who have had an unsuccessful stapedectomy operation in the past, associated with loss of hearing.

Fortunately relatively few patients are seriously afflicted by tinnitus and appropriate aids and adequate reassurance should control the symptoms in most cases.

DISORDERS OF BALANCE (see Table 24.5)

The patient's description of the problem may require careful interpretation. Light-headedness, faintness, giddiness, floating, a sensation of swimming, ataxia and vertigo may all be used to describe the sensation of imbalance. Dizziness is a common complaint in the elderly and by the age of 65 over 30% of people will have experienced episodes of dizziness (Roydhouse, 1974) but by 80 years two-thirds of women and one-third of men will have reported episodes of vertigo (Sheldon, 1948).

TABLE 24.5 OTOLOGICAL CAUSES OF DIZZINESS IN THE ELDERLY

Chronic middle ear disease
  (A) Result of cholesteatoma
  (B) Failed previous surgery
Otosclerosis
Ramsay Hunt syndrome
Menière's disease
Vestibular neuronitis
Malignant tumours of nasopharynx or middle ear
Acoustic neuroma

Loss of balance is a symptom that the elderly find frightening and it may consequently immediately curtail their way of life as well as arouse their suspicion of a serious brain lesion such as a tumour or an impending stroke.

Maintaining balance requires the integration in the central nervous system of sensory information from the visual, superficial sensory, proprioceptive and vestibular systems and this means that there are many possible causes of loss of balance. Dysfunction in the generation, integration or modulation of sensory stimuli may result in dizziness or vertigo, and Drachman and Hart (1972) have emphasized the importance of sensory deficits in the elderly.

The most common causes of loss of balance are related to cardiovascular, in particular cerebrovascular impairment, cervical disease, post-traumatic syndromes, vestibular dysfunction, neoplastic and iatrogenic induced conditions. Other less common causes arise out of haematological, metabolic, visual and psychogenic disorders.

Cardiovascular

Transient cardiac dysrhythmias are a common cause of episodic dizziness and are discussed in Chapter 28.

Cerebrovascular Disease

The peripheral vestibular system and the central vestibular connections in the brain stem are supplied by the vertebrobasilar vessels and interference to the circulation in this system may result in vestibular symptoms as the vestibular nuclei, in the lateral brain stem, are affected. These areas according to Gillilan (1964) are particularly susceptible to the effect of a reduction in blood flow from the basilar artery.

Vertigo and dizziness have been reported as the most frequent symptoms of vertebrobasilar insufficiency and conversely vertebrobasilar ischaemia is probably the commonest cause of dizziness in an elderly population (Luxon, 1980).

The pathology of vertebrobasilar ischaemia has been extensively studied (Naritomi *et al.*, 1979). The diagnosis of vertebrobasilar ischaemia in an elderly person is usually made easily—sometimes too easily—but if the presenting symptom is the isolated one of dizziness, it may be forgotten. It is generally agreed that sudden episodic vertigo is more likely to be due to a peripheral vestibular lesion while vertigo associated with a central lesion is more usually of gradual onset and continuous when established. Barber and Dionne (1971) have emphasized that vertebrobasilar ischaemia is usually accompanied by deafness and tinnitus and other signs of brain stem ischaemia.

Vertebrobasilar ischaemia may in addition affect the midbrain, pons, medulla, and cerebellum—all areas important in maintaining balance.

Cervical Disease

The neck has for a long time been implicated in the aetiology of disordered balance, although the exact mechanisms are unknown. There are three main theories of the role played by the degeneration of structures in the neck in the elderly.

1. Sympathetic irritation resulting in vertebrobasilar ischaemia (Barre, 1926).
2. Intermittent vertebral artery compression by osteophytes due to cervical spondylosis (Sheehan *et al.*, 1960).
3. Deranged somatosensory output from cervical kinaesthetic receptors (Wyke, 1979).

A history of neck pain, especially if it is associated with cervical root symptoms, may point to the neck as the cause of dizziness.

Post-traumatic

It is well known that impairment of balance may occur after a head injury (Rubin, 1973). This may occur following a fracture through a temporal bone or local damage to the brain and eighth nerve within the cranial cavity but even mild trauma may upset the control of balance. It is no longer thought that post-traumatic causes of dizziness are psychological. Trauma may be followed by episodes usually of benign positional vertigo of the paroxysmal type. These may delay functional recovery, especially in the elderly. When the injury involves the temporal bone itself the patient will classically face towards the affected side with spontaneous nystagmus whose quick phase is to the uninjured side.

Psychogenic

Dizziness is a common symptom in psychiatric clinics. Blumenthal and Davie (1980) found that in 100 psychiatric patients studied, over 40% had episodes of dizziness. The most common cause, however, was thought to be tricyclic antidepressants.

Neurological

Of neurological symptoms occurring in the elderly, Parkinson's disease often presents with a sensation of imbalance. Over 30% of patients presenting with neurosyphilis were over the age of 60 (Luxon *et al.*, 1979) and dizziness was a common problem. Epilepsy, especially temporal lobe attacks, may have dizziness, followed by a loss of balance, as a symptom (see Chapter 15).

Neoplastic

Dizziness is a common symptom in intracerebellar and, more especially, extracerebellar posterior fossa tumours. Carcinomatous encephalitis may involve the vestibular nerve.

Impairment of the Vestibular Apparatus

Most research into the pathology of the ear has been directed towards the hearing mechanisms and consequently our knowledge of the vestibular apparatus is comparatively poor. The three semicircular canals and the cochlea are linked and sensory information is carried by the eighth nerve which has both cochlear and vestibular compartments.

Schuknecht (1974) has suggested that degeneration of the vestibular apparatus may be divided as shown below. This classification is somewhat speculative as pathological correlations are lacking.

1. *Cupulolithiasis* is caused by the presence of a deposit on the cupula of the posterior semicircular canal rendering it unduly sensitive to gravitational force and head movement. It is associated with postural vertigo.
2. *Ampullary disequilibrium* causes momentary vertigo and is thought to be a result of degenerative change in the ampullary mechanism.
3. *Macular disequilibrium* results in dizziness when the head position is changed and is thought to be due to changes in the sensory epithelia of the utricle.

Pathologically, Johnson and Hawkins (1972) have shown an age-related degeneration of the saccule; Rosenhall and Rubin (1975) showed a reduction of hair cells of the cristae ampullares.

Vestibular Ataxia

Degeneration, for whatever reason, of the vestibule of the labyrinth and vestibular nuclei gives rise to constant unsteadiness on ambulation.

Chronic middle ear disease is a very common condition in the elderly and in any patient with dizziness it is important to exclude the ear as the cause of the problem. Many patients forget to inform the doctor that they have or have had ear trouble: it may have been a part of their life for so long that it is forgotten. Perforations of the tympanic membrane are very common and apart from causing a conductive deafness, a small amount of water in the middle ear may give rise to persisting middle ear infection and possibly a cholesteatoma.

Although malignant tumours are rare, the presence of an acoustic neuroma must not be overlooked merely on account of the patient's age, for Morrison (1975) found that 20% of presenting acoustic neuromas were over the age of 60. Anyone with unilateral deafness, tinnitus and vertigo must have the necessary investigations to exclude the disease.

Paget's disease and otosclerosis are two diseases where local vestibular pathology may give rise to dizziness. Autoimmune diseases including Wegener's granulomatosis, temporal arteritis (Kinmont and McCallum, 1965), Behçet's syndrome (Hughes and Lehner, 1979), and relapsing polychondritis (McCadan *et al.*, 1976) have all been implicated in vestibular dizziness.

Iatrogenic

Mastoid surgery used to be very common. Mastoidectomy exposes the bone covering the labyrinth and any local infection at a later date may irritate this system. Operation on the middle ear, particularly in the presence of disease, may give rise to a perilymph fistula.

Most elderly people are receiving medication and many drugs may have adverse effects on vestibular function. Aminoglycosides, salicylates and diuretics may be ototoxic, especially in the elderly, in view of age-related changes in drug handling leading to higher blood levels. This is particularly important with diuretics and aspirin. Drug-induced hypotension and cardiac dysrhythmias may also cause a sensation of imbalance.

Management

Dizziness, vertigo or imbalance are multifactoral problems and the cause is often difficult to establish. Elderly patients frequently find it difficult to distinguish between non-specific dizziness and a 'hallucination of movement' which is the main manifestation of a disordered vestibular system. Moreover, it is rarely easy to evaluate the effects of treatment when one is dealing with subjective symptoms. Medical treatment is the mainstay of the management of the problem except in those cases where specific middle ear disease has been diagnosed. After a detailed history, full examination and appropriate investigations, any treatable underlying causes may be corrected. Medication, in particular, should be reviewed as this is likely to be a contributory cause.

All drugs used in the treatment of imbalance are liable to produce side-effects. Benzodiazepines in small doses have been found to be of some help probably because they change the threshold of response of the vestibular receptors (Yatsu & Smith, 1984). Unfortunately they are particularly prone to adverse effects in the elderly. Phenothiazines are not recommended because of their extrapyramidal side-effects. The antihistamines reduce the reactivity of the vestibular system and may also have a central effect. The most commonly used are cinnarizine and betahistine. Prochlorperazine is an antiemetic very commonly used and may be effective in a severe attack of vertigo. It probably acts on the brain stem. This, like many other drugs, however, should not be used in non-specific giddiness or on a chronic basis as it frequently has adverse effects, especially in the elderly, in whom it is probably the commonest cause of drug-induced parkinsonism. Anticholinergic drugs diminish the activity of the vestibular nucleus neurones and suppress the spontaneous firing of the vestibular nerve and may also be used in cases of acute vertigo.

'Labyrinthic' exercises have been found to be effective especially in treating those whose dizziness is related to trauma. They may be helpful in any case where there is unilateral labyrinthine dysfunction. Following injury, the intact vestibular system has to compensate for the loss of the other vestibular apparatus. Exercises that trigger vertigo stimulate the development of compensatory functions. These exercises, which are known to most physiotherapy departments, were first described by Cawthorne (1945).

The presence of nystagmus, whether persistent or positional, is often the main objective indicator as to whether or not medical treatment has worked. Unfortunately, the amount of nystagmus recorded polygraphically does not correlate with the severity of the disease.

Surgery may be indicated in some cases. Mastoid surgery must be carried out for persisting aural disease, labyrinthitis, abscess and to stop further bone disease. The risk of operation and the possibility of deterioration in hearing must be taken into account when surgery is contemplated. The management of acoustic neuroma is discussed in Chapter 16 but it is worth reiterating that, despite the morbidity and mortality from early surgery, active treatment is preferable to a wait-and-see policy based upon the hope that the patient will outlive the disease.

Various operations have been described for vestibular disease. These are best carried out in specialist centres; even then the results in the elderly are not generally as good as in younger patients. Residual dizziness is common. Intractable positional vertigo is best treated either by total labyrinthectomy (Cawthorne, 1956) or by division of the vestibular nerve itself (Glasscock *et al.*, 1980). Endolymphatic sac surgery, sacculotomy, cervical sympathectomy, vestibular destruction (Angell-James, 1969) have all been described but postoperative compensation breakdown, stimulation of the vestibular nerve and persisting vestibular dysfunction make surgeons reluctant to operate on elderly patients. Ocular problems including cataracts may be corrected surgically and this will often help rehabilitation.

The neck, which is often considered to be the cause of the problem, may be treated locally with heat or immobilized with a collar. Muscle relaxants, such as diazepam, and physiotherapy have all been shown to help. However, benzodiazepines may do more harm than good in the elderly. Psychological and social factors must also be taken into account. A giddy patient may suffer severe anxiety and there will be a self-fulfilling expectation that he or she is condemned to remain indoors for the rest of his or her life. There is the additional worry of not being able to call for assistance in the case of falls. Vestibular dysfunction, like deafness, may lead to a vicious circle of increasing isolation and loneliness.

Sudden audiological and vestibular failure is an emergency and management should include urgent referral to an experienced otorhinolaryngologist.

REFERENCES

Angell-James, J. (1969) Menière's Disease—Treatment with Ultra Sound. *J. Laryngol.*, **83**, 771–85.

Barber, A.O., and Dionne, J. (1971). Vestibular Findings in Vertebro-Basilar Ischaemia. *Ann. Otol.*, **80**, 805–12.

Barre, J.A. (1926). Sur un syndrome sympathique cervicale postérieure et sa cause fréquente, l'arthrite cervicale. *Rev. Neurol.*, **33**, 1246–52.

Blumenfeld, V.G., Bergman, M., and Miller, E. (1969). Speech discrimination in an ageing population. *J. Speech Hearing Res.*, **12**, 210–17.

Blumenthal, M., and Davie, J.W. (1980). Dizziness and falling in elderly psychiatric outpatients. *Am. J. Psychiatry*, **137**, 203–6.

Caird, F.I., Andrews, G.R., and Kennedy, R.D. (1973). Effect of posture on blood pressure in the elderly. *Br. Heart J.*, **35**, 527–30.

Calearo, C., and Lazzaroni, A. (1957). Speech intelligibility in relation to the speed of the message. *Laryngoscope*, **67**, 427–9.

Cawthorne, T.E. (1945). Vestibular injuries. *Proc. Roy. Soc. Med.*, **39**, 270–2.

Cawthorne, T.E. (1956). Menière's Disease. *J. Laryngol.*, **70**, 695–700.

Drachman, D.A., and Hart, C. (1972). An approach to the dizzy patient. *Neurology*, **22**, 323–34.

Dublin, W.B. (1976). *Fundamentals of Sensorineural Auditory Pathology*, Thomas, Springfield, Illinois.

Feldman, R., and Reger, S. (1967). Relations among hearing reaction Time and Age. *J. Speech Hearing Res.*, **10**, 479–95.

Gaeth, J. (1948). A study of Phonemic Regression in Relation to Hearing Loss. Unpublished Doctoral Dissertation. Northwestern University of Chicago, USA.

Gilhome-Herbst K.R., and Humphrey, C.M. (1980). Hearing impairment and mental state in the elderly living at home. *Br. Med. J.* **281**, 903–5.

Gillilan, L.A. (1964). The correlation of the blood supply to the human brainstem with clinical brainstem lesions. *J. Neuropathol Exp. Neurol.*, **23**, 78–108.

Glasscock, M.E., Davis, W.E., Hughes, G.B., and Jackson, C.G. (1980). Labyrinthectomy versus middle fossa vestibular nerve section in Menière's disease. *Ann. Otol. Rhinol. Laryngol.*, **89**, 318–24.

Goldstein, D.P., and Stephens, D.G. (1981). Audiological Rehabilitation. Management model 1. *Audiology*, **20**, 432–52.

Haggard, M. (1980). Epidemiology of Tinnitus. Paper read at meeting of British Society of Audiology, Nottingham, July 1980.

Hansen, C.C., and Reske-Neilson, E. (1965). Pathological studies in presbyacuses: cochlear and central findings in 12 aged patients. *Arch. Otolaryngol.*, **82**, 115–32.

Hinchcliffe, R. (1962). The anatomical locus of presbyacusis. *J. Speech Hearing Dis.*, **27**, 301–10.

Hughes, R.A.C., and Lehner, T. (1979). Neurological aspects of Behçet's syndrome. In: Lehnert, T., and Barnes, P. (eds.) *Behçet's Syndrome*, Academic Press, London.

Humphrey, C., Gilhome-Herst, K., and Farugi, A. (1981). Some characteristics of the hearing impaired who do not present themselves for rehabilitation. *Br. J. Audiol.*, **75**, 25–30.

Johnson, L.G., and Hawkins, J.E. (1972). Sensory and neural degeneration with ageing as seen in micro dissection of the human ear. *Ann. Oto-Rhino-Laryngol.*, **81**, 179–93.

Kaplan, B.M., Langendorf, R., Lev, M., and Pick, M. (1973). Tachycardia–bradycardia syndrome pathology, mechanisms and treatment. *Am. J. Cardiol.*, **31**, 497–508.

Kay, D.W.K., Beamish, P., and Roth, M. (1964). Old age mental disorders in Newcastle Upon Tyne—Pt II a study of possible social and medical causes. *Br. J. Psychiatry*, **129**, 207–15.

Kinmont, P.D.C., and McCallum, D. (1965). The aetiology, pathology and course of giant cell arteritis. *Br. J. Dermatol.*, **77**, 193–202.

Kirikae, J., Sato, J., and Shitata, T. (1964). Study of hearing in advanced age. *Laryngoscope*, **74**, 205–20.

Konigsmark, B.N., and Murphy, E.A. (1972). Volume of the ventral cochlear nucleus in man: its relationship to neuronal population and age. *J. Neuropathol. Exp. Neurol.*, **31**, 304–16.

Luxon, L.M. (1980). *Vertigo*, John Wiley & Sons, Chichester.

Luxon, L.M., Lees, A.J., and Greenwood, R.J. (1979). Neurosyphilis today. *Lancet*, **i**, 90–3.

McAdam, L.P., O'Hanlan, M.A., Bluestone, R., and Pearson, C.M. (1976). Relapsing polychondritis. *Medicine*, **55**, 193–215.

Morrison, A. (1975). *Management of Sensorineural Deafness*, Butterworths, London.

Naritomi, H., Sakai, F., and Meyer, J.S. (1979). Pathogenesis of transient ischaemia attacks within the vertebrobasilar arterial system. *Arch. Neurol.*, **36**, 121–8.

Rosenhall, U., and Rubin, W. (1975). Degenerative changes in the human vestibular sensory epithelium. *Acta Otolaryngol.*, **79**, 69–81.

Roydhouse, N. (1974). Vertigo and its treatment. *Drugs*, **7**, 297–309.

Rubin, W. (1973). Whiplash with vestibular involvement. *Arch. Otolaryngol.*, **97**, 85–7.

Schuknecht, H.F. (1974). *Pathology of the Ear*, Harvard University Press, Cambridge, Mass.

Sheehan, S., Bauer, R.B., and Meyer, J.A. (1960). Vertebral artery compression in cervical spondylosis. *Neurology*, **10**, 968–86.

Sheldon, J.A. (1948). *The Social Medicine of Old Age*, Oxford University Press, London.

Wood, P.H.N. (1975). Classification of Impairments and Handicaps. Paper presented to the International Conference for the Ninth Revision of the International Classification of Diseases. WHO, Geneva, WHO/ICDGI Rev. Conf. 75, 15.

Wyke, B. (1979). Cervical articular contributions to posture and gait. Their relation to senile dysequilibrium. *Age Ageing*, **8**, 251–8.

Yatsu Smith, J.D. (1984). Neurological aspects of vertigo. In: Ballantyne, J., and Groves, J. (eds.) *Scott Brown's Diseases of the Ear, Nose and Throat*, Butterworths, London, p. 861.

Zwardemaker, A. (1899). Der Verlust an hohen Tonen mit zunchmendem Alter: em neues Gesetz. *Arch. Ohren Heilkunde*, **47**.

Chapter 25

Neurological Diseases Usually Acquired Earlier in Life

James Howe

Consultant Physician in Medicine for the Elderly, Airedale General Hospital, Steeton, Keighley, West Yorkshire, UK

The diagnosis and treatment of most diseases of the nervous system in the elderly does not differ from that in the young, and few neurological diseases spare the elderly, rather the opposite. The two disorders considered in this chapter, multiple sclerosis (MS) and myasthenia gravis (MG), are often thought to be exclusive to the young. In fact, MS is being recognized more frequently in older patients, though the use of the term 'elderly' in the neurological literature for people in their 50s and 60s might raise a smile among geriatricians (Noseworthy *et al.*, 1983). Myasthenia gravis (MG) can occur at any age (Penn and Rowland, 1984) and the Lambert–Eaton myasthenic syndrome (LEMS) when associated with carcinoma is more likely to affect older people.

MULTIPLE SCLEROSIS

The diagnostic term 'multiple sclerosis' brings to mind an image of a severely disabled, middle-aged woman. Although the peak age of onset is in the early 30s and in perhaps 95% of patients the illness begins between the ages of 10 and 50 (Paty and Poser, 1984), geriatricians will certainly see cases and may be seeing more than they realize. Patients with MS may come to a geriatrician in three ways. First, because of the lack of facilities for the younger disabled and the commitment of geriatricians to long-term care, victims of MS under the age of 70 are

being cared for in many geriatric departments in the UK. Secondly, as many as 20% of MS sufferers have a benign illness with survival into the 70s (McAlpine, 1964; McKay and Hirano, 1967) and two-thirds of patients with MS will still be walking 25 years after onset (Confayreux *et al.*, 1980). These patients will carry their disease into old age with the added problems of senescence and multiple pathology. Thirdly, it is becoming clear that the first manifestations of MS can present later in life, both first attacks and first presentation (Noseworthy *et al.*, 1983). When this happens MS may not be recognized or may even be dismissed.

Until recently the diagnostic criteria which were widely accepted for trials and studies of MS recommended the exclusion of cases where the initial symptoms occurred over age 50 (Schumacher *et al.*, 1965; Rose *et al.*, 1976; McDonald and Halliday, 1977). In 1982, new diagnostic criteria were drawn up at a workshop in Boston on the diagnosis of MS. The age of onset was extended to 59, and supportive laboratory data were included in the definitions (Poser *et al.*, 1983). The participants emphasized the fact that the diagnosis of MS is still clinical because no reliable, specific diagnostic test yet exists (Rudick *et al.*, 1986).

It is also better appreciated that the spectrum of disease activity ranges from the completely unexpected and totally asymptomatic case found at autopsy to a few with rapid deterioration and death only months after onset (Herndon and Rudick, 1983). Two recent autopsy studies reported unsuspected MS with a frequency which suggests that the disease may be twice as common as currently given (Gilbert and Sadler, 1983; Castaigne *et al.*, 1981). In these two reports six of the nine patients were over 60 and four were over 70. In the UK the prevalence of MS is approximately 100/100 000 (Williams and McKeran, 1986; Shepherd and Downie, 1978). For information on the worldwide prevalence the reviews of Acheson (1985) and Kurtzke (1983) should be consulted.

Diagnosis of MS in the Elderly

The spectrum of clinical symptoms and signs that are now recognized as caused by MS is very wide and it has been called 'the great imitator' in neurological disease (Paty and Poser, 1984). The diagnosis of MS can be difficult at any age but perhaps more so in older patients where it is rarely considered and other diseases may coexist. A recent study (Noseworthy *et al.*, 1983) demonstrated that MS presenting after age 50 was not rare and it was often misdiagnosed by neurologists. In an 8 year period, 79 patients with first presentation after age 50 were found among 838 patients seen at an MS clinic in London, Ontario. Forty patients had onset of the disease, so far as the authors could tell, after age 50. MS was considered to be the most likely initial diagnosis in only 27 of the 79 patients. Spondylotic myelopathy was most often put first, while vascular disease, motor neurone disease, hereditary spinocerebellar degeneration, familial paraplegia, tumour, subacute combined degeneration of the cord, post-infectious encephalomyelitis and normal pressure hydrocephalus were thought most likely in other cases.

Relapsing and remitting disease afflicts up to 70% of young patients with MS (Paty and Poser, 1984) whereas a chronic progressive course appears to be more common in older patients and to carry a worse prognosis at any age (Paty and Poser, 1984; Noseworthy *et al.*, 1983). It is this group of patients in whom diagnosis is most difficult. The majority have a progressive, chronic spinal syndrome, though

cerebral (dementing) and cerebellar syndromes are also seen.

In trying to establish a diagnosis in an older patient with a chronic, progressive neurological disease, careful enquiry to elicit typical and reliable symptoms of MS in the past may clearly demonstrate 'historical' dissemination of lesions. The most useful symptoms are typical optic neuritis, Lhermitte's symptom (sudden, brief 'electric shock' or tingling sensations radiating down the spine and limbs on flexion of the neck), acute transverse myelitis with recovery, trigeminal neuralgia occurring under age 40, horizontal diplopia on gaze to either side with minimal or no diplopia in the primary position, suggestive of inter-nuclear ophthalmoplegia, and a sensory useless hand (Poser, 1984). Sometimes patients have forgotten completely about such episodes until their memory is prompted; in one personal case a myelogram reminded a 70 year old man that he had had a lumbar puncture 50 years before for blindness in one eye which had recovered.

When historical evidence of second lesions cannot be obtained, laboratory evidence can help. Cerebrospinal fluid immunoglobulin abnormalities, evoked potential measurements and computed tomography (CT) have all been studied in younger patients, but the abnormalities revealed are not absolutely specific to MS and their significance in the over 70s, so far as MS is concerned, is not yet clear.

Cerebrospinal fluid immunoglobulins

The most useful supporting evidence for MS is the presence of oligoclonal banding on agarose gel electrophoresis of CSF (Ebers and Paty, 1980). If electrophoresis is not available the next best test seems to be the CSF IgG index (Hershey and Trotter, 1980). More than 90% of patients with clinically definite MS have oligoclonal banding, while only 8% of non-MS neurological diseases show this phenomenon (Ebers and Paty, 1980). The CSF IgG index is abnormal in approximately 90% of clinically definite cases (Hershey and Trotter, 1980). Unfortunately these tests are not available in every district general hospital. CSF IgG abnormalities are also seen in infections and other immunologically mediated diseases of the nervous system such as

Guillain–Barré syndrome, systemic lupus erythematosus, sarcoidosis and neurosyphilis (Hershey and Trotter, 1980).

Evoked potentials

The recording of evoked potentials is now very popular because they are relatively inexpensive, completely harmless and can reveal clinically unsuspected lesions and so provide supporting evidence of dissemination in space. The pattern shift visual evoked potential is the most widely available and the characteristic abnormality in MS is a delay in the major positive wave (P100) with a preserved wave form. All evoked potentials show a delay with ageing (Katzman and Terry, 1983). Guidelines for interpreting visual evoked responses in the elderly have been put forward (Celesia and Daley, 1977). The presence of multiple pathology will make the interpretation of these tests difficult apart from the effects of ageing.

Computed tomography

Because it is non-invasive and harmless, though the injection of contrast material is not, CT scanning is now a routine investigation in suspected MS in the USA. CT scans in MS patients may reveal generalized atrophy (Cala *et al.*, 1978) or hypodense areas, some of which enhance with contrast (Lebow *et al.*, 1978). Enhancement appears to correlate with disease activity (Ebers *et al.*, 1984). The technique of 'double dosing' with contrast to demonstrate more lesions needs care in the elderly because of renal impairment and possible volume overload (Ebers *et al.*, 1984). These abnormalities need to be interpreted with caution as similar lesions can be seen in brain metastases, multicentric gliomas, cerebral lymphomas ('micro-glioma'), sarcoidosis and systemic lymphoma with cerebral involvement (Abbott *et al.*, 1982; Sagar *et al.*, 1982).

Magnetic resonance imaging

This technique reveals MS lesions with great clarity (Young *et al.*, 1981) but it is unlikely to become widely available in the UK in the near future. It may become the best test (Gebarski *et al.*, 1985).

Without definite evidence of dissemination of lesions myelography is still needed to investigate patients with progressive spinal cord syndromes. It is neither safe nor correct to examine the CSF without doing a myelogram in such cases. Spinal cord swelling seen at myelography cannot be assumed to be due to intramedullary tumour as a similar appearance has been reported in MS (Feasby *et al.*, 1981).

Aetiology and Pathogenesis

The cause of MS is unknown, but both cause and pathogenesis appear to be multifactorial. The best hypothesis at present is that an environmental agent, or agents, affects a genetically susceptible human of the right age and gender. The most likely agent is a virus that either persists in the nervous system or induces autoimmunity and disappears (Ellison *et al.*, 1984). The pathological process in MS appears to be immunologically mediated, with involvement of the humoral and cell mediated immune systems (Arnason, 1983).

There are age-related changes in the regulation of the immune response which may determine the clinical course of late onset MS. Observations in animals suggest that the ability to mount an effective immune response declines with age, and deficiencies have been observed both in vivo and in vitro in bone marrow derived (B-cell) and thymus derived (T-cell) function (Makinodan and Kay, 1980). Relapses of MS and progressive disease are associated with an absolute decline in suppressor T-cells (Weiner and Hauser, 1982). If there is a decline in the number and function of suppressor T-cells with ageing in MS patients, this could permit continued disease activity, prevent remissions and so result in the chronic progressive clinical picture which is typical of late onset MS and the later stages of the disease (Noseworthy *et al.*, 1983).

Management

Therapeutic nihilism is not confined to the care of the elderly; it also afflicts younger patients with MS, presumably because of its exaggerated reputation as an incurable, crippling and depressing disease. While at present there is no cure, a great deal can be done to relieve the symptoms and help patients and carers cope.

Matthews (1984) has comprehensively reviewed the present position on treatment. ACTH is believed to shorten the duration of relapses (Rose *et al.*, 1970), though many neurologists use oral steroids for convenience (Tourtelotte 1983). The demonstration by Snyder *et al.* (1981) that ACTH-induced cortisol production in MS patients could be extremely variable lends support to the use of steroids. There is no evidence that long-term ACTH is of any value (Millar *et al.*, 1967). Trials of immunosuppressive regimens including plasmapheresis have been slightly encouraging but are hazardous (Hughes, 1983). A reduction in the relapse rate has been reported with intrathecal interferon (Jacobs *et al.*, 1982, 1985), and oral linoleic acid reduces the severity and duration of relapses (Dworkin *et al.*, 1984).

Currently there is a vogue for hyperbaric oxygen but benefit has not been demonstrated (Barnes *et al.*, 1985; Fischer *et al.*, 1983). Spinal cord stimulation has been used as an experimental procedure in MS. Spasticity can be reduced and bladder control improved in some patients. The long-term possibilities have not been worked out and further study is needed before this procedure will be more than experimental (Matthews, 1984).

The general rehabilitation of older MS patients does not differ from the guidelines elsewhere in this book (Section 4). The most prominent problems in the later stages of MS are spasticity and weakness, ataxia and tremor, incontinence, cognitive impairment and depression. Just recognizing that someone has MS may help by removing uncertainty and enabling puzzling and uncomfortable symptoms to be explained and treated. For instance, a rise in body temperature can produce striking deterioration in MS patients and has been used as a diagnostic test (Davis, 1984).

Paroxysmal symptoms and pain

While not common, these may be incorrectly labelled, especially in older patients, and then not handled in the best way. These symptoms can be disturbing and sometimes lead to accusations of hysteria or manipulation. In a study of Lhermitte's symptom 10% of patients who had experienced it had never told a doctor about it because they thought the symptom was too strange (Khanchandani and Howe, 1982). Anticonvulsants in standard doses can relieve many of these paroxysmal episodes, such as painful tonic seizures, paroxysmal sensory disturbances including trigeminal neuralgia and epilepsy, which also occurs in MS. In older patients, or those with ataxia who are intolerant of carbamazepine or phenytoin, benzodiazepine anticonvulsants such as clobazam or clonazepam are effective. Pain is not often mentioned in standard books on MS but Clifford and Trotter (1984) found clinically significant pain occurred in nearly 30% of a group of 317 MS patients. The pains were of various types and the incidence of pain was greater in patients who had had the disease for 20 years or more. Careful attention to the type of pain and possible pathophysiological mechanisms led to a rational choice of therapy with benefit for most patients. They found tricyclic antidepressants particularly helpful for chronic unpleasant sensory disturbances and headaches, whether there was depression or not.

Weakness and spasticity

Weakness is almost always of upper motor neurone type and associated with spasticity, clonus and involuntary spasm. In addition MS patients tend to be easily fatigued and weak from disuse and despair—and this is not helped by the negative reinforcement of 'ageism', either personal or provided by those who deal with the patient.

Inactivity leads to contractures, pressure sores, infections and venous thrombosis (though the latter seems less common in people with severe spasticity). Therefore it would seem reasonable to assume that activity should delay or prevent these complications and it also has a beneficial effect on morale. Activity to the point of fatigue can be encouraged with instruction from a physiotherapist, reinforced by explanation of the benefits from the doctor.

Spasticity (stiffness of the extremities and hyperreflexia), is common in the later stages of MS; it may enable a patient with severe weakness to stand and pivot when transferring, but increases the energy cost of movement as the agonist must overcome the spastic response in the antagonist.

Active and passive stretching, massage and external cold packs can be helpful. Infections, painful ulcers and rectal or bladder distension aggravate spasticity. Drugs can be of help when used with care, and combinations may be more effective (Young and Delwaide, 1981). Starting with low doses of diazepam (2 mg), baclofen (5 mg) or dantrolene (25 mg) twice a day and building slowly, by adding doses every third day, helps to avoid side-effects. Drowsiness, weakness and light-headedness are the most common side-effects. Diazepam must be withdrawn slowly as seizures can be precipitated by abrupt withdrawal. Hepatotoxicity has been reported with dantrolene and the manufacturers recommend periodic liver function tests and discontinuation of treatment if no benefit is seen after 2 weeks at the maximum recommended dose of 100 mg four times daily.

Where spasticity is more severe or contractures are beginning to interfere with comfort and nursing care, physical measures can be used. Nerve blocks with phenol, intrathecal phenol (Dimitrijevic and Sherwood, 1980) or section of tendons may be needed in extreme cases, though patients with MS may react badly to operations. These problems are more likely to be found in patients with progressive and long-standing disease.

Ataxia and tremor

It is difficult to relieve these problems. Aids and adaptations, carefully selected and given with instruction in their use, can help. Stereotactic thalamotomy can transform the care of patients disabled by violent tremor (Samra *et al.*, 1970). However, these authors recommend that patients in the terminal stages of the disease should not be selected for operation.

A speech therapist can advise on ways to improve communication in patients with severe dysarthria. There are many types of aid available; careful selection and training can help enormously (Milward, 1984). The distress of hunger and thirst in patients who cannot swallow can be relieved with microbore tube feeding or percutaneous gastrostomy (Russell *et al.*, 1984).

Incontinence

This is a common and distressing symptom in MS at all ages. For a clear and authoritative account of the aids and appliances available, the monograph by Mandelstam (1986) is excellent.

The physiology of the bladder is complex and physiological investigations not widely available. A simple approach based on a classification into failure to store or failure to empty is useful. An attempt can then be made to convert storage problems into failure to empty and the bladder emptied mechanically (Parsons, 1983). Anticholinergic drugs are widely used and combinations are worth trying when single drugs fail. Intermittent self-catheterization could perhaps be used more, even in older patients (Lapides *et al.*, 1974). Bladder neck resection can help difficulty in emptying but has also been recommended for detrusor instability (Jakobsen *et al.*, 1973). It should be remembered that patients with MS are not immune to other diseases and prostatic enlargement, bladder stones and metabolic causes of a diuresis may need treatment.

Cognitive impairment

Although not always recognized, cognitive impairment is common in MS (Peyser *et al.*, 1980; Rabins *et al.*, 1986). This is hardly surprising since ventricular dilatation is the commonest radiological finding. Depression is also common (McIvor *et al.*, 1984; Rabins *et al.*, 1986; Schiffer and Babigian, 1984; Whitlock and Siskind, 1980), and seems to be more common in older patients. Depression is often overlooked and neglected in medical patients but can be treated successfully even in the disabled and elderly (Mayou and Hawton, 1986). This additional cause of suffering should be sought and relieved as energetically as possible (Rodin and Voshart, 1986). Recognition of cognitive impairment leads to a better assessment of the patient's needs and those of his carers and much can be done to help them cope (Gilleard, 1984). Pathological laughing and crying in patients with bilateral forebrain lesions is a very distressing symptom for sufferer and carers alike; full explanation helps. It may respond to amitriptyline (Schiffer *et al.*, 1985).

The cause of MS is still unknown and it cannot yet be cured. It is clear that it does affect older people but this is not widely appreciated. Management (physical, psychological and social) is improved by correct diagnosis and thorough assessment. When effective palliative therapy of MS becomes available, and current research suggests that this is not too far away (Ellison *et al.*, 1984), it will be even more important to recognize MS in the elderly.

MYASTHENIA GRAVIS

Typical myasthenia gravis (MG) may begin at any age but it is said to be uncommon before age 10 or after age 65 (Penn and Rowland, 1984). However, there are reported series with up to 45% of patients presenting after 60 years of age (Osserman *et al.*, 1958; Herishanu *et al.*, 1976; Evoli *et al.*, 1983). MG is a rare disease with a prevalence of 3/100 000; two-thirds of patients are women though in the older age group the sexes seem to be equally affected (Penn and Rowland, 1984).

Although myasthenia gravis is rare, it is important because increased awareness could prevent months or years of misdiagnosis, 13 years in one reported case (Vellodi and Tallis, 1988). It is an autoimmune disease in which tremendous advances in understanding and treatment have been made since Simpson (1960) first suggested antibodies to the motor end plate could be involved.

MG is a disorder of neuromuscular transmission caused by a loss of functional acetylcholine receptors (AChR) at the postsynaptic membrane of the neuromuscular junction. Newsom-Davis (1984) has provided an up-to-date and authoritative account of current knowledge on the pathophysiology and immunology. Myasthenia may also be a prominent component of the weakness occurring in polymyositis (Johns *et al.*, 1971) and features suggesting myasthenia may be seen in motor neurone disease and some polyneuropathies (Simpson, 1966).

Clinical Patterns

Myasthenia is not a homogeneous disorder. Apart from neonatal myasthenia due to transplacental transfer of antibody, there are also rare congenital forms (Newsom-Davis, 1984). In some patients myasthenia remains confined to the ocular muscles and in generalized acquired myasthenia there seem to be three distinct clinical patterns (Compston *et al.*, 1980). These patterns have important therapeutic implications. Firstly, generalized myasthenia gravis may be associated with thymoma. There is no clear HLA association in Caucasians, but high titres of antibodies to AChR are found, and 90% of thymoma patients have anti-striated muscle antibodies. The peak age of onset is from 30 to 50 but thymic tumours can be found at any age and the sexes are equally affected. Secondly, it may be associated with thymus atrophy. The onset of myasthenia is then usually after the age of 40 and there is an association with HLA3, B7 and DR2. Titres of antibodies to AChR are low but 60% have anti-striated muscle antibody and males are affected three times as often as females. Thirdly, it may be associated with thymic hyperplasia with onset usually under the age of 40. There is an association with HLA1, B8 and DR3. These patients often have other autoimmune diseases and anti-AChR antibody titres are highest in this group. Only 20% have antibody to striated muscle and females are affected three times as often as males (Table 25.1).

Clinical Recognition

The recognition of myasthenia gravis is difficult at any age, with an average time to diagnosis of 2 years (Scadding and Havard, 1981) most patients (and especially women) being labelled anxious or hysterical. As usual, in older patients, there will be increased diagnostic difficulty because of possible associated conditions such as cerebrovascular and cardiopulmonary disease (Herishanu *et al.*, 1976) and the common tendency to call every cranial nerve disorder in the elderly 'vertebrobasilar insufficiency'.

There are three general characteristics that, together, provide a diagnostic combination (Penn

TABLE 25.1 MYASTHENIA GRAVIS: CLINICAL PATTERNS*

	Generalized			Ocular
Thymus pathology	Hyperplasia	Thymoma	Atrophy	?
Age of onset	<40	Peak 30–50	>40	Wide range
Sex ratio (M:F)	1:3	1:1	3:1	3:1
Anti-AChR titre	High	Intermediate	Low	Very low
Anti-striated	20%	90%	60%	30%

* Adapted from Newsom-Davis (1984), with permission.

and Rowland, 1984). The fluctuating nature of the weakness is unlike any other disease, varying markedly throughout each day and from day to day. Penn and Rowland (1984) challenge the use of the term 'excessive fatigability' (Leading Article, 1986). Patients with MG almost never complain of 'fatigue' or of symptoms that might be thought of as fatigue. The symptoms are always due to weakness: for example, double vision, difficulty chewing or swallowing with choking, inability to raise the arms high enough to comb hair or hang out washing, falls and so on. Patients describe a difficulty which varies in severity but which is always due to muscle weakness.

The second characteristic of myasthenia gravis is the distribution of weakness. Ocular muscles are affected first in about 40% of patients and ultimately in about 85% (Penn and Rowland, 1984). Drooping eyelids and double vision, which can lead to feelings of instability and complaints of dizziness, result. Other common symptoms are weakness of facial and oropharyngeal muscles with slurred speech and difficulty swallowing and chewing, often accompanied by choking over liquids and solids. Oropharyngeal and ocular weakness cause symptoms in virtually all patients with myasthenia gravis at any age. The limbs are almost never affected alone. Proximal limb muscles are affected more than distal and the weakness may be asymmetrical. The muscle stretch reflexes are usually present even with marked weakness. Some patients may present with breathing difficulty in association with apparently trivial chest infection or prolonged ventilatory failure after general anaesthesia; this is also seen in the Lambert–Eaton myasthenic syndrome (see Chapter 21).

The third characteristic of myasthenic weakness is the response to cholinergic drugs, most usually seen with a positive edrophonium (Tensilon) test (Osserman and Genkins, 1966). False negative responses may occur in association with severe weakness especially if there is muscle wasting (Simpson, 1958). However, muscle wasting is unusual, occurring in less than 10% of patients (Oosterhuis, 1981; Oosterhuis and Bethlem, 1973). Malnutrition due to dysphagia can also contribute to wasting. Intravenous atropine is recommended prior to the injection of edrophonium to block parasympathetic side-effects like bradycardia and nausea, but in the elderly care is needed with cholinergic drugs because of central side-effects, possible glaucoma or prostatic obstruction. In patients over 75 years of age less than 0.6 mg of atropine is safer, followed by 1 mg of edrophonium as a test and then 5–10 mg. Facilities for resuscitation must be available and it is preferable for two doctors to be present in case of transient worsening in very weak patients.

The differential diagnosis therefore includes all diseases that are accompanied by weakness of ocular, oropharyngeal or limb muscles, such as motor neurone disease, muscular dystrophies, metabolic and inflammatory myopathies, transient ischaemic attacks and minor strokes, and even cardiac or respiratory failure (Herishanu *et al.*, 1976).

Myasthenia gravis can also develop as a result of penicillamine therapy particularly in patients with rheumatoid arthritis but it usually remits when the drug is stopped (Bucknall *et al.*, 1975). If myasthenia remains restricted to the ocular muscles for approximately 1 year, and certainly if it is restricted after 2 years, it very rarely becomes generalized (Bever *et al.*, 1983).

Pathology

About 70% of thymus glands from adults with myasthenia gravis are not involuted. Lymphoid hyperplasia is seen with numerous lymphoid follicles containing germinal centres. These contain B-cells. Normal and myasthenic glands contain alpha-thymosin, a hormone important for T-cell maturation (Penn and Rowland, 1984).

Thymomas occur in up to 10% of patients and contain lymphoepithelial tissue and T-cells. The tumour may invade locally but almost never spreads to other organs (Rowland, 1980). At the neuromuscular junction there is loss of the postsynaptic folds and the synaptic cleft is widened. Immunocytochemical studies have shown antibody-like structures, IgG and complement components 3 and 9 on the residual synaptic folds (Engel, 1980; Sahashi *et al.*, 1980; Santa *et al.*, 1972).

Immunology

Anti-AChR antibodies are detectable in about 90% of patients with generalized myasthenia. True biological false positives are found in first degree relatives of myasthenia patients (Vincent and Newsom-Davis, 1985) and in elderly patients with other autoimmune disease (Robb *et al.*, 1985). Anti-AChR antibodies are also found in patients with penicillamine-induced myasthenia (Compston *et al.*, 1980). Some patients with generalized myasthenia have no anti-AChR antibodies. Some have a non-autoimmune congenital myasthenia and in others there is clear evidence of immunoglobulin mediated impairment of neuromuscular transmission by antibodies that are thought to bind to non-AChR determinants on the postsynaptic membrane (Mossman *et al.*, 1986). Anti-AChR antibodies may also be absent early in the disease and in ocular myasthenia antibodies are found in much lower incidence (50%) and titre.

Antibody titres have a broad inverse relationship with muscle strength in individual patients. The physiological abnormalities in myasthenia seem to be at least partly caused by antibody and complement mediated lysis of the postsynaptic membrane. Accelerated AChR degradation and direct blocking of the receptor by antibody may also be involved (Drachman *et al.*, 1978; Newsom-Davis, 1984).

Other autoantibodies may be detected and those to striated muscle are of importance, being found in 90% of patients with a thymoma (Compston *et al.*, 1980). There is an increased incidence of other autoimmune diseases in MG patients and their first degree relatives.

Neurophysiology

Impairment of neuromuscular transmission can be demonstrated in up to 90% of patients by an abnormal decremental response of the compound muscle action potential to repetitive nerve stimulation (Ozdemir and Young, 1976). Single fibre electromyography can also demonstrate faulty transmission by an increased variation in activation time or 'jitter' between the action potentials of two muscle fibres of the same motor unit or 'blocking' when one action potential fails completely (Stalberg *et al.*, 1976; Sanders *et al.*, 1979). Even when symptoms are confined to the ocular muscles, electrophysiological abnormalities are found in skeletal muscle (Stalberg *et al.*, 1976). Standard needle electromyography and nerve conduction studies usually show no abnormality, though occasionally a myopathic pattern may be seen (Penn and Rowland, 1984).

Radiology

Plain X-rays are usually enough to show thymic tumours which seem to be commoner in older patients but computed tomography may be needed (Fon *et al.*, 1982).

Treatment

Anticholinesterase drugs and plasmapheresis provide symptomatic relief. Immunosuppression and thymectomy affect the disease process.

Anticholinesterases

Of the drugs available, pyridostigmine is the most popular because of its slightly longer duration of action and slightly less severe muscarinic side-effects. The drug needs to be given 4 or 3 hourly, depending on response. Abdominal colic and diarrhoea can be blocked with small doses of atropine or propantheline but after a time few patients need these. There is no evidence that any one anticholinesterase is more effective than the others or that combinations are better than any one alone. In generalized disease anticholinesterases actually mask the underlying disease process and do not return function to normal. The risk of crisis persists and there are experimental findings which suggest these drugs may cause a loss of functional acetylcholine receptors (Engel *et al.*, 1973; Chang *et al.*, 1973). Benefit is unlikely with doses of pyridostigmine greater than 120 mg 2 hourly and if such doses are needed this is an indication for some other form of therapy.

Thymectomy

This is now standard treatment for generalized myasthenia gravis in the under 40s. Retrospective studies indicate that 60 to 80% of patients without a thymoma improve and 20 to 25% go into complete remission (Newsom-Davis, 1984). With an experienced team the operation is safe. It is also recommended at any age to remove thymic tumours which may be locally invasive but the myasthenia is less likely to benefit. According to Newsom-Davis (1984) there is no clear evidence that thymectomy benefits patients with onset of myasthenia after age 40. There are reports of thymectomy in patients over 50 (Slater *et al.*, 1978) and over 60 (Evoli *et al.*, 1983; Olanow *et al.*, 1982; Monden *et al.*, 1985). These reports, from retrospective analysis of small numbers, claim that thymectomy is both beneficial and safe and should be considered in the presence of severe myasthenia if the patient is fit for surgery. They emphasize the possible adverse effects of steroids on coexisting diseases in older patients. Postoperative radiotherapy is sometimes given with locally invasive tumours.

Immunosuppression

Steroids and azathioprine are more widely used nowadays and have even been recommended for ocular myasthenia. However, ocular myasthenia is not life-threatening, pyridostigmine can usually alleviate ptosis and an eyepatch will abolish double vision. The introduction of steroids may be accompanied by transient worsening of symptoms so patients should be admitted to hospital and prednisolone introduced gradually. An alternate day, single morning dose with up to 100 mg of prednisolone is the most popular regimen (Newsom-Davis, 1984). A decline in anti-AChR antibody which correlates with the clinical response can be expected (Oosterhuis *et al.*, 1983). Dose reductions should be made slowly at no more than 5 mg per month to avoid relapse (Newsom-Davis, 1984).

Azathioprine was first used by Mertens *et al.* (1981) and a dose of 2.5 mg/kg body weight is recommended. Clinical improvement and a reduction in antibody levels occurs more slowly than with steroids, maximum benefit not appearing in under 6 months. In Mertens' report, the response to azathioprine was more favourable in older patients (greater than 35 years) and in those with thymoma or thymic hyperplasia.

Plasmapheresis

Since the first report (Pinching *et al.*, 1976) this technique has also become more widely used. It seems to induce a brief remission typically lasting 3 to 5 weeks and is mainly used to prepare patients for thymectomy, shorten a myasthenic crisis or control a sudden deterioration following the start of steroids. The technique can safely be used in older patients but care is needed to avoid fluid overload and, in this respect, continuous flow exchange is better (A. Robinson, personal communication). Patients with ischaemic heart disease or cardiac rhythm disturbances should probably be monitored during exchange.

Myasthenic Crisis

The need for assisted ventilation seems to occur most often in patients with oropharyngeal or respiratory muscle weakness. It can be provoked by respiratory infection or surgery including thymectomy, but may occur without apparent provocation. Some drugs may aggravate myasthenia. Bulk laxatives reduce the absorption of pyridostigmine and of course myasthenic patients are more sensitive to neuromuscular blocking drugs. Antiarrhythmic agents reduce muscle membrane excitability and probably inhibit neuromuscular transmission so quinine, quinidine, procainamide, lignocaine and beta blockers should be avoided. Aminoglycoside antibiotics impair neuromuscular transmission by inhibiting the release of acetylcholine so streptomycin, gentamicin, kanamycin, neomycin and polymyxin should be avoided. Central nervous system depressant drugs such as morphine must be used with caution and hypokalaemia avoided (Scadding and Havard, 1981).

Protection of the airway and ventilatory support in an intensive care unit has reduced the mortality. Anticholinesterases may be stopped once a patient is on a ventilator and other forms of therapy introduced or altered to speed recovery. Whether a patient has a cholinergic or myasthenic crisis is often debated but is irrelevant. If aspiration is likely or ventilatory failure developing, a cuffed endotracheal tube and ventilator support are needed before, not after, total collapse (Rowland, 1980). The aim is to maintain vital functions and nutrition and avoid or treat complications of immobility until the patient recovers, in a few days or weeks. Intensive care unit staff who are used to dealing with unconscious patients may need to be reminded that their myasthenic patient, while unable to move, is completely alert. Anticholinergics need not be reintroduced until the patient is breathing without assistance.

Clinicians are faced with a choice of five types of therapy. In the elderly the place of thymectomy is controversial; although recommended for patients with tumours, the myasthenia is less likely to benefit. These tumours do not usually metastasize, and rarely spread locally and as Rowland (1980) has observed the reason for thymectomy when a tumour is present is the hope of improvement in the myasthenia.

For all elderly patients, anticholinesterases can be prescribed and in those with a good stable result nothing more need be recommended. In a crisis or with continued life-threatening or disabling generalized symptoms, plasmapheresis with immunosuppression using alternate day steroids and azathioprine can be used and thymectomy reserved for patients with tumours who are fit for surgery, or patients who fail to respond to all other measures.

REFERENCES

Multiple Sclerosis

Abbott, R.J., Howe, J.G., Currie, S., and Holland, I. (1982). Multiple sclerosis plaque mimicking tumour on computed tomography. *Br. Med. J.*, **285**, 1616–17.

Acheson, E.D. (1985). The epidemiology of multiple sclerosis, the pattern of the disease. In: Matthews, W.B., Acheson, E.D., Batchelor, J.R., and Weller, R.D., (eds.) *McAlpine's Multiple Sclerosis*, Churchill Livingstone, Edinburgh, pp. 3–26.

Arnason, B.G.W. (1983). Immunology of multiple sclerosis. *Clin. Immunol. Update*, **4**, 235–59.

Barnes, M.P., Bates, D., Cartlidge, N.E., French, J.M., and Shaw, D.A. (1985). Hyperbaric oxygen and multiple sclerosis: short term results of a placebo controlled double blind trial. *Lancet*, **1**, 297–300.

Cala, L.A., Mastaglia, F.L., and Black, J.L. (1978). Computerised tomography of brain and optic nerve in multiple sclerosis. *J. Neurol. Sci.*, **36**, 411–20.

Castaigne, P., Lhermitte, F., Escourolle, R., Hauw, J.J., Gray F., and Lyon-Caen, O. (1981). Les scléroses en plaqués asymptomatiques. *Rev. Neurol.*, **137**, 729–39.

Celesia, G.C., and Daley, R.F. (1977). Effects of ageing on visual evoked responses. *Arch. Neurol.*, **34**, 403–7.

Clifford, D.B., and Trotter, J.L. (1984). Pain in multiple sclerosis. *Arch. Neurol.*, **41**, 1270–2.

Confayreux, C., Aimard, G., and Devic, M. (1980). Multiple sclerosis in Rochester, Minnesota: a 60 year appraisal of course and prognosis assessed by the computerised data processing of 349 patients. *Brain*, **103**, 281–300.

Davis, F.A. (1984). The hot bath test. In: Poser, C.M., Paty, D.W., McDonald, W.I., Ebers, G.C., and Scheinberg, L. (eds.) *The Diagnosis of Multiple Sclerosis*, Thieme-Stratton, New York, pp. 44–8.

Dimitrijevic, M.R., and Sherwood, A.M. (1980). Spasticity: medical and surgical treatment. *Neurology*, **30**, 19–27.

Dworkin, R.H., Bates, D., Millar, J.H., and Paty, D.W. (1984). Linoleic acid and multiple sclerosis: a re-analysis of 3 double blind trials. *Neurology*, **34**, 1441–5.

Ebers, G.C., and Paty, D.W. (1980). CSF electrophoresis in 1000 patients. *Can. J. Neurol. Sci.*, **7**, 275–80.

Ebers, G.C., Vinuela, F.V., Feasby, T.E., and Bass, B.H. (1984). Multi-focal CT enhancement in multiple sclerosis. *Neurology*, **34**, 341–6.

Ellison, G.W., Visscher, B.R., Graves, M.C., and Fahey, J.L. (1984). Multiple sclerosis. *Ann. Intern. Med.*, **101**, 514–26.

Feasby, T.E., Paty, D.W., Ebers, G.C., and Fox, A.J. (1981). Spinal cord swelling in multiple sclerosis. *Can. J. Neurol. Sci.*, **8**, 151–3.

Fischer, B.H., Marks, M., and Reich, T. (1983). Hyperbaric oxygen treatment of multiple sclerosis: a randomised placebo controlled double blind study. *N. Engl. J. Med.*, 181–6.

Gebarski, S.S., Gabrielsen, T.O., and Gilman, S. (1985). The initial diagnosis of multiple sclerosis: clinical impact of magnetic resonance imaging. *Ann. Neurol.*, **17**, 469–74.

Gilbert, J., and Sadler, M. (1983). Unsuspected multiple sclerosis. *Arch. Neurol.*, **40**, 533–6.

Herndon, R.M., and Rudick, R.A. (Editorial). (1983). Multiple sclerosis: the spectrum of severity. *Arch. Neurol.*, **40**, 531–2.

Hershey, L.A., and Trotter, J.L. (1980). The use and abuse of the cerebro-spinal fluid IgG profile in the adult: a practical evaluation. *Ann. Neurol.*, **8**, 426–34.

Hughes, R.A.C. (1983). Immunological treatment of multiple sclerosis. *J. Neurol.*, **230**, 73–80.

Jacobs, L., O'Malley, J., Freeman, A., Murawski, J., and Ekes, R. (1982). Intrathecal interferon in multiple sclerosis. *Arch. Neurol.*, **39**, 609–15.

Jacobs, L., O'Malley, J., Freeman, A., Murawski, J., and Ekes, R. (1985). Intrathecal interferon in the treatment of multiple sclerosis. Patient follow up. *Arch. Neurol.*, **42**, 841–7.

Jakobsen, B.E., Pedersen, E., and Gruynderup, V. (1973). Bladder neck resection in multiple sclerosis. *Urologica Internationalis*, **28**, 109–20.

Kanchandani, R., and Howe, J.G. (1982). Lhermitte's sign in multiple sclerosis: a clinical survey and review of the literature. *J. Neurol. Neurosurg. Psychiatry*, **45**, 308–12.

Katzman, R., and Terry, R. (1983). In: Katzman, R., and Terry, R. (eds.) *The Neurology of Ageing*, F.A. Davis, Philadelphia, pp. 32–4.

Kurtzke, J.F. (1983) The epidemiology of multiple sclerosis. In: Hallpike, J.F., Adams, C.W.M., and Tourtelotte, W.W. (eds.) *Multiple Sclerosis. Pathology, Diagnosis and Management*, Chapman and Hall, London, pp. 47–95.

Lapides, J., Diokno, A.C., Lowes, B.G., and Alish, M.D. (1974). Follow up on unsterile intermittent self-catheterisation. *J. Urol.*, **111**, 184–7.

Lebow, S., Anderson, D.C., Mastry, A., and Larson, D. (1978). Acute multiple sclerosis with contrast enhancing plaques. *Arch. Neurol.*, **35**, 435–9.

McAlpine, D. (1964). The benign form of multiple sclerosis: results of a long term study. *Br. Med. J.*, **ii**, 1029–32.

McDonald, W.I., and Halliday, A.M. (1977). Diagnosis and classification of multiple sclerosis. *Br. Med. Bull.*, **33**, 4–8.

McIvor, G.P., Rikland, M., and Resnikoff, M. (1984). Depression in multiple sclerosis as a function of length and severity of illness, age, remissions and perceived social support. *J. Clin. Psychol.*, **40**, 1028–33.

McKay, R.P., and Hirano, A. (1967). Forms of benign multiple sclerosis. *Arch. Neurol.*, **17**, 588–600.

Makinodan, T., and Kay, M.M.B. (1980). Age influence on the immune system. *Adv. Immunol.*, **29**, 287–330.

Mandelstam, D. (1986). *Incontinence and its Management*, 2nd edn, Croom-Helm, Kent.

Matthews, W.B. (1984). The treatment of multiple sclerosis. In: Matthews, W.B., and Glaser, G.H. (eds.) *Recent Advances in Clinical Neurology*, No. 4. Churchill Livingstone, Edinburgh, pp. 179–98.

Mayou, R., and Hawton, K. (1986). Psychiatric disorder in the General Hospital. *Br. J. Psychiat.*, **149**, 172–90.

Millar, J.H.D., Vas, C.J., Noronha, M.J., Liversedge, L.A., and Rawson, M.D. (1967). Long term treatment of multiple sclerosis with corticotrophin. *Lancet*, **ii**, 429–31.

Milward, S. (1984). Practical help in multiple sclerosis. *Br. Med. J.*, **289**, 1441–2.

Noseworthy, J., Paty, D., Wonnacott, T., Feasby, T., and Ebers, G. (1983). Multiple sclerosis after age 50. *Neurology (Cleveland)*, **33**, 1537–44.

Parsons, L. (1983). The Bladder in Multiple Sclerosis. In: Hallpike, J.F., Adams, C.W.M., and Tourtelotte, W.W. (eds.) *Multiple Sclerosis—Pathology, Diagnosis and Management*, Chapman and Hall, London, pp 597–602.

Paty, D.W., and Poser, C.M. (1984). Clinical symptoms and signs of multiple sclerosis. In: Poser, C.M., Paty, D.W., McDonald, W.I., Ebers, G.C., and Scheinberg, L. (eds.) *The Diagnosis of Multiple Sclerosis*, Thieme-Stratton, New York, pp. 27–43.

Peyser, J.M., Edwards, K.R., Poser, C.W., and Filskov, S.B. (1980). Cognitive function in patients with MS. *Arch. Neurol.*, **37**, 577–9.

Poser, C.M. (1984). The diagnostic process in multiple sclerosis. In: Poser, C.M., Paty, D.W., McDonald, W.I., Ebers, G.C. and Scheinberg, L. (eds.) *The Diagnosis of Multiple Sclerosis*, Thieme-Stratton, New York, pp. 3–13.

Poser, C.M., Paty, D.W., Scheinberg, L., McDonald, W.I., Davis, F.A., Ebers, G.C., Johnson, K.P., Sibley, W.A., Silberberg, D.H., and Tourtelotte, W.W. (1983). New diagnostic criteria for multiple sclerosis: guidelines for research protocols. *Ann. Neurol.*, **13**, 227–31.

Rabins, P.V., Brooks, B.R., O'Donnell, P., Pearlson, G.D., Moberg, P., Jubelt, B., Coyle, P., Dalos, N., and Folstein, M.F. (1986). Structural brain correlates of emotional disorder in multiple sclerosis. *Brain*, **109**, 585–97.

Rodin, G., and Voshart, K. (1986). Depression in the medically ill: An overview. *Am. J. Psychiatry*, **143**, 696–705.

Rose, A.S., Kuyma, J.W., and Kurtzke, J.F. (1970). Co-operative study in the evaluation of therapy in multiple sclerosis: ACTH versus placebo. Final report. *Neurology (Minneapolis)*, **20** (Suppl.), 1–59.

Rose, A.S., Ellison, G.W., Myers, L.W., and Tourtelotte, W.W. (1976). Criteria for the clinical diagnosis of multiple sclerosis, *Neurology (Minneapolis)*, **26**(2), 20–2.

Rudick, R.A., Schiffer, R.B., Schwetz, K.M., and Herndon, R.M. (1986). Multiple sclerosis. The problem of incorrect diagnosis. *Arch. Neurol.*, **43**, 578–83.

Russell, T.R., Brotman, M., and Forbes, N. (1984). Percutaneous gastrostomy, a new simplified and cost-effective technique. *Am. J. Surg.*, **148**, 132–5.

Sagar, H.J., Warlow, C.P., Sheldon, P.W., and Esiri, M.M. (1982). Multiple sclerosis with clinical and radiological features of cerebral tumour. *J. Neurol. Neurosurg. Psychiatry*, **45**, 802–8.

Samra, K., Walts, J.M., Riklan, M., Koslow, M., and Cooper, I.S. (1970). Relief of intention tremor by thalamic surgery. *J. Neurol. Neurosurg. Psychiatry*, **33**, 7–15.

Schiffer, R.B., and Babigian, H.M. (1984). Behavioural disorders in multiple sclerosis, temporal lobe epilepsy and amyotrophic lateral sclerosis: An epidemiological study. *Arch. Neurol.*, **41**, 1067–9.

Schiffer, R.B., Herndon, R.M., and Rudick, R.A. (1985). Treatment of pathological laughing and weeping with amitriptyline. *N. Engl. J. Med.*, **312**, 1480–2.

Schumacher, G.A., Beebe, G., Kibler, R.F., Kurland, L., Kurtzke, J.F., McDowell, F., Nagler, B., Sibley, W.A., Tourtelotte, W.W., and Willman, T.L. (1965). Problems of experimental trials of therapy in multiple sclerosis: report by the panel on the evaluation of experimental trials of therapy in multiple sclerosis. *Ann. N.Y. Acad. Sci.*, **122**, 552–68.

Sears, E.S., McCammon, A., Bigelow, R., and Heymann, L.A. (1982). Maximising the harvest of contrast enhancing lesions in multiple sclerosis. *Neurology (N.Y.)*, **32**, 815–20.

Shepherd, D.I., and Downie, A.W. (1978). Prevalence of MS in North-East Scotland. *Br. Med. J.*, **ii**, 314–16.

Snyder, B.D., Lakutua, D.J., and Doe, R.P. (1981). ACTH induced cortisol production in multiple sclerosis. *Ann. Neurol.*, **10**, 388–9.

Tourtelotte, W.W. (1983). Comprehensive management of multiple sclerosis. In: Hallpike, J.F., Adams, C.W.M., and Tourtelotte, W.W. (eds.) *Multiple Sclerosis—Pathology, Diagnosis and Treatment*, Chapman and Hall, London, pp. 513–78.

Weiner, H.L., and Hauser, S.L. (1982). Neuro-immunology: immuno regulation in neurological disease. *Ann. Neurol*, **11**, 437–49.

Whitlock, F.A., and Siskind, M.M. (1980). Depression as a major symptom of multiple sclerosis. *J. Neurol. Neurosurg. Psychiatry*, **43**, 861–5.

Williams, E.S., and McKeran, R.O. (1986). Prevalence of multiple sclerosis in a South London borough. *Br. Med. J.*, **293**, 237–9.

Young, I.R., and Delwaide, B.J. (1981). Drug therapy. Spasticity. *N. Engl. J. Med.*, **304**, 28–33 and 96–9.

Young, I.R., Hall, A.S., and Pallis, C.A. (1981). Nuclear magnetic resonance imaging of the brain in multiple sclerosis. *Lancet*, **ii**, 1063–6.

Myasthenia Gravis

Bever, C.T., Abdias, V.A., Penn, A.S., Lovelace, R.E., and Rowland, L.P. (1983). Prognosis of ocular myasthenia. *Ann. Neurol.*, **14**, 516–19.

Bucknall, R.C., Dixon, A. StJ., Glick, E.N., Woodland, J., and Zutushi, D.W. (1975). Myasthenia gravis associated with penicillamine treatment for rheumatoid arthritis. *Br. Med. J.*, **i**, 600–2.

Chang, C.C., Cheng, T.E., and Chuang, S.T. (1973). Influence of chronic neostigmine treatment on the number of acetylcholine receptors and the release of acetylcholine from the rat diaphragm. *J. Physiol. (Lond).*, **230**, 613–18.

Compston, D.A.S., Vincent, A., Newsom-Davis, J., and Bachelor, J.R. (1980). Clinical, pathological, HLA antigen and immunological evidence for disease heterogeneity in myasthenia gravis. *Brain*, **103**, 570–601.

Drachman, D.B., Angus, C.W., Adams, R.N., Michelson, J.D., and Hoffman, G.J. (1978). Myasthenic antibodies cross-link AChR to accelerate degradation. *N. Engl. J. Med.*, **298**, 1116–22.

Engel, A. (1980). Morphologic and immunopathologic findings in myasthenia gravis and in congenital myasthenic syndromes. *J. Neurol. Neurosurg. Psychiat.*, **43**, 577–89.

Engel, A.G., Lambert, E.H., and Santa, T. (1973). Study of long term anticholinesterase therapy. *Neurol. (N.Y.).*, **23**, 1273–81.

Evoli, A., Tonali, P., Scoppetta, C., and David, P. (1983). Myasthenia gravis in the elderly: report of 37 cases. *J. Am. Geriatr. Soc.*, **31**, 352–5.

Fon, G.T., Bein, M.E., Mancuso, A.A., Keesey, J.C., Lupetin, A.R., and Wong, W.S. (1982). Computed tomography of the anterior mediastinum in myasthenia gravis. *Radiology*, **142**, 135–46.

Herishanu, Y., Abramsky, O., and Feldman, T. (1976). Myasthenia gravis in the elderly. *J. Am. Geriatr. Soc.*, **24**, 228–31.

Johns, T.R., Crowley, W.J., Miller, J.Q., and Campa, J.F. (1971). The syndrome of myasthenia and polymyositis with comments on therapy. *Ann. N.Y. Acad. Sci.*, **183**, 64–71.

Leading Article (1986). *Lancet*, **i**, 658–60.

Mertens, H.G., Hertel, G., Reuther, P., and Ricker, K. (1981). Effect of immunosuppressive drugs (azathioprine). *Ann. N.Y. Acad. Sci.*, **377**, 691–8.

Monden, Y., Nakahara, K., Fuji, Y., Hasimoto, J., Ohno, K., Masaoka, A., and Kawashima, Y. (1985). Myasthenia gravis in elderly patients. *Ann. Thorac. Surg.*, **39**, 433–6.

Mossman, S., Vincent, A., and Newsom-Davis, J. (1986). Myasthenia gravis without acetyl-choline receptor antibody: a distinct disease entity. *Lancet*, **i**, 116–19.

Newsom-Davis, J. (1984). Myasthenia. In: Matthews,

W.B., and Glaser, G.H. (eds.) *Recent Advances in Clinical Neurology, No. 4*, Churchill Livingstone, Edinburgh, pp. 1–18.

Olanow, C.W., Lane, R.J.M., and Rose, A.D. (1982). Thymectomy in late onset myasthenia gravis. *Arch. Neurol.*, **39**, 82–3.

Oosterhuis, H.J.G.H. (1981). Observations in the natural history of myasthenia gravis and the effect of thymectomy. *Ann. N.Y. Acad. Sci.*, **377**, 678–89.

Oosterhuis, H.J.G.H., and Bethlem, J. (1973). Neurogenic muscle involvement in myasthenia gravis: a clinical and histopathological study. *J. Neurol. Neurosurg. Psychiatry*, **36**, 244–54.

Oosterhuis, H.J.G.H., Limburg, P.C., Hummel-Tappel, E., and The, T.H. (1983). Anti-acetyl-choline receptor antibodies in myasthenia gravis: clinical and serological follow up of patients. *J. Neurol. Sci.*, **58**, 371–85.

Osserman, K.E., and Genkins, G. (1966). Critical reappraisal of the use of edrophonium chloride (Tensilon) test in myasthenia gravis and significance of clinical observation. *Ann. N.Y. Acad. Sci.*, **135**, 312–26.

Ozdemir, C., and Young, R.R. (1976). The results to be expected from electrical testing in the diagnosis of myasthenia gravis. *Ann. N.Y. Acad. Sci.*, **274**, 203–22.

Penn, A.S., and Rowland, L.P. (1984). Neuromuscular junction. In: Rowland, L.P. (ed.) *Merritt's Textbook of Neurology*, seventh edition, Lea and Febiger, Philadelphia, pp. 561–7.

Pinching, A.J., Peters, D.K., and Newsom-Davis, J. (1976). Remission of myasthenia gravis following plasma exchange. *Lancet*, **ii**, 1373–6.

Robb, S.A., Vincent, A., McGregor, M.A., McGregor, A.N., and Newsom-Davis, J.M. (1985). Acetyl-choline receptor antibodies in the elderly and in Down's syndrome. *J. Neuroimmunol.*, **9**, 139–46.

Rowland, L.P. (1980). Controversies about the treatment of myasthenia gravis. *J. Neurol. Neurosurg. Psychiatry*, **43**, 644–59.

Sahashi, K., Engel, A.G., Lambert, E.H., and Howard, F.M. (1980). Ultra-structural localisation of the terminal and lytic 9th component of complement at the motor end plate in myasthenia gravis. *J. Neuropathol. Exp. Neurol.*, **39**, 160–72.

Sanders, D.B., Howard, J.F., and Johns, T.R. (1979). Single fibre electromyography in myasthenia gravis. *Neurology*, **29**, 68–76.

Santa, S., Engel, A.G., and Lambert, E.H. (1972). Histometric study of neuromuscular junction ultrastructure. 1. Myasthenia gravis. *Neurology*, **22**, 71–82.

Scadding, G.K., and Havard, C.W.H. (1981). Pathogenesis and treatment of myasthenia gravis. *Br. Med. J.*, **283**, 1008–12.

Simpson, J.A. (1958). An evaluation of thymectomy in myasthenia gravis. *Brain*, **81**, 112–14.

Simpson, J.A. (1960). Myasthenia gravis: a new hypothesis. *Scot. Med. J.*, **5**, 419–36.

Simpson, J.A. (1966). Applied electrophysiology in nerve and muscle disease. Disorders of neuromuscular transmission. *Proc. Roy. Soc. Med.*, **59**, 993–8.

Slater, G., Papatestas, A.E., Genkins, G., Kornfeld, P., and Horowitz, S.A. (1978). Thymectomy in patients more than 40 years of age with myasthenia gravis. *Surg. Gynecol. Obstet.*, **146**, 54–6.

Stalberg, E., Trontelj, J.V., and Schwartz, M.S. (1976). Single muscle fibre recording of the jitter phenomenon in patients with myasthenia gravis and in members of their families. *Ann. N.Y. Acad. Sci.*, **274**, 189–202.

Vellodi, C., and Tallis, R.C. (1988). An unusual case of myasthenia gravis in an elderly patient with severe muscular atrophy. *Gerontology*, **34**, 209–11.

Vincent, A., and Newsom-Davis, J. (1985). Acetyl-choline receptor antibody as a diagnostic test for myasthenia gravis: results in 153 validated cases and 1967 diagnostic assays. *J. Neurol. Neurosurg. Psychiatry*, **48**, 1246–52.

The Clinical Neurology of Old Age
Edited by R. Tallis
© 1989 John Wiley & Sons Ltd

Chapter 26

Drug-induced Neurological Disease

Cameron Swift

Professor of Health Care of the Elderly, King's College School of Medicine and Dentistry, London, UK

INTRODUCTION

The Central Nervous System as an Age-modified Target Organ

Drugs may act on the brain in a manner which is specific (i.e. related to a defined molecular interaction with a given receptor system) or non-specific (i.e. related to several molecular mechanisms). Specificity may decrease at higher doses and may also depend on other factors, such as: permeation of the diffusional barrier between blood and brain; regional distribution within the brain; the numbers and integrity of receptor sites; the binding affinity of a drug for the receptors; and the structural and functional integrity of the target organ itself (Bloom, 1985). It will be apparent that the intensity of drug effects on the brain (also governed by these factors), the range of actions of a particular drug, and the relationship of beneficial to adverse drug effects may all theoretically be altered by structural and functional changes in the brain occurring with advancing age.

The macroscopic and microscopic histological changes in cerebral morphology which occur with ageing are described in detail elsewhere in this text. These include atrophic gyral changes and decline in brain volume with preferential loss of white matter and, at a microscopic level, the well-known features of neurofibrillary tangles, argyrophilic plaques, lipofuscin deposition (especially in medulla and hippocampus) granulovacuolar degeneration (also a

hippocampal finding) and altered dendritic morphology. These changes show marked interindividual variation.

Changes in neurotransmitter function with age are non-uniform, with variation from one neurotransmitter to another, and between different regions of the brain. Problems of post-mortem study are similar to those encountered in studies of morphology. They include the effects on neurotransmitter levels of drugs administered prior to death and of processes occurring at or after death. Consequently synthetic or degradative enzymes are commonly measured rather than the neurotransmitters per se, which tend to be more unstable.

Assay of such enzymes appears to be little affected by a post-mortem interval of up to several hours (McGeer, 1978). Information on cholinergic transmission has been obtained from the extensive study of the marker enzyme, choline acetyltransferase (CAT) which has arisen from the possible involvement of this system in memory processes and dementia (Davies and Maloney, 1976; Perry et al., 1977; Spillane et al., 1977). The effect of normal ageing may be a reduction of CAT activity in some but not all areas of the cortex and limbic system (Bowen et al., 1979; Rossor et al., 1981; McGeer, 1978). Cell loss from the nucleus basalis of Meynert, where the cell bodies of the cortical cholinergic nerve terminals lie, is substantial in Alzheimer's disease, but not in normal ageing (Whitehouse et al., 1983).

By contrast, catecholaminergic cells appear particularly susceptible to age changes. Considerable decline in the activities of the synthetic enzymes tyrosine hydroxylase and DOPA decarboxylase is found in some regions of brain, although most of this occurs in early adult life (McGeer, 1978). The decline is paralleled by loss of dopaminergic neurones in the substantia nigra (McGeer *et al.*, 1977). Noradrenergic synthetic activity also declines in keeping with the reported loss of neurones from the locus coeruleus (Vijayashanker and Brody, 1979) and in addition the activity of the catecholamine degradative enzyme, monoamine oxidase, increases, especially in the globus pallidus, hippocampus and substantia nigra (Gottfries *et al.*, 1975).

There are regional differences in the changes described for levels of 5-hydroxytryptamine (5-HT), e.g. an increase in the brain stem, but a decrease in the hippocampus. The synthetic enzyme for gamma-aminobutyric acid (GABA), glutamic acid decarboxylase, declines with age, particularly in earlier life. Reliable information on neuropeptides and neurohumoral transmission in old age awaits further study.

For recent reviews of this topic see also Selko and Kosik (1984), Wilcock (1985).

Pharmacokinetic Considerations

While changes occurring in the ageing brain itself may be an important source of altered drug effects with increasing age, changes in drug handling by the body (pharmacokinetics) may result in increased concentrations of drug reaching the target organ. There have been many recent extensive reviews of this topic (Crooks *et al.*, 1976; Vestal, 1978; Greenblatt *et al.*, 1982; Swift and Triggs, 1987).

Increased bioavailability (amount of administered dose reaching the systemic circulation) may occur for some orally administered drugs which are extensively extracted by the liver on passage through the portal circulation (first pass effect), since this effect declines with age (e.g. propranolol; see Castleden and George, 1979). The bioavailability of levodopa is increased in the elderly, probably as a result of reduced dopa decarboxylase activity in the gastric wall (Evans *et al.*, 1981). Changes in body composition with age, notably the increased ratio of

fat to lean body mass and body water, result in altered distribution of some drugs to the tissues leading to an increase or decrease in plasma concentrations and to changes in elimination half-life after single dosage. Reduced protein binding due to the decline in plasma albumin levels with age (Woodford-Williams *et al.*, 1964) may lead to increased concentrations of free (unbound) drug, which is the pharmacologically active portion, reaching the target organ. Many centrally acting drugs are highly lipophilic. Their elimination from the body involves metabolism in the liver, commonly via oxidative pathways, such as demethylation and hydroxylation, to more polar, water soluble compounds capable of renal or biliary excretion. Such metabolites may themselves be pharmacologically active and require further metabolic breakdown to inactive substances prior to elimination. Clearance of oxidatively metabolized drugs, including a group of the benzodiazepines and their metabolites and many tricyclic and related antidepressants, is slower in the elderly, resulting in the potential for accumulation of higher steady-state concentrations on repeated dosage.

Such pharmacokinetic factors have undoubtedly contributed, along with changes in the structure, function and responsiveness of the target organ to the epidemiology of drug-induced neurological disease in the elderly. Much of this disease has been attributable to dose-related factors, although the overall high level of prescribing contributes in addition.

Epidemiology

Investigation of the epidemiology of adverse drug reactions (ADR) in the elderly has been largely confined to hospital based studies. The general increase in susceptibility to ADR with advancing age was initially demonstrated by Seidl *et al.* (1966), and Hurwitz (1969). More specifically in relation to the CNS, a study of 236 patients admitted to a psychogeriatric service documented adverse reactions to psychotropic drugs in 27 (16%) and inferred that such effects probably contribute to over 20% of admissions in this category (Learoyd, 1972). Three studies from the Boston Collaborative Drug Surveil-

TABLE 26.1   CONTRIBUTION OF CENTRAL NERVOUS SYSTEM AND CARDIOVASCULAR (CVS) DRUGS TO ADVERSE DRUG REACTIONS (ADR) IN THE ELDERLY

	Total recipients	Number (%) with reported ADR	Hospitalization attributed to drug	
			Sole or contributory cause	Sole cause
All drugs	1625	248 (15.3%)	—	—
CNS (Main groups)	1017	103 (10.1%)	90 (8.1%)	36 (3.2%)
Antidepressants	473	57 (12.1%)	48 (10.1%)	11 (2.3%)
Hypnotics/sedatives	444	33 (7.4%)	31 (7.0%)	18 (4.1%)
Ridigity/tremor control	100	13 (13.0%)	11 (11.0%)	7 (7.0%)
CVS (Main groups)	1255	120 (9.6%)	95 (7.6%)	18 (1.4%)
Diuretics	747	60 (8.4%)	42 (5.6%)	4 (0.5%)
Digitalis	407	46 (11.5%)	39 (9.7%)	9 (2.2%)
Hypotensives	107	14 (13.12%)	14 (13.1%)	5 (4.7%)

Modified from data of Williamson and Chopin (1980).

lance Program demonstrated a clear dose-related increase with age in the frequency of unwanted effects (principally oversedation) from the benzodiazepine drugs (Boston Collaborative Drug Surveillance Program, 1973; Greenblatt *et al.*, 1977; Greenblatt and Allen, 1978). The contribution of centrally acting drugs to ADR in elderly hospital patients is also shown in data from a UK multicentre study (Williamson and Chopin, 1980) (see Table 26.1). Reported adverse effects were predominantly from CNS and cardiovascular preparations. In more than three out of 100 patients, the hospital admission was attributed solely to the effects of drugs acting on the brain. Anti-parkinsonian compounds were particularly singled out.

Such epidemiological evidence, though now requiring reinvestigation in the light of increased awareness of drug problems in the elderly, has drawn attention to the sensitivity of the ageing brain to CNS drugs, though a proportion of drug-induced neurological disease is due to compounds targeted at other systems. Some of the commoner drug-induced clinical neurological problems in the elderly will now be discussed with reference, where appropriate, to the general considerations outlined above.

DISTURBANCES OF CONSCIOUS LEVEL

Disturbances of conscious level are common in the medicine of old age and it is important diagnostically to consider the possibility of drugs in therapeutic use as a primary cause. The commonest problems are those of oversedation and transient loss of consciousness.

Interindividual variability in responsiveness to sedative, anxiolytic and hypnotic drugs is probably even greater in later life than in youth. However, several studies have shown that sensitivity to these preparations increases with age. The measured sedative effects of single doses of diazepam (Cook *et al.*, 1984; Swift *et al.*, 1985a), nitrazepam (Castleden *et al.*, 1977), temazepam (Swift *et al.*, 1981), loprazolam (Swift *et al.*, 1985b) and chlormethiazole (Hockings *et al.*, 1982) have been shown to be accentuated with age in controlled studies comparing groups of young and elderly subjects. Corresponding plasma concentrations showed no significant differences between the groups; thus a pharmacodynamic mechanism appears most probable.

The specificity of action of the benzodiazepines is known to be high at therapeutic concentrations, through the identification of receptors localized within a supramolecular complex in the subsynaptic fraction of GABA-ergic neurones within the brain (Braestrup and Squires, 1977; Möhler and Okada, 1977). Increased numbers and/or binding affinity of benzodiazepine receptors with age might offer theoretical, if rather unlikely, explanations for the accentuated response; but preliminary studies in animals have shown no change in either measurement, suggesting that changes in post-receptor mechanisms are involved. This view is supported by the findings of a similar change in responsiveness to chlormethiazole (Hockings *et al.*, 1982) which has less specificity of action, possibly involving direct effects on chloride channel permeability.

Drowsiness, stupor and even deep daytime sleep may occur in elderly patients, especially the very old and those of slight build, if standard adult doses of benzodiazepines are administered. This is particularly likely on initial dosage. Slow-clearance oxidatively metabolized benzodiazepines (e.g. diazepam, desalkylflurazepam) are more slowly eliminated by the elderly so that increased accumulation is likely and presents an additional risk of oversedation on repeated administration. This will not occur with chlormethiazole, which is rapidly metabolized, or with the more rapidly cleared benzodiazepines, such as temazepam and triazolam, but care is still required with dosage if unwanted sedation is to be avoided.

Oversedation occurs readily in the elderly with sedative antidepressants such as amitriptyline, mianserin and trazodone. Central histamine receptors

mediate at least some of the sedative effect, though there is no clear evidence for pharmacodynamic accentuation of this response with age. The serious practical significance of such oversedation for an elderly person should not be underestimated. A pharmacokinetic explanation (reduced plasma clearance with prolongation of action and accumulation) is probable in most cases.

The risks of oversedation with antipsychotic drugs are self-evident, well recognized and higher in the elderly, though the mechanisms are less clear. Other compounds requiring caution include the antihistamines, anticonvulsants, antiemetics and centrally acting antihypertensive and analgesic drugs. It should also be remembered that alcohol gives rise to summation of sedative effect with any of these compounds. The key to avoiding such unwanted effects is in recognition of the increased risk, avoidance of unnecessary prescription, care in the choice of compound, invariable use of reduced initial dosage, and careful surveillance during treatment.

Drugs which influence metabolism, thermoregulation or endocrine function are also potential precipitants of metabolic stupor or coma but will not be considered in this context.

Transient loss of consciousness due to failure of maintenance of cerebral blood flow may be caused by drugs which directly affect cardiac rhythm and output but is commonly caused by drugs influencing blood pressure control via mechanisms within the central nervous system or in the autonomic nervous system. Morphine-induced orthostatic hypotension, for example, is due to reduction in baroreceptor sensitivity (Petty and Reid, 1982) which is centrally mediated (Zelis *et al.*, 1974). Reduction in the apparent volume of distribution of morphine with age (Owen *et al.*, 1983) leading to increased plasma concentrations after single dosage may increase the likelihood of this effect in elderly recipients. Impaired baroreceptor function is a well-known example of impaired homeostatic reserve in the elderly and numerous drugs which directly affect this mechanism via blockade of alpha receptors (e.g. the phenothiazines, tricyclic antidepressants and several vasodilators) or place it under 'stress' via other mechanisms including venodilatation and reduction in plasma volume (e.g. diuretics) are frequent and well-known causes of syncope amongst older patients.

DISTURBANCE OF HIGHER MENTAL FUNCTION

The classification of drug-induced organic brain syndromes (OBS) presents similar difficulties to those encountered with specific disease entities. Except for certain compounds, such as ethanol, detailed description of the cerebral dysfunction produced by drugs is generally lacking. Clinicians tend to think in general of delirium (one of the commonest disorders) or more loosely of 'confusional states' but most, if not all, of the syndromes defined in the Diagnostic and Statistical Manual of Mental Disorder (DSM III; American Psychiatric Association, 1980) may be caused by drugs, usually with some overlap of diagnostic presentation (Table 26.2).

Drug-induced OBS may result from:

1. Interference with CNS neurotransmitters or their associated receptors.
2. Non-specific CNS stimulation or depression.
3. Indirect effects via reduced cerebral perfusion or oxygenation, or via metabolic disturbance.
4. Direct reversible or irreversible brain cell toxicity.
5. Withdrawal mechanisms.

TABLE 26.2 DIAGNOSTIC AND STATISTICAL MANUAL OF MENTAL DISORDER (DSM III) CLASSIFICATION OF ORGANIC BRAIN SYNDROMES (OBS)

Relatively global cognitive impairment
Delirium
Dementia

Relatively selective cognitive impairment
Amnestic syndrome
Organic hallucinosis

Predominantly non-cognitive features
Organic delusional syndrome
Organic affective syndrome
Organic personality syndrome

As with disturbances of conscious level (which may often be a contributory factor) susceptibility may be increased in the elderly by pharmacokinetic and pharmacodynamic changes, by the underlying structural and physiological changes of cerebral ageing and by concurrent disease processes. Discussion will be confined to drugs recognized as common precipitants of OBS in the elderly in 'therapeutic' dosage.

Drugs Predominantly Affecting Neurotransmission or Specific Receptor Function

Effects on monoamines or their receptors

The CNS effects of the catecholamines (e.g. adrenaline, noradrenaline, dopamine) tend to be slight because these compounds do not readily cross the blood–brain barrier. However, the indirectly acting sympathomimetic drugs, notably the amphetamines, methylphenidate and, to a lesser extent, ephedrine, readily permeate the central nervous system, where most of the central stimulatory actions are considered to be due to the release of catecholamines from nerve terminals. This is particularly true of the psychic and behavioural effects. The latter are to some extent dose-related but hyperexcitability, mental confusion or the complete syndrome of delirium may readily be precipitated in susceptible individuals, particularly the elderly. Noradrenergic, serotonergic and dopaminergic aspects of neurotransmission may all be involved.

Similarly, the selective beta$_2$ agonists, terbutaline and salbutamol, used in the treatment of obstructive airways disease may be more prone to cause CNS effects than the catecholamine, isoprenaline. These compounds may produce hyperexcitable states in the elderly associated with mental confusion and often accompanied by pronounced coarse tremor. These phenomena are usually an indication of excessive dosage beyond the requirement for effective relief of airways obstruction.

Mental and behavioural disturbances are well recognized as a central side-effect of the treatment of parkinsonism with levodopa. Such effects are directly attributed to increased dopaminergic activity and are at least as common with the combined preparations (containing levodopa and extracerebral decarboxylase inhibitor) as with levodopa alone. They are also reported with compounds considered to have dopaminergic agonist activity, such as amantadine. As well as cognitive impairment, hallucinations, paranoia, manic states, insomnia, anxiety, nightmares and emotional depression occur. These effects are more common in patients with coexisting parkinsonism and dementia. Differentiation from the mental disturbances of the underlying disease process may be difficult unless an adequate pretreatment assessment has been undertaken. The prevalence of dementia in Parkinson's disease has been variably estimated between 8–10% and 60% in studies using various diagnostic criteria (e.g. Pollock and Hornabrook, 1966; Markham *et al.*, 1974; Loranger *et al.*, 1972). Paradoxically, improvement in both mood and mental performance is often a feature of satisfactory treatment with levodopa. The central side-effects have been said to be more common in elderly patients (Yahr, 1975); most reports, however, emerged when levodopa was given in high initial dosage and it is likely that these effects are dose-related. As mentioned above, the gastric activity of the synthetic enzyme dopa-decarboxylase is reduced in the elderly thus leading to a marked increase in the bioavailability of the drug (Evans *et al.*, 1981). Low initial dosage is therefore mandatory in elderly parkinsonian patients. The need for caution is even greater in those who have pretreatment evidence of mental impairment, since the therapeutic response is often less satisfactory and the likelihood of central side-effects much increased. A much publicized occurrence of hypomanic states (a component of which may be inappropriate or excessive sexual behaviour) is extremely rare.

The centrally acting antihypertensive agent clonidine is generally considered to produce its hypotensive effect by stimulation of pre- and post-synaptic alpha$_2$ receptors in the CNS. Similarly, methyldopa is also thought to act as an indirect alpha$_2$ agonist. Both drugs may cause sedation and impairment of mental functions, as well as mood disturbances including insomnia, nightmares, depression and anxiety. The action of reserpine in depleting many organs, particularly the brain, of catecholamines and 5-hydroxytryptamine, with the risk of severe depressive illness, is now legendary; the drug is contraindicated for the treatment of hypertension in the elderly.

A number of beta adrenergic blocking agents, particularly those of high lipophilicity, penetrate the blood–brain barrier in significant amounts. Reported CNS effects include lassitude, sleep disturbance, hallucinations and depression (Greenblatt and Shader, 1972). The specific relationship of these symptoms to beta blockade is doubtful, however; they may reflect an adverse 'placebo' response or the effects of blood pressure control on cerebral perfusion, rather than blockade of central beta receptors.

Anticholinergic effects

Although the role of the noradrenergic system in cognitive function continues to be debated, the existence of a cholinergic link in the transition from short-term (or primary) to long-term (secondary) memory has been clearly established (for reviews see Crow *et al.*, 1982). Significant effects on learning tasks of the anticholinergic compounds, hyoscine and atropine, have been demonstrated in experimental studies (Crow *et al.*, 1976). In clinical practice, therefore, compounds with anticholinergic actions have been readily implicated in drug-induced organic brain syndromes, including delirium.

Anticholinergic agents used in the treatment of parkinsonism, such as orphenadrine and benzhexol, have in the past been a frequent cause of disabling drug-induced confusion in older patients, but the incidence is probably declining along with the use of these agents.

Anticholinergic mechanisms probably play a major part in confusional states induced by both tricyclic antidepressants and phenothiazines. The problems tend to be pronounced during the early stages of treatment with both types of drug and, as already indicated, are likely to have a pharmacokinetic basis. Most of the tricyclic drugs are metabolized via oxidative routes, such as demethylation and hydroxylation, so that the potential for accumulation of toxic concentrations of some tricyclics is increased in the elderly because of reduced metabolic clearance. It is now standard practice to give smaller doses of these drugs and to monitor carefully for such side-effects or, alternatively, to use 'second generation' compounds with less anticholinergic activity. The pharmacokinetics of the phenothiazines have been less carefully studied, but similar mechanisms probably apply.

Effects on other neurotransmitter systems

Antihistamines (H_1 receptor antagonists) are well known to cause CNS depression, with diminished alertness, prolonged reaction times and drowsiness. A direct effect on CNS H_1 receptors seems the likeliest mechanism, since there is high specific receptor binding of these drugs. The degree of CNS depression varies between drugs in the class and some compounds are less specific, also exhibiting anticholinergic effects.

The H_2 receptor antagonist, cimetidine, has been linked to case reports of CNS disturbances particularly affecting the elderly. These include drowsiness, impaired orientation and cognitive function, agitated states, hallucinations and even epilepsy. The mechanism of the effects is unclear. Compared with the extensive use of the drug they are comparatively rare occurrences and appear even more so with the alternative compound, ranitidine, which exhibits less penetration of the blood–brain barrier.

The benzodiazepine compounds, although acting on specific receptors, have a mode of action closely linked to GABA transmission in the CNS. GABA is an inhibitory neurotransmitter. Other hypnotics with less specific modes of action, such as the barbiturates, also produce some of their sedative effect through enhancement of GABA-ergic transmission. In general, confusional states caused by these compounds are secondary to their sedative and anxiolytic effects. Under certain circumstances, however, paradoxical states of excitement, agitation, sleep disturbance and nightmares occur in some individuals, particularly with the barbiturates and with benzodiazepines containing a nitro group (e.g. nitrazepam).

Drugs Acting Via Non-specific Mechanisms

The acute effects of alcohol administration result from depression of inhibitory control mechanisms. Mental processes dependent on training and previous experience are impaired initially, followed by coordination, memory, concentration and insight. There is some evidence for inhibition of neuronal reuptake of catecholamines (Eisenhofer *et al.*, 1983).

Elderly patients with respiratory disease are probably more likely to develop central nervous side-effects from methylxanthine compounds (theophylline, aminophylline), than their younger counterparts. The metabolic clearance of theophylline is reduced in old age, leading to the potential for accumulation of toxic concentrations of the drug (Antal *et al.*, 1981).

In general, the methylxanthines exert their effects through inhibition of the cyclic nucleotide, phosphodiesterase, and by inhibition of adenosine receptors. The precise mode of action in the CNS is not clear but the respiratory stimulation induced by theophylline can be accentuated by dopaminergic antagonists. The toxic effects of theophylline on the CNS are related to dose and plasma concentration, so that caution with dosage and monitoring of plasma theophylline concentrations (preferably free concentrations) may be desirable in some elderly recipients. Some preliminary evidence suggests that central nervous sensitivity to the effects of methylxanthines may be enhanced in the elderly (Swift and Tiplady, 1988).

Unwanted CNS effects via non-specific mechanisms may occur with several cardiovascular drugs if given to elderly individuals in too high a dosage. The Class 1 antiarrhythmic compound, quinidine, may cause cinchonism (tinnitus, deafness and blurred vision), but full scale delirium may occur at more toxic levels. Mental disturbances are a well-recognized component of digitalis toxicity in the elderly. Lignocaine often causes sedation or agitation, disorientation or dissociated feelings, particularly in elderly subjects.

The unwanted CNS effects of anticonvulsant compounds are substantially dose-related and can be prevented by appropriate therapeutic monitoring.

The combination of sedation, mental confusion and cerebellar dysfunction is characteristic of both phenytoin and carbamazepine toxicity. In general these effects are less commonly seen with sodium valproate.

Drugs Affecting Cerebral Function via Metabolic and Other Indirect Mechanisms

The possibility that restlessness, aggression or delirium may be due to hypoglycaemia induced by one or other of the oral antidiabetic preparations should always be borne in mind where a patient is known or suspected to be receiving these compounds. The pharmacokinetics of both the sulphonylureas and biguanides are poorly documented in the elderly but the likelihood is that the renal clearance of metformin and the metabolites of chlorpropamide, along with the metabolism of most of the sulphonylureas, is to some extent impaired in the elderly. The effects of corticosteroid compounds on the CNS are poorly understood. Mental changes may be in part due to the effects of steroids on blood volume, glucose, and electrolyte homeostasis, but there are probably also direct CNS effects as well. Steroid-induced cerebral dysfunction may include mood changes (euphoria, depression or psychosis), sleep disturbance, restlessness or agitation. Many of these are reversible if the steroids are appropriately withdrawn.

Mental disturbances have also been reported in patients receiving diuretics, probably resulting from the effects of these compounds on electrolyte transport.

Organic Brain Syndrome due to Direct CNS Toxicity

Ethyl alcohol is the main example in this category. The literature on the aetiology of presenile dementia implicates alcohol in some 7% of patients (Marsden and Harrison, 1972; Freeman, 1976). In older patients its contribution to the epidemiology of dementia will naturally be proportionately smaller, but remains significant.

Evaluation of the mental disorders of alcoholism has changed somewhat in recent years. They are now probably divisible into four main categories, some or all of which may coexist.

1. Acute Korsakoff's syndrome associated with Wernicke's encephalopathy. The Korsakoff defect is a specific disorder of both recent and short-term memory function, coupled with loss of drive and apathy. This is somewhat different from the global picture of dementia. It is well known traditionally to occur in the context of Wernicke's encephalopathy, which includes mental confusion, ophthalmoplegia, nystagmus and ataxia, specifically linked to deficiency of vitamin B_1 in nutritionally deprived alcoholics (Victor *et al.*, 1971).

2. Korsakoff's syndrome of gradual onset without vitamin B_1 deficiency. This specific disorder has been defined by Cutting (1978). Its existence implies a direct toxic effect of ethyl alcohol on the central nervous system and is associated with cortical atrophy demonstrable both at post-mortem and on computed tomography (CT) (Lishman *et al.*, 1980).

3. 'Alcoholic dementia'. Here there is a more global deterioration in cognitive function than exhibited by patients with Korsakoff's syndrome.

4. Mental disturbance due to deficiency states and complications of alcoholism. This group of disorders will include the encephalopathy of hepatocellular failure, other vitamin deficiencies and the consequences of alcoholic cardiomyopathy.

Differentiation of these effects of alcoholism is important, since some may be amenable to improvement or treatment. For a fuller review see Alexander and Geschwind (1984).

Withdrawal Effects of Drugs

Drug withdrawal syndromes in elderly patients are most commonly encountered in long-term users of alcohol, benzodiazepines and non-benzodiazepine hypnotics, such as barbiturates, meprobamate, methaqualone, glutethimide, and chloral hydrate. Of these the alcohol withdrawal syndrome is the most fully described. For assessment purposes, four stages or categories of disturbance are defined, (1) predelirium tremens, (2) withdrawal seizures, (3) hallucinosis, and (4) delirium tremens.

1. Predelirium tremens. This is characterized by gastrointestinal symptoms (anorexia and nausea) sweating, hyporeflexia, pyrexia, hypertension and a state of anxious depressed restlessness with sleep disturbance. The severity of the reaction varies with both the extent and duration of preceding alcohol exposure (Sellers and Kalant, 1982). Symptoms usually appear within a few hours after withdrawal and abate within 48 hours.

2. Withdrawal seizures. Such grand-mal fits may be isolated, multiple or even status epilepticus and probably represent one of the more severe manifestations of alcohol withdrawal. They are commonly a part of the full picture of delirium tremens.

3. Hallucinosis. Hallucinations may occur in the absence of disorientation or tremor but are more commonly associated with other manifestations.

4. Delirium tremens. The diagnosis depends on the combined presence of tremor, disorientation and hallucinations. It is commonly the culmination of a progressive syndrome encompassing the symptoms described above and reaching its peak some 72 hours after withdrawal. In practice there is much overlap between the timing and occurrence of the symptom patterns. Delirium tremens carries a significant mortality. For this reason careful clinical observation and monitoring during the period of withdrawal are essential. The overall description has changed little since the account of Victor and Adams (1953). As with the effects of withdrawal from other general CNS depressants, the precise mechanisms involved are not clear. A high index of suspicion of this disorder should always be maintained with elderly patients who develop acute organic brain syndromes, since the prevalence of alcohol abuse in the elderly is quite significant (Wattis, 1981).

Withdrawal symptoms occurring with prescribed central sedative medication follow a fairly standard pattern common to most of the drugs involved,

including the benzodiazepines. These include rebound increases in rapid eye movement (REM) sleep, paroxysmal EEG abnormalities, rebound insomnia and/or anxiety. With greater severity there is tremulousness and weakness, progressing to tonic/clonic fits and delirium (Jaffe, 1985). With barbiturates, the severity of symptoms, in particular the likelihood of withdrawal convulsions, increases in proportion to the scale of previous regular dosage. The clinical presentation is very similar for meprobamate, glutethimide and methaqualone. Withdrawal from tricyclic antidepressants may cause peripheral cholinergic hyperactivity, insomnia, extrapyramidal symptoms and acute psychiatric disturbances, including delirium or acute psychoses (*Drug and Therapeutics Bulletin*, 1986).

The subject of withdrawal from benzodiazepines has generated considerable debate. There have been no specific studies in the elderly. There is, however, reasonable circumstantial evidence that a form of dependence occurs in long-term users of benzodiazepine hypnotics (Swift *et al.*, 1984). Severe withdrawal effects are probably uncommon except in those who have taken large doses for long periods and particularly those with a previous history of dependence on other drugs or alcohol. Milder forms of benzodiazepine withdrawal have probably been quite common in the elderly, presenting with agitated anxiety, insomnia and sometimes agitated confusion. The effects may be delayed and less severe with slowly eliminated compounds, whereas with intermediate or rapid clearance benzodiazepines (e.g. temazepam, triazolam) the onset may be more abrupt and pronounced (Kales *et al.*, 1979). Both dependence and withdrawal may possibly be more marked with benzodiazepines of high receptor binding affinity (and potency) such as lorazepam.

DISTURBANCES OF MOVEMENT AND BALANCE

Postural Instability and Falls

Maintenance of the upright position depends on local anticipatory reflexes, proprioceptive, visual and vestibular input, and central processing of information from these sources. Postural stability has commonly been quantified by measurement of body sway using a variety of methods. Sway increases with advancing age (Sheldon, 1963; Overstall et al., 1977), and elderly patients presenting with non-accidental falls have been found to exhibit greater sway than their normal healthy counterparts.

Postural sway has also been found to be a relatively sensitive indicator of drug-induced sedation (Swift, 1984). The effect on sway of a sedative dose of a benzodiazepine hypnotic, such as temazepam or diazepam (Swift and Stevenson, 1983; Swift et al., 1985a) is accentuated in the elderly, probably as a result of pharmacodynamic mechanisms. The finding is not specific to the benzodiazepines. It might be anticipated, therefore, that elderly patients receiving hypnotic drugs are prone to postural instability. One study reported a clear association between nocturnal femoral fracture and the use of night-time barbiturate sedation (MacDonald and MacDonald, 1977), but this finding has not been substantiated. A further study showed that a higher proportion of elderly people who fell had taken tranquillizers (but not hypnotics) compared with non-fallers (Prudham and Evans, 1981). Overstall et al. (1977), however, failed to demonstrate a relationship between increased postural sway and hypnotic use, and Swift et al. (1984) showed no increase in postural sway in elderly long-term users of flurazepam and nitrazepam. It is likely that postural instability due to sedative/hypnotic drugs occurs on acute dosage or during the first few days of therapy before pharmacodynamic 'tolerance' has begun to develop. The causes of falls due to transient loss of consciousness are dealt with above (see 'Disturbances of Conscious Level').

Cerebellar Ataxia

A reversible cerebellar syndrome is a well-recognized feature of acute toxicity with barbiturate and hydantoin anticonvulsant compounds. Associations have also been found between a chronic, irreversible cerebellar syndrome and long-standing anticonvulsant therapy (Munoz-Garcia et al., 1982). However, difficulty is experienced in establishing a causal relationship to drugs, rather than to effects of recurrent seizures.

Cerebellar ataxia is, of course, a well-recognized syndrome of Wernicke's encephalopathy in alcoholism. Thiamine deficiency is an important component of this syndrome and folate deficiency may play a part in anticonvulsant-induced cerebellar syndromes.

Tremor, Parkinsonism and Related Movement Disorder

Several drugs may cause simple tremor in the elderly, notably central stimulant drugs, adrenoceptor agonists, such as isoprenaline, salbutamol and ephedrine, methylxanthines (e.g. theophylline), lithium and tricyclic antidepressants. A mild, reversible tremor which develops gradually and is to some extent dose-related, occurs with sodium valproate therapy (Davidson 1983).

The complete parkinsonian syndrome (bradykinesia, rigidity and tremor of variable anatomic situation) is one of a range of movement disorders which may be caused by drugs which block central dopamine (D_2) receptors. The drugs most commonly implicated are the antipsychotic agents, namely, the phenothiazines, thioxanthenes and other heterocyclic compounds, such as haloperidol, timozide, molindone, loxapine and clozapine. Metoclopramide, though possessing only weak antipsychotic activity and not, therefore, classified as an antipsychotic, also blocks D_2 receptors and may exhibit similar side-effects.

Drug-induced parkinsonism is probably under-diagnosed (Murdoch and Williamson, 1982). It is important to realize that the clinical features may persist for many months after discontinuing the causative agent. Hence, failure to obtain a careful enough drug history may result in an erroneous diagnosis of idiopathic Parkinson's disease. Drug-induced parkinsonism may to some extent, however, act as a precipitant of the idiopathic form if there is already an existing trend to cerebral dopamine depletion (Rajput et al., 1982; Goetz and Klawans, 1983).

A study of 3775 subjects receiving antipsychotic drugs identified parkinsonism as a complication in 15% (Ayd, 1961). Female gender and older age were both found to be predisposing factors. Other workers have suggested that susceptibility to drug-induced parkinsonism may have a familial basis (Myrianthopoulos *et al.*, 1962, 1969). Drug-induced parkinsonism persisting for more than 2 years after discontinuing the D_2 receptor blocker is generally accepted as indicating the presence of idiopathic Parkinson's disease.

In the treatment of drug-induced parkinsonism the use of anticholinergic compounds is traditional on the grounds that levodopa is rendered ineffective by competition from the dopamine receptor blocker for receptor sites and that it exacerbates the underlying psychotic disorder (Yaryura-Tobias *et al.*, 1970). This assumption is now questioned. Anticholinergic compounds often produce an unsatisfactory response particularly in the elderly, for whom both the central and peripheral anticholinergic side-effects are poorly tolerated. Furthermore, the receptor blockade may be overcome by large doses of levodopa.

Other reversible neurological side-effects of D_2 receptor blocking drugs include acute dystonia, acute akathisia and the neuroleptic malignant syndrome.

The acute dystonic reaction is an early complication of treatment with D_2 receptor blocking drugs, occurring between 1 and 5 days after initiating therapy. There is spasm of the muscles of the face, jaw, tongue and neck leading to sustained grimacing and torticollis. The trunk and limbs may be involved producing bizarre postures and torsion spasms of the limbs. Sustained ocular deviation resembling oculogyric crises may occur. The syndrome may be mistaken for hysteria. It is a well-recognized side-effect of treatment with metoclopramide, as well as with the antipsychotic preparations.

Withdrawal of the causative drug is followed by rapid resolution within a few hours but the condition is often distressing and there is occasionally risk of upper airways obstruction. Immediate administration of parenteral diphenhydramine, anticholinergic preparations, intravenous diazepam or possibly methylphenidate almost invariably produces relief and can be diagnostic of the disorder; this suggests that central anticholinergic activity plays a part in the mechanism of the syndrome, although it has never been fully explained. Most antipsychotic compounds have both anticholinergic and antidopaminergic activity and it has been suggested that an imbalance between the two actions during the elimination phase of plasma concentrations after

administration may be responsible (Garver *et al.* 1976). Predisposing factors to drug-induced acute dystonia include younger age and male gender (Ayd, 1961). Metoclopramide is a particularly common causative agent (Kris *et al.*, 1983).

Akathisia is a syndrome of motor restlessness which is quite distinct from anxiety or agitation. The patient feels jittery and has a compulsion to move about, often rising from a chair and pacing about, crossing and uncrossing legs, rocking the body, fidgeting, or marking time. Recognition of the diagnosis is important, since akathisia may be profoundly distressing and an increase in antipsychotic dosage may otherwise be erroneously recommended. The condition is the commonest motor complication of antipsychotic medication, usually occurring between 4 or 5 days to 8 weeks after the initiation of therapy. There are no particular predisposing factors, including age. Management may include a reduction in dosage, and/or the use of anticholinergic compounds, benzodiazepines or non-selective beta blockers (e.g. propranolol in low dosage, 20–60 mg daily). For a recent review, see Szabadi (1986).

The neuroleptic malignant syndrome (NMS) is a rare idiosyncratic reaction to antipsychotic drugs characterized by autonomic disturbance (pyrexia, dyspnoea, swings of heart rate and blood pressure), muscular spasm or dystonia, and agitation, confusion or catatonia. The condition carries a significant mortality rate and may occur at any time during antipsychotic therapy. Laboratory findings are consistent with idiosyncratic systemic illness, including elevation of white cell count, creatine kinase and hepatic enzymes. The body temperature may rise as high as 42 °C. Treatment is directed at reducing the body temperature by supportive means together with the combination of dantrolene (60 mg intravenously, 8 hourly) and bromocriptine (up to 60 mg orally daily) (Granato *et al.*, 1983).

Of the late onset or delayed (tardive) neurological complications of treatment with D_2 receptor blocking drugs, the most important and troublesome is the syndrome of *tardive dyskinesia*. The term is specific to this category of drug. The involuntary movements produced are rapid, brief and chorea-like, but differ from chorea in their repetitive (stereotypical) nature. Tardive dystonia and tardive akathisia are variants of the disorder which sometimes coexist with it. Tardive dyskinesia is characteristically persistent; resolution may occur after several months or it may become permanently established if untreated. Very occasionally the onset may be earlier during treatment.

The face and mouth are particularly affected, leading to repetitive sucking, chewing or lip-smacking movements and protrusion of the tongue (fly catching). The movements may be voluntarily suppressed, and disappear during sleep. The repetition pattern is a most important distinguishing feature particularly in relation to the oral dyskinesia of Huntington's chorea. Limb involvement typically consists of repetitive movements of the extremities, such as 'piano playing' or lateral and tapping movements of the feet. Rocking movements of the trunk may occur. The patient is most likely to be aware of, and to complain of, these symptoms when they are accompanied by akathisia.

Older age is an undoubted predisposing factor to tardive dyskinesia and the likelihood of spontaneous remission also declines with age (Smith and Baldessarini, 1980; Kane et al., 1983). Other risk factors include female gender (Smith et al., 1978), interruption of drug therapy (Jeste et al., 1979) and possibly pre-existing cerebral damage or long-standing psychotic disease process.

Post-mortem studies have failed to define consistent pathological changes, as have studies in animals exposed to high doses of D_2 receptor blocking drugs. Attempts have been made to define the underlying mechanisms in terms of neurotransmission, but studies of dopamine metabolites in CSF have also produced inconsistent findings.

The most widely held hypothesis is that longstanding dopamine receptor blockade leads to a compensatory increase in the numbers or sensitivity of postsynaptic dopamine receptors in the corpus striatum. This hypothesis, however, fails to explain the necessity for prolonged treatment, the persistence or permanence of the condition, or the increased susceptibility of the elderly. Tardive dyskinesia is improved by increasing the dose of the antipsychotic drug or of metoclopramide, but the improvement is only temporary. Withdrawal of the drug exacerbates the condition and is sometimes the

mechanism whereby mild reversible variants (withdrawal emergent dyskinesias) are revealed.

No satisfactory drug treatment for tardive dyskinesia has so far emerged in spite of trials with a wide variety of agents, including antidopaminergic, dopaminergic, cholinergic, GABA-ergic and various other miscellaneous compounds. The prevalence of the condition has caused wide concern and emphasized the importance of a preventative approach. The rules of thumb are basically as follows:

1. Avoid inappropriate or non-essential use of antipsychotic drugs, for example, in the management of anxiety, aggressive behaviour or insomnia.
2. Avoid long-term use of metoclopramide.
3. When dopamine receptor-blocking agents are essential, use low doses for the shortest possible time, especially in the elderly.
4. Monitor closely for signs of tardive dyskinesia and lower the dose of antipsychotic drug if and when symptoms first appear.
5. Avoid routine prescription of anticholinergic compounds to 'prevent' drug-induced parkinsonism, since they may mask tardive dyskinesia.

The reader is referred to recent more extensive reviews of this topic (Fahn, 1984; *Drug and Therapeutics Bulletin*, 1986). The differential diagnosis includes the various forms of chorea, dystonia, myoclonus, tics and tremor.

DRUG-INDUCED NEUROPATHY AND MYOPATHY

The effects of age on the structure, integrity and function of peripheral nerves and of muscles are described elsewhere in this volume. These agerelated changes may cause some difficulty in the clinical diagnosis of drug-induced syndromes and electrophysiological techniques are often important in reaching a conclusion and deciding whether particular drugs should be continued or discontinued.

Drugs in many categories are known to be causally related to peripheral neuropathy or myopathy but the epidemiology is poorly documented. It is difficult to say with certainty whether or not age is a predisposing factor. The relationship to drug treatment may not be suspected and subclinical forms of both neuropathy and myopathy may be commoner than is generally recognized.

The subject of *drug-induced neuropathy* has been reviewed by Argov and Mastaglia (1979). The pathogenesis is commonly an axonal degeneration, though segmental demyelination may occur with certain drugs such as perhexiline. Mechanisms involved include direct neurotubule toxicity, production of B vitamin deficiencies, interference with lipid metabolism and ischaemic damage due to arthritis or vasospasm. Pharmacogenetic and pharmacokinetic factors may increase predisposition so that for some drugs the elderly may be more at risk.

Antimicrobial Agents

Mixed sensory and motor neuropathy may be caused by several antituberculous agents (isoniazid, ethambutol, streptomycin), by nitrofurantoin and by metronidazole. Isoniazid neuropathy may be prevented by supplementation with vitamin B_6. Nitrofurantoin neuropathy may be related to dose and the rate of renal elimination. Other causative agents include chloramphenicol (sensory), colistin and nalidixic acid.

Cytotoxic Drugs

Vincristine is the best known example, with peripheral neuropathy and painful proximal myopathy developing in a high proportion of long-term recipients. The autonomic system may be involved, with the development of postural hypotension and constipation.

Cardiovascular Drugs

The anti-anginal agent perhexiline causes neuropathy of varying severity depending on dosage. Cranial nerve involvement is well recognized. As mentioned above, the mechanism appears to be segmental demyelination. Neuropathies have also been recognized with hydralazine, amiodarone, disopyramide and propranolol.

Centrally Acting Compounds

There have been reports of neuropathic symptoms in patients treated with the hypnotic methaqualone and the antidepressants, imipramine and amitriptyline. Phenytoin is the only anticonvulsant known to cause peripheral nerve damage, the clinical presentation (when present) being predominantly sensory.

Antirheumatic Drugs

Gold therapy is a well-recognized cause of a rather acute polyneuropathy, which may involve the facial nerves and mimic acute ascending polyneuritis. There are reports of mixed neuropathies caused by indomethacin, chloroquine, phenylbutazone and penicillamine.

TABLE 26.3   DRUG-INDUCED MYOPATHIES

Myopathic disorder	Causative agent
Focal myopathy	Intramuscular injections
Fibrotic contractures	Pethidine Antibiotics Chlorpromazine Paraldehyde } intramuscularly
Acute or subacute painful proximal myopathy	Vincristine Other cytotoxics Drugs lowering serum potassium[a] Metolazone Cimetidine Lithium Alcohol
Subacute or chronic painless proximal myopathy	Corticosteroids (especially fluorinated) Drugs lowering serum potassium[a] Alcohol
Myasthenic syndrome	Aminoglycosides Tetracyclines Succinylcholine D-Penicillamine Beta-blockers Phenytoin Chlorpromazine } precipitate pre-existing myasthenia gravis Procainamide Colchicine

[a] Creatine kinase levels elevated.
Modified from the classification of Lane and Mastaglia (1978).

Other Drugs

Sulphonylurea oral hypoglycaemic agents (tolbutamide, chlorpropamide), ergotamine, lithium and cimetidine are all agents which may give rise to neuropathy in the elderly.

The *drug-induced myopathies* in man have been reviewed, classified and tabulated by Lane and Mastaglia (1978). Several agents, in particular alcohol, may cause different categories of myopathy simultaneously and there may also be associated neuropathy. Electromyographic assessment may yield the definitive diagnosis and with some disorders elevated creatine kinase levels may be helpful, though this finding lacks specificity. Table 26.3 shows some of the main disorders relevant to the elderly. The commonest is probably chronic painless proximal myopathy due to corticosteroid therapy. This is particularly prone to occur with the fluorinated steroids, triamcinolone, betamethasone and dexamethasone. The diagnosis is important, since the condition can sometimes be reversed by substituting prednisolone. Rarer disorders include the potentially fatal severe necrotizing myopathy (acute rhabdomyolysis) which may develop with alcohol abuse, and the occurrence of myotonia either in association with other drug-induced neuropathy or myopathy or through precipitation of an existing myotonic disorder (suxamethonium, beta blockers).

REFERENCES

Alexander, M.P., and Geschwind, N. (1984). Dementia in the elderly. In: Albert M.L. (ed.) *Clinical Neurology of Aging*, Oxford University Press, New York, pp. 254–76.

Antal, E.J., Kramer, P.A., Mercik, S.A., Chapron, D.J., and Lawson, I.R. (1981). Theophylline pharmacokinetics in advanced age. *Br. J. Clin. Pharmacol.*, **12**, 637–45.

Argov, Z., and Mastaglia, F.L. (1979). Drug-induced peripheral neuropathies. *Br. Med. J.*, **i**, 663–6.

Ayd, F.J. (1961). A survey of drug-induced extrapyramidal reactions. *J.A.M.A.*, **175**, 1054–60.

Bloom, F.E. (1985). Neurohumoral transmission and the central nervous system. In: Gilman, A.G., Goodman, L.S., Rall, T.W., and Murad, F. (eds) *Goodman and Gilman's The Pharmacological Basis of Therapeutics*, seventh edition, Macmillan, New York, pp. 236–59.

Boston Collaborative Drug Surveillance Program (1973). Clinical depression of the CNS due to diazepam and chlordiazepoxide in relation to cigarette smoking and age. *N. Engl. J. Med.*, **288**, 277–80.

Bowen, D.M., White, P., Spillane, J.A., Goodhardt, M.J., Curzon, G., Iwangoff, P., Meier-Ruge, W., and Davison, A.N. (1979). Accelerated ageing of selected neuronal loss as an important cause of dementia. *Lancet*, **i**, 11–14.

Braestrup, C., and Squires, R.F. (1977). Brain specific benzodiazepine receptors in rats characterized by high affinity 3H-diazepam binding. *Proc. Natl Acad. Sci. USA*, **74**, 3805–9.

Castleden, C.M., and George, C.F. (1979). The effect of ageing on the hepatic clearance of propranolol. *Br. J. Clin. Pharmacol.*, **7**, 49–54.

Castelden, C.M., George, C.F., Marcer, D., and Hallet, C. (1977). Increased sensitivity to nitrazepam in old age. *Br. Med. J.*, **1**, 10–12.

Cook, P.J., Flanagan, R., and James, I.M. (1984). Diazepam tolerance: effect of age, regular sedation and alcohol. *Br. Med. J.*, **289**, 351–3.

Crooks, J., O'Malley, K., and Stevenson, I.H. (1976). Pharmacokinetics in the elderly. *Clin. Pharmacokinet*, **1**, 280–96.

Crow, T.J., Grove-White, I.G., and Ross, D.G. (1976). The specificity of the action of hyoscine on human learning. *Br. J. Clin. Pharmacol.*, **2**, 367–8P.

Crow, T.J., Cross, A.J., Grove-White, I.G., and Ross, D.G. (1982). Central neurotransmitters, memory and dementia. In: Wheatley, D. (ed.) *Psychopharmacology of Old Age*, Oxford University Press, Oxford.

Cutting, J. (1978). The relationship between Korsakoff's syndrome and "alcoholic dementia". *Br. J. Psychiatry*, **132**, 240–51.

Davidson, D.L.W. (1983). A review of the side-effects of sodium valproate. *Br. J. Clin. Practice*, Symposium supplement, **27**, 79–85.

Davies, P., and Maloney, A.J. (1976). Selective loss of central cholinergic neurones in Alzheimer's disease. *Lancet*, **ii**, 1403.

Drug and Therapeutics Bulletin (1986). **24**, 27–28.

Eisenhofer, G., Lambie, D.G., and Johnson, R.H. (1983). Effects of ethanol on plasma catecholamines and norepinephrine clearance. *Clin. Pharmacol. Ther.*, **34**, 143–7.

Evans, M.A., Broe, G.A., Triggs, E.J., Cheung, M., Creasey, H., and Paull, P.D. (1981). Gastric emptying rate and the systemic availability of levodopa in the elderly parkinsonian patient. *Neurology (N.Y.)*, **31**, 1288–94.

Fahn, S. (1984). The tardive dyskinesias. In: Matthews, W.B., and Glaser, H. (eds) *Recent Advances in Clinical Neurology*, Churchill Livingstone, London, pp. 229–60.

Freeman, F.R. (1976). Evaluation of patients with progressive intellectual deterioration. *Arch. Neurol.*, **33**, 658–9.

Garver, D.L., Davis, J.M., Dekermejian, H., Erickson, S., Gosenfeld, L., and Haraszti, J. (1976). Dystonic reactions following neuroleptics: time course and proposed mechanisms. *Psychopharmacology*, **47**, 199–210.

Goetz, C.G., and Klawans, H.L. (1982). Controversies in animal models of tardive dyskinesia. In: Marsden, C.D., and Fahn, S. (eds.) *Movement Disorders*, Butterworth Scientific, London, pp. 263–76.

Gottfries, C.G., Orland, L., Wiberg, A., and Winblad, B. (1975). Lowered monoamine oxidase activity in brains from alcoholic suicides. *J. Neurochem.*, **25**, 667–73.

Granato, J.E., Stern, B.J., Ringel, A., Karim, A.H., Krumholz, A., Coyle, J., and Adler, S. (1983). Neuroleptic malignant syndrome; successful treatment with dantrolene and bromocriptine. *Ann. Neurol.*, **14**, 89–90.

Greenblatt, D.J., and Allen, M.D. (1978). Toxicity of nitrazepam in the elderly: a report from the Boston Collaborative Drug Surveillance Program. *Br. J. Clin. Pharmacol.*, **5**, 407–13.

Greenblatt, D.J., Allen, M.D., and Shader, R.I. (1977). Toxicity of high-dose flurazepam in the elderly. *Clin. Pharmacol. Ther.*, **21**, 355–61.

Greenblatt, D.J., Sellers, E.M., and Shader, R.I. (1982). Drug disposition in old age. *N. Engl. J. Med.*, **306**, 1081.

Greenblatt, D.J., and Shader, R.I. (1972). On the psychopharmacology of beta-adrenergic blockade. *Curr. Ther. Res.*, **14**, 615–25.

Hockings, N., Stevenson, I.H., and Swift, C.G. (1982). Hypnotic response in the elderly—single dose effects of chlormethiazole and dichloralphenazone. *Br. J. Clin. Pharmacol.*, **14**, 143P.

Hurwitz, N. (1969). Predisposing factors in adverse reactions to drugs. *Br. Med. J.*, **1**, 536–40.

Jaffe, J.H. (1985). Drug addiction and drug abuse. In: Gilman, A.G., Goodman, L.S., Rall, T.W., and Murad, F. (eds) *Goodman and Gilman's The Pharmacological Basis of Therapeutics*, seventh edition, Macmillan, New York, pp. 532–81.

Jeste, D.V., Potkin, S.G., Sinha, S., Feder, S., and Wyatt, R.J. (1979). Tardive dyskinesia—reversible and persistent. *Arch. Gen. Psychiatry*, **36**, 585–90.

Kales, A., Scharf, M.B., Kales, J.D., Constantin, R., and Soldatos, R. (1979). Rebound insomnia. A potential hazard following withdrawal of certain benzodiazepines. *J.A.M.A.*, **24**, 1692–5.

Kane, J.M., Woerner, M., Weinhold, K., Kinon, B., Leiberman, J., and Wagner, J. (1983). Epidemiology of tardive dyskinesia. *Clin. Neuropharmacol.*, **6**, 109–15.

Kris, M.G., Tyson, L.B., Gralla, R.J., Clark, R.A., Allen, J.C., and Reilly, L.K. (1983). Extrapyramidal reactions with high dose metoclopramide. *N. Engl. J. Med.*, **309**, 433.

Lane, R.J.M., and Mastaglia, F.L. (1978). Drug-induced myopathies in man. *Lancet*, **ii**, 562–6.

Learoyd, B.M. (1972). Psychotropic drugs and the elderly patient. *Med. J. Aust*, **1**, 1131–3.

Lishman, W.A., Ron, M.A., and Acker, W. (1980). Computed tomography and psychometric assessment of alcoholic patients. In: Richter, D. (ed.) *Addiction and Brain Damage*, Croom Helm, London, pp. 215–27.

Loranger, A.W., Goodell, H., McDowell, F.H., Lee, J.E., and Sweet, R.D. (1972). Intellectual impairment in Parkinson's syndrome. *Brain*, **95**, 405–12.

MacDonald, J.B., and MacDonald, E.T. (1977). Nocturnal femoral fracture and continuing widespread use of barbiturate hypnotics. *Br. Med. J.*, **ii**, 483–5.

McGeer, E.G. (1978). Aging and neurotransmitter metabolism in human brain. In: Katzman, R., Terry, R.D., and Bick, K.L. (eds.) *Alzheimer's Disease: Senile Dementia and Related Disorders*, Raven Press, New York, pp. 427–40.

McGeer, P.L., McGeer, E.G., and Suzuki, P.S. (1977). Aging and extrapyramidal function. *Arch. Neurol.*, **34**, 33–5.

Markham, C.H., Treciokas, L.J., and Diamond, S.G. (1974). Parkinson's disease and levodopa. *West J. Med.*, **121**, 188–206.

Marsden, C.D., and Harrison, M.J.G. (1972). Outcome of investigation of patients with pre-senile dementia. *Br. Med. J.*, **ii**, 249–52.

Möhler, H., and Okada, T. (1977). Benzodiazepines receptor: demonstration in the central nervous system. *Science*, **198**, 849–51.

Munoz-Garcia, D., Del Ser, T., Bermejo, F., Portera, A. (1982). Truncal ataxia in chronic anticonvulsant treatment. Association with drug-induced folate deficiency. *J. Neurol. Sci.*, **55**, 305–11.

Murdoch, P.S., and Williamson, J. (1982). A danger in making the diagnosis of Parkinson's disease. *Lancet*, **i**, 1212–13.

Myrianthopoulos, N.C., Kurland, A.A., and Kurland, L.T. (1962). Hereditary predisposition in drug-induced parkinsonism. *Arch. Neurol.*, **6**, 5–12.

Myrianthopoulos, N.C., Waldrop, F.N., and Vincent, B.L. (1969). A repeat study of predisposition in drug-induced parkinsonism. In: Barbeau, A., and Brunette, J.R. (eds) *Progress in Neuro-Genetics*. Excerpta Medica International Congress Series, Amsterdam No. 175, pp. 486–91.

Overstall, P.W., Exton-Smith, A.N., Imms, F.J., and Johnson, A.L. (1977). Falls in the elderly related to postural imbalance. *Br. Med. J.*, **i**, 261–4.

Owen, J.A., Sitar, D.S., Berger, L., Brownell, L., Duke, P.C., and Mitenko, P.A. (1983). Age-related morphine kinetics. *Clin. Pharmacol. Ther.*, **34**, 364–8.

Perry, E.K., Perry, R.H., Blessed, G., and Tomlinson, B.E. (1977). Necropsy evidence of central cholinergic deficits in senile dementia. *Lancet*, **i**, 189–90.

Petty, M.A., and Reid, J.L. (1982). The effect of opiates on arterial baroreceptor reflex function in the rabbit. *Naunym-Schmiedeberg's Arch. Pharmacol.*, **319**, 206–11.

Pollock, M., and Hornabrook, R.W. (1966). The prevalence, natural history and dementia of Parkinsonism. *Brain*, **89**, 429–48.

Prudham, D., and Evans, J.G. (1981). Factors associated

with falls in the elderly: a community study. *Age Ageing*, **10**, 141–6.

Rajput, A.H., Rozdilsky, B., Hornykiewicz, O., Shannak, K., Lee, T., and Seeman, P. (1982). Reversible drug-induced parkinsonism: Clinicopathologic study of two cases. *Arch. Neurol.*, **39**, 644–6.

Rossor, M.N., Iversen, L.L., Johnson, A.J., Mountjoy, C.Q., and Roth, M. (1981). Cholinergic deficit in frontal cerebral cortex in Alzheimer's disease is age dependent. *Lancet*, **ii**, 1422.

Seidl, L.G., Thornton, G.F., Smith, J.W., and Cluff, L.E. (1966). Studies on the epidemiology of adverse drug reactions. 111 Reactions in patients on a General Medical Service. *Johns Hopkins Hosp. Bull.*, **119**, 299–315.

Selko, D., and Kosik, K. (1984). Neurochemical changes with aging. In: Albert, M.L. (ed.) *Clinical Neurology of Aging*, Oxford University Press, New York, pp. 53–75.

Sellers, E.M., and Kalant, H. (1982). Alcohol withdrawal and delirium tremens. In: Pattison, E.M., and Kaufman, E. (eds.) *Encyclopedic Handbook of Alcoholism*, Gardner Press, New York, pp. 147–66.

Sheldon, J.H. (1963). The effect of age on the control of sway. *Gerontol. Clin.*, **5**, 129–38.

Smith, J.M., and Baldessarini, R.J. (1980). Changes in prevalence, severity and recovery in tardive dyskinesia with age. *Arch. Gen. Psychiatry*, **37**, 1368–73.

Smith, J.M., Oswald, W.T., Kucharski, L.T., and Waterman, L.J. (1978). Tardive dyskinesia age and sex differences in hospitalised schizophrenics. *Psychopharmacology*, **58**, 207–11.

Spillane, J.A., White, P., Goodhardt, M.J., Flack, R.H.A., Bowen, D.M., and Davison, A.N. (1977). Selective vulnerability of neurones in organic dementia. *Nature*, **266**, 558–9.

Swift, C.G. (1984). Postural instability as a measure of sedative drug response. *Br. J. Clin. Pharmacol.*, **18**, 87S.

Swift, C.G., and Stevenson, I.H. (1983). Benzodiazepines in the elderly. In: Costa, E. (ed.) *The Benzodiazepines: from Molecular Biology to Clinical Practice*, Raven Press, New York, pp. 225–36.

Swift, C.G., and Tiplady, B. (1988). Effects of caffeine on psychomotor performance in young and elderly volunteers. *Psychopharmacology* (in press).

Swift, C.G., and Triggs, E.J. (1987). Clinical pharmacokinetics. In: Swift, C.G. (ed.) *Clinical Pharmacology in the Elderly*, Marcel Dekker, New York.

Swift, C.G., Haythorne, J.M., Clarke, P., and Stevenson, I.H. (1981). The effect of ageing on measured responses to single doses of oral temazepam. *Br. J. Clin. Pharmacol.*, **11**, 413–14.

Swift, C.G., Swift, M.R., Hamley, J., Stevenson, I.H., and Crooks, J. (1984). Side effect 'tolerance' in elderly long-term recipients of benzodiazepine hypnotics. *Age Ageing*, **13**, 335–43.

Swift, C.G., Swift, M.R., Ankier, S.I., Pidgen, A., and Robinson, J. (1985b). Single dose pharmacokinetics and pharmacodynamics of oral loprazolam in the elderly. *Br. J. Clin. Pharmacol.*, **20**, 119–28.

Szabadi, E. (1986). Akathisia—or not sitting. *Br. Med. J.*, **292**, 1034–5.

Vestal, R. (1978). Drug use in the elderly: A review of problems and special considerations. *Drugs*, **16**, 358.

Victor, M., and Adams, R.D. (1953). The effect of alcohol on the nervous system. *Res. Publ. Assoc. Nerv. Ment. Dis.*, **32**, 526–73.

Victor, M., Adams, R.D., and Colling, G.H. (1971). *The Wernicke–Korsakoff Syndrome*, F.A. Davis, Philadelphia.

Vijayashanker, N., and Brody, H. (1979). A quantitative study of the pigmented neurones in the nucleus locus coeruleus and subcoeruleus as related to ageing. *J. Neuropathol. Exp. Neurol.*, **38**, 490–7.

Wattis, J.P. (1981). Alcohol problems in the elderly. *J. Am. Geriatr. Soc.*, **29**, 131–4.

Whitehouse, P.J., Parhad, I.M., Hodreen, J.C., Clark, A.W., White, C.L., Struble, R.G., and Price, D.L. (1983). Integrity of nucleus basalis of Meynert in normal ageing. *Neurology*, **33** (Suppl. 2), 159.

Wilcock, G.K. (1985). Neurochemistry of ageing and disease in the central nervous system. In: Hildick-Smith, M. (ed.) *Neurological Problems in the Elderly*, Baillière Tindall, Eastbourne, pp. 7–20.

Williamson, J., and Chopin, J.M. (1980). Adverse reactions to prescribed drugs in the elderly: A multicentre investigation. *Age Ageing*, **9**, 73.

Woodford-Williams, E., Alvarez, A.S., Webster, D., Landless, B., and Dixon, M.P. (1964). Serum protein patterns in 'normal' and pathological ageing. *Gerontologia*, **10**, 86–99.

Yahr, M.D. (1975). Levodopa. *Ann. Intern. Med.*, **83**, 677–82.

Yaryura-Tobias, J.A., Wolpert, T.A., Dana, L., and Merlis, S. (1970). Action of L-dopa in drug-induced extrapyramidalism. *Dis. Nerv. Sys.* **31**, 60–63.

Zelis, R., Mansour, E.J., Capone, R.J., and Mason, D.T. (1974). The cardiovascular effects of morphine. *J. Clin. Invest.*, **54**, 1247–58.

Chapter 27

Dementia

John Wattis

Senior Lecturer and Consultant in the Psychiatry of Old Age, St James' University Hospital, Leeds, UK

Until recently, dementia has been rather neglected, falling in the no-man's-land between neurology and psychiatry. Lately, however, the rising prevalence of dementia in old age has stimulated both the provision of specialist psychiatric services for old people (Wattis *et al.*, 1981; Wattis and Arie, 1984) and major research into the aetiology and management of dementia worldwide (World Health Organization, 1986).

Dementia has been defined in many ways. The Royal College of Physicians' definition (1982) is widely used. This describes dementia as 'The acquired global impairment of higher cortical functions, including memory, the capacity to solve the problems of day to day living, the performance of learned perceptuo-motor skills, the correct use of social skills, all aspects of language and communication and the control of emotional reactions in the absence of gross clouding of consciousness. The condition is often progressive, though not necessarily irreversible.'

There is some debate as to whether the term dementia does or should imply irreversibility. For this reason, alternatives such as chronic brain syndrome or brain failure (Livesley, 1978) have been proposed.

However we define it, the fact remains that the developed nations, especially in north-western Europe are suffering an epidemic of dementia (Leading Article, 1978). This epidemic is related to the age structure of the population and Britain has one of the most aged societies within north-western Europe which in turn leads the so-called 'ageing societies' of south and east Europe, North America, Japan, Australia and New Zealand (Grundy, 1983).

Before long, the developing countries will go through a similar experience. The British experience in this area is therefore of interest to the whole world. Table 27.1 shows the changing age structure of our society. Although the proportion of the population over 65 years old in the UK will remain steady and even decline marginally towards the end of the century, the proportion of very old people will continue to rise. Table 27.2 gives the age-specific prevalence rates for dementia of all types, showing that it is very old people who are most vulnerable to the disease. Recent studies have also shown that the natural history of dementia is changing with increased survival of those admitted to hospital with the disease (Blessed and Wilson, 1982). This is probably due to the fact that Alzheimer's disease, the commonest of the dementias of old age, pursues a more benign course in very old people (Roth, 1986).

Very old people suffer from multiple disadvantages. They are more likely to be living alone (see Table 27.3), often in substandard housing, they are more likely to be poor and they are more likely to have multiple medical problems often presenting in non-specific ways. The size of the problem is thus potentially enormous and a feeling of hopelessness in the face of this 'Rising Tide' (Dick, 1982) of dementia can lead to indifference. Already the

TABLE 27.1 OLD PEOPLE AS A PERCENTAGE OF THE POPULATION OF THE UK

	Over 65	75–84 years	85 years and over
1901	4.7	1.2	0.2
1951	11.0	3.1	0.5
1981	15.1	4.8	1.0
2001	14.3	5.0	1.5

Source: Adapted from Wells (1979).
Reproduced from Wattis and Church (1986) by permission of Croom Helm.

TABLE 27.2 AGE-SPECIFIC PREVALENCE RATES FOR DEMENTIA

Age	Percentage of 'chronic brain syndrome'
65–69	2
70–74	3
75–79	6
80+	22

Source: Kay *et al.* (1970).
Reproduced from Wattis and Church (1986) by permission of Croom Helm.

TABLE 27.3 WHERE OLD PEOPLE LIVE

With spouse in two-person household	41%
Alone	28%
In other types of household	13%
With children	12%
In residential/hospital accommodation	6%

Source: Adapted from Wells (1979).
Reproduced from Wattis and Church (1986) by permission of Croom Helm.

medical and social services in the UK are unequal to the task of providing enough good quality care of demented people and there is evidence of a fall in planned local authority provision of residential care (Grundy and Arie, 1982) together with unplanned, but largely publically funded growth in the private sector (Laing, 1985).

ETHICAL ISSUES

One of the more negative responses to the problem of dementia has been the suggestion that euthanasia should be 'offered' to old people who become demented. In another context Gillon (1986) has argued that the killing of a newborn baby with Down's syndrome might be justified on the grounds that such an infant is not fully a person. One can see how this argument, used already to justify the liberalization of the abortion laws, could be extended to those who had lost their right to be regarded as a person by becoming demented. This view that people can be deprived of their personhood has been challenged elsewhere (Wattis, 1986). It is, of course, an economically tempting solution.

Another argument that has been used in favour of euthanasia is the poor 'quality of life' of those who are severely demented. Much of this poor quality of life is, however, not the result of dementia, but of chronic under-investment in community services and institutional care. There is a tendency amongst doctors to concentrate on the personal and negative aspects of ethics ('thou shalt not kill') rather than on the social and positive aspects of our ethical duty to provide good quality assessment and management (including long-term care where necessary) for all groups in the population including mentally ill old people. It is true that some of the issues are outside the direct control of doctors, but as those most aware of the problems, we can take a lead in campaigning for a better deal for old people.

TYPES OF DEMENTIA IN OLD AGE

Much early research work on dementia was confounded by the failure to distinguish between different types of dementia despite evidence from the natural history (Roth, 1955) and pathology (Blessed *et al.*, 1968) of dementia sufferers that there were at least two main types of dementia in old age. Pathological studies (based on a group dying as psychiatric inpatients and therefore not free from bias) suggest that senile dementia of the Alzheimer type (SDAT) is responsible for 50% of dementia in old age, multi-infarct dementia (MID) accounts for about a further 20%, mixed SDAT/MID accounts for approximately another 20% and the remaining 10% is due to a variety of causes.

Epidemiological studies suggest that in some areas at least, MID is more common than SDAT (Henderson, 1986). There are several possible reasons for this: it may be that the original pathological studies were based on an atypical population; some studies may have used inadequate criteria for differential diagnosis; there may be cultural pressures in favour of diagnosing MID; or, of course, there may be a genuine difference in prevalence.

Alzheimer's Disease

This disease was first described histologically by the pathologist whose name it bears (Alzheimer, 1907). For many years it was seen as a form of 'presenile' dementia distinct from senile dementia itself. Over the years it became clear that the pathology of senile dementia was virtually identical with that of presenile Alzheimer's disease and so the term senile dementia of the Alzheimer type was coined. Pathologically, the chief findings are an atrophied brain with widened sulci and enlarged ventricles (Figure 27.1). Despite this, because of the overlaps with the normal and functionally ill populations, the distinction between SDAT and other mental disorders in old age cannot reliably be made on computed tomography (CT), though there is hope that newer scanning techniques will be more helpful (McGeer, 1986). Microscopically, the characteristic changes of SDAT are neurofibrillary tangles and large numbers of senile plaques (Figure 27.2). The plaque count has been correlated with the degree of clinical impairment before death and a threshold effect has been demonstrated in that dementia only becomes evident when a certain density of plaque formation is present (Blessed *et al.*, 1968). More recently, biochemical correlations have been established, espe-

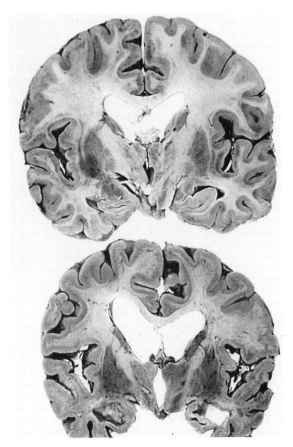

Figure 27.1. Alzheimer's disease compared with normal brain (*courtesy of Dr J. M. MacKenzie*).

cially with the cholinergic neurotransmitter system (Perry *et al.*, 1978) and more recently still, two different forms of Alzheimer's disease have been delineated pathologically and biochemically (Bondareff, 1983; Rossor *et al.*, 1984). The first of these, which occurs in older people, is clinically less aggressive and has relatively localized neuropathological changes affecting chiefly the cholinergic neurotransmitter system. The second type tends to affect younger people and is clinically more aggressive, shortening life expectancy and producing more generalized pathological changes involving several different neurotransmitter systems.

The genetics of Alzheimer's disease are still far from clear. Females seem to be affected more commonly than men, even allowing for the greater

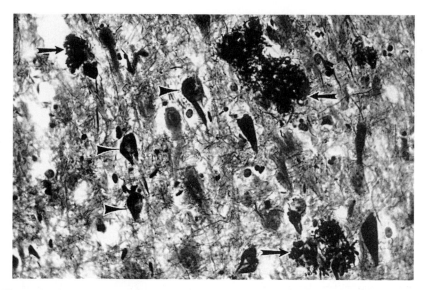

Figure 27.2. Histology of Alzheimer's disease (*courtesy of Dr J. M. MacKenzie*).
(Key: arrowheads=neurofibrillary tangles; arrows=senile plaques.)

proportion of women surviving into extreme old age. Some family pedigrees suggest an autosomal dominant inheritance with reduced penetrance, but other features of the disease, including the falling genetic risk with increasing age, are more suggestive of polygenic inheritance. In the majority of late onset cases, the risk for relatives is probably only slightly higher than for the general population. For some relatives of earlier onset cases, the risk is higher.

HLA markers have so far been found to have only a weak relationship with Alzheimer's disease (Renvoize, 1984). The genetics of Alzheimer's disease have recently been reviewed in some detail by Kay (1986).

By analogy with Creutzfeld–Jakob disease and kuru in man and with scrapie, a transmissible neurological degenerative disease of sheep, the possibility of a transmissible agent for Alzheimer's disease has been argued, but a recent review by Corsellis (1986) suggests that on present evidence, this seems unlikely. The presence of amyloid material in senile plaques has led to a theory that the disease might have an autoimmune component, but this has yet to be demonstrated. The association of aluminium with neurofibrillary degeneration in the Guam Parkinson-dementia syndrome has led to an interest in aluminium as a possible causative agent. Recently, this

theory has been supported by the finding of aluminium–silicon complexes at the heart of human senile plaques (Candy *et al.*, 1986). The possibility that these complexes are a secondary accumulation in already damaged tissues remains but the aluminium hypothesis has now been restored as a front runner in the search for aetiological agents. Alzheimer's disease, in addition to central nervous system damage, has been associated with more generalized changes such as a slowing in peripheral nervous conduction (Levy, 1975) and with generalized wasting despite apparently adequate nutritional intake (Aspland *et al.*, 1981). Although acute confusional states in old people have been related to thiamine deficiency (Older and Dickerson, 1982) and an association has been demonstrated between dementia and low serum B12 levels (Droller and Dosset, 1959), no causal association has yet been demonstrated between vitamin deficiency and Alzheimer's dementia. Kemm and Ancill (1985) have recently comprehensively reviewed the subject of vitamin deficiency in old people.

The clinical course of Alzheimer's disease is characterized by an insidious onset of memory problems. Often friends and relatives find it very difficult to give a date for the onset of memory problems, especially as they may initially be confused with normal ageing. Bergmann (1981) has discussed how neurosis in old people is slow to present because we have relatively low expectations of old people. The same probably applies to memory impairment. We are too ready to dismiss them: 'What can you expect at your age?' Certainly many cases of dementia are unknown to general practitioners (Williamson *et al.*, 1964). One way of improving the accuracy of a relative's reporting of the time course of the illness is to use time landmarks such as the previous Christmas, the last birthday or some major national event. When memory difficulties are first experienced, the sufferer, especially if there have been previous paranoid personality traits, may rationalize the problem by accusing others of stealing or hiding lost items. This may alienate relatives and helpers who perhaps do not recognize this as a sign of disease; an explanatory word from the doctor can be helpful here. Often, in a partially successful attempt to contain their disability, sufferers will develop rigid lifestyles and a resistance to change which may initially prevent them from accepting appropriate and necessary help. Again, in the early stages of the disease, those with pre-existing tendencies to depression may develop a secondary depressive illness which in itself increases disability and perceived memory impairment. Gradually memory impairment leads to an inability to organize the tasks of daily living. Disruption of visuo-spatial ability, topographical disorientation, dyspraxias, dysphasia, left–right disorientation and other signs of cortical damage emerge. In practical terms these can lead to the sufferer wandering out and being unable to find her way home, to difficulties in dressing and with communication and even to a failure to recognize husband or wife. Ability to manage household affairs will be impaired and this is especially important for those living alone. Eventually the sufferer will need assistance to maintain continence and personal hygiene and useful verbal communication will become impossible though generally some ability at non-verbal communication will be retained. As dementia progresses, so the dependence of the sufferer on her surroundings will increase and the provision of appropriate environmental support become more important. Incontinence, which develops relatively late in the disease, is often related to an inability to find the toilet without help rather than to true loss of bladder control. Early incontinence is probably due to problems such as poor mobility or local causes such as urinary infection or constipation. Alternatively, it may be a pointer to a different diagnosis, such as normal pressure hydrocephalus (Adams *et al.*, 1965) or parasagittal meningioma. At first, simple memory prostheses, such as notes left by relatives, direct or telephoned verbal prompts can be of great assistance. As time goes on and the disease progresses, regular help, especially for those living alone, is essential. This can take the form of home help, a daily warden, the provision of meals on wheels or day centre attendance to provide a structure that permits the sufferer and her family to carry on coping. Especially if the sufferer lives alone, such community services, however extensive, will eventually have to give way to 24 hour care, often in an old people's home or other institution, but sometimes in a surrogate family.

Recently, attempts have been made to produce a clinical staging for Alzheimer's disease for descriptive and research purposes, but unfortunately, not all patients with Alzheimer's disease show the same temporal relationship between the deterioration of different functions. Cole (1988) proposed that each function deteriorates in a hierarchical way, a mirror image of Piaget's developmental stages, and devised a series of hierarchical tests which enable one to build a composite picture of the patient's functions in different areas. This approach is attractive from both the research and clinical viewpoint. Numerous instruments have been developed for psychometric assessment of dementia. For a discussion of some of the different methods, their value and limitations, see Huppert and Tym (1986).

Multi-Infarct Dementia (MID)

This is clinically distinguished from SDAT by a sudden onset of confusion often with a partial recovery and sometimes associated with a stroke. The disease tends to progress in a stepwise fashion with plateaus of no deterioration punctuated by periods of sudden worsening again, often with partial recovery (Birkett, 1972). The differences between the time courses of SDAT and MID are summarized

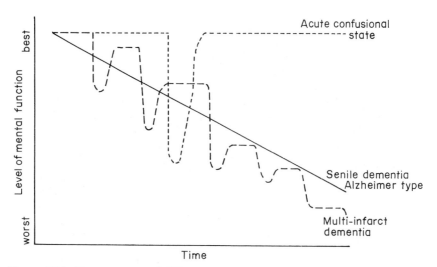

Figure 27.3. Time courses of different causes of confusion. (*Reproduced from Wattis and Church (1986, Chapter 5) by permission of Croom Helm.*)

in Figure 27.3. The dementia tends to be more patchy than in SDAT and insight is often relatively well preserved. Occasionally a stroke may produce a degree of productive aphasia so severe as to lead to the erroneous conclusion that the patient is demented. The patient's frustration at this state of affairs can then lead to aggression which can be seen as confirmation of the erroneous diagnosis. Ability to respond well to non-verbal communication and preservation of other functions as well as the history of sudden onset can help in this important differential diagnosis. Once the condition is recognized, appropriate management, including speech therapy, can often produce a major improvement in the patient. Such dysphasia can also occur in people who have other impairments sufficient to justify a diagnosis of dementia, but even in these cases, attention to such focal neuropsychological functions can be useful (Wattis and Church, 1986, Chapter 9). Depressed mood and loss of emotional control are common and can be very disabling even to those whose cognitive functions are otherwise well preserved. Loss of control over aggressive impulses can make life especially difficult for the sufferer and caregivers. Frequently there will be a history of hypertension or other signs of vascular disease including focal neurological signs or ECG changes. Hachinski and his colleagues (1975) have made these

TABLE 27.4   ISCHAEMIC SCORE

Feature	Score
Abrupt onset	2
Stepwise deterioration	1
Fluctuating course	2
Nocturnal confusion	1
Relative preservation of personality	1
Depression	1
Somatic complaints	1
Emotional incontinence	1
History of hypertension	1
History of strokes	2
Evidence of associated atherosclerosis	1
Focal neurological symptoms	2
Focal neurological signs	2

Patients scoring 7 and above may be classified as having multi-infarct dementia, and patients scoring 4 and below may be classified as having primary degenerative dementia.

Source: Hachinski *et al.* (1975).
Reproduced from Wattis and Church (1986) by permission of Croom Helm.

clinical features the basis for an 'Ischaemic score' (Table 27.4) which can help distinguish between the SDAT and MID.

This scale has now been confirmed and refined in a small scale post-mortem study by Rosen *et al.* (1980).

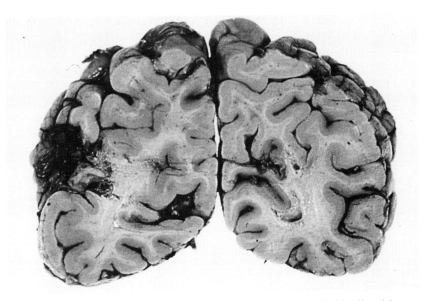

Figure 27.4. Multi-infarct dementia (*courtesy of Dr J. M. MacKenzie*).

A much larger study by the Newcastle group (Blessed *et al.*, 1968; Tomlinson *et al.*, 1970) based on Roth's operational definitions of 'senile psychosis' (SDAT) and 'arteriosclerotic psychosis' (MID) demonstrated not only the pathological differences between SDAT and MID, but also was able to show a relationship between the volume of cerebral infarction ('softening') and the clinical degree of dementia and behavioural impairment. Macroscopically, the brain of a patient may show large or small cerebral infarctions or a mixture of both (Figure 27.4). Microscopically, there is neuronal loss and gliosis. Some sufferers from MID may have changes in platelet stickiness similar to those found in some stroke victims (Szanto, 1972) and this presents a possible avenue for a therapeutic or preventative approach.

Mixed SDAT/MID

Pathologically and clinically this condition is intermediate between SDAT and MID, and the work of Blessed *et al.* (1968) suggested that there was a summation of effect between the two pathologies in producing clinically discernible damage.

Other Causes of Dementia

Though individually rare, these other causes are important because some of them are potentially reversible. Normal pressure hydrocephalus (Adams *et al.*, 1965) is a good example of such a syndrome. Clinically characterized by the triad of confusion, gait disturbance and disproportionate incontinence, this diagnosis can be confirmed by CT and direct neurosurgical pressure studies following which a shunt can be inserted if appropriate. In some patients this can produce a dramatic recovery, though doubt has recently been thrown on this (Briggs *et al.*, 1981).

The metabolic dementias (see Chapter 20) share some features in common. They tend to present with marked cognitive slowing similar to and sometimes mistaken for depressive retardation. There is a lack of cortical signs though this may be masked by the cognitive slowing and apparent lack of cooperation. When examining the patient for memory deficit, the interviewer will often feel that the patient has encoded memories but is unable to locate them, a state described by some as 'forgetfulness'. In such cases, the patient's performance can often be markedly improved by giving them more time or by providing 'cues'. This picture has been described in more detail elsewhere (Cummings and Benson, 1983) and has been called 'subcortical dementia'. The concept has been challenged by others (Whitehouse, 1986). Clinically, it does sometimes seem possible to distinguish such a syndrome and it helps for teaching purposes to think of these features as 'subcortical' although the neuroanatomical and neurophysiological bases are probably more complicated. In vitamin B12 deficiency, the prevalence of which increases with increasing age, there will often be subjective complaints of tiredness or accusations from relatives of 'laziness'. There may be factors in the history which contribute to the diagnosis such as partial gastrectomy or previous history of pernicious anaemia, the treatment for which has lapsed following a change of doctor. Sometimes the picture will be complicated by a previous history of depressive illness or the coincidental presence of this illness or SDAT. Appropriate haematological investigations will usually reveal the underlying deficiency. There is controversy about whether a B12 induced dementia can coexist with a normal blood film. Certainly, dementia, low serum B12 and normal haemoglobin and marrow can co-exist (Droller and Dossett, 1959) though the direction of causality is uncertain. While the controversy persists, it is probably worth estimating the serum B12 level in any early case of dementia which show features of the 'subcortical syndrome' even in the presence of a normal haemoglobin and blood film. Grossly abnormal B12 results present no problems of interpretation (provided, if a biological assay is used, the patient has not been on antibiotics) but marginal results may well be secondary to chronic subnutrition in a patient with a primary depressive illness or dementia. Droller and Dossett (1959) suggested that in old people, an intermediate range of B12 results might not be clinically significant.

Thyroid deficiency, as well as presenting with the 'subcortical syndrome' will usually present with some of the other features of thyroid deficiency such as coarsening of the hair, deepening of the voice or bradycardia. It may also be associated with other manifestations of autoimmune disease, including B12 deficiency. The clinical diagnosis can be confirmed by appropriate laboratory investigations. There may be difficulty in interpreting investigation results in old people where the 'normal ranges' may

be different from those found in younger people.

Folic acid deficiency has been suggested as a potential cause of dementia in old people. Serum folate levels are rapidly sensitive to dietary intake and low serum levels are a frequent coincidental finding in old people with SDAT (MacLennan, 1985). Such deficiency is not costly to correct, but it is rare to see any appreciable effect on the patient's mental state.

Alcohol is a potent cause of acute and chronic confusion in old people. The myth that alcohol abuse is a self-limiting disease, rarely seen in old age (Drew, 1968) has now been exposed (Rosin and Glatt, 1971) and some epidemiological evidence suggests that whereas the prevalence of alcoholism for men does peak in the fifth decade, for women, rates, though much lower, continue rising into the 70s (Edwards *et al.*, 1973). The risk for alcoholic dementia rises with increasing age and it may well be that the role of alcohol in the genesis of dementia in old age has been underestimated. Alcohol abuse is closely related to cultural patterns of drinking and it may be that an increase in the prevalence of alcoholic dementia will be seen in Britain and other countries as drinking habits change under the pressures of modern marketing. Chronic alcohol abuse appears to damage the brain in at least two ways. First, there is a cerebral shrinkage which appears to be a direct neurotoxic effect of alcohol and which is at least partly reversible in many cases provided there is total abstention from alcohol (Lishman, 1981). Secondly, there may be the effects of malnutrition. Some cases diagnosed as Korsakoff's syndrome have features of alcoholic dementia and it is possible that Korsakoff's pathology may contribute to alcoholic dementia (Cutting, 1978). It may be that there is a threshold effect, with summation of the effects of different pathologies, although this has yet to be demonstrated. In this context, it is worth noting that hypertension, a risk factor for MID, is sometimes related to heavy alcohol consumption.

Korsakoff psychosis itself is sometimes found in old people. Characterized by apparent inability to encode new memories and consequent confabulation with otherwise relatively well-preserved mental ability and not therefore in the terms of the Royal College of Physicians' definition strictly a dementia, Korsakoff psychosis is accompanied by pathological changes in the mamillary bodies and the periaque-ductal grey matter. This disease, once established, is irreversible. It is due to thiamine deficiency and its acute stage, Wernicke's encephalopathy, presents with a triad of acute confusion, ophthalmoplegia and ataxia. Intravenous thiamine given at, or preferably before, this stage may abort the development of the chronic condition. Any patient with an unexplained acute confusional state should be checked to make sure they are not suffering from Wernicke's encepha-lopathy and if there is any doubt, thiamine should be given. An unexplained acute confusional state deve-loping shortly after admission to hospital may be due to an alcohol withdrawal syndrome, carrying the double risk of delirium tremens, itself a potentially fatal condition, and, if there is associated thiamine deficiency, of a Wernicke–Korsakoff syndrome. Often, initial histories do not contain the necessary information to enable this diagnosis to be made with confidence (Barrison *et al.*, 1980) and the rule again should be to treat if in doubt, until the situation can be clarified, using an appropriate sedative regimen (such as decreasing doses of chlormethiazole) and thiamine. A fuller account of the condition can be found in Cutting (1982).

Confabulation, a feature of Korsakoff psychosis, is also found in Alzheimer's disease, though in this condition, it is usually more fragmentary as the cortical damage superimposes a poverty of thought which does not permit the wild embellishments of the Korsakoff syndrome (Berlyne, 1972). Thiamine defi-ciency itself is not unique to alcoholism (see Chapter 20). In the elderly patient it may be the result of chronic poor diet and Older and Dickerson (1982) have correlated thiamine levels in elderly ortho-paedic patients with the degree of postoperative confusion. They also found that thiamine levels were more likely to be low in patients admitted for fractured neck of femur than for patients admitted for elective surgery. Other vitamins have an effect on mental function and the role of vitamins in old age has recently been comprehensively reviewed by Kemm and Ancill (1985). In the present state of knowledge about thiamine, it is probably best to err on the side of unnecessary treatment rather than run the risk of irreversible subcortical brain damage in any old person subject to major trauma whose nutritional status is uncertain.

Infective dementias are thankfully rare. Creutz-feld–Jakob disease is characterized by a prodromal flu-like illness and a subsequent rapid onset of dementia with focal neurological signs often termi-nating fatally within a few weeks or months. It has apparently been transmitted from man to man by corneal transplant and by the use of penetrating electrodes. (See Corsellis, 1986, for a full discussion of the transmissibility of dementia.) Neurosyphilis which once was responsible for many cases of mental illness is now rare, largely due to success in treating the earlier stages of the disease, but still occurs (Luxon *et al.*, 1978). Loss of social judgement and inhibitions are often early signs of the disease which then progresses to a more generalized dementia with focal neurological signs including the well-known Argyll Robertson pupils.

Genetically Determined Dementias

There is a genetic component to Alzheimer's disease, probably more marked in the earlier onset cases. Pick's disease is probably inherited by a single autosomal dominant gene, possibly modified by other genes. Pick's disease is relatively rare in old age though geographical pockets of increased prevalence can be found. It may be under-diagnosed because of the overwhelming prevalence of Alzheimer's disease in this age group. Pathologically, it is characterized by selective shrinking of the frontal and temporal lobes of the brain and microscopically by neuronal loss, astrocytic proliferation and gliosis. The patho-logy is reflected in the clinical presentation with disinhibition, impaired judgement and psychomotor perseveration, all characteristic of frontal lobe damage, as relatively early signs.

Huntington's chorea (Lishman, 1978, Chapter 10), which is inherited as an autosomal dominant, mainly has its onset in young or middle life, though rarely late onset cases are seen. Sufferers usually have the characteristic choreiform movement disorder though rare cases are found where dementia is the presenting symptom. The movement disorder may also be preceded by personality changes or a schizophreniform psychosis. Suicide is common in the early stages of the disease. As the disease progresses, damage, largely at the subcortical level, renders communication increasingly difficult. Though there is probably an element of true dementia, one of the most disturbing aspects of this disease is that those who work intimately with sufferers, even at an advanced stage of the disease, often form the impression that they have quite a good grasp of their surroundings. Care should therefore be taken in looking after these sufferers not to treat them as though they were without comprehension of their plight. Unfortunately, in many cases, such patients are relegated to the back wards of mental hospitals where their needs may not be properly understood. Huntington's chorea also raises major questions about genetic counselling. If a marker for those who are going to develop the disease is found, then sufferers will be faced with the choice of blindly having children who may be sufferers, of discovering definitely whether they are personally going to develop the disease or of not having children.

Space-occupying lesions can also produce dementia. Malignant tumours, whether primary or secondary, can present with confusion often accompanied by headache and focal neurological signs. The rapid progression of symptoms and the focal signs usually lead to diagnosis which can be confirmed by finding a primary tumour site in the case of metastatic lesions or by CT. Prognosis for survival is usually poor though a primary tumour may rarely be operable if discovered early. Non-malignant space-occupying lesions usually present with headaches and focal neurological signs and symptoms. Rarely a deep seated lesion, such as a parasagittal meningioma, may present with vague symptoms of confusion and disinhibition. Gait apraxia and disproportionate incontinence can help in establishing this diagnosis which can be confirmed by CT. The symptoms of chronic subdural haematoma may be diffuse and non-specific (Brocklehurst, 1972). Headache and focal neurological signs and symptoms are useful if present, but not essential to the diagnosis and in some cases there is no clear history of head injury (Meadows, 1980). Clinically, one of the best diagnostic pointers is a mental state with level of consciousness fluctuating rather more slowly than in acute confusional state due to other causes. There also tends to be psychomotor slowing. In cases of doubt, CT

should be performed as subdural haematoma is a condition with good prognosis given the appropriate neurosurgical treatment.

Acute confusional states (see Chapter 30), characterized by rapid onset and fluctuating level of consciousness, often with associated visual hallucinations and perplexed or irritable mood, are seen in association with many physical illnesses in old age, presumably due to a combination of decreased cerebral reserve and a reduced capacity of the ageing body to maintain homeostasis. They are not forms of dementia, though some may progress to irreversible damage if not appropriately treated; however, they are discussed briefly here because of their importance in differential diagnosis. The commonest causes of such disorders are infections (especially chest and urinary infections), heart failure and medication (especially benzodiazepines and drugs with anticholinergic actions) (Jenike, 1985, Chapter 8), but many other causes are possible.

For a fuller description of some of the rarer causes of dementia in old age, the reader is referred to more detailed texts (Lishman, 1978; Cummings and Benson, 1983).

THE MANAGEMENT OF DEMENTIA

Dementia often presents as a crisis (Arie, 1986). Earlier detection would enable appropriate intervention to prevent many such crises and could occasionally enable the early treatment of reversible cases. Doctors, social workers, other carers and ultimately the public at large need to be educated not to accept intellectual decline in old age as inevitable and to assume that 'nothing can be done about it'. In fact, a careful assessment, even if not strictly 'objective' (Muir-Gray, 1978), can be of substantial help to most dementia sufferers and their relatives.

History and Examination

The demented patient rarely presents directly to the doctor. Usually relatives, friends or neighbours seek help from medical or social services because they have become aware of the problem. The usual complaint is of memory loss, difficult behaviour or self neglect, often summed up in the general complaint that the patient is 'confused'. This, however, is not an acceptable medical diagnosis and the first step in management is to establish the cause.

As with most other aspects of medicine, the key to diagnosis is a clear and detailed history. Almost always this will have to be obtained from someone other than the sufferer. Usually this will be a relative, friend, home help or neighbour, but sometimes, with isolated old people, the story will have to be pieced together from a variety of sources, often most conveniently over the telephone. Vital questions must be answered about the mode of onset and the time course of the disease. A sudden onset, within the previous few days, of mental confusion and disturbed behaviour points to a diagnosis of acute confusional state. A sudden onset in the more distant past may indicate a subacute confusional state or may have been the first in a series of mild acute confusional states punctuated by periods of partial recovery characteristic of multi-infarct dementia. Figure 27.3 summarizes graphically the time course of SDAT, MID and acute confusional state. A patient with a depressive pseudo-dementia will often have a shorter history than a patient with SDAT with an apparently equivalent degree of confusion. In addition, the patient with depression will often have an initial history of loss of interest rather than loss of memory. A detailed personal history from the patient will often reveal previous episodes of depression or obvious precipitants or vulnerability factors (Murphy, 1982). In depressive pseudo-dementia and other conditions, a family history of a similar disease will help to establish the diagnosis. A history of hypertension, vascular disease or diabetes may point towards a diagnosis of multi-infarct dementia, but in the last case, complications of the diabetes and its treatment will also be considered.

Mental State Examination

The setting for mental state examination is crucial. Few surgeons would consider performing a major operation on the kitchen table or in Victorian conditions, but it is amazing how often doctors make the mistake of thinking they can perform an adequate mental state examination in a noisy, busy or disorientating casualty department. The Scottish Health Education Council have produced an excellent video* on the disorientating effects of a badly managed acute admission to hospital for an elderly patient which graphically illustrates this. The ideal place to conduct an initial interview and mental state examination is in the patient's own home where the discomfort, disorientation and sheer inconvenience of being taken to a busy outpatient clinic are avoided. If an interview must be conducted in hospital, then every attempt must be made to secure a quiet, distraction-free environment and to put the patient at ease. Patients may have prejudices about the doctor thinking, for example, that the doctor has come to 'put them away' in the local workhouse. This confusion is not helped by the fact that many doctors in the field are operating out of Victorian workhouses which elderly people often remember by their old names. The doctor will need to spend time introducing himself and explaining what help he has to offer. Then, ideally, after getting a brief history from a friend or relative, the doctor can begin to assess the patient's mental state whilst taking the history. The patient should not be talked over and her wishes must be consulted as to whether or not any friend or relative remains in the room whilst the interview proceeds. The order in which the history is taken will vary from patient to patient but in many people with memory loss it is kindest to begin a personal history with a conversational opening such as 'tell me about yourself, were you born around here?' Whilst the history is being taken, checks of memory can be introduced by asking the patient's current age, date of birth, year of leaving school, year of marriage, years of important external events (e.g., World Wars) and checking for internal consistency or correlation with a relative's account of the patient's history. The interviewer must try to appreciate the patient's experience of the interview including any problems caused by sensory impairment. During the interview the patient's memory, level of awareness, attention and concentration, general appearance and behaviour and mood can all be assessed. Headings under which the mental state

* 'Mental Confusion in the Elderly'. Available from Skyline Film and TV Productions Ltd, 1st Floor, 24 Scala Street, London, W1P 1LU.

TABLE 27.5 MNEMONIC MENTAL STATE EXAMINATION

Awareness	—level of consciousness, fluctuation, attention and concentration
Behaviour	—general appearance of the patient (and his house) as well as behaviour during interview. Standardized form.
Affect	—depression, elation, anxiety, perplexity. Suicide risk. Somatic changes (e.g. sleep pattern, constipation, appetite, weight loss in depression; palpitations, tremor, churning stomach in anxiety).
Thought and talk	—form, speed, content, dysarthria, dysphasia, perseveration
Hallucinations, delusions, obsessions, illusions	
Orientation	—time, place and person
Memory	—remote, ability to encode new information, forgetfulness
Apraxia	—in everyday tasks (e.g. dressing, feeding). Constructional tasks.
Nominal aphasia	—everyday objects in order of increasing difficulty
Judgement and insight	
Other cognitive functions (e.g. arithmetic, proverbs)	
Educational level must be taken into account.	

Reproduced from Wattis and Church (1986) by permission of Croom Helm.

examination can be recorded are summarized in mnemonic form in Table 27.5.

Level of awareness is hard to describe as it is perceived indirectly by noting fluctuations in performance, attention and concentration. Gross impairment of the level of consciousness, as in stupor, is easy to detect but lesser degrees require more practice. Rapid fluctuation in the level of consciousness is found in acute confusional states and a slower fluctuation may be seen in subdural haematoma. General appearance and behaviour includes not only the patient's appearance, but also the state of the home. If a person has developed an acute confusional state, the home will often appear basically clean and tidy, but with a recent overlay of disruption due to the patient's fragmented behaviour. A similar picture may be produced by hypomania. In someone with a more gradual onset of dementia living alone, the home will be more chronically disorganized and dirty. Clothes worn inappropriately may be a sign of dressing apraxia, apathy, memory problems or perseveration in dressing. The state of the home, especially safety factors, is also important to planning management. Behavioural rating scales have now been designed which can assist in measuring the patient's overall disability and in highlighting areas of special behavioural need (e.g. Robinson, 1961; Pattie and Gilleard, 1979). A useful sourcebook of geriatric assessment (Israel *et al.*, 1984) contains these and many other standard assessment instruments. Behavioural rating scales are usually filled in by carers. They help ensure that important areas of behaviour are covered, enable comparison between disability levels in different care settings (Wilkin *et al.*, 1978) and help in the evaluation of treatments and management problems. Such scales take little time and can be applied as part of the routine clinical assessment.

Affect or mood involves not only what the patient reports, but also what the interviewer observes through the patient's facial expression and general demeanour. Disorders of mood along the manic–depressive continuum may be associated with manic–depressive illness, but both depression (Hendrickson *et al.*, 1979; Jacoby *et al.*, 1981) and hypomania (Shulman and Post, 1980) may in some cases be symptomatic of organic brain damage. Loss of emotional control is sometimes associated with stroke or multi-infarct dementia and can pose serious management problems. Whenever depressed mood is found, in whatever context, it is essential to enquire whether the patient has any thoughts of suicide. A useful probe is to ask whether the patient has ever felt so bad that life didn't seem to be worth living. If the patient responds positively, then further questions can be asked to clarify the situation. If the patient responds negatively and the doctor wishes to pursue the subject further, the patient can be asked why he wants to continue living. An appreciable suicide risk indicates hospital admission and observation. Reference must be made to a standard text of psychiatry (e.g. Trethowan and Sims, 1983) for a more detailed discussion.

Hallucinations can be briefly defined as perceptions without an external stimulus. In organic states they are usually visual. Though auditory hallucinations are characteristic of schizophrenia or severe affective psychoses, they can occur in dementia. Olfactory hallucinations are relatively rare, but sometimes found in depressive illness. Complex visual and olfactory hallucinations sometimes occur in temporal lobe epilepsy. Sometimes, visual hallucinations are found in people with eye disease who otherwise appear mentally well (Berrios and Brook, 1984).

Another situation where hallucinations, auditory or visual, may occur in a mentally well person is during a bereavement reaction (Parkes, 1985, 1986). Sensory deprivation, in whatever modality, predisposes to hallucination and hearing loss in particular is also a risk factor for developing paranoid illness (Cooper *et al.*, 1974).

A delusion is briefly described as a false, unshakeable belief incompatible with a person's culture and education. Fragmentary delusions are found in dementia and acute confusional states. They may be held with great vigour, though usually transient. Systematized and complicated delusional systems are generally more characteristic of schizophrenia, though sometimes found in early dementia, especially where there is a pre-existing paranoid personality. Illusions, false interpretations of real perceptions, are common in acute confusional states and account for some of the disturbed behaviour seen in many patients with acute confusion. Some people prefer the term 'delirium' when an acute confusional state is accompanied by such 'productive' symptoms.

Memory and its assessment is at the heart of most concepts of dementia. Although memory for more distant events is characteristically better than for recent events in demented subjects, even this remote memory is far from perfect. Memory for recent events and ability to encode new information may seem virtually non-existent. However, different aspects of memory behave differently and memory for faces may, for example, be retained even when names are forgotten. This can be applied practically in planning patient care. Some patients may refuse to cooperate in attending the day hospital if the ambulance driver is not a familiar face and many will find constant changes of staff difficult to cope with. Ability to learn new material can be assessed both in

TABLE 27.6   10 ITEM MEMORY-INFORMATION SCORE

1 Age
2 Time (to nearest hour)
3 Address for recall at end of test—this should be repeated to make sure the patient has heard it correctly: 42 West Street
4 Year
5 Name of hospital (or address of place seen)
6 Recognition of two people
7 Date of birth
8 Years of First World War
9 Name of present Monarch
10 Count backwards from 20 to 1

Source: Hodkinson (1972).
Reproduced from Wattis and Church (1986) by permission of Croom Helm.

terms of immediate memory span (e.g., digit span) and of the encoding of new material (e.g. remembering a name and address over several minutes). The memory difficulty in 'subcortical syndrome' is characterized by a subjective feeling in the interviewer that the patient has encoded the memory but is unable to retrieve it and this feeling can be confirmed by the rapid location of the memory if a memory cue is provided. When asked the name of the Prime Minister, the subject may not be able to remember, but told the sex or the first name, may rapidly remember the rest of the name. Given an address to remember over 2 minutes, the patient may not be able to retrieve the memory, but if prompted by the first part of the address, the remainder will be rapidly remembered.

Orientation is a function closely related to memory. The main dimensions of orientation are time, place and person. Some questions are more difficult than others and this hierarchical principle has been used in the construction of tests (Cole, 1988). The exact date is more difficult than the year, a familiar person easier to recognize than a relative stranger and so on. Many short lists of items to test memory have been devised. One of the most scientifically valid of these is the ten item Royal College of Physicians' scale (Table 27.6) devised by Hodkinson (Hodkinson, 1972) from the pathologically verified scale of Blessed *et al.* (1968).

Visuo-spatial ability and constructional apraxia can be assessed by getting the patient to copy standardized figures on a sheet of unlined paper. The author commonly uses a square, a triangle and a simple outline of a house for this purpose. Psychologists are beginning to recognize common patterns of abnormal performance in such tests (Moore and Wyke, 1984). Many such tests are not 'pure' but are influenced by other aspects of cognitive function. Perseveration, for example, may cause the patient to repeatedly draw a square or write his own name when he should have moved on to another task.

Nominal aphasia is best assessed on a standard range of objects of increasing difficulty. Several standard sets of objects exist but, especially for home assessment, objects normally carried by the doctor such as a wrist watch, its strap and smaller parts are convenient. Nominal aphasia and constructional apraxia have been chosen from the other tests of cortical function because they are relatively easy and quick to perform. If they are abnormal, they suggest more widespread brain damage than is implied by loss of memory alone and probably imply poorer prognosis (Hare, 1978).

Judgement and insight are rather abstract concepts, but they are of vital importance in the management of demented patients. Has the patient the capacity to manage her own financial affairs? If she is refusing admission to residential care, is this founded on a sound appreciation of her situation and the alternatives before her or on an irrational belief in her own capacity to look after herself? Respect for the autonomy of the individual may be carried too far if she is allowed to die unhappy and hypothermic in her own house when she could be living happily in a residential home. This is especially the case if she has refused simply because her dementia makes her afraid of change or causes her to assume the home will be run like an old fashioned workhouse. Hard pressed workers with inadequate resources at their command may consciously or unconsciously rationalize the neglect they are almost forced to inflict on the sufferer as respect for her autonomy.

Judgement may be affected directly, especially by lesions of the frontal lobe, or indirectly if made on the basis of faulty memory or abnormal mood. Insight, the degree to which the patient recognizes she is ill, is

mercifully limited in most dementia sufferers but is relatively preserved in MID and possibly in Huntington's chorea.

Other tests of neuropsychological function are dealt with in more specialized texts (Lishman, 1978; Cummings and Benson, 1983). Frontal lobe dysfunction is commonly associated with disinhibition and there may be problems of motor sequencing. The patient may be able to perform all the individual components of a given task but may be unable to fit them together into a coherent whole. She may show perseveration. Disorders of motor sequencing can be revealed by asking the patient to repeat a demonstrated series of movements and perseveration can be directly observed in speech, in motor tasks and in simple drawing tasks.

The interpretation of neuropsychological evaluation is often difficult. Although certain functions can be localized to certain brain areas, the pathways are so complicated that a lesion in one area may produce signs appropriate to another area and recently, theorists have moved away from the idea of localized function to the concept of interlocking physiological systems with complicated interactions, which make attempts at precise 'phrenological' localization irrelevant (Wexler, 1986). Constructional apraxia may, for example, be difficult to demonstrate or interpret if there is marked perseveration. Some psychologists working in this area have stressed that evaluation is generally not useful unless it concentrates on functions that are *retained* and how to make the best of them (Church and Wattis, 1988).

The patient's educational and cultural background has to be considered in evaluating the results of neuropsychological and general mental state examination. Some standard neuropsychological batteries include tests like drawing a representation of a three dimensional cube that have never been within the educational achievement of many old people. Some immigrants from Third World countries may never have known their date of birth or the years of the First World War. Some families do not talk about emotion and people who have been brought up in such a tradition may deny emotions or express them in concrete physical terms. Depression may thus be expressed as a 'heavy head' or some other somatic complaint and the verbalized observation that the patient is near to tears may lead to sudden intensification of physical complaints of pain in the neck and elsewhere.

Physical Examination

A thorough physical examination is a vital part of the investigation of any patient with dementia. The doctor will be looking not only for signs of hypertension, neurological, metabolic or other systemic disease which might be causing the dementia, but also for incidental illnesses which might be causing a temporary worsening of the patient's condition ('acute on chronic confusional state'). Patients will often only come to medical attention following a sudden deterioration and so there is always the possibility of finding an exacerbating physical problem, whether it is something mundane like constipation or something more dramatic like pneumonia. The physical evaluation of the elderly patient has been described in more detail by Caird and Judge (1979).

Investigations

In a patient with early dementia, it is important to exclude potentially treatable conditions. How far investigation should go depends on the stage of the dementia and its clinical characteristics. A patient with an advanced dementia that had developed gradually over several years and with a history and mental state examination typical of Alzheimer's disease might not merit any further investigation because the probability of finding a treatable lesion would be too low. On the other hand, a dementia of relatively recent origin with pronounced slowing and a memory difficulty marked by 'forgetfulness' would justify investigation with appropriate tests to exclude a 'metabolic dementia'. The dilemma in this area is compounded by the fact that though potentially treatable dementias are excessively rare, when they are found the impact on the individual is enormous. Even on cost–benefit grounds it can be argued that the saving on cost of community and institutional care for those few cases of reversible dementia might compensate for the costs of an extensive investigation of all patients. A recent retrospective study of 'routine' investigations in elderly psychiatric patients (Colgan and Philpott, 1985) has suggested that these should be limited to full blood count, urea and electrolytes, serum folate and urine culture, with other investigations only when specifically indicated, but this study only looks indirectly at the question of costs. Extensive analysis of costs and benefits is needed to clarify this issue and it is better not to take a dogmatic stance at present.

Computed tomography is not of much help in diagnosing SDAT because of the overlap between the general population, those with other mental illness and those with SDAT (Jacoby *et al.*, 1980; Jacoby and Levy, 1980a, 1980b). However, CT can detect cerebral infarction and a variety of space-occupying lesions including subdural haematoma. It can also indicate the likelihood of normal pressure hydrocephalus, though it is not in itself diagnostic of that condition. In cases where there is an atypical presentation or where an experienced clinician feels uneasy about the diagnosis, then a scan should probably be carried out as, in these circumstances, even negative findings can be useful in planning the patient's long-term management.

The Social Assessment

A full social assessment is the province of the specialized social worker. However, a brief social assessment is an important part of the initial medical contact with any demented old person since management is going to depend, in most cases, more on the social circumstances than on the precise diagnosis. As dementia increases, so does the sufferer's dependence on the external environment. The doctor is therefore interested in the support network the patient enjoys and how this might be improved. A social network diagram (Capildeo *et al.*, 1976) is a useful way of summarizing this. A modified version of this is presented in Figure 27.5. The box represents the patient's dwelling and should contain the patient's name and age, the names and ages of any other occupants and a brief description of the type of dwelling. Down one side are listed all visits from family and friends and down the other, visits from the helping services. The bottom of the box is used to

Friends and relatives   Services

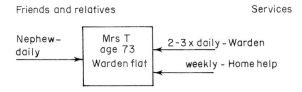

Figure 27.5. Social network diagram. (*Reproduced from Wattis and Church (1986) by permission of Croom Helm.*)

list all visits out by the patient. A glance at such a diagram can reveal the important gaps in social support and can help in the planning of any intervention.

As well as quantitative aspects of social support, it is necessary to note the quality of relationships which will often depend on the sufferer's premorbid personality. People who have had a generous spirit are more likely to meet a generous response to their own need than those who have been hostile, over-dependent or critical in their relationships. Sometimes there will be overt family pathology such as a tendency to encourage over-dependence in the sufferer or the 'fallen dictator' or 'power reversal' described by Bergmann *et al.* (1978). Sometimes the carer may be victim of over-dependent or frankly hostile behaviour from a patient whose behaviour in hospital is exemplary. This 'Jekyll and Hyde syndrome' (Boyd and Woodman 1978) is a good illustration of the fact that behaviour depends on environment and interpersonal interactions as well as on personality attributes. Some families may become over-involved in trying to provide personal care for a demented relative and may feel guilty when the old person has to accept help from outside the family. More difficult for most professional carers are those 'disengaged' families who provide little care themselves, but stridently and anxiously insist on help from the services.

Analysing the Problems

Collecting the necessary data is only the first step to helping the patient. Those data then have to be sorted in a way that will define the problems that need to be tackled to bring benefit to the sufferer. The traditional medical way of doing this is to form a

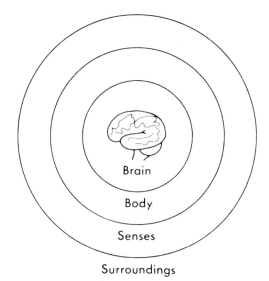

Figure 27.6. An interactive model of confusion. (*Reproduced from Wattis and Church (1986, Chapter 5) by permission of Croom Helm.*)

diagnosis. In the case of the demented patient, this is necessary but not sufficient. Where the medical diagnosis defines a curable or potentially curable disorder like B12 deficiency, subdural haematoma or alcoholic dementia, then that is obviously the single most important fact in the patient's management. Where, however, the diagnosis defines a chronic condition likely to follow a deteriorating course, like SDAT or MID, other factors become more important in management. These factors must be considered systematically to ensure that each problem receives its proper attention at the proper time. The use of a problem list often helps in this.

Figure 27.6 provides a model for analysing the range of problems found in most cases of dementia and can be used as a basis for a problem list. Working from the inside out we start with processes intrinsic to the brain. These include not only structural problems like SDAT and MID, but also biochemical and potentially reversible problems like depression and the patient's learned abilities to cope or not cope with life (personality assets and deficits). The inner circle represents factors in the patient's physical health which might have a bearing on management. A nutritional deficiency may be primary or secondary. It still needs to be corrected. A simple problem

TABLE 27.7 DRUGS THAT MAY CAUSE CONFUSION

Digoxin	Diuretics
Barbiturates	Indomethacin and other non-steroidal anti-inflammatory drugs
Short- and long acting benzodiazepines	
Tricyclic antidepressants	Anti-parkinsonian drugs
Steroids	
Antihistamines	

Reproduced from Wattis and Church (1986) by permission of Croom Helm.

like constipation can cause a major increase in agitation. Prescribed drugs, particularly the longer-acting benzodiazepines and drugs with marked anticholinergic actions (Table 27.7), can also contribute to confusion at this level as can the readily available CNS depressant, alcohol. The next circle in Figure 27.6 represents the special senses. Difficulties here can magnify any underlying dementia. A simple step like clearing wax from the ears, supplying a hearing aid or bringing the patient's spectacles into hospital may improve communication to such an extent that the patient appears less confused. Occasionally, people who become profoundly deaf in old age can be so cut off that they are mistakenly diagnosed as demented. A powerful portable hearing aid such as the SEEL 'Easi-com'* can be a useful tool to the examining doctor. Some old people, whether or not they are demented, will find it hard to adapt to a new aid, but whenever possible, staff should persevere in demonstrating the usefulness of the aid. When cataracts are present, the possible benefits of operation in a demented patient should be weighed against the risk of increased confusion secondary to the operation with its attendant sensory deprivation. Confusion can be minimized by careful nursing in the pre- and postoperative period.

The outermost circle in Figure 27.6 represents the environment including interpersonal relationships. Rapid environmental change of the kind involved in bringing a patient into hospital or residential care can increase confusion in the dementia sufferer.

*Available from: The Seel Co. Ltd, 3 Young Square, Livingstone, Scotland.

Some protection against this can be given by careful preparation for the move whenever possible and by a familiar person travelling with the patient and reminding her constantly what is happening and where she is. The environment that makes it possible for a demented patient to stay in the community often depends on friends and relatives and they may need a great deal of support to carry on coping. This will usually include practical support with cleaning, meals on wheels, day care and respite admission as well as emotional support, perhaps offered through a voluntary group such as Alzheimer's Disease Society, who publish a book on Alzheimer's disease for relatives of sufferers, as well as through members of the multidisciplinary team. One problem frequently seen is 'living bereavement' (Wattis and Church 1986, Chapter 5). Here, the relative may experience the anger, depression and despair of bereavement reaction for the sufferer whilst at the same time being frustrated by constant efforts to communicate with and help the sufferer. The services available to relatives vary from one part of the country to another, but will often include home help, meals on wheels, a daily neighbourhood warden, nursing services, incontinence and mobility aids, day care and respite care. In some areas voluntary groups also provide specialized day care, sitting services or support groups. Bergmann *et al.* (1978) have argued that these services should be concentrated not on old people living alone with dementia, but on those living with relatives. The argument is advanced that people living alone with more severe levels of disability can soak up services and still be at risk. These people need 24 hour care. Patients living with families can, however, be kept at home even when quite disabled by the provision of good community services. This is not to suggest that patients with milder degrees of dementia living alone should receive no help, only that it must be recognized when the point is reached where care in a residential or hospital situation is safer, cheaper and more humane than trying to support the patient in her own home.

In dementia, the environment can also be used in a prosthetic way to compensate for loss of memory. The simplest example of a memory prosthesis, used by most of us, is the writing of shopping lists. Family and friends can leave notes to remind the old person to lock the door before going to bed or only to cook a meal for one. Phone calls can also be used to remind people to get ready for transport to the day centre or as a cue for some other important event. These straightforward 'common sense' approaches are discussed in detail by Holden and Woods (1982). Such measures must be individually tailored to take advantage of an individual's residual capabilities. At a more general level, the design of facilities for old people must take into account the fact that many will have problems with mobility, sensory impairment and memory. Buildings should generally be on one level with doors wide enough to permit wheelchair access. Toilets should be clearly signposted and clear colour-coding of doors used to make them more readily identifiable and memorable (Wattis and Church, 1986, Chapter 9). A dementia sufferer who is initially unable to find the toilet may learn to do so over several weeks with help from the staff and environmental cues.

The importance of the model in Figure 27.6 is that it represents an interactive system. Deficits can be additive across more than one area. Thus a person with poor eyesight and hearing will be more susceptible to the confusing effects of environmental change. It is possible to have several patients all presenting with the same level of confusion but with each case having a unique combination of causative factors. This is represented schematically in Figure 27.7. In this illustration, subject A's confusion is mostly due to dementia, but the additional impairments superimposed by constipation and an under-stimulating, under-structured environment at home contribute significantly to the overall level of disability and if these problems are tackled, then a functional improvement will occur even though the underlying dementia is unaffected. In subject B with the same overall level of confusion, there is relatively little dementia, but heart failure is producing a superadded acute confusional state compounded by the problems of emergency hospital admission in a patient with relative sensory deprivation. An assessment of this subject at this point in time might suggest that she is too confused for home care, when in fact, after all treatable problems have been dealt with, the patient is quite capable of living alone with

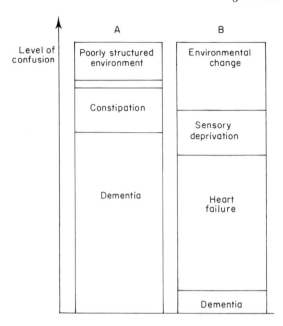

Figure 27.7. Components of confusion.

intermittent support. In analysing the patient's problems, we have therefore to go beyond a single diagnosis, to list and deal with all the problems systematically and in the right order. The list should include not only the diagnosis, but also relevant problems in physical health, sensory impairment and the environment, including family factors and any recent changes. Such a problem list can be the foundation for rational and efficient treatment.

Planning Treatment

The main forms of dementia in old age are not susceptible to conventional medical treatment with vasodilators (Leading Article, 1979), and although the cholinergic hypothesis offers some hope for the future (Hollander *et al.*, 1986) other approaches, such as the use of hyperbaric oxygen, CNS stimulants and high potency vitamins have yet to be shown to have any clinically significant effect (Kopelman and Lishman, 1986). Occasionally, drugs may be of marginal benefit, but in most cases, apart from symptomatic use of tranquillizers or treatment of coincidental depression, drugs will have little part to play. In MID there is some cause for hope in the finding that low dose aspirin in men can produce a reduction in recurrent episodes of stroke. Research into other antiplatelet drugs for stroke may also bear fruit useful in MID. Since hypertension is linked to MID, the early detection and treatment of high blood pressure might bring about a reduction in the incidence of MID. Some of the rarer dementias, especially vitamin B12 deficiency and thyroid deficiency, are amenable to specific treatment. There is no specific treatment for genetic disease such as Huntington's chorea, though genetic counselling may have a preventative role. Cerebrovascular syphilis may respond to an appropriate course of antibiotics (see Chapter 19). When an antidepressant is used to treat a coincidental depression in a demented patient, it is best to choose an antidepressant relatively free from anticholinergic side-effects (e.g. mianserin), as the more strongly anticholinergic antidepressants, such as amitriptyline, may provoke increased confusion. The drug should be started in low doses and built up over several weeks to the highest permissible dose that the patient can tolerate without unacceptable side-effects. After 3–4 weeks at this dose, the antidepressant should be discontinued unless there is definite benefit.

Neuroleptics (major tranquillizers) are often used for symptomatic control of wandering, agitation or aggression. Theoretically very low doses of a drug with little or no anticholinergic action such as haloperidol are preferable to drugs like thioridazine (Jenike, 1985) with inbuilt anticholinergic action but in practice both types of drug are used with some success. The problem in the use of any of these drugs is adjusting the dose so that the desired symptom relief is achieved without unacceptable side-effects. In many cases alternatives to drugs such as the provision of more day care, the increase of caring staff numbers or a better environment and range of activities may render the use of these drugs unnecessary. There is an ethical problem here. If powerful medications are used to sedate patients simply because enough staff are not available to provide proper care, this is an abuse (though sometimes a necessary one) and should be recognized as such.

In most cases of dementia, psychoactive drugs are not a central part of the management strategy. Using the model of Figure 27.6, problems can be systematically defined and tackled. In the physical area an adequate diet with a reasonable amount of fibre can help prevent secondary vitamin deficiencies and constipation, though a laxative may also sometimes be needed for the latter problem. Other aspects of physical health should be kept under review and sensory impairment treated when appropriate. Once the diagnosis is established, however, management will focus on the external environment and supporting caring relatives and friends with appropriate services. This requires a multifaceted, multidisciplinary approach.

If the patient lives alone, special attention will have to be paid to making the home safe. This may mean fitting foolproof gas appliances or substituting safer electrical ones. Fire hazards will need to be minimized by the removal of highly inflammable furnishings, discouraging smoking when possible and even fitting smoke detector fire alarms. At the other extreme, the risk of death from hypothermia can be reduced by external or automatic control of heating. Given this kind of common-sense approach and the regular stimulus and structure of a daily visit from a neighbour or neighbourhood warden and appropriate services such as meals on wheels, home help and day centre attendance, many demented old people can be kept happy in the community for some years even though they live alone. Seven out of every eight demented people in Great Britain live at home at present and it is unlikely, given adequate community services, that we will need a major increase in age-related provision. On the other hand it is unlikely that the community services could begin to cope with the burden if the provision of 24 hour institutional care is reduced as it recently appears to have been (Grundy and Arie, 1982). As has been previously discussed, this fall has been accompanied by a parallel rise in private sector provision (Laing, 1985).

Sometimes the need for 24 hour care is not recognized by the family or by the authorities and a demented old person is neglected. Alternatively, the family or authorities may recognize the need but the patient refuses the care offered. Here family and professional helpers will face the difficult decision as to how far they are justified in over-riding the patient's autonomy. Many demented old people do not realize what they are really refusing and given patience may be won over. This will depend to some extent on professional skills in building relationships as well as on the patient's personality. Often it is impossible, in the public sector, to guarantee a place in a specific home. This is because there is no surplus of places. In these circumstances it is difficult for the helping professional to gently introduce the idea of residential care through visits as it is impossible to know which home to show the patient. The quality of care in both the public and private sector is very variable and the doctor may sometimes be faced with the unenviable task of persuading an old person to go into care when he has grave reservations about the quality of that care. At present, because of shortages, most admissions to local authority care occur in emergency situations where there is little time to respect the sufferer's autonomy or to prepare her for the move. Other problems may occur when the demented person has a pet to which she is extremely attached and the home is unable to accept animals. The family or professional carer in these situations will be faced with difficult ethical decisions which are made more difficult by current lack of resources. Rarely it will be necessary to use the powers of the 1983 Mental Health Act to compel a sufferer to come into hospital or (where local authorities will respect their responsibilities under this act) to use the guardianship powers of the Mental Health Act to compel a sufferer to live in residential care. Some of the general issues concerning this act are discussed by Bluglass (1983) and, with special reference to old people, by Wattis and Church (1986, Chapter 10). The National Assistance Act (1948) also provides, under Section 47, for magistrates to order compulsory admission to a place of safety for old people on public health grounds. The power to apply for admission under this act rests with community physicians and is rarely used. The Court of Protection and the enduring power of attorney provide legal means of looking after the finances of demented people.

For those elderly demented people who live with their spouses, the vital issue is usually to provide sufficient practical and emotional support to enable the carer to carry on coping. The range of services that can be provided has already been described. Without a properly planned package of practical support the offer of emotional support is of relatively little value. At the same time the doctor should be frank about deficiencies in the locally available facilities. It is no use offering what cannot be provided.

CONCLUSION

The diagnosis of dementia must be made with care. In most cases the underlying pathology will be fundamentally beyond the scope of present medical treatment but it is vital to recognize those few cases due to potentially remediable causes. A careful history of the evolution of the disease and a detailed mental state examination will be sufficient for this task in most cases. The issue of routine screening tests, especially the more expensive investigations like computed tomography, is difficult. The possibility of economic savings by a decreased need for institutional care in those few with clinically unsuspected but potentially treatable causes has to be weighed against the cost of the investigations. Probably the best balance at present is to perform simple inexpensive investigations in early cases of dementia, and in later cases where a specific finding in the history of mental state suggests it, but to reserve the more expensive investigations to those patients where there are definite indications. Though direct medical treatment of SDAT and MID is not yet possible, for MID at least some prevention may be possible by treatment of hypertension early in life and by the use of appropriate antiplatelet drugs in selected patients. For most patients with these diseases, however, the judicious use of drugs for symptomatic treatment and the treatment of associated medical conditions together with the arrangement of appropriate practical and emotional support will be the best the doctor can offer. Delivering this support depends on a positive attitude to the problems of demented old people, a capacity to work smoothly with professionals of other disciplines and an ability to rise above the frustrations imposed by grossly inadequate resources. Since the quality of a civilization can be judged by the care it gives its dependent members, this effort is supremely worth-while.

REFERENCES

Adams, R.D., Fisher, C.M., Hakim, S. Ojemann, R.G., and Sweet, W.H. (1975). Symptomatic occult hydroce-phalus with "normal" cerebrospinal fluid pressure. A treatable syndrome. *N. Engl. J. Med.*, **273**, 117–26.

Alzheimer, A. (1979). (On a peculiar disease of the cerebral cortex) 1907. Translation: Wilkins, R.H., Brody, I.A. Alzheimer's disease. *Arch. Neurol.*, **21**, 109–10.

Arie, T. (1986). Management of dementia: A review. *Br. Med. Bull.*, **42**(1), 91–6.

Aspland, K., Normark, M., and Peterson, V. (1981). Nutritional assessment of psychogeriatric patients. *Age and Ageing*, **10**, 87–94.

Barrison, I.G., Viola, L., and Murray-Lyon, I.M. (1980). Do housemen take an adequate drinking history? *Br. Med. J.*, **281**, 1040.

Bergmann, K. (1981). Neurosis in old age. In: Arie, T. (ed.) *Health Care of the Elderly*, Croom Helm, London.

Bergmann, K., Foster, E.M., Justice, A.W., and Mat-thews, V. (1978). Management of the demented elderly patient in the community. *Br. J. Psychol.*, **132**, 491–9.

Berlyne, N. (1972). Confabulation. *Br. J. Psychiatry*, **120**, 31–9.

Berrios, G.F., and Brook, P. (1984). Visual hallucinations and sensory deprivation in the elderly. *Br. J. Psychiatry*, **144**, 662–4.

Birkett, D.P. (1972). The psychiatric differentiation of senility and arteriosclerosis. *Br. J. Psychiatry*, **120**, 321–5.

Blessed, G., Tomlinson, B.E., and Roth, M. (1968). The association between quantitative measures of dementia and senile changes in the grey matter of elderly people. *Br. J. Psychiatry*, **114**, 797–811.

Blessed, G., and Wilson, I.D. (1982). The contemporary natural history of mental disorder in old age. *Br. J. Psychiatry*, **141**, 59–67.

Bluglass, R. (1983). *A Guide to the Mental Health Act*, Churchill Livingstone, London.

Bondareff, W. (1983). Age and Alzheimer's disease. *Lancet*, **1**, 1447.

Boyd, R.V., and Woodman, J.A. (1978). The Jekyll and Hyde syndrome. *Lancet*, **ii**, 671–2.

Briggs, R.S., Castleden, G.M., and Alvarez, A.S. (1981). Normal pressure hydrocephalus in the elderly: A treat-able cause of dementia? *Age and Ageing*, **10**, 254–8.

Brocklehurst, G. (1982). Diagnosis not to be missed: Subdural haematoma. *Br. J. Hosp. Med.*, **27**, 170–4.

Caird, F.I., and Judge, T.G. (1979). *Assessment of the Elderly Patient*. Pitman Medical Publishing, Tunbridge Wells.

Candy, J.M. *et al.* (1986). Aluminosilicates and senile plaque formation in Alzheimer's disease. *Lancet*, **ii**, 354–7.

Capildeo, R., Court, C., and Rose, F. (1976). Social network diagram. *Br. Med. J.*, **i**, 143–4.

Church, M., and Wattis, J.P. (1987). In: Wattis, J.P., and Hindmarch, (eds.) *Psychological Assessment of Old People*, Churchill Livingstone, London (in press).

Cole, M.G., (1988). Measuring levels of disability—an hierarchical approach. In: Wattis, J.P., and Hind-march, I. (eds.) *Psychological Assessment of Old People*, Churchill Livingstone, London.

Colgan, J., and Philpot, M. (1985). The routine use of investigations in elderly psychiatric patients. *Age and Ageing*, **14**, 163–7.

Cooper, A.F., Curry, A.R., Kay, D.W.K., Garside, K.F., and Roth, M. (1974). Hearing loss in paranoid and affective psychoses in the elderly. *Lancet*, **ii**, 851–4.

Corsellis, J.A.N. (1986). The transmissibility of dementia. *Brit. Med. J.*, **42**(1): 111–14.

Cummings, J.L., and Benson, D.F. (1983). *Dementia—a Clinical Approach*, Butterworth, Boston.

Cutting, J. (1978). The relationship between Korsakov's syndrome and alcoholic dementia. *Br. J. Psychiatry*, **132**, 240–51.

Cutting, J. (1982). Neuropsychiatric complications of alcohol. *Br. J. Hosp. Med.*, 27/4, 342–55.

Dick, D.H. (1982). The rising tide: Developing services for mental illness in old age. NHS Advisory Service, Sutton.

Drew, L.R.H. (1968). Alcoholism as a self-limiting dis-order. *Q. J. Stud. Alcohol*, **29**, 956–67.

Droller, H., and Dosset, J.A. (1959). Vitamin B12 levels in senile dementia and confusional states. *Geriatrics*, 367–73.

Edwards, G., Hanker, L., Hensmay, C., Peto, J., and Williamson, V. (1973). Alcoholics known or unknown to agencies: Epidemiological studies in a London suburb. *Br. J. Psychiatry*, **123**, 169–83.

Gillon, R. (1986). Philosophical medical ethics. *Br. Med. J.*, **292**, 543–5.

Grundy, E. (1983). Demography and old age. *J. Am. Geriatr. Soc.*, **31**, 325–32.

Grundy, E., and Arie, T.H.D. (1982). Falling rate of provision of residential care for the elderly. *Br. Med. J.*, **284**, 799–802.

Hachinski, V.C. *et al.* (1975). Cerebral blood flow in dementia. *Arch. Neurol.*, **32**, 632–7.

Hare, M. (1978). Clinical check list for the diagnosis of dementia. *Br. Med. J.*, **ii**, 266–7.

Henderson, A.S. (1986). The epidemiology of Alzheimer's disease. *Br. Med. Bull.*, **42**(1), 3–10.

Hendrickson, E., Levy, R., and Post, F. (1979). Average evoked responses in relation to cognitive and affective state of elderly psychiatric patients. *Br. J. Psychiatry*, **134**, 494–500.

Hodkinson, H.M. (1972). Evaluation of a Mental Test Score for assessment of mental impairment in the elderly. _Age Ageing_, **1**, 223–8.

Holden, U.P., and Woods, R.T. (1982). _Reality Orientation. Psychological Approaches to the Confused Elderly_. Churchill Livingstone, Edinburgh.

Hollander, E., Mohs, R.C., and Davis, K.L. (1986). Cholinergic approaches to the treatment of Alzheimer's disease. _Br. Med. Bull._, **42**, 97–100.

Huppert, F.A., and Tym, E. (1986). Clinical and neuro-psychological assessment of dementia. _Br. Med. Bull._, **42**, 1–18.

Israel, L., Kozarevic, D., and Sartorius, N. (1984). A Sourcebook of Geriatric Assessment, Karger/WHO, Basle.

Jacoby, R.J., and Levy, R. (1980a). Computed tomography in the elderly. 2. Senile dementia, diagnosis and functional impairment. _Br. J. Psychiatry_, **136**, 256–9.

Jacoby, R.J., and Levy, R. (1980b). Computed tomography in the elderly. 3. Affective disorder. _Br. J. Psychiatry_, **136**, 270–5.

Jacoby, R.J., Levy, R., and Bird, J.M. (1981). Computed tomography and the outcome of affective disorders: A follow-up study of elderly patients. _Br. J. Psychiatry_, **139**, 288–92.

Jacoby, R.J., Levy, R., and Dawson, J.M. (1980). Computed tomography in the elderly: 1. The normal population. _Br. J. Psychiatry_, **136**, 249–55.

Jenike, M.A. (1985). _Handbook of Geriatric Psychopharmacology_, PSG Publishing Company, Littleton, Massachusetts.

Kay, D.W.K. (1986). The genetics of Alzheimer's disease. _Br. Med. Bull._, **42**(1), 19–23.

Kay, D.W.K., Bergmann, K., Foster, E.M., McKechnie, A.A., and Roth, M. (1970). _Comprehensive Psychiatry_, **ii**, 26–35.

Kemm, J.R., and Ancill, R.J. (eds). (1985). _Vitamin Deficiency in the Elderly_, Blackwell Scientific Publications, Oxford.

Kopelman, M.D., and Lishman, W.A. (1986). The pharmacological treatments of dementia (non cholinergic). _Br. Med. Bull._, **42**(1), 101–5.

Laing, W. (1985). _Private Health Care_, Office of Health Economics, London.

Lay, C., and Woods, B. (1984). _Caring for the Person with Dementia_, Alzheimer's Disease Society, London.

Leading Article (1978). Dementia: The quiet epidemic. _Br. Med. J._, **1**, 1–2.

Leading Article (1979). Vasodilators in senile dementia. _Br. Med. J._, **ii**, 511–12.

Levy, R. (1975). The neurophysiology of dementia. In: Silverstone, T., and Barraclough, B. (eds.) _Contemporary Psychiatry_, Royal College of Psychiatrists, London.

Lishman, W.A. (1978). _Organic Psychiatry_, Blackwell Scientific Publications, Oxford.

Lishman, W.A. (1981). Cerebral disorder in alcoholism: syndromes of impairment. _Brain_, **104**, 1–20.

Livesley, B. (1978). The treatment and prevention of brain failure. _Age and Ageing_, **7**, 27–34.

Luxon, L., Lees, A.J., and Greenwood, R.J. (1979). Neurosyphilis today. _Lancet_, **i**, 90–3.

McGeer, P.L. (1986). Brain imaging in Alzheimer's disease. _Br. Med. Bull._, **42**(1), 24–8.

MacLennan, W.J. (1985). Clinical assessment of nutritional status in the elderly. In: Kemm and Ancill (eds.) _Vitamin Deficiency in the Elderly_, Blackwell Scientific Publications, Oxford.

Meadows, J. (1980). Subdural haematoma: Recognising the chronic form. _Geriatr. Med._, **12**, 42–8.

Moore, V., and Wyke, M.A. (1984). Drawing disability in patients with senile dementia. _Psychological Medicine_, **14**(1), 97–105.

Muir-Gray, J.A. (1978). The myth of objective assessment. _Community Care_, **3**, 21–3.

Murphy, E. (1982). Social origins of depression in old age. _Br. J. Psychiatry_, **141**, 135–42.

Older, M.W.J., and Dickerson, J.W.T. (1982). Thiamine and the elderly orthopaedic patient. _Age and Ageing_, **11**, 101–7.

Parkes, C.M. (1985). Bereavement. _Br. J. Psychiatry_, **146**, 11–17.

Parkes, C.M. (1986). _Bereavement: Studies of Grief in Adult Life_, second edition, Pelican, London.

Pattie, A.H., and Gilleard, C.J. (1979). _Manual of the Clifton Assessment Procedure for the Elderly (CAPE)_, Hodder and Stoughton, Kent.

Perl, D.P., and Brody, A.R. (1980). Alzheimer's disease; X-ray spectrometric evidence of aluminium accumulation in neurofibrillary tangle-bearing neurones. _Science_, **208**, 297–8.

Perry, E.K., Tomlinson, B.E., Blessed, G., Bergmann, K., Gibson, P.H., and Perry, R.H. (1978). Correlations of cholinergic abnormalities and mental test scores in senile dementia. _Br. Med. J._, **ii**, 1457–9.

Renvoize, E.B. (1984). An HLA and family study of Alzheimer's disease. _Psychol. Med._, **14**, 515–20.

Robinson, R.A. (1961). Some problems of clinical trials in elderly people. _Gerontol. Clin._, **3**, 247–57.

Rosen, W.A., Terry, R.D., Fuld, P.A., Katzman, R., and Peck, A. (1980). Pathological verification of ischaemic score in differentiation of dementias. _Ann. Neurol._, **7**(5), 486–8.

Rosin, A.J., and Glatt, M.M. (1971). Alcohol excess in the elderly. _Q. J. Stud. Alcoholism_, **32**, 53–9.

Rossor, M.N., Iverson, L.L., Reynolds, G.P., Mountjoy, C.Q., and Roth, M. (1984). Neurochemical characteristics of early and late onset types of Alzheimer's disease. _Br. Med. J._, **288**, 961–4.

Roth, M. (1955). The natural history of mental disorder in old age. _J. Mental Sci._, **101**, 281–301.

Roth, M. (1986). The association of clinical and neurological findings and its bearing on the classification and aetiology of Alzheimer's disease. *Br. Med. Bull.*, **42**, 42–50.

Royal College of Physicians (1982). Organic mental impairment in the elderly. Implications for research, education and the provision of services: A report of the Royal College of Physicians by the College Committee on Geriatrics, London.

Shulman, K., and Post, F. (1980). Bipolar affective disorder in old age. *Br. J. Psychiatry*, **136**, 26–32.

Szanto, S. (1972). Blood platelet behaviour in primary neuronal and vascular dementia. *Age and Ageing*, **1**, 207–12.

Tomlinson, B., Blessed, G., and Roth, M. (1970). Observations on the brains of demented old people. *J. Neurol. Sci.*, **11**, 205–42.

Trethowan, W.H., and Sims, A.C.P. (1983). *Psychiatry*, fifth edition, Baillière Tindall, London.

Wattis, J.P. (1986). Step by step along the road to euthanasia. *Geriatr. Med.*, **16**, 1.

Wattis, J., and Arie, T. (1984). Further developments in psychogeriatrics in Britain. *Br. Med. J.*, **289**, 778.

Wattis, J.P., and Church, M. (1986). *Practical Psychiatry of Old Age*, Croom Helm, London.

Wattis, J., Wattis, L., and Arie, T. (1981). Psychogeriatrics: A national survey of a new branch of psychiatry. *Br. Med. J.*, **282**, 1529–33.

Wells, N.E.J. (1979). *Dementia in Old Age*, Office of Health Economics, London.

Wexler, B.E. (1986). A model of brain function and its implications for psychiatric research. *Br. J. Psychiatry*, **148**, 357–62.

Whitehouse, R.J. (1986). The concept of sub-cortical and cortical dementia: Another look. *Ann. Neurol.*, **19**, 1–6.

Wilkin, D., Jolley, D., and Masiah, T. (1978). Changes in behavioural characteristics of elderly populations in Local Authority Homes and Long Stay Hospital wards, 1976–77. *Br. Med. J.*, **ii**, 1274–6.

Williamson, J., Stokoe, I.H., Gray, S. *et al.* (1964). Old people at home: Their unreported needs. *Lancet*, **i**, 1117–20.

World Health Organization (1986). Dementia in later life: Research and action. *Technical Report Series*, 730 WHO, Geneva.

SECTION THREE

Some Common Neurological Symptoms in the Elderly

The Clinical Neurology of Old Age
Edited by R. Tallis
© 1989 John Wiley & Sons Ltd

Chapter 28

'Funny Turns', Episodic Loss of Consciousness, and Falls

Brian Livesley

The University of London's Professor of the Care of the Elderly (Geriatrics), Charing Cross Hospital and Westminster Medical School, London, UK

INTRODUCTION

Direct questioning of old people during systematic evaluation after their admission to hospital shows that the majority of falls go unreported. They are simply accepted as a 'normal' accompaniment of old age. Recent random surveys of old people living at home have confirmed the pioneer findings of Sheldon (1960) and shown that some 20% of men and 40% of women have experienced a fall during previous months (Exton-Smith, 1977; Prudham and Evans, 1981). Furthermore, the frequency of falling increases with age (Campbell *et al.*, 1981; Prudham and Evans, 1981). Despite our ageing society, however, falls are not a new phenomenon. Although serious falls in the home occur at any age, they occur more commonly in the old (Archer, 1985). Indeed, accidents in the home due to falls were reported to affect all ages at an annual rate of 16.8 per 1000 population over 30 years ago (Castle, 1950); while, in 1962, it was noted that of 3200 people who died in England and Wales as a result of injuries due to falls indoors, 89% were older than 64 years (Backett, 1965). These facts underline the importance of more recent evidence that *at all ages*, but particularly in the old, some people have a tendency to fall. In an investigation, within an acute care hospital in the USA, patients who had already fallen once had a subsequent fall rate of 91.7 per 1000 patients

compared with an overall fall rate of 18.7 for the first time fallers (Morgan *et al.*, 1985). Rates were highest for patients aged over 65 and for those admitted with mental disorders.

Falls associated with fractures of the femur in elderly and aged patients have been shown to accompany 'a poorer physical state' (Brocklehurst *et al.*, 1978) and falls among institutionalized women with Alzheimer's disease appeared 'to be related to the process of decline in vigour' (Brody *et al.*, 1984). These observations add weight to the suggestion made several years ago that repeated falls in the elderly are a symptom requiring further investigation (Livesley and Atkinson, 1974), or, as stated more recently, a sign requiring as much explanation as anaemia (Duthie and Gambert, 1983). Certainly, these last authors do not overestimate the size of the problem when they point out that in the USA alone fractures resulting from either accidents or falls cost approximately $1 billion annually.

INITIAL PRESENTATION

One of the common questions that has to be answered by physicians responsible for old people is: did the patient trip, slip on some object or fall down for no good environmental reason? So many body systems are concerned in the maintenance of posture it is not surprising that the multiple disorders accompanying ageing produce not one but several weak links in the control of balance, precipitating a fall. Moreover, an accumulation of environmental hazards can so complicate the clinical presentation, it may be difficult to tease out the actual factors responsible for the fall. This becomes a particular problem if, as has been pointed out (Chipman, 1981), patients try to pass off the incident by claiming 'I must have slipped (or tripped)' when what they really mean is 'I don't really know what happened—so, I must have slipped'. Under these circumstances it is easy to overlook remedial but masked organic factors that may precipitate another fall producing injury or unexpected death.

The key question for the practitioner to answer is: 'Has this been a one-off event or have there been previous falls?'

INCIDENTAL FALLS, ACCIDENTAL FALLS, AND ILLNESSES

Repeated falls at any age are associated with organic factors. Careful questioning of the patient, and if possible an unbiased observer, is a prerequisite to accurate diagnosis, effective prevention, and appropriate management. If there is no obvious or serious injury the practitioner should determine first whether the event was due to an incident, an accident, or an illness while bearing in mind that obvious or masked illness can make its own contribution to both incidental and accidental falls. Until the true nature of the event is apparent, it is important to use the term *incident* and thereby avoid merely labelling the event an accident. This is particularly essential within long-stay institutions where incidental falls are more likely to occur during changes in posture or position, notably while using the toilet or transferring between bed and chair. Moreover, the medico-legal implications of such events, with the distraction of 'accident forms', may distort interpretations and divert carers from recognizing that the patient is developing an increasing dependency, due to physical and mental decline, and now requires more careful protection.

Once an incidental fall has been excluded, it is next important to determine if the event was actually an accidental fall due to preventable hazards

(including not only environmental factors but also visual deterioration and unwanted drug effects) and masked illness. Here specific questions are needed: did the patient genuinely trip or slip; was the patient 'giddy', light-headed, or pale prior to or after the event? or was the fall one of a short series of spontaneous but unobserved events that now require further investigation?

Additional, useful information can be obtained by finding out what was happening immediately prior to the fall (Livesley and Atkinson, 1974). For example, if the fall occurred during standing from the sitting or lying position it may have been precipitated by postural hypotension. If it occurred during walking it may have been associated with a properly identifiable trip-or-slip event to which the patient may have been predisposed because of drug side-effects, ageing-associated infirmity, or organic disease. Whereas, if the fall occurred unexpectedly while the patient was standing or walking, the effects of several factors may have summated with erstwhile silent illnesses to produce apparently spontaneous falls as will be discussed later. In many cases, and particularly in advanced old age, the problems are compounded because it is difficult to obtain a clear-cut account of events.

ACCIDENTAL FALLS

Various environmental hazards, including slippery surfaces, loose or defective rugs and carpets, loose objects, poor lighting, and doorsteps have been found to be responsible for accidental falls (Lucht, 1971). Moreover, one-third of falls sustained by old people at home have been described as accidental (Sheldon, 1960) and unlit stairs featured high on the list. An additional 10% of these patients tripped producing an overall accidental fall rate of 45% which compares well with the 47% tripping rate found 17 years later (Overstall *et al.*, 1977). Sheldon (1960) was one of the first to observe that old people trip because they do not lift their feet high enough. In patients aged 65 to 74 years tripping features more prominently as the cause of falls than it does in those aged over 75 years (Exton-Smith, 1977; Brocklehurst *et al.*, 1978). This is perhaps because those aged 65–74 years have yet to appreciate that mobility carries risks literally related to the failure to pick up feet. Studies on gait have since shown that elderly fallers have gait characteristics different from elderly non-fallers. Slow speed, short step length, narrow stride width, wide range of stepping frequency, and large variability of step length have all been identified as characteristics reflecting loss of gait automaticity in hospitalized fallers (Guimaraes and Isaacs, 1980). These changes, however, may only indicate increased frailty, poor general health, and impaired postural control, as has been pointed out elsewhere (Campbell *et al.*, 1981).

Impaired postural control in the aged with an increased tendency to sway was also first observed by Sheldon (1963) and has since been confirmed in a retrospective study (Overstall *et al.*, 1977). Although postural sway has been accepted as an indicator of the tendency to fall, the difference in sway between fallers and non-fallers in a prospective investigation was less than expected and there was no correlation of increasing postural sway with increased frequency of falls (Fernie *et al.*, 1982). While a close relationship between increased sway and impaired vibration sense in the legs has been noted (Brocklehurst *et al.*, 1982) this was not correlated with proprioceptive changes and only in 'the very old' (6% of patients studied) was there evidence of vestibular impairment. This contrasts with the 25% incidence of falls 'associated with vertigo' reported by Sheldon (1948) in patients aged from 65 to over-85 years; but compares with the 7% incidence he reported later when half of those affected were over 80 years of age (Sheldon, 1960). Furthermore, Brocklehurst and his colleagues found only a limited relationship between falls in the previous year and both sway and proprioceptive changes.

What has not been given sufficient consideration, however, is the importance of vision in maintaining stance. Visual cues provide important proprioceptive information. Although partial sightedness was an important factor in falls due to loss of balance (Brocklehurst *et al.*, 1978) there is another interesting aspect to the problem. Fallers, who are more likely to be elderly, have been found to have a significantly increased error ($P < 0.01$) of visual perception of both the vertical and the horizontal compared with non-fallers (Tobis *et al.*, 1981). This phenomenon

may be particularly important in the elderly when impoverished ankle–foot proprioception is associated with frailty.

FALLS AS AN INDICATOR OF ILL-HEALTH

Although falls are common in the elderly and aged they do not occur all the time. Other events are needed, if only to aggravate the patient's tendency to sway and actually precipitate the fall. In the elderly (aged 65–74 years) such factors are more likely to be extrinsic or environmental and associated with trip-or-slip falls; whereas, in the aged (aged over-75 years) intrinsic factors associated with illness-and-disability assume greater importance (Exton-Smith, 1977; Brocklehurst *et al.*, 1978; Morfitt, 1983). Despite this, in the majority of instances, obvious environmental hazards may distract all but the more alert practitioner from discovering the silent and intrinsic factors impairing health that have really predisposed to, if not actually precipitated, the fall. Good examples here include: the unwanted actions of frequently unnecessary drug therapies (especially sedatives, hypnotics, tranquillizers, alcohol, too potent hypotensives, and diuretics), as well as the earlier but unspoken development of a sensory stroke or tremor-free, but bradykinetic, Parkinson's disease. These, together with almost any acute illness (commonly pneumonia, myocardial infarction, mild stroke, and urinary tract infection) may subtly interfere with the patient's usual perception and mobility so that frailty is aggravated and hazards are not appreciated.

In a prospective study of accidental falls and resulting injuries in the home among elderly people, intrinsic organic factors accounted for 55% of falls (Lucht, 1971). These included dizziness, sudden malaise, confusion, fainting, and senile dementia. Regretfully, this and the many other studies on falls do not help us to determine the exact cause or likely nature of spontaneous falls in individual elderly and aged patients. This is because, by the very nature of the problem, the majority of epidemiological studies of falls have been either retrospective or have assessed readily available populations of patients (viz., the elderly at home (Sheldon, 1948; Droller, 1955; Exton-Smith, 1977) or in a high-rise apartment (Perry, 1982); 100 healthy elderly people observed for one year (Gabell *et al.*, 1985); a non-random mixture of patients (Overstall *et al.*, 1977); outpatient or accident-and-emergency populations (Seiler and Ramsay, 1954; Sheldon, 1960; Macqueen, 1960; Waller, 1974; Morfitt, 1983); patients treated for a fractured femur (Brocklehurst *et al.*, 1978; Sloan and Holloway, 1981); female patients treated for a fractured femur (Clark, 1968); patients admitted to a geriatric unit because of a fall (Naylor and Rosin, 1970; Guimaraes and Isaacs, 1980); patients referred to a geriatric unit and who were then found to have fallen (Livesley and Atkinson, 1974); patients who were observed to fall in a geriatric unit (Fine, 1959; Sehested and Severin-Neilsen, 1977; Morgan *et al.*, 1985); all inpatient accidents in a city's hospitals (Uden, 1985); and other elderly institutionalized populations (Rodstein, 1964; Rodstein and Camus, 1973; Margulec *et al.*, 1970; Gryfe *et al.*, 1977; Ashley *et al.*, 1977; Kalchthaler *et al.*, 1978; Pablo, 1977; Miller and Elliott, 1979; Berry *et al.*, 1981; Fernie *et al.*, 1982; Woodhouse *et al.*, 1983; Brody *et al.*, 1984)). Only two recent surveys of geographically defined populations aged over-65 years who were subject to falls have been found in the literature (Prudham and Evans, 1981; Campbell *et al.*, 1981).

INTERPRETING EPIDEMIOLOGICAL SURVEYS

'The basic assumption underlying the work of all epidemiologists is that the phenomena they study are not randomly distributed among the general population. By identifying the nature of such nonrandom distribution we can obtain important information about why one group may be more affected than another' (Waller, 1974). In an important retrospective community investigation of 2793 respondents aged 65 and over (Prudham and Evans, 1981) the estimated annual rate of falls was 28%. This case-control comparison showed that fallers: (a) had been in more recent contact with their general practitioner; (b) had a higher prevalence of problems with mobility and daily living; (c) had a more frequent history of stroke and heart disease, more episodes of non-rotatory vertigo, double vision, faints and black-

outs, and episodes of weakness or numbness; and (d) were more likely to be taking diuretics and tranquillizers. Of the 660 respondents experiencing one or more falls in the 12 months preceding interview, 50% fell because of tripping, more than 20% were unable to give any reason, 11% reported falls due to dizziness or vertigo or loss of consciousness, and almost 10% reported their legs giving way. Almost half of those affected had had falls on more than one occasion.

While acknowledging that the majority of falls in old age result from a combination of factors, a comparison of descriptive and diagnostic classifications of 'falling syndromes' (Campbell *et al.*, 1981) has produced some interesting results and indirectly shown how difficult it is to determine precisely why old people fall. In this investigation a positive response to the question 'Do you get a feeling of dizziness or unsteadiness when you stand up suddenly after lying down?' did not correlate with either the presence of postural hypotension or with falls in 74 of 553 fallers who demonstrated a drop of 20 mmHg or more of systolic pressure on rising. In only fourteen subjects could the cause of the fall be definitely attributed to postural hypotension. Although this may have been due to the care taken on rising by many elderly patients who would otherwise have experienced symptoms, it may also be explained on the basis of adequate cerebral autoregulation of pressure as cerebral blood flow began to fall at the onset of postural hypotension. Indeed, variation in cerebral autoregulation have been shown to explain why only some elderly patients develop brain dysfunction during postural hypotension (Wollner *et al.*, 1979; see also Chapter 14). During the measurement of cerebral flow rates in eleven patients, symptoms of postural hypotension occurred only in the seven patients who had failure (four bilaterally and three unilaterally) of cerebral autoregulation. This may explain why only some elderly patients develop brain dysfunction leading to falls, strokes, confusion, or brain failure when they have impaired cardiac performance because of myocardial infarction or transient cardiac dysrhythmia. It may also explain why not all elderly patients are susceptible to the cerebral effects of hypovolaemia due to dehydration induced by diuretics, diarrhoea and vomiting, newly diagnosed or uncontrolled diabetes mellitus, and the relative hypovolaemia induced by methyldopa and other potent hypotensive agents.

Unfortunately, epidemiological studies tell us little about the pathophysiology of falls. Indeed, the transient nature of both the event and the phenomena precipitating the fall commonly leave for detection only the residuum of secondarily or even unassociated anatomical changes. It is not surprising, therefore, in the presence of only minimal external upset, falls have been assessed as arising 'primarily from a disorder of balance or postural stability in the subject' (Campbell *et al.*, 1981) and that discriminant analysis of these results could only show the principal effective 'predictors' of repeated falls in men and women consisted of persisting functional disability and the need for support services.

Against this background what practical advice can be given to doctors faced with the problem of an elderly patient who has had more than one fall in the previous 12 months?

DIAGNOSIS

Falls can be assessed in two ways, one descriptive and the other diagnostic. The former literally describes the circumstances leading up to and accompanying the fall. The latter seeks out the specific precipitating and aggravating factors that prompted particular falls. The descriptive approach can point the way towards diagnosis. Examples here include falls associated with symptoms of postural hypotension or obvious environmental hazards causing accidents as described earlier. This approach, however valuable initially, should not allow the physician to overlook equally important secondary and tertiary conditions that may summate with extrinsic factors to provoke a fall (e.g. unexpected disorientation associated with a silent or missed pneumonia). The golden rule here, as with any diagnosis in the elderly and aged, is not merely to look for a single cause but to determine how the summating effects of multiple pathology are each making a contribution and what needs to be done to tackle each one and manage the patient as a whole. For example, drug-induced parkinsonism

predisposing to a pneumonia that has triggered atrial fibrillation may result in not only silent myocardial infarction and one fall but also cerebral hypoperfusion causing confusion and further falls. The contribution of each of these several factors needs to be resolved before any superimposed and complicating lack of confidence can be corrected to enable the patient to become safely active.

All patients who have recently experienced two or more unexpected falls should have a complete physical examination supported by appropriate ancillary investigation to determine the full extent and implications for effective management of both clinically obvious and masked illnesses. Those aged over 65 years who live at home have on average 3.5 chronic diseases (Williamson *et al.*, 1964). Armed with this knowledge the doctor will not be too distracted by the patient's frailty due to underlying chronic conditions and overlook the acute and subacute illnesses that may have precipitated the patient's falls. The doctor's dilemma, however, is that any acute illness in the elderly, and particularly the aged, may predispose to, if not actually precipitate, a fall. Many such illnesses are otherwise asymptomatic or are associated with vague or non-specific symptoms. Repeated falls associated with an aged patient's failure to thrive may be dismissed as being simply due to old age complicated by 'social problems'. Under such circumstances insufficient consideration will be given to identifying and correcting underlying disease.

Falls and 'Funny Turns'

The ageing patient who is overtaken by a fall is frequently unable to give a coherent account of the event. This is not only because of the frequently sudden and unexpected nature of the episode but also because the resulting alarm and anxiety and/or the presence of confusion makes it difficult for the patient (as an untrained observer) to give the details necessary for accurate diagnosis. Moreover, after 'drop attacks' the patient may genuinely not know what happened and simply state, 'I just went down'; 'I do not know what came over me'; 'I found myself on the floor'; 'I came over queer'; or 'I had a funny turn'. If the patient's sensorium is impaired before or during the falls the terms 'giddiness', 'dizziness', or 'blackout' may be used. These need to be interpreted with caution since the patient (and even the untrained observer) may be making a rationalization that is coloured with hindsight or even proffering terms that they think most helpful to the doctor. Furthermore, patients who are susceptible to episodic losses of consciousness may not know or be able to recall that the event has occurred. There are obvious diagnostic difficulties if the patient lives alone and repeated falls are only signalled by facial bruises whose significance is lost in the absence of an alert observer. Unfortunately, the causes of 'drop attacks' and 'funny turns' are rarely found despite extensive and careful medical evaluation. It is tempting to suggest they are due to transient cerebral or brain stem ischaemia but there is no evidence for this; certainly, as an alternative diagnosis, true vertigo is a rare cause of falls in the elderly.

Episodic Losses of Consciousness
(see also Chapter 15)

Epilepsy causes only a minority of falls in the elderly. On the other hand, transient ischaemia affecting blood flow along the carotid and vertebral arteries commonly occurs in patients susceptible to falls, and, for the reasons stated above, can be difficult to recognize. While cough, micturition, and defecation syncope are easily identifiable causes of loss of consciousness, they are more likely to occur in susceptible younger patients who can more readily raise their intrathoracic pressure and impede central venous filling. The age-related pathophysiological changes predisposing to the effects of transient ischaemia and syncope in the elderly and their evaluation have been well reviewed by Lipsitz (1983); (see also Chapter 14). The role of transient ischaemia and syncope in producing falls is often overlooked because either the doctor is distracted by the presence of more obvious pathology (e.g., a stroke or a fractured femur) or an account of a classical vasovagal attack is sought and other causes of transient cerebral ischaemia are not considered. Without producing syncope, brief periods of ischaemia due to paroxysmal cardiac dysrhythmias or

other factors can produce serious transient or lingering effects in the elderly whose compensatory mechanisms may be already compromised by anaemia, cardiac disease, or a drugged cardiovascular system. The diagnosis may also be difficult because of the interrelationships between paroxysmal cardiac dysrhythmias and myocardial and cerebral ischaemia (Livesley, 1975). Prolonged ambulatory cardiographic monitoring to determine the precipitating factor for falls, syncope and dizziness in a geriatric institutional setting showed one-third of 37 falling patients had previously undetected cardiac dysrhythmias contributing to their falls and these dysrhythmias had not been picked up by standard 12-lead electrocardiography (Gordon *et al.*, 1982). This is comparable to the more than one-third incidence of previously unknown episodic arrhythmias that were severe enough to cause 'dizzy spells' and syncope in 58 consecutive aged patients admitted to hospital for fracture of the upper end of the femur (Abdon and Nilsson, 1980); and to the 50% incidence of falls due to unstable rhythm reported previously in geriatric inpatients (Livesley and Atkinson, 1974). In none of these reports were the patients investigated stated to be representative of the elderly population as a whole and the figures for falls due to paroxysmal dysrhythmias may be too high for patients living at home. If there is any doubt about the diagnosis, however, prolonged cardiographic monitoring can be very helpful in detecting remediable paroxysmal dysrhythmias as has been shown by others (McCarthy and Wollner, 1977). Atrial fibrillation occurring in the absence of recognizable cardiac disease is common in the elderly and has been regarded as benign. Recent evidence now suggests otherwise (Leading Article, 1986). Prolonged cardiac pauses have been observed even in patients with asymptomatic atrial fibrillation (Pitcher *et al.*, 1986). Whether these pauses are responsible for producing falls and other cerebral symptoms in those elderly patients with impaired cerebral autoregulation has yet to be established but it should not be forgotten that the cerebral effects of dysrhythmias may be compounded by coincidental anaemia and valvular heart disease requiring specific treatment as well as already established drug therapy which may require review.

Additional Predisposing and Precipitating Factors

Drugs

Although the immediate and hangover effects of sedatives, hypnotics, tranquillizers, and alcohol may all produce added intellectual impairment predisposing to falls, more fallers than non-fallers have been found to be taking tranquillizers but not hypnotics (Prudham and Evans, 1981). Hypoglycaemia due to chlorpropamide or insulin is an uncommon but easily correctable cause of falls. Inappropriate hypotensive therapy is a well-recognized cause of falls from postural hypotension. It is interesting to note that hypotensive therapy not associated with overt side-effects in 1002 elderly and aged ambulatory patients who were followed for almost 4 years was not reported as being correlated with falls (Stegman, 1983). The variables strongly associated with falling by these patients were reports of weakness, dizziness, and/or orthostatic hypotension. It seems distinctly possible that these symptoms were attributable to the hypotensive therapy. This consisted of diuretics only in 45% and diuretics and alpha or beta blockers in 32% of fallers. This speculation is supported by the report elsewhere that more fallers than non-fallers had been taking diuretics (Prudham and Evans, 1981).

Illness

As stated above, a fall may be the presenting feature of any acute illness and a careful examination is essential for accurate diagnosis and effective management. Repeated falls are common in patients with toxic confusional states. These may be due to drug side-effects; drug withdrawal effects (classically, alcohol but also barbiturates and diazepam); and acute infections (commonly of the respiratory and urinary tracts). Parkinson's syndrome (particularly when this is primarily of the tremor-free bradykinetic type that is common in the elderly), stroke, and peripheral neuropathy may each aggravate the frailty of the ageing and predispose to falls. Moreover, as has been reviewed by Botez and Hausser (1982), orthostatic hypotension can be associated with parkinsonian syndromes, olivopontocerebellar atrophy, and diabetic neuropathy. Falls may also be associated with normal pressure hydrocephalus and cerebral tumours including the rare colloid cyst of the third ventricle.

COMPLICATIONS OF FALLS

Injury and death are obvious and common complications of falls. In an investigation covering 2000 square miles and a population of 1.6 million people, two-thirds of fatal accidents among the elderly resulted from falls at home, the chief cause of death was head injury, and most deaths occurred within 2 weeks of admission to hospital (Copeland, 1985). It is not surprising, therefore, that falls are a source of concern not only to patients who have fallen and who think they may fall again but also to those responsible for them. This poses particular problems in institutions where, for example, 59% of 201 residents in social service (Part III) homes have been found to have one or more falls in a year and 22% of these resulted in some form of injury (Woodhouse *et al.*, 1983). Falls may not only cause fractures but also be the result of them. Stress fractures of the neck of the femur were considered to be the cause of the patient's fall in almost one-quarter of 54 consecutive patients (age range 52 to 90 years, mean 76.7 years). These patients were quite emphatic they had fallen because their hip had given way and it was considered that they had had stress fractures which later became displaced (Sloan and Holloway, 1981). These are probably related to another major problem associated with ageing—osteoporosis. The problem of falls and fractures has several components with different kinds of preventive action possible (Gloag, 1988).

CONCLUSION

Further studies on falls are essential and should be population based as has been suggested by Perry (1982). Until these results are available what advice can be offered about the strategies that might be used to reduce the risk of morbidity from falls in individuals and the investigations that should be carried out in those not seriously injured? The need—still widely unrecognized—for health care of the elderly at home is even more important now than when it was described 20 years ago (Williamson *et al.*, 1964) but the amount of work required need not be excessive if simple primary preventative care is placed in the hands of an interested and informed practice nurse or health visitor. Screening to discover and treat diseases of eyes, ears and feet should be accompanied by advice on avoiding home accidents.

An unexplained fall in old age may be associated with a fracture of the femur (Leading Article, 1978; Sloan and Holloway, 1981) or be the presenting feature of any acute illness. If there is no obvious or serious injury the practitioner should first determine whether the event was due to an accident, an incident, or an illness. Accidents may be due to preventable hazards including visual deterioration and drug effects. Incidents are common in institutions during changes in posture or position, notably while using the toilet or transferring between bed and chair, and may be the early sign of an inevitably increasing dependency from unavoidable physical and mental decline. Unexpected falls, however, require investigation. Obvious acute illness indicates its own treatment, but in other cases remediable precipitating factors should be sought carefully. These include postural hypotension (arguably the most important indication for using the sphygmomanometer in the very elderly), transient cardiac arrhythmias, and drug effects (Berry *et al.*, 1981).

Secondary prevention after a fall may require adjustments to the home (adequate and accessible lighting, particularly of stairs and toilets used at night) as well as physiotherapy assessment with a view to correcting easily acquired disuse atrophy of those muscle groups responsible for controlling posture and gait. The simple, but equally important, use of kind and optimistic reassurance to restore confidence after a fall frequently plays a major role in restoring independence (Livesley, 1984).

APPENDIX: GUIDELINES FOR THE MANAGEMENT OF FALLS

The key to successful management is to determine if specific precipitating, aggravating, and predisposing factors can be identified and prevented.

Questions to Ask to Assist Diagnosis

Did the patient trip, slip, or just fall down?
Has this been a one-off event or have there been previous falls?
Was the event due to (a) an incident, (b) an accident, or (c) an illness?

Action points

(a) Incidents commonly occur in chronically frail elderly people who are simply changing their bodily position or posture.
(b) Accidents are commonly associated with preventable environmental hazards (unlit stairs, slippery surfaces, loose carpets, etc.); *but* the effects of these may be aggravated by impaired perception due to drugs, alcohol, masked acute illness, mental confusion.
(c) Acute illness in the elderly and particularly the aged is commonly masked by an obvious inability to cope with the normal activities of daily living. Under these circumstances too much attention may be paid to the obvious bruise or fracture associated with the fall, and the predisposing acute pneumonia, myocardial infarction, transient cardiac dysrhythmia, stroke, etc., may be overlooked; as may *continuing illness* due to failing eyesight and inappropriate drug therapies (including diuretics, too potent hypotensive agents, hypoglycaemic agents, etc.).

Questions to Ask to Assist Management

After a fall what treatment may be required?
What aftercare is necessary?

Action points

Clinical management of the underlying illnesses.
Physiotherapy including management of strokes and other acquired gait abnormalities.
Occupational therapy assessment followed by simple practical advice to improve safety of normal activities of daily living.
Social casework if appropriate with advice to patients and family about the options for future social supports (including services available at home and, if necessary, alternative types of accommodation).
Review to modify and, as appropriate, withdraw drug therapies, physiotherapy and occupational therapy, and social services that are no longer required.

REFERENCES

Abdon, N.J., and Nilsson, B.E. (1980). Episodic cardiac arrhythmia and femoral neck fracture. *Acta Med. Scand.*, **208**, 73–6.

Archer, V. (1985). *Home Accident Data for the Use in Junior Schools*, Consumer Safety Unit, Department of Trade and Industry, London.

Ashley, M.J., Gryfe, C.I., and Amies, A. (1977). A longitudinal study of falls in an elderly population. II. Some circumstances of falling. *Age Ageing*, **6**, 211–20.

Backett, E.M. (1965). *Domestic Accidents*, WHO, Geneva.

Berry, G., Fisher, R.H., and Lang, S. (1981). Detrimental incidents, including falls, in an elderly institutional population. *J. Am. Geriatr. Soc.*, **29**, 322–4.

Botez, M.I., and Hausser, H.O. (1982). Falls. *Br. J. Hosp. Med.*, **28**, 494–503.

Brocklehurst, J.C., Robertson, D., and James-Groom, P. (1982). Clinical correlates of sway in old age—sensory modalities. *Age Ageing*, **11**, 1–10.

Brocklehurst, J.C., Exton-Smith, A.N., Lempert Barber, S.M., Hunt, L.P., and Palmer, M.K. (1978). Fracture of the femur in old age: A two-centre study of associated clinical factors and the cause of the fall. *Age Ageing*, **7**, 7–15.

Brody, E.M., Kleban, M.H., Moss, M.S., and Kleban, F. (1984). Predictors of falls among institutionalized women with Alzheimer's Disease. *J. Am. Geriatr. Soc.*, **32**, 877–82.

Campbell, A.J., Reinken, J., Allen, B.C., and Martinez, G.S. (1981). Falls in old age: A study of frequency and related clinical factors. *Age Ageing*, **10**, 264–70.

Castle, O.M. (1950). Accidents in the home. *Lancet*, **1**, 315–19.

Chipman, C. (1981). What does it mean when a patient falls? Part I: Pinpointing the cause. *Geriatrics*, **36**, 83–5.

Clark, A.N.G. (1968). Factors in fracture of the female femur: A clinical study of the environmental, physical, medical and preventative aspects of this injury. *Gerontol. Clin.*, **10**, 257–70.

Copeland, A.R. (1985). Fatal accidental falls among the elderly—the Metro Dade County experience. *Med. Sci. Law*, **25**, 172–5.

Droller, H. (1955). Falls among elderly people living at home. *Geriatrics*, **10**, 239–44.

Duthie, E.H., and Gambert, S.R. (1983). Accident and fall prevention in the elderly. *Wiscon. Med. J.*, **82**, 23–5.

Exton-Smith, A.N. (1977). Functional consequences of ageing: clinical manifestations. In: Exton-Smith, A.N., and Evans, J.G. (eds.) *Care of the Elderly: Meeting the Challenge of Dependency*. Academic Press, London, pp. 47–9.

Fernie, G.R., Gryfe, C.I., Holliday, P.J., and Llewellyn, A. (1982). The relationship of postural sway in standing to the incidence of falls in geriatric subjects. *Age Ageing*, **11**, 11–16.

Fine, W. (1959). An analysis of 277 falls in hospital. *Gerontol. Clin.*, **1**, 298–300.

Gabell, A., Simons, M.A., and, Nayak, U.S.L. (1985). Falls in the healthy elderly: Predisposing causes. *Ergonomics*, **28**, 965–75.

Gloag, D. (1988). Strategies for accident prevention: a review. In: Livesley, B. (ed.) *Strategies for Accident Prevention: a Colloquium*, HMSO, London, p. 74.

Gordon, M., Huang, M., and Gryfe, C.I. (1982). An evaluation of falls, syncope, and dizziness by prolonged ambulatory cardiographic monitoring in a geriatric institutional setting. *J. Am. Geriatr. Soc.*, **30**, 6–12.

Gryfe, C.I., Amies, A., and Ashley, M.J. (1977). A longitudinal study of falls in an elderly population. I. Incidence and morbidity. *Age Ageing*, **6**, 201–10.

Guimaraes, R.M., and Isaacs, B. (1980). Characteristics of the gait in old people who fall. *Int. Rehab. Med.*, **2**, 177–80.

Kalchthaler, T., Bascon, R.A., and Quintos, V. (1978). Falls in the institutionalised elderly. *J. Am. Geriatr. Soc.*, **26**, 424–8.

Leading Article (1978). Falls and femoral fractures. *Br. Med. J.*, **ii**, 522.

Leading Article (1986). Is lone atrial fibrillation really benign? *Lancet*, **i**, 305–6.

Lipsitz, L.A. (1983). Syncope in the elderly. *Ann. Intern. Med.*, **99**, 92–105.

Livesley, B. (1975). The resolution of the Heberden-Parry controversy. *Med. Hist.*, **19**, 158–71.

Livesley, B. (1984). Falls in older age. *Br. Med. J.*, **289**, 568.

Livesley, B., and Atkinson, L. (1974). Repeated falls in the elderly. *Mod. Geriatr.*, **4**, 458–67.

Lucht, U. (1971). A prospective study of accidental falls and resulting injuries in the home among elderly people. *Acta Soc. Med. Scand.*, **2**, 105–20.

McCarthy, S.T., and Wollner, L. (1977). Cardiac dysrhythmias: A treatable cause of transient cerebral dysfunction in the elderly. *Lancet*, **ii**, 202–3.

Macqueen, I.A. (1960). *Home Accidents in Aberdeen*, Livingstone, London.

Margulec, I., Librach, G., and Schadel, M. (1970). Epidemiological study of accidents among residents of homes for the aged. *J. Gerontol.*, **25**, 342–6.

Miller, M.B., and Elliott, D.F. (1979). Accidents in nursing homes: Implications for patients and administrators. In: Miller, M.B. (ed.) *Current Issues in Clinical Geriatrics*, Tiresias Press, New York, pp. 97–137.

Morfitt, J.M. (1983). Falls in old people at home: Intrinsic versus environmental factors in causation. *Public Health Lond.*, **97**, 115–20.

Morgan, V.R., Mathison, J.H., Rice, J.C., and Clemmer, D.I. (1985). 'Hospital falls: A persistent problem', *Am. J. Public Health*, **75**, 775–7.

Naylor, R., and Rosin, A.J. (1970). Falling as a cause of admission to a geriatric unit. *Practitioner*, **205**, 327–30.

Overstall, P.W., Exton-Smith, A.N., Imms, F.J., and Johnson, A.L. (1977). Falls in the elderly related to postural imbalance. *Br. Med. J.*, **1**, 261–4.

Pablo, R.Y. (1977). Patient accidents in a long-term-care facility. *Can. J. Public Health*, **68**, 237–47.

Perry, B.C. (1982). Falls among the elderly: A review of the methods and conclusions of epidemiologic studies. *J. Am. Geriatr. Soc.*, **30**, 367–71.

Pitcher, D., Papouchado, M., James, M.A., and Rees, J.R. (1986). Twenty four hour ambulatory electrocardiography in patients with chronic atrial fibrillation. *Br. Med. J.*, **292**, 594.

Prudham, D., and Evans, J.G. (1981). Factors associated with falls in the elderly: A community study. *Age Ageing*, **10**, 141–6.

Rodstein, M. (1964). Accidents among the aged: incidence, causes, and prevention. *Chron. Dis.*, **17**, 515–26.

Rodstein, M., and Camus, A.S. (1973). Interrelation of heart disease and accidents. *Geriatrics*, **28**, 87–96.

Sehested, P., and Severin-Neilsen, T. (1977). Falls by hospitalised elderly patients: Causes, prevention. *Geriatrics*, **32**, 101–8.

Seiler, H.E., and Ramsay, C.B. (1954). Home accidents. *Practitioner*, **172**, 628–36.

Sheldon, J.H. (1948). *The Social Medicine of Old Age*, Oxford University Press, London, pp. 96–104.

Sheldon, J.H. (1960). On the natural history of falls in old age. *Br. Med. J.*, **ii**, 1685–90.

Sheldon, J.H. (1963). The effects of age on the control of sway. *Gerontol. Clin.*, **5**, 129–38.

Sloan, J., and Holloway, G. (1981). Fractured neck of the femur: the cause of the fall? *Injury*, **13**, 230–2.

Stegman, M.R. (1983). Falls among elderly hypotensives—Are they iatrogenic? *Gerontology*, **29**, 399–406.

Tobis, J.S., Nyak, L., and Hoehler, F. (1981). Visual perception of verticality and horizontality among elderly fallers. *Arch. Phys. Med. Rehab.*, **62**, 619–22.

Uden, G. (1985). Inpatient accidents in hospitals. *J. Am. Geriatr. Soc.*, **33**, 833–41.

Waller, J.A. (1974). Injury in aged: Clinical and epidemiological implications. *N.Y. State J. Med.*, **74**, 2200–8.

Williamson, J., Stokoe, I.H., Gray, S., Fisher, M., Smith, A., McGhee, A., and Stephenson, E. (1964). Old people at home: Their unreported needs. *Lancet*, **i**, 1117–20.

Wollner, L., McCarthy, S.T., Soper, N.D.W., and Macy, D.J. (1979). Failure of cerebral autoregulation as a cause of brain dysfunction in the elderly. *Br. Med. J.*, **i**, 1117–18.

Woodhouse, P.R., Briggs, R.S., and Ward, D. (1983). Falls and disability in old people's homes. *J. Clin. Exp. Gerontol.*, **5**, 308–21.

Chapter 29

Headaches and Facial Pain

James Howe

Consultant Physician in Medicine for the Elderly, Airedale General Hospital, Steeton, Keighley, West Yorkshire, UK

People seem to complain less about headache as they grow older. Zeigler *et al.* (1977) found that only 1% of the population over 65 which they sampled had started to complain of severe headache in the previous year and only 18% of the men and 29% of the women over 65 complained of disabling or severe headaches. However, there are three causes of head pain which become more common with increasing age: temporal arteritis (TA), trigeminal neuralgia (TN) and post-herpetic neuralgia (PHN); and the elderly are not immune to pain caused by other pathological processes in the head and neck.

In many studies, the prevalence of both migraine and headache declines after middle age (Goldstein and Chen, 1982) and it is interesting to note that Leviton *et al.* (1974) reported a slightly higher risk of death before age 70 for migraine sufferers. The generally accepted interpretation is that migraine is a self-limiting disorder and gradually disappears after middle age. It does not disappear altogether, for Whitty and Hockaday (1968) reviewed a group of patients with migraine who had attended a hospital outpatient clinic up to 20 years before and found that half of them were still having migraine attacks after the age of 65.

Headache may be less common in the elderly, but it is not unknown and presents a diagnostic challenge which can generally be solved with a careful history. Blau (1982) and Lance (1978) have provided helpful articles on taking a history from headache patients.

When attempting a differential diagnosis of headache and facial pain, two things are of most practical value: a simple mental picture of the pain sensitive structures in the head and the sensory pathways; and an analysis of the time course of the pain. It is particularly helpful to imagine and review all the tissues and organs in the solid part of the head that would be sliced off by a cut from the vertex to the chin, remembering that they are all innervated by the trigeminal nerve (Figure 29.1) (DeMyer, 1980). In fact, all structures above the tentorium cerebelli are innervated by the trigeminal nerve (Figure 29.2). For a complete review of the pain pathways and mechanisms of headache, the reader is referred to Lance (1982).

INTRACRANIAL PAIN

The brain itself, the ependymal lining of the ventricles, the choroid plexus and much of the dura and pia-arachnoid are insensitive to pain. Distortion of cranial nerves which carry pain fibres will give rise to pain, but the most important structures inside the head which register pain are the blood vessels: the proximal parts of the cerebral and dural arteries and the large veins and venous sinuses. Distortion of, traction on, or inflammation in, these vessels gives rise to sensations of pain. Thus expanding lesions, expansion of the ventricles, cerebral oedema or low lumbar CSF pressure with subsequent shifting of the

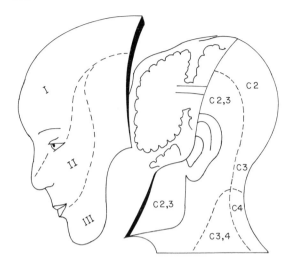

Figure 29.1. All structures in the part sliced off send impulses via the trigeminal nerve. (*Reproduced from DeMeyer (1980) by permission of McGraw-Hill Book Company.*)

brain when the body is upright can all cause pain. Because of this vascular origin, all forms of intra-cranial head pain tend to throb with the pulse and are made worse by any sudden jolt, coughing, sneezing or straining.

Pain from supratentorial structures is referred to the anterior two-thirds of the head via the trigeminal nerve and pain from infratentorial structures is referred to the back of the head and top of the neck via the upper cervical roots (Figure 29.2), (Lance, 1982).

PAIN FROM EXTRACRANIAL ARTERIES

The scalp arteries are also sensitive to stretching and inflammation and pain is felt in the immediate neighbourhood.

PAIN FROM THE SKULL, SINUSES, EYES, TEETH AND NECK

The cranial periosteum is sensitive and pain is usually felt locally. Pain from the eyes, sinuses and teeth is felt locally at first but may then be referred to the appropriate division of the trigeminal nerve and, if severe, overflow to other divisions. If local pain

continues, diffuse headache from contraction of head and neck muscles follows. Degenerative changes, inflammation or neoplasia in the upper cervical spine may affect structures innervated by the first, second and third cervical nerve roots with reference of pain to the back of the head. Stimulation of the first, inconstant, cervical nerve root can give rise to frontal and orbital pain in man but stimulation of the second cervical root does not do so (Kerr, 1961).

As well as reviewing possible causes of head pain anatomically, analysis based on the time pattern of the pain is most useful in any age group (Lance, 1978).

ACUTE SINGLE EPISODES OF HEADACHE

Subarachnoid haemorrhage, meningitis and encephalitis, sinus and middle ear infection present in this way. The pain from an acute attack of closed angle glaucoma is usually localized to the eye but is referred to surrounding areas and may be overlooked if mistings of vision and pupillary changes are not sought (Behrens, 1976).

The headache that follows a head injury must be distinguished from the pain due to cerebral compression and distortion by extradural or subdural haematoma. Progressive impairment of consciousness and unilateral third nerve palsy, with pupillary dilatation, are signs of transtentorial herniation which must not be missed if neurosurgical action is to be initiated in time. The use of the Glasgow Coma Scale should help to prevent this (Teasdale and Jennett, 1974).

An attack of herpes zoster can cause severe pain before the rash appears, but the rash usually follows quickly.

ACUTE RECURRENT EPISODES OF HEAD PAIN

In the elderly these are much less likely to be due to migraine or 'tension headache' than in younger age groups. More than one episode of meningitis should prompt a search for CSF leakage, particularly from the nose. Repeated episodes of subarachnoid haemorrhage due to angiomas rather than aneurysms may occur and lead to hydrocephalus with

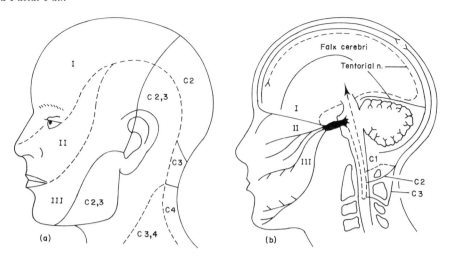

Figure 29.2. (a) Cutaneous distribution of the trigeminal nerve to the face and anterior two-thirds of the scalp, showing the watershed with the cervical nerves above the ear line (after Cunningham). (b). Schematic representation of the three divisions of the trigeminal nerve, the gasserian ganglion and the upper cervical nerve roots. Attention is drawn to three interrupted lines. One line indicates the path taken by the spinal tract and nucleus of the trigeminal nerve as it descends into the upper cervical segments of the cord. Afferent fibres from the first, second and third cervical nerve roots and the trigeminal pathway converge upon the same cells in the posterior horns of the spinal cord, thus permitting referral of pain from neck to head and vice versa. The crossed second-order neurones pass upwards to the thalamus. Another interrupted line indicates the course of the tentorial nerve. The first cervical nerve root is represented by an interrupted line because it is inconstant. (*Reproduced from Lance (1982) by permission of Butterworth.*)

walking difficulty, cognitive impairment, clouding of consciousness and incontinence.

Intermittent hydrocephalus due to an intraventricular tumour is a very rare cause of headache at any age. The headache is usually severe and accompanied by vomiting, collapse and impaired consciousness and may occur with sudden change of position.

Trigeminal and glossopharyngeal neuralgia have such a unique pattern there is usually little difficulty in recognizing them and they are discussed in more detail below.

The pattern of 'cluster headache' is also distinct, with unilateral, severe pain around an eye, lasting from approximately 15 minutes to 2 hours each day, though it can occur more than once a day and continue daily in bouts lasting for a few weeks at a time. Watering of the eye and nasal blockage on the affected side are characteristic and though this condition is usually seen in younger patients, it can occur in the elderly.

In patients with ischaemic stroke or transient ischaemic attacks, headache sometimes occurs but is usually mild, and focal neurological symptoms and signs will be much more prominent (Edmeads, 1979a; Lance, 1981; Grindal and Toole, 1974). The pain of myocardial ischaemia can be referred to the neck and face.

HEADACHES OF SUBACUTE ONSET

Progressively severe head pain in someone who is not usually subject to it raises the possibility of a space-occupying lesion inside the head. When accompanied by progressive signs pointing to a single lesion, a space-occupying lesion must be presumed until excluded. Primary and secondary tumours, abscesses and subdural collections of blood, all occur in older patients. Forty three per cent of patients with subdural haematoma in one series had headache (Cameron, 1978). In the elderly, headache and papilloedema are not such prominent features in the presentation of intracranial tumours. Godfrey and Caird (1984) found only 10% of their patients with tumours had headache and only 2.5% had papilloedema. Tumours and osteomyelitis involving the bones of the skull and cervical spine must also be considered. Headache is a prominent feature in meningeal involvement with tumour, often combined with cranial nerve signs and mental changes (Wasserstrom *et al.*, 1978). Nasopharyngeal tumours can also present with pain in the face and may be accompanied by cranial nerve signs, particularly involvement of the fifth and sixth cranial nerves and epistaxis.

Paget's disease of the skull can also cause head pain, as well as involvement of cranial nerves, most commonly producing deafness. Craniovertebral distortion due to basilar invagination in Paget's disease can also cause progressive ataxia and spasticity, but the diagnosis is usually obvious (Friedman *et al.*, 1971).

Temporal arteritis presents with a gradually progressive headache and will be discussed more fully below, as will post-herpetic neuralgia.

Intracranial vasodilatation such as occurs in carbon dioxide retention in chronic obstructive airways disease or with vasodilator drugs, such as nifedipine, can produce headache, sometimes severe. Any febrile disorder may be accompanied by headache, but this is usually mild.

Carbon monoxide poisoning causes headache and confusion progressing to coma and old people who live in poorly ventilated rooms with old or poorly maintained gas appliances are at risk. Hyperbaric oxygen should be given even if there is a delay in starting treatment (Danel and Barret, 1984; James, 1984; Ziser *et al.*, 1984).

Pain from eye disease has been mentioned in connection with acute glaucoma. Pain from uveitis is usually clearly localized to the eye, though it may also radiate over the forehead (Behrens, 1976).

It is usually obvious that a dentist is needed to deal with pain from infected teeth or retained roots, but occasionally dental pain may be mistaken for trigeminal neuralgia. With dental infection there is usually a continuous background of pain and tapping the tooth rather than touching the gum will trigger pain in dental disease but is unlikely to do so in trigeminal neuralgia.

Pain in the temporomandibular joint is very rarely due to rheumatoid or degenerative arthritis. Pain on moving the jaw as in eating or talking is more likely to be due to temporal arteritis ('jaw claudication'), trigeminal neuralgia, dental infection or suppurative parotitis (Cawson, 1984). Parotitis can cause severe distress and dehydrated, ill, elderly people, particularly when on anticholinergic drugs such as tricyclic antidepressants, are particularly at risk (Hodkinson and Gunther, 1972).

Degenerative arthropathy in the neck is universal in older people, yet they seem to complain very little about neck pain. When severe neck pain does occur in an elderly person, secondary carcinoma should be excluded (Edmeads, 1979a).

Finally, some depressed patients complain of headache. Depression in the elderly is more likely to generate somatic complaints, being associated with an increase in hypochondriasis (*Lancet*, 1984).

INVESTIGATION

After a careful history and clinical examination, the necessary tests should be carried out. The erythrocyte sedimentation rate (ESR) should be done in all elderly patients with headache and plain X-rays of the skull, sinuses or neck bones may be needed. Computed tomography (CT) should not be ruled out on grounds of age alone as palliative treatment of tumours and hydrocephalus is successful in the elderly, subdural haematomas can be removed, infections cured and Paget's disease treated (Graham and Caird, 1978; Godfrey and Caird, 1984; Cameron, 1978).

It is beyond the scope of this chapter to discuss in detail the management of all the causes of head pain, but the three conditions which are particularly important in the elderly will be discussed in detail.

TEMPORAL ARTERITIS (see also Chapter 12)

This is a collagen vascular disease that occurs most often in people over 55 years of age. Women are affected four times as frequently as men and the approximate annual incidence is 6/100 000 rising to 55/100 000 in those over 80 (Murray, 1977; Hauser *et al.*, 1971; Huston *et al.*, 1978; Jonasson *et al.*, 1979; Bengtsson and Malmvall, 1981).

It is a granulomatous form of arteritis which affects medium-sized vessels and the temporal and ophthalmic arteries are usually involved bilaterally. Any of the branches of the aorta may be involved, including the coronary, sub-clavian and renal arteries (Wilkinson and Russell, 1972). The inner layers of the media are infiltrated by lymphocytes, plasma cells, eosinophils, macrophages and the characteristic giant cells. Necrosis and connective tissue repair are seen in lesions. Although the vessel may be totally occluded, recanalization can occur. The temporal artery is usually affected throughout its length, but lesions may involve only short sections (Klein *et al.*, 1976) giving negative biopsy results if too short a piece of artery is removed.

Immunoglobulin deposition has been demonstrated in affected arteries but its significance is not clear and the aetiology of the condition is unknown (Liang *et al.*, 1974).

The clinical picture is well known: Patients with temporal arteritis look and feel dejected and unwell. There may be low grade pyrexia and the course is one of progressive deterioration. Huston *et al.* (1978) found headache in 90% of sufferers, tenderness of the temporal artery in 70% and generalized muscle aching, stiffness and mild weakness (polymyalgia) in 50%. In this series, 70% of patients complained of pain in the masseter and temporal muscles during talking and eating—'jaw claudication'. Weight loss was noted in 55%. The temporal artery pulse was absent in only 40%. They recorded visual symptoms in 40% of patients, but the risk of visual impairment in untreated patients is said to be as high as 50% (Murray, 1977). Despite early diagnosis and corticosteroid treatment, visual impairment still occurs in up to 13% of sufferers (Klein *et al.*, 1976).

The ESR is usually high, often over 100 mm/hour, but an ESR of less than 40 mm/hour was found in nearly 30% of biopsy positive cases in one series (Kansu *et al.*, 1976).

Temporal artery biopsy is recommended in all suspected cases since steroid treatment will be needed for a long time. A generous section of artery should be taken. Treatment must be started immediately because of the risk to vision. Allison and

Gallagher (1984) found that 60% of biopsies were still positive after 7 days of steroid treatment. However, the same workers found 18% of biopsies were negative before treatment in clinically typical cases with a high ESR. The risk of blindness, the occurrence of biopsy proven cases with a normal ESR and negative biopsies in clinically definite cases make a high index of suspicion for temporal arteritis essential in any elderly patient with headache, general malaise or polymyalgia.

Temporal artery biopsy in patients who have only polymyalgia rheumatica is said to show arteritis in up to 50% (Fauchald *et al.*, 1972). The development of clinically apparent arteritis in patients with polymyalgia whose symptoms were relieved by non-steroidal anti-inflammatory drugs has been recorded (Easterbrook *et al.*, 1976).

Loss of vision is usually sudden and complete and can be bilateral. Both temporal arteritis and polymyalgia rheumatica require urgent treatment and prednisone 60 mg daily for 5 days will usually control symptoms. Hunder *et al.* (1975) compared daily and alternate day regimens and found that alternate day treatment was less satisfactory in controlling symptoms. If symptoms are completely controlled after 5 days, the dose of prednisone can be reduced to 45 mg daily for 2 weeks and then by 5 mg every 2 weeks to a maintenance dose of 10 to 15 mg daily, depending on the clinical response and the ESR. Relapse is common when steroids are stopped and maintenance treatment should be continued for at least 2 years (Huston *et al.*, 1978; Hunder *et al.*, 1975). The management of temporal arteritis when visual loss has already occurred is discussed in Chapter 23.

TRIGEMINAL NEURALGIA
(see also Chapter 22)

This is a common cause of severe pain and distress which becomes more common in older age groups (Lance, 1981). Irritation of the trigeminal nerve at the point where it enters the pons causes sudden, brief, intolerable stabbing pains. The lightning explosions of pain are often triggered by minimal cutaneous stimuli at particular places, a light touch on the cheek, a breath of wind, food touching the gum, blowing the nose. Triggering of pain like this will prevent a patient with trigeminal neuralgia washing, shaving or eating properly during an episode. The pain rarely attacks all three sensory divisions of the nerve and the first division is less often affected than the other two (Fromm *et al.*, 1984). The presence of sensory loss or motor weakness should arouse suspicion of a progressive structural lesion affecting the nerve or nucleus.

Glossopharyngeal neuralgia is much rarer. The pattern of pain is similar to trigeminal neuralgia though triggered and felt in the throat, sometimes radiating to the ear. Involvement of vagal fibres may cause autonomic symptoms such as syncope or bradycardia (Rushton *et al.*, 1981).

Dandy (1934) was first to draw attention to lesions distorting the trigeminal nerve and noted that the superior cerebellar artery was most often responsible. Janetta (1976) using microsurgical techniques during posterior fossa craniotomy in patients with trigeminal neuralgia concluded that all trigeminal neuralgia is symptomatic rather than 'idiopathic'. In 100 consecutive patients he found six tumours, vascular compression in 88 and evidence of multiple sclerosis in six (trigeminal neuralgia in patients under age 40 is most often due to multiple sclerosis (Paty and Poser, 1984)). Progressive elongation and tortuosity of arterial loops with advancing age seems to account for the increased prevalence in old age.

The pain of trigeminal neuralgia can be suppressed with anticonvulsant drugs such as carbamazepine, phenytoin and clonazepam (Lance, 1981). The present author has found clobazam effective and easier to use in frail, elderly patients who are intolerant of the other drugs because of ataxia. Baclofen has also been used with some success (Fromm *et al.*, 1980).

In the elderly a low starting dose and gradual increases in dose are essential if dangerous ataxia is to be avoided with carbamazepine and phenytoin.

When drugs are ineffective, microvascular decompression of the trigeminal nerve is effective in over 90% of patients (Janetta *et al.*, 1976; Richards *et al.*, 1983). However, this requires a posterior fossa craniotomy. For patients too frail or unwilling to undergo this procedure, thermocoagulation of the ganglion is a faster and simpler procedure and is successful in relieving neuralgia in approximately 90% of patients, though approximately 2% are left with troublesome dysaesthesia (Sweet and Wepsic, 1974).

POST-HERPETIC NEURALGIA
(see also Chapters 19 and 22)

Not only does the incidence of herpes zoster rise exponentially with increase in age, affecting half of those who reach age 85 (Hope-Simpson, 1965) but the number of patients still suffering pain one year after the acute attack follows the same trend. More than 60% of those aged over 70 with involvement of the trigeminal nerve, which is the dermatome most commonly affected, and nearly 50% of those over 70 who have shingles elsewhere on the body report persisting pain one year after the acute attack (de Moragas and Kierland, 1957). The pain is felt in the dermatome affected by the rash. It can be agonizing and persistent, usually described as 'burning' with increased, painful and abnormal sensitivity to any stimulus in the affected area. Stabbing neuralgic type pain may also occur and sufferers quickly become demoralized and depressed. The severity and duration of pain is worse in the elderly (Rogers and Tindall, 1971). Since the number of patients who continue to suffer pain after the skin lesions have healed gradually declines, the duration of pain that marks the transition from acute to post-herpetic neuralgia is arbitrary, but important, so that therapeutic regimens can be compared (Portenoy *et al.*, 1986). These authors suggest that pain continuing 2 months after the onset of the rash should be labelled post-herpetic neuralgia. Their paper provides an authoritative and up to date account of the pathophysiology and management of this condition.

Recently, oral and intravenous acyclovir have been shown to speed resolution and reduce the pain of the acute attack and studies are in progress to see if this treatment also reduces post-herpetic neuralgia (McKendrick *et al.*, 1986). Acyclovir should certainly be used in all elderly patients with trigeminal herpes zoster and possibly in all elderly patients with shingles.

It is not clear whether corticosteroids should be used at the time of the acute attack. Elliot (1964) first suggested this and Portenoy *et al.* (1986) recommend it. The only controlled study by Eaglstein *et al.* (1970) showed that the number of patients with pain persisting at 1 year was the same whether given steroids or not, though fewer had pain at 2 months. Worries about the use of steroids were raised by reports of dissemination of the rash in steroid treated patients, but this seems to have been reported only in seriously immunocompromised patients already on steroid treatment (Merselis *et al.*, 1964). My own practice is to give steroids and acyclovir to patients with ophthalmic herpes, those with severe pain, extensive skin lesions and motor or autonomic involvement.

In the patient with established post-herpetic neuralgia, a comprehensive and straightforward treatment plan has been laid out by Portenoy *et al.* (1986) and their scheme can be readily implemented at a day hospital. They recommend the simultaneous prescription of a tricyclic antidepressant (Watson *et al.*, 1982), physical therapy to increase activity, build confidence and improve function and transcutaneous electrical nerve stimulation (TENS). The response to TENS is variable and different electrode placements and stimulation protocols should be tried before abandoning it. Small portable stimulators are inexpensive, reliable and useful in other pain syndromes and should be available in every geriatric department.

If dysaesthesia or triggering of painful paroxysms are features, then anticonvulsants are helpful (Killian and Fromm, 1968). Portenoy *et al.* (1986) emphasize the importance of psychological, functional and social approaches to management from the start. Putting the patient back in control of at least some aspect of his disorder is helpful in this as in other chronic disorders. Teaching methods of relaxation and distraction and encouraging and measuring increasing levels of physical and social activity by using a diary are recommended. The provision of an anaesthetic spray with instructions on 'counter-irritation' by brisk rubbing of the affected area or a TENS apparatus to use at home are ways in which the patient can regain some control over the symptoms. Portenoy *et al.* conclude that neurolytic techniques should be avoided in post-herpetic neuralgia and that surgical measures are also generally unhelpful.

CONCLUSION

Head pain may not be common in the elderly and diagnosis may be made more difficult by problems with communication and multiple pathology, but successful treatment is possible in most patients. Pain developing over a short period and increasing in severity, especially if associated with neurological signs, demands immediate investigation. The pattern of pain in the more common conditions is usually characteristic and effective treatment is available.

REFERENCES

Allison, M.C., and Gallaher, P.J. (1984). Temporal artery biopsy and corticosteroid treatment. *Ann. Rheum. Dis.*, **43**, 416–17.

Behrens, M.M. (1976). Headaches and head pains associated with diseases of the eye. *Res. Clin. Stud. Headache*, **4**, 18–36.

Bengtsson, B.A., and Malmvall, B.E. (1981). The epidemiology of giant cell arteritis including temporal arteritis and polymyalgia rheumatica: incidences of different clinical presentations and eye complications. *Arthritis Rheum.*, **24**, 899–904.

Blau, J.N. (1982). How to take a history of head or facial pain. *Br. Med. J.*, **285**, 1249–51.

Cameron, M.M. (1978). Chronic subdural haematoma: A review of 114 cases. *J. Neurol. Neurosurg. Psychiatry*, **41**, 834–9.

Cawson, R.A. (1984). Pain in the temporomandibular joint. *Br. Med. J.*, **288**, 1857–8.

Dandy, W.E. (1934). Concerning the cause of trigeminal neuralgia. *Am. J. Surg.*, **24**, 447–55.

Danel, V., and Barret, L. (1984). Late sequelae of carbon monoxide poisoning. *Lancet*, **ii**, 637–8.

de Moragas, J.M., and Kierland, R.R. (1957). The outcome of patients with herpes zoster. *Arch. Dermatol.*, **75**, 193–6.

DeMyer, W. (1980). *Technique of the Neurologic Examination*, third edition, McGraw-Hill, New York, p. 291.

Eaglstein, W.H., Katz, R., and Brown, J.A. (1970). The effects of early corticosteroid therapy on the skin eruption and pain of herpes zoster. *J.A.M.A.*, **211**, 1681–3.

Easterbrook, W.M., Baxter, D.W., and Martin, J.R. (1967). Temporal arteritis developing during indomethacin therapy of polymyalgia rheumatica. *Can. Med. Assoc. J.*, **97**, 296.

Edmeads, J. (1979a). Headaches and head pains associated with diseases of the cervical spine. *Med. Clin. North Am.*, **62**, 533–44.

Edmeads, J. (1979b). The headaches of ischaemic cerebrovascular disease. *Headache*, **19**, 345–9.

Elliot, F.A. (1964). Treatment of herpes zoster with high dose prednisone. *Lancet*, **ii**, 610–11.

Fauchald, P., Rygvold, O., and Oystese, B. (1972). Temporal arteritis and polymyalgia rheumatica: Clinical and biopsy findings. *Ann. Intern. Med.*, **77**, 845–52.

Friedman, P., Sklaver, N., and Klawans, H.L. (1971). Neurological manifestations of Paget's disease of the skull. *Dis. Nerv. Syst.*, **32**, 809–17.

Fromm, G.H., Terrence, G.F., and Maroon, J.C. (1984). Trigeminal neuralgia: Current concepts regarding aetiology and pathogenesis. *Arch. Neurol.*, **41**, 1204–7.

Fromm, G.H., Terrence, G.F., Chatta, A.S., and Glass, J.D. (1980). Baclofen in the treatment of refractory trigeminal neuralgia. *Arch. Neurol.*, **37**, 768–71.

Godfrey, J.B., and Caird, F.I. (1984). Intracranial tumours in the elderly: Diagnosis and treatment. *Age Ageing*, **13**, 152–8.

Goldstein, M., and Chen, T.C. (1982). The epidemiology of disabling headache. In: Critchley, M., Friedman, A.P., Gorini, S., and Sicuteri, F. (eds) *Headache, Advances in Neurology*, Vol. 33, Raven Press, New York, pp. 377–90.

Graham, K., and Caird, F.I. (1978). High dose steroid therapy of intracranial tumour in the elderly. *Age Ageing*, **7**, 146–50.

Grindal, A.B., and Toole, J.F. (1984). Headache and transient ischaemic attacks. *Stroke*, **5**, 603–6.

Hauser, W.A., Ferguson, R.H., and Holley, K.E. (1971). Temporal arteritis in Rochester, Minnesota, 1951–1967. *Mayo Clin. Proc.*, **46**, 597.

Hodkinson, H.M., and Gunther, H.N.C. (1972). Drug factors in acute suppurative salivary gland infection. *Age Ageing*, **1**, 38.

Hope-Simpson, R.E. (1965). The nature of herpes zoster: a long-term study and a new hypothesis. *Proc. R. Soc. Lond. (Biol.)*, **58**, 9–20.

Hunder, G.G., Sheps, S.G., Allen, G.I., and Yoyce, J.W. (1975). Daily and alternate day corticosteroid regimens in treatment of giant cell arteritis: Comparison in a prospective study. *Ann. Intern. Med.*, **82**, 613–18.

Huston, K.A., Hunder, G.G., and Lie, J.T. (1978). A 25 year epidemiologic, clinical and pathological study in temporal arteritis. *Ann. Intern. Med.*, **88**, 162–7.

James, P.B. (1984). Carbon monoxide poisoning. *Lancet*, **ii**, 810.

Janetta, P.J. (1976). Treatment of trigeminal neuralgia by

sub-occipital and transtentorial cranial operations. *Clin. Neurosurg.*, **24**, 538–49.

Jonasson F., Cullen, J.F., and Elton, R.A. (1979). Temporal arteritis: a 14-year epidemiological, clinical and prognostic study. *Scottish Med. J.*, **24**, 111–17.

Kansu, T., Corbett, J.J., Savino, P., and Schatz, N.J. (1977). Giant cell arteritis with normal sedimentation rate. *Arch. Neurol.*, **34**, 624–5.

Kerr, F.W.L. (1961). A mechanism to account for frontal headache in cases of posterior fossa tumour. *J. Neurosurg.*, **18**, 605.

Killian, J.M., and Fromm, G.H. (1968). Carbamazepine for the treatment of neuralgia. *Arch. Neurol.*, **19**, 129–36.

Klein, R.G., Campbell, R.J., and Hunder, G.G. (1976). Skip lesions in temporal arteritis. *Mayo Clin. Proc.*, **51**, 504–10.

Lance, J.W. (1978). Outpatient problems: Headache. *Br. J. Hosp. Med.*, **19**, 377–8.

Lance, J.W. (1981). Headache. *Ann. Neurol.*, **10**, 1–10.

Lance, J.W. (1982). *The Mechanism and Management of Headache*, fourth edition, Butterworth, London.

Lancet (1984). Headache and depression (Leading article.). **i**, 495.

Leviton, A., Malvea, B., and Graham, J.R. (1974). Vascular disease, mortality and migraine in the parents of migraine patients. *Neurology*, **24**, 669–72.

Liang, G.C., Simkin, P.A., and Mannik, M. (1974). Immunoglobulins in temporal arteritis. An immunofluorescent study. *Ann. Intern. Med.*, **81**, 19–24.

McKendrick, M.W., McGill, J.I., White, J.E., and Wood, M.J. (1986). Oral acyclovir in acute herpes zoster. *Br. Med. J.*, **293**, 1529–32.

Merselis, J.G., Kaye, D., and Hook, E.W. (1964). Disseminated herpes zoster: Report of 17 cases. *Arch. Intern. Med.*, **113**, 679–86.

Murray, J.J. (1977). Temporal arteritis. *J. Am. Geriatr. Soc.*, **25**, 450–3.

Paty, D.W., and Poser, C.M. (1984). Clinical symptoms and signs of multiple sclerosis. In: Poser, C.M., Paty, D.W., McDonald, W.I., Ebers, G.C., and Scheinberg, L. (eds) *The Management of Multiple Sclerosis*. Thieme-Stratton, New York, pp. 27–43.

Portenoy, R.K., Duma, D., and Foley, K.M. (1986). Acute herpetic and post-herpetic neuralgia: Clinical review and current management. *Ann. Neurol.*, **20**, 651–64.

Richards, P., Shawdon, H., and Illingworth, R. (1983). Operative findings on microsurgical exploration of the cerebello-pontine angle in trigeminal neuralgia. *J. Neurol. Neurosurg. Psychiatry*, **46**, 1098–101.

Rogers, R.S., and Tindall, J.P. (1971). Geriatric herpes zoster. *J. Am. Geriatr. Soc.*, **19**, 495–503.

Rushton, J.G., Stevens, J.C., and Miller, R.H. (1981). Glossopharyngeal (vagoglossopharyngeal) neuralgia: A study of 217 cases. *Arch. Neurol.*, **38**, 201–5.

Sweet, W.H., and Wepsic, J.G. (1974). Controlled thermocoagulation of trigeminal ganglion and rootlets for differential destruction of pain fibres 1. Trigeminal neuralgia. *Adv. Neurol.*, **4**, 665–72.

Teasedale, G., and Jennett, B. (1974). Assessment of impaired consciousness and coma: A practical scale. *Lancet*, **ii:** 81–4.

Wasserstrom, W.R., Glass, J.P., and Posner, J.B. (1978). Diagnosis and treatment of leptomeningeal metastases from solid tumours. *Cancer*, **49**, 759–72.

Watson, C.P., Evans, R.J., Reed, K., Merskey, H., Goldsmith, L., and Walsh, J. (1982). Amitriptyline versus placebo in post-herpetic neuralgia. *Neurology*, **32**, 671–3.

Whitty, C.W.M., and Hockaday, J.M. (1968). Migraine: A follow up study of 92 patients. *Br. Med. J.*, **i**, 735–6.

Wilkinson, I.M.S., and Russell, R.W.F. (1972). Arteries of the head and neck in giant cell arteritis. *Arch. Neurol.*, **27**, 378–91.

Zeigler, D.K., Hassanein, R.S., and Couch, J.R. (1977). Characteristics of life headache histories in a non-clinical population. *Neurology*, **27**, 265–9.

Ziser, A., Shupak, A., Halpern, P., Gozal, D., and Melamed, Y. (1984). Delayed hyperbaric oxygen for acute carbon monoxide poisoning. *Br. Med. J.*, **289**, 960.

Chapter 30

Recurrent Acute Confusional States

Robin Philpott

Consultant Psychogeriatrician, Royal Liverpool Hospital, Liverpool, UK

INTRODUCTION

Recurrent acute confusional states are amongst the commonest yet least recognized disorders in the elderly (Lipowski, 1980). With the continuing rise in the elderly and the very elderly population recurrent confusional states will be encountered with increasing frequency (Kay and Bergman, 1980). Up to 40% of patients may develop delirium on general medical wards and 10–15% postoperatively on surgical and orthopaedic wards (Robinson, 1956; Lowry *et al.*, 1973). Delirium or acute confusion is most commonly found in geriatric and psychogeriatric patients. Despite their ubiquity, recurrent confusional states have merited little serious study. They are not regarded as the responsibility of any medical specialty, and their transience and variable clinical presentation result in under-diagnosis and make comprehensive study or description difficult (Lipowski, 1983).

Confusional states often present with disturbed, disinhibited and frightening behaviour which may cloud the judgement of medical and nursing attendants (Wolanin and Philips, 1981). Minor confusional episodes in the elderly living in their own homes, may not be reported. The medical condition causing a confusional state may be treated appropriately without the secondary confusional state being recognized.

The term 'acute confusional state' or its descriptive alternatives, is not a diagnosis in itself nor does it,

of necessity, lead to effective action. It implies: global psychological disturbance; acuteness of onset; medical causation; and reversibility (Lishman, 1978).

Most medical textbooks include a description of acute confusional states, but often use alternative terminology such as delirium, toxic confusional state, acute organic brain syndrome or even reversible dementia. The standard clinical description may be misleading to those dealing with the old and very old. Even texts dealing specifically with the elderly may contain descriptions of acute confusional states that are more commonly seen in younger patients.

Several factors, therefore, contribute to the problems of defining recurrent acute confusion in old age, assessing its frequency, describing its phenomenology and thus optimizing management strategies.

DEFINITIONS

The numerous synonyms for acute confusion reflect genuine difficulties in the classification, descriptive psychopathology and conceptualization of confusional states, even though the need to recognize the major patterns of mental disorder has been realized for some time (Roth, 1955).

The development of the American Psychiatric Association's *Diagnostic and Statistical Manual of Mental Disorders* (DSM) illustrates some of the problems involved. DSM-I in 1952 emphasized the differentiation of acute from chronic brain disorder; DSM-II in

1968, emphasized the difference between psychotic and non-psychotic forms of the disorder; and DSM-III in 1980 attempted to introduce reliable operational definitions to describe organic brain syndromes, dependent on the dominant psychopathology (Committee on Nomenclature and Statistics of the American Psychiatric Association, 1952, 1968, 1980).

In the UK the term 'acute confusional state' still holds sway but even so differences in diagnostic style may affect its use. General medical specialties and most undergraduate teaching emphasizes a system of unitary exclusive diagnoses. In geriatric medicine the problem orientated medical record is often used to encompass the multiplicity of related medical, psychological and social problems found in elderly patients (Weed, 1971). Psychiatrists may use a diagnostic formulation. Other health care professionals respond to different professional and theoretical values: nurses may use the nursing process (McFarlane and Castledine, 1982); psychologists may use behavioural analysis (Lieberman, 1972); and remedial therapists an analysis of daily living activities.

The care of the elderly requires the contribution of many disciplines, but the multiplicity of diagnostic languages they use may erect a Tower of Babel around the confused patient (Simpson, 1984).

THE INCREASED SUSCEPTIBILITY OF THE AGED TO ACUTE CONFUSION

The range of normal widens in old age. Moreover, the elderly are a diverse population spanning four decades. They take with them into old age widely differing levels of physical and psychological health. Elderly individuals age at different rates and chronological age can be only an approximate indicator of biological ageing. Their cultural and social values may differ from those younger persons who are responsible for their treatment. Defects of vision and hearing become increasingly common in the eighth and ninth decades and will predispose elderly subjects to confusional symptoms (Storand, 1986). Minor degrees of disorientation may occur in the absence of any progressive brain pathology (Kral, 1962).

ACUTE ON CHRONIC CONFUSION

In clinical practice recurrent confusional states are most often encountered in the very old, those who have an established dementia, and those with multiple or severe physical illnesses (Kay, 1972). During senescence, physiological, biochemical and morphological changes occur within the brain which will reduce the reserve of cerebral capacity available to the individual (see Chapter 1). These include reduced blood flow (Thomas *et al.*, 1979), loss of neurones, and reduction of some enzymic activity and neurotransmitters (Bowen and Davison, 1982). Abnormal structures proliferate such as senile plaques and neurofibrillary tangles (Corsellis, 1962).

The very elderly thus have more limited cerebral reserve to protect them from the effects of systemic illness. Patients with established dementia are even more likely to be affected by minor illness as they function with no cerebral reserve (Engel and Romano, 1959). Subjects with physical illnesses such as chronic heart failure or renal failure may be prone to acute exacerbations whose severity overwhelms normal brain function. Many very elderly patients have both diminished or absent cerebral reserve and several physical disorders which render them particularly prone to recurrent confusional states.

RECURRENT ACUTE ON CHRONIC CONFUSION

Recurrent confusional episodes are most likely to occur in those with pre-existing dementia. The presence of dementia may dramatically affect the clinical manifestations of acute confusion. Some consideration is required of the common types of dementia, their pathological processes and clinical manifestations (see also Chapter 27).

The prevalence of dementia increases from 3% in the young elderly (aged 65–70) to over 20% in those over 80 (Kay *et al.*, 1964; Gurland *et al.*, 1983); 50–60% of all dementias in old age are attributed to senile dementia of the Alzheimer type (SDAT). A further 30% are attributed to either arteriosclerotic dementia (ASD) as the sole pathological process or in combination with SDAT. The remaining 10% of dementing disorders are due to a variety of aetiologies such as alcoholism, hypoxia and space-occupying lesions (Tomlinson, 1977).

SENILE DEMENTIA OF THE ALZHEIMER TYPE (Lishman, 1978)

Senile dementia of the Alzheimer type (SDAT) usually presents to the clinician only after 12–24 months' progression. The onset is insidious with disturbances initially of memory and of conceptual thinking. In the middle stages language disturbances, expressive and receptive, and parietal lobe dysfunction become prominent. In those few who survive to the final stages, mobility may be lost and the patient becomes totally dependent on 24 hour nursing care. Disturbed behaviour is seen frequently in the early and middle stages of the disease including marked affective disturbance, and secondary delusions, but as the disease progresses the residual conceptual abilities of the dementing brain become diminished (Roth, 1959; Kral, 1972). The brain's ability to elaborate complex behaviours, particularly hallucinations and delusions, is lost (Robinson, 1956; Simon and Cahan, 1962) and affective disturbances, though still present, are usually short lived and labile. This failure of the severely demented brain to elaborate and hold disturbed behaviour and affect is crucial in understanding the presentation of acute confusional states in the presence of severe dementia.

ARTERIOSCLEROTIC (MULTI-INFARCT) DEMENTIA (Lishman, 1978)

Patients with arteriosclerotic dementia (ASD) are most likely to present as an acute neuropsychiatric event. ASD may present in the early stages of the disease as recurrent acute confusional states (Roth, 1959; Lipowski, 1983). In the initial phases of the disease, patients are particularly prone to disturbed behaviour, visual hallucinations and affective lability and vascular incidents may resemble recurrent acute confusional episodes. The disease progresses in a chaotic and unpredictable fashion. Occasionally, islands of normal brain function and behaviour continue despite extreme deficits in other areas. In the final stages reduction in all brain function occurs as in SDAT and the ability to elaborate hallucinations and delusions, as well as complex disturbed behaviour, may be lost. In end state ASD, as in SDAT, intellectual and emotional responses are so diminished that acute confusional episodes may manifest in an attenuated form.

In some elderly patients, several processes may contribute to a dementing disorder thus increasing the heterogeneity of presentation and progression; SDAT and ASD occur together in 15% of elderly dements (Tomlinson, 1977). Repeated hypoxia due to recurrent heart or respiratory failure may exacerbate the cerebral deficits of patients with SDAT or ASD.

SYMPTOMS OF ACUTE CONFUSION IN OLD AGE

The signs and symptoms of recurrent acute confusion may be subdivided into: florid or positive acute confusional symptoms which commonly occur in mentally preserved individuals; and negative or attenuated confusional symptoms which are more likely to occur in patients with pre-existing dementia (Table 30.1). The sub-division is artificial in that the descriptions apply to the ends of a symptom spectrum.

Florid or Positive Confusional Symptoms

These are the symptoms traditionally associated with acute confusion (Engel and Romano, 1959; Kral, 1972). The patient rapidly becomes disorientated for time, place and person. Thinking is fragmentary and disorganized. Mood is labile with prominent anxiety, fear and mistrust. Misinterpretations, illusions and hallucinations, especially visual, are commonly present and worsen at night. These abnormal beliefs may give rise to behaviour disturbance. Restlessness and repetitive behaviour, often related to the patient's past life style, is common.

Attenuated or Negative Confusional Symptoms

Demented patients and the very elderly are more likely to show attenuated symptoms of confusion.

TABLE 30.1   PRESENTATION OF ACUTE
             CONFUSIONAL STATES

Positive/florid	Negative/vegetative
Obvious attention and concentration deficits	Reduced attention and concentration may be difficult to elicit
Fear/agitation	Apathetic
Overactive	Retarded
Overtalkative with perseveration and confabulation	Reduced speech or mute
Goal-directed restlessness (occupational delirium)	Aimless, stereotyped activity
Delusions, hallucinations, misinterpretations and illusions prominent	Rarely prominent
Basic skills usually preserved	Loss of basic skills of daily living, anorexia, impaired mobility

Disturbance of memory and thinking will exacerbate existing disorientation. The patient may suddenly no longer remember relatives or care attendants previously well recognized, or lose orientation in a previously familiar environment. Impairment of intellect may result in the loss of skills such as dressing, toileting, feeding and continence. Reduced comprehension may precipitate transient illusions, delusions or hallucinations recognizable by the disturbed behaviour patterns they cause, rather than the patient's poorly verbalized complaints. The patient may show sudden loss of drive with marked apathy or inactivity. In profoundly demented patients the major effects of acute physical illness may be anorexia, loss of mobility and a general 'failure to thrive'. In these patients only intimate attendants, such as relatives or nurses, may notice the sudden decline in the patient's residual mental function.

Most of these negative symptoms are, of course, found during the inevitable decline of progressive dementia. It is the suddenness with which they occur or progress which differentiates an acute confusional episode from the slow decline of dementia.

It is worthwhile stating some general principles:

1. Acute confusion may be a reversible condition if diagnosed and treated effectively.
2. Any confused patient should be assumed to be in an acute confusional state unless a clear history of long-standing confusion is available from a reliable informant.
3. In patients with established chronic confusion any sudden change in their behaviour or levels of ability should be assumed to be an acute confusional state.
4. Each episode of recurrent acute confusion in the elderly must be diagnosed and treated as a new event.

CAUSES OF ACUTE RECURRENT CONFUSION

Almost any medical illness afflicting the elderly may be responsible for causing an acute confusional state (Bedford, 1959; Dunn and Arie, 1972; Liston, 1982; Lipowski, 1983), but some aetiological agents are more likely to cause recurrent confusion (Table 30.2). The mechanisms by which acute confusion is mediated are unknown. Attempts to reduce the mechanisms to a single process have generally been unsuccessful (Kral, 1972). It is likely that several mechanisms are involved.

Intracranial causes of acute confusion may have direct anatomical or physiological effects on brain function. Systemic illnesses are likely to exert their influence via hypoxia, hypostasis, bacterial endotoxaemia or the accumulation of toxic metabolites. Drugs may have direct toxic affects on brain function (Greenblatt and Shader, 1982; see also Chapter 26) or may exert their effect on brain function when withdrawn (Foy *et al.*, 1986). Electrolyte imbalance will affect the intraneuronal environment of the brain. Hypothermia or hyperthermia have direct effects on brain function.

Some aetiological agents are particularly likely to be recurrent and may cause recurrent confusion in the non-elderly. Transient ischaemic attacks and late onset epilepsy may present as recurrent confusion (see Chapter 15). Elderly patients with chronic obstructive airway disease are at risk of recurrent acute or chronic chest infections. Similarly, unstable diabetics may become hyperglycaemic or iatrogenically hypoglycaemic.

TABLE 30.2   COMMON CAUSES OF RECURRENT ACUTE CONFUSION

	Onset	Confirmed by	Additional information
Neurological			
Transient ischaemic attacks		History and	
Strokes	Sudden	physical examination	May contribute to
Epilepsy	Post epilepsy	EEG	arteriosclerotic dementia
Cardiovascular			
Atrial fibrillation	Sudden	Physical	May contribute to
Recurrent conduction		examination	hypoxic brain damage
disorders		Cardiac enzymes	or arteriosclerotic dementia
Emboli		ECG	
Recurrent congestive cardiac			
failure	Hours/days		
Myocardial infarction		Chest X-ray	
Respiratory			
Recurrent infections	Hours/days	Physical	May contribute to
		examination	hypoxic brain damage
		Chest X-ray	
		Sputum	
Hormonal			
Myxoedema	Months	Thryoid function tests	Pre-existing mental
Hyperglycaemia	Days	Blood sugar	disorders. Dementia
Hypoglycaemia	Sudden/hours		and depression may cause the patient to omit treatment
Drugs			
Alcohol	Usually	Medical history	Drug and alcohol
(includes delirium	hours/days	Physical	abuse may be concealed
tremens)		examination	
Benzodiazepines			
Psychotropics			
Analgesics			
Anti-parkinsonian			
Diuretics			
Digoxin			
Urinary tract infection	Days	History of incontinence	May occur in mentally clear or
		Pyrexia sometimes	chronically confused
		Urine culture	
Affective disorder	Weeks/months	Psychiatric history and examination	
Constipation	Days/weeks	Rectal examination	Most common cause of acute exacerbation in chronically confused
Relocation	After relocation	Medical and psychiatric history	May exacerbate chronic confusion

Recurring cardiac abnormalities may precipitate perplexing confusional states (Livesley, 1977; Jonas *et al.*, 1977). Supraventricular tachycardias, heart block, or atrial fibrillation may be intermittent and these abnormalities may not be detected until long-term cardiac monitoring is undertaken. Patients known to be in atrial fibrillation may discharge emboli to the cerebral circulation and those who have diminished cardiac reserve may repeatedly slip into congestive cardiac failure (Caird *et al.*, 1976). Conversely, overtreatment of apparent cardiac failure may cause confusion (Editorial, 1978).

Patients prone to recurrent urinary tract infections, due to genitourinary pathologies such as prostatic outflow obstruction or recurrent pyelonephritis are at risk of recurrent confusion.

Drug intoxications are a particularly potent cause of recurrent confusional episodes in the elderly, both those with established dementia and those who are normally mentally clear (Liston, 1982). They include: long-acting benzodiazepines, barbiturates, drugs used in the treatment of Parkinson's disease, analgesics and many psychotropic drugs, particularly those with anticholinergic effects (Greenblatt and Shader, 1982). Patients may conceal their use of tranquillizers, analgesics and alcohol. Alcohol abuse may result in recurrent confusional symptoms in old age with prominent visual hallucinosis or paranoia.

Patients with recurrent depression may present predominantly with symptoms of dementia. A personal and family history of affective disorder, psychomotor retardation and depressed facial expression are of particular diagnostic significance (Mahendra, 1985).

Some aetiological factors are more likely to precipitate recurrent acute confusional states in those already suffering from dementia. Constipation is probably the single most common cause of recurrent confusional state in those with an established dementia. Volume depletion and/or dehydration have been implicated (Seymour *et al.*, 1980). Recurrent urinary tract infections are the next most common medical cause of confusion in those who are already demented. Demented patients respond poorly to relocation from home to hospital and between wards or hospitals. The practice of frequent respite admissions or attendance at day hospitals may exacerbate

confusional symptoms, sometimes causing relatives to abandon this form of care (Smith, 1986; Rai *et al.*, 1986). Patients with dementia are particularly prone to the side-effects of hypnotics, major tranquillizers and tricyclic antidepressants. Unfortunately their behavioural deficits commonly require the use of these drugs. Patients with dementia may also develop affective disturbances which result in subacute worsening of symptoms over weeks or months. This possibility should be considered in demented patients who become anorexic, restless, frightened or who have depressive thought content.

Many patients presenting with recurrent confusional states have multiple causes for their confusion. In addition to the primary cause of confusion, be it infection, stroke or cardiac disease, they may have developed secondary problems such as dehydration, electrolyte imbalance and uraemia. The patient is then further susceptible to infection or circulatory collapse (Seymour *et al.*, 1980).

The symptoms of confusion may be of little guide to the aetiological agent, presentation being more related to the patient's predominant mental state prior to the development of symptoms rather than the aetiological agent itself. Even so, the mode of presentation may be helpful (Post, 1971). Confusional states that are of extremely sudden onset are most likely to be related to vascular incidents, either cerebral or cardiac, or to epileptic fits which may be non-convulsive (see Chapter 15). Infective agents usually produce confusional states that evolve in hours or at most days. Drug intoxications and confusional states due to constipation usually evolve over days or weeks. Depression develops over weeks or months.

ASSESSMENT

The assessment of recurrent confusional states in the elderly requires skills in medical and psychiatric history taking, physical and mental state examination and assessment of the patient's social background and current support networks. It must be remembered that an adequate history cannot be taken from a patient who is confused. Considerable time may be saved in history taking, as well as undue credibility being put on unreliable information from the patient, if, when confusional states are suspected in the elderly, a brief assessment of orientation is made at an early stage. It would be appropriate to perform simple tests of orientation, such as asking the patient's age and date of birth, checking to see if they tally, and asking the patient the current date and day of the week. A simple learning test can be undertaken by establishing whether the patient can learn the doctor's name, and retain this information for 5 minutes. If after three to four attempts the patient still fails then a confusional state is likely. Almost invariably, patients with recurrent acute confusional states will show abnormalities of orientation but in very rare circumstances patients with all the stigmata of acute confusion may remain well orientated. All attempts should be made to take a history from an independent witness.

Two major questions need to be asked in relation to the patient's medical and psychiatric history. The general form of development of symptoms and the time span will indicate whether the patient is suffering from an acute confusional state, having been previously mentally normal, or whether this is a sudden deterioration in confusional symptoms which were already present (Post, 1971). Detailed history taking may also indicate that other acute exacerbations have occurred in the past. This ability to identify sudden deterioration in the psychological state of the patient is a skill that is required by all health professionals who work with the elderly.

The doctor, however, has a specific responsibility to undertake a detailed analysis of other symptoms that may lead to a more accurate diagnosis of the underlying medical condition. The mode of onset may give some clues as to the likely underlying medical condition (see above). The type of psychological symptom present, confusional, delusional, or hallucinatory, will probably not contribute to diagnosis. It is useful to have a checklist of medical symptoms which should be enquired into such as febrile illness, sudden collapse, minor (especially lateralized) neurological symptoms, speech and language deficits, symptoms of cardiac or respiratory distress or increasing ankle oedema. Major symptoms of depression such as appetite and weight loss, early morning wakening, profound mood change

and suicidal thoughts or acts should be sought.

The patient's past medical and past psychiatric history may be of considerable importance, particularly when this includes a history of repeated cerebrovascular incidents, cardiac disease, chronic pulmonary disease, alcoholism or drug problems. A long-standing previous history of affective disorder, whether this is depressive or bipolar, may be of value.

A detailed physical examination is essential in all cases and disturbed patients may require repeated examinations. Signs of dehydration and recent weight loss and the patient's general nutritional state should be noted. The temperature should be taken, if necessary rectally, in winter months to exclude hypothermia (Irvine, 1974). Signs of cyanosis, anaemia and lymphadenopathy should be noted. The patient's skin condition and general cleanliness may give some indication of the duration of symptoms. A thorough examination of the cardiovascular system is essential with particular emphasis on detecting abnormalities of rhythm or heart failure and abnormalities in the peripheral circulation. Tachypnoea, dyspnoea and crepitations may suggest a chest infection, though negative respiratory signs may be misleading. Examination of the gastrointestinal tract may reveal hepatomegaly, bowel distension or simple constipation and a rectal examination is essential.

The patient should be observed for signs of facial asymmetry, tongue or palate deviation. Pupillary size and reflexes as well as ocular movements should be ascertained. Complete examination of reflexes, motor and sensory function may be difficult in patients with confusion, and only a general impression of strength, coordination and simple reflexes may be achieved. Observation of facial expression, posture and gait may be more valuable than a formal neurological examination. Attempts at fundoscopy should be made but may again prove difficult.

The patient's mental state should be examined in detail and methodically. Does the patient look ill or dishevelled? Is there evidence of long-standing personal neglect? Has the patient been recently incontinent? Patients may be friendly, bemused or stunned in manner. Conversely they may be guarded, frightened and distrustful of their examining doctor. Speech may be either rapid, incoherent and garbled, with evidence of perseveration and confabulation, or markedly reduced in both quantity and complexity. Simple tests of comprehension of simple commands, such as 'close your eyes', 'put out your tongue' may be useful. Expressive speech may show syntactic errors, paraphrasias and neologisms as well as nominal dysphasia on specific testing. In apparently uncooperative patients, response to non-verbal cues such as simple physical prompting and guiding may be helpful.

There may be complex abnormalities of mood, with depressive, euphoric and paranoid features occurring simultaneously or during short time periods. The thought content of the confused elderly patient is said to be characterized by transient and often very frightening misinterpretations. These may be simple perceptual abnormalities, memory deceptions or frank delusions and hallucinations. Some patients, particularly those with established confusion, may become increasingly apathetic, inert and lacking in conceptual ability.

Cognitive function assessments should be undertaken but may be difficult. Attention and concentration are probably best assessed by the patient's general response to the interview rather than specific responses to tests such as Serial 7's, Serial 3's or repetition of the Babcock sentence. These tests are in any case influenced by social class and educational status (Hinton and Withers, 1971). Simple tests of orientation such as age, date of birth, current date, day of week and being able to learn and retain the identity of the doctor may be the best simple test available. Other short validated tests include the Mini-Mental State (Folstein *et al.*, 1975) and Abbreviated Mental Test Score (Hodkinson, 1972; Vardon and Blessed, 1986). Whatever tests are chosen should be brief and easily administered; they should also be administered in the least threatening way.

There should be a detailed assessment of current social support, particularly when the patient is assessed at home or in the accident and emergency department. Social assessment should include the composition of the patient's household. The presence of a caring spouse or child in the household or the ability to recruit support in the community may determine whether treatment can be carried out in

the home or requires admission to hospital or another treatment environment. This support may be informal via friends or neighbours, or by the statutory services or home helps or district nurses. Admission to hospital may also be averted if there is the immediate availability of attendance at an effective geriatric or psychogeriatric day hospital. When the assessment is complete the doctor should be able to complete the checklist in Table 30.3.

INVESTIGATIONS (Table 30.4)

Investigations will vary considerably from patient to patient. Thus a profoundly demented patient, who is well known to the geriatric or psychogeriatric services and is prone to constipation, will require few investigations (Colgan and Philpot, 1985). A patient who has had one previous confusional episode may require the full investigations that would normally be undertaken in any case of undiagnosed acute confusion.

MANAGEMENT AND TREATMENT

Patients should be treated at home whenever possible. This decision will be influenced by the medical diagnosis, treatability of the underlying condition, the severity of disturbed behaviour and the degree of support available from the family and the community. Resources need to be rapidly made available to patients with acute confusional states. A brief period of very intensive nursing care in the community may prevent hospitalization and the deficits and damages that can occur to elderly patients as a result of hospitalization. Accurate diagnosis of the underlying medical condition will help in predicting the duration of nursing care and support that may be required by a patient in the community. It may be possible to negotiate a brief period of intensive home treatment with a caring family.

Some patients will require admission to hospital. Hospitalization should be undertaken with the minimum of disruption to the patient. A relative or friend should if possible stay with the patient to reduce the more distressing effects of hospitalization in the first few hours of admission. Once admitted, the patient should not be moved from ward to ward or within

TABLE 30.3   CHECKLIST FOR ASSESSMENT OF RECURRENT CONFUSION

1   *Is the patient confused?*
    Perform simple tests of orientation, attention and concentration.

2   *How long has the patient been confused?* (An independent account is required.)
    Is this an acute event?
    Was the patient previously mentally normal or chronically mentally impaired?
    Have there been previous acute episodes? If so what was the cause?

3   *Is the patient physically ill?*
    An acute decline in mental function almost certainly indicates physical illness.
    A detailed and methodical history, examination and routine investigations are required.

4   *Is the patient confused by the environment?*
    Has the patient been moved recently? Particularly multiple moves.

5   *Are emotional factors involved?*
    Is the patient depressed?
    Are fear and anxiety exacerbating the patient's confusion?

6   *Are sensory or other neurological factors involved?*
    Deafness
    Blindness
    Dysphasia

7   *What social supports are available?*
    Household composition
    Availability of informal carers
    Availability of statutory services

8   *What legal/ethical issues are involved?*
    What are the previously expressed views of the patient?
    What are the wishes of the patient's family?

TABLE 30.4   INVESTIGATION OF RECURRENT CONFUSION

Routine investigations
1   Haemoglobin white cell count, film, ESR
2   Urea and electrolytes
3   Liver function tests
4   Blood sugar
5   Serological test for syphilis
6   Chest and skull X-ray
7   Mid-stream specimen of urine
8   ECG and cardiac enzymes are required in patients with very sudden onset confusion particularly in the presence of other cardiovascular symptoms.
9   Patients who are known to abuse alcohol or drugs should be screened for alcohol or the presence of barbiturates or benzodiazepines or other drugs.

Non-routine investigations (as indicated)
1   B12, folate
2   Further biochemistry, e.g. serum calcium
3   Further radiography (contrast studies etc.)
4   Computed tomography
5   Electroencephalogram

ward areas. Nursing staff with both psychiatric and physical experience are needed in the management of these patients, but the majority of these patients are admitted to medical, surgical, geriatric or orthopaedic wards, where psychiatrically trained staff are unlikely to be available. Very disturbed patients may require transfer to psychiatric or psychogeriatric wards as these patients have combined psychiatric and physical illness, often complicated by social problems. They are ideally admitted to a psychogeriatric assessment unit (DHSS, 1971) or a department of health care of the elderly (Arie, 1983), where geriatric and psychiatric needs can both be met.

Treatment of the underlying condition causing the patient's confusional state is the most important medical priority. Some drugs used in treatment may cause confusional symptoms and these should be avoided. The need for sedation may be avoided by good nursing care, but if required then clear guidelines and policy decisions should be made by medical and nursing attendants as to its appropriate use. Night sedation may be required and would be best undertaken with hypnotics with very short metabolic half-lives such as chlormethiazole, chloral or short-acting benzodiazepines (Swift, 1982). If daytime sedation is required it is best to ensure effective sedation, rather than ineffective or intermittent sedation resulting in an even more confused, semimobile and accident prone patient. There is little agreement on choice of drugs in these patients. Regular small doses of chlormethiazole in subhypnotic doses has been recommended. Haloperidol is less prone to cause postural hypertension (Lipowski, 1983) but it may cause acute and possibly irreversible neurological problems in the elderly. Promazine and thioridazine remain popular drugs for elderly confused patients due to their relative lack of parkinsonian side-effects compared with other neuroleptics. Occasionally very disturbed elderly patients may require chlorpromazine.

The need for sedative medication will be considerably reduced by good nursing practice. Attention to the patient's general bodily functions including elimination, hydration and nutrition are of great importance with specific care to ensure minimal physical or emotional distress. Nursing the patient in a single room with the least possible changes of attendants will be particularly beneficial. Subdued lighting, the avoidance of glare and potential sensory misinterpretations are important. The confused patient will probably benefit from the presence of nurses wearing uniform (Wolanin and Philips, 1981).

Rehabilitation should begin as soon as the initial phase of acute confusion passes. Early mobilization will avoid the accumulation of secondary deficits due to prolonged bed rest. Regular assessments should be made of the patient's remaining mental deficits and these should be actively rehabilitated by dressing practice, a graded toilet retraining regimen, social skills retraining, small group activities, and reminiscence and reality orientation (RO). Patients should receive 24 hour RO care in which they are constantly reminded of their personal identity, whereabouts and the activities that are required of them (Woods and Holden, 1982; see also Chapter 33).

Recurrent confusional states should be carefully monitored in hospital to ensure that a further acute confusional state induced by treatment does not occur during the recovery phase.

If the patient has been hospitalized, discharge arrangements are best made by negotiations between medical, nursing, rehabilitation staff, social worker and the patient's relatives (Horrocks, 1986). It is essential that the elderly who are predisposed to confusion have adequate discharge arrangements made to prevent rapid relapse. Decisions will need to be taken as to the patient's optimum long-term medical treatment, but the patient may be discharged from hospital quite appropriately before full rehabilitation has been undertaken. Rehabilitation may be best completed at home rather than in hospital. Suitable arrangements will then be required for the patient's management at home by the district nursing services or attendance at an appropriate day centre or day hospital. In all circumstances the general practitioner should be forewarned of discharge.

The patient may require social support from home help or meals on wheels services or by voluntary agencies. Agreements should be reached by all team members who are responsible for the patient's care, including doctors, nurses, social workers and the patient's main carer before discharge is undertaken. A key worker should be identified who will supervise and manage the patient on a regular basis in the community. This may be hospital based medical staff, social worker or community psychiatric nurse, or in primary care, the general practitioner or district nurse. Patients who suffer from recurrent confusional states should receive regular medical supervision, either from hospital or primary care services. The frequency of follow-up will depend upon individual cases but should be lifelong. Relatives should be warned of the likelihood of recurrence of confusional symptoms and advised on action they should take.

OUTCOME

There are no studies of outcome in patients with recurrent confusional states. It seems likely that the long-term outcome for patients with recurrent confusion will be worse than those suffering from a single acute confusional episode. Thirty-five per cent of all confused patients are discharged home in 4 weeks (Hodkinson, 1973); mortality may be as high as 50% at 6 months (Roth, 1955). In patients with recurrent confusional states complicating dementia, the prognosis will be worse than the outcome for uncomplicated dementia, dementia and physical illness together being predictors of poor survival (Blessed and Wilson, 1982; Black, 1985). Disappointingly there has been no apparent improvement in survival in elderly patients with acute confusional episodes in the last 30 years (Blessed, 1982).

LEGAL CONSIDERATIONS

Patients with confusion are often non-volitional and are unable to give valid consent to their treatment (Norman, 1980; Age Concern, 1986). To give valid consent it is necessary for the patient: to be given adequate information on the nature of the treatment and the likely effects of treatment; to be able to understand this information; and to give consent without duress or deception. Patients who are suffering from confusional states are unlikely to be able to fulfil the second of these requirements, that of

comprehension. The patient's supervising doctor may then be faced with a legal dilemma. Any physical treatment of a patient who cannot give consent may be regarded legally as a trespass against the person. Even though legal action is unlikely, the issue should be borne in mind when treatment is undertaken on behalf of a confused patient. Common law also requires that doctors and nurses have a duty of care to a patient who is clearly in danger of death or irreversible damage without active treatment. These two aspects of the common law leave many grey areas both clinically and legally (Gostin, 1983). The doctor responsible for the patient should act in the patient's interests, consult with other doctors as to optimal treatment and take account of the views of the relatives and of other health professionals, particularly when working in multidisciplinary teams (DHSS, 1985). Formal powers of detention under the 1983 Mental Health Act should be avoided unless the patient persistently refuses treatment or other care essential to maintain life, safety or the safety of others.

RESEARCH, HEALTH DELIVERY AND EDUCATION

There is little information on elderly patients with recurrent acute confusional states (Royal College of Physicians, 1982; Lipowski, 1983, 1984). Non-recurrent confusional states in the elderly receive disproportionately sparse attention in medical, geriatric or psychogeriatric texts. Their incidence in the elderly population at large is unknown.

The nature of recurrent and non-recurrent confusional states makes adequate study difficult. They are short lived and protean in their manifestations. Operational definitions of acute confusion in the mentally preserved are unlikely to encompass acute confusion in demented patients even though the medical precipitant is the same.

Cross-sectional epidemiological surveys have usually failed to pick up acute confusional episodes (but see Freedman *et al.*, 1967). Incidence studies in medical settings showed wide discrepancies reflecting differences in medical style and admission criteria rather than intrinsic variance in acute confusional states.

Acute confusion in old age has not yet attracted the interest of biological scientists, but the increase in research into progressive dementias such as SDAT seems likely to have spin-off effects in the understanding of the acute reversible confusions.

Three avenues of research seem particularly valuable: long-term incidence studies of elderly populations at home (previous prevalence studies have failed to detect acute confusional states); long-term follow-up studies of at risk individuals (the very old and/or demented); and the use of new imaging techniques such as positron emission tomography (PET) or nuclear magnetic resonance (NMR) brain scanning. These may shed some light on the incidence/frequency and outcome/prognosis and define populations at risk of recurrent acute confusion. They may also help to elucidate the neurophysiology and neuropsychology of confusional states.

However, whilst these advances in knowledge are awaited it is essential to utilize what knowledge we have of acute confusional states and our more extensive knowledge of gerontology and health care delivery of the elderly. Where effective geriatric and psychogeriatric services exist and, hopefully, cooperate then they should jointly be able to respond to the crises caused by recurrent acute confusional states (DHSS, 1970). Home assessment, day hospital and readily available acute inpatient care are essential for the diagnosis and early management of these illnesses. Rehabilitation and longer-term supervision will require the usual skills of multidisciplinary team work, and the likelihood of sudden and unpredictable relapse demands effective communication between hospital staff, general practice staff, the patient and importantly the patient's relatives.

Few existing staff in either medical, psychiatric or social services have adequate training in the skills of caring for the confused elderly (Arie, 1983). Recurrent acute confusional states may present in the patient's own home, in private, voluntary or local authority homes, in acute medical and surgical wards and in specialist geriatric and psychogeriatric specialties. The task of teaching the skills of assessment and treatment of all types of confusional states in the elderly, is massive and involves all professional groups: doctors, nurses, social workers, paramedical staff and both qualified and unqualified staff, and

not least the relatives of the elderly. This task is now beginning to be addressed by the increasing number of clinical and academic geriatric and psychogeriatric departments of health (Arie, 1983; Wattis and Arie, 1984).

The simple message that should be imparted to all those who care for the elderly is:

> any sudden deterioration in the patient's mental function should always be regarded as an emergency, demanding prompt medical intervention.

REFERENCES

Age Concern (1986). *The Law and Vulnerable Elderly People*, Eyre and Spottiswoode, Andover.

Arie, T. (1983). Organisation of services for the elderly: Implications for education and patient care—experience in Nottingham. In: Bergener, M. (ed.) *Geropsychiatric Diagnosis and Treatment*, Springer, New York.

Bedford, P.D. (1959). General medical aspects of confusional states in elderly people. *Br. Med. J.*, ii, 185–8.

Black, D.W. (1985). The Iowa record-linkage study: excess mortality in patients with organic mental disorder. *Arch. Gen. Psychiatry*, 42(1), 78–81.

Blessed, G., and Wilson, I.D. (1982). The contemporary natural history of mental disorder in old age. *Br. J. Psychiatry*, 141, 56–67.

Bowen, D.M., and Davison, A.N. (1982). The biochemistry of the ageing brain. In: Caird, F.I. (ed.) *Neurological Disorders and the Elderly*, John Wright, Bristol.

Caird, F.I., Dall, J.L.C., and Kennedy, R.D. (1976). *Cardiology in Old Age*, Plenum Press, New York.

Colgan, J., and Philpot, M. (1985). The routine use of investigations in elderly psychiatric patients. *Age Ageing*, 14, 1263–7.

Committee on Nomenclature and Statistics of the American Psychiatric Association (1952). *Diagnostic and Statistical Manual of Mental Disorders*, ed. 1 (DSMI), Washington DC.

Committee on Nomenclature and Statistics of the American Psychiatric Association (1968). *Diagnostic and Statistical Manual of Mental Disorders*, ed. 2 (DSMII), Washington DC.

Committee on Nomenclature and Statistics of the American Psychiatric Association (1980). *Diagnostic and Statistical Manual of Mental Disorders*, ed. 3 (DSMIII), Washington DC.

Corsellis, J.A.N. (1962). *Mental Illness and the Ageing Brain*, Oxford University Press, London.

DHSS (1970). Psychogeriatric Assessment Units HM(70)11.

DHSS (1985). Mental Health Act 1983: draft code of practice HC (85) 32.

Dunn, T., and Arie, T. (1972). Mental disturbances in the ill old person. *Br. Med. J.*, **ii**, 413–16.

Editorial (1978). Diuretics in the elderly. *Br. Med. J.*, **i**, 1092–3.

Engel, G.L., and Romano, J. (1959). Delirium, a syndrome of cerebral insufficiency. *J. Chronic Dis.*, **9**, 260.

Folstein, M., Folstein, S.E., and McHugh, P.R. (1975). "Mini-Mental state" a practical method for grading the cognitive state of patients for the clinician. *J. Psychiatr. Res.*, **12**, 189–98.

Foy, A., Drinkwater V., March, S., and Mearrick, P. (1986). Confusion after admission to hospital in elderly patients using Benzodiazepines. *Br. Med. J.*, **293**, 1072.

Freedman, D.K., Troll, L., Mills, A.B., and Baker, P. (1967). *Acute Organic Disorder Accompanied by Mental Symptoms*, Dept of Mental Hygiene, Sacramento, California.

Gostin, L. (1983). *A Practical Guide to Mental Health Law*, Mind Publications, London.

Greenblatt, D.J., and Shader, R. (1982). Drug therapy: Drug disposition in old age. *N. Engl. J. Med.*, **306**, 1081–8.

Gurland, B., Copeland, J., Kuriansky, J., Kelleher, M., Sharpe, L., and Dean, L.L. (1983). *The Mind and Mood of Ageing*, The Haworth Press, New York.

Hinton J., and Withers, E. (1971). The usefulness of the clinical tests of the sensorium. *Br. J. Psychiatry*, **119**, 9–18.

Hodkinson, H.M. (1972). Evaluation of a mental test score for the assessment of mental impairment in the elderly. *Age Ageing*, **1**, 233–8.

Hodkinson, H.M. (1973). Mental impairment in the elderly. *J. Roy. Coll. Phys. Lond.*, **7**, 305–17.

Horrocks, P. (1986). The components of a comprehensive district health service for elderly people—a personal view. *Age Ageing*, **15**, 321–42.

Irvine, R.E. (1974). Hypothermia in old age. *Practitioner*, **213**, 795–800.

Jonas, S., Klein, I., and Dimant, J. (1977). Importance of Holter monitoring in patients with periodic cerebral symptoms. *Ann. Neurol.*, **1**, 470–4.

Kay, D.W.K. (1972). Epidemiological aspects of organic brain disease in the aged. In *Ageing and the Brain*, Plenum Press, New York.

Kay, D.W.K., Beamish, P., and Roth, M. (1964). Old age mental disorders in Newcastle upon Tyne part 1, A study of prevalence. *Br. J. Psychiatry*, **110**, 146–58.

Kay, D.W.K., and Bergman, K. (1980). Epidemiology of mental disorder in the community. In: Birren, J.E., and Sloane, R.B. (eds.) *Handbook of Mental Health and Ageing*, Prentice-Hall, Englewood Cliffs.

Kral, V.A. (1962). Senescent forgetfulness. Benign and malignant. *Can. Med. Assoc. J.*, **86**, 257–60.

Kral, V.A. (1972). Senile dementia and normal ageing. *Can. Psychiatry Ass. J.*, **17**, 25–30.

Lieberman, R.P. (1972). *A Guide to Behavioural Analysis and Therapy*, Pergamon Press, New York.

Lipowski, Z.J. (1980). *Delirium: Acute Brain Failure in Man*, Charles C. Thomas, Illinois.

Lipowski, Z.J. (1983). Transient cognitive disorders (delirium, acute confusional states) in the elderly. *Am. J. Psychiatry*, **140**(11), 1426–36.

Lipowski, Z.J. (1984). Organic brain syndromes: New classification concepts and prospects. *Can. J. Psychiatry*, **29**(3), 198–204.

Lishman, W. (1978). *Organic Psychiatry: The Psychological Consequences of Cerebral Disorder*, Blackwell Scientific Publications, Oxford.

Liston, E.H. (1982). Delirium in the aged. In: Jarvik, L.F., and Small, G.W. (eds.) *The Psychiatric Clinics of North America*, W.B. Saunders, Philadelphia.

Livesley, B. (1977). The pathogenesis of brain failure in the aged. *Age Ageing* (Suppl.) **6**, 9–19.

Lowry, F.M., Engelsman, F., and Lipowski, Z.J. (1973). Study of cognitive functioning in a medical population. *Comprehensive Psychiatry*, **14**, 331–8.

McFarlane, J.K., and Castledine, G. (1982). *The Practice of Nursing Using the Nursing Process*, G.V. Mosby, London.

Mahendra, B. (1985). Depression and dementia: The multi faceted relationship. *Psychol. Med.*, **15**, 227–36.

Norman, J.A. (1980). *Rights and Risks*, Centre for Policy on Ageing, Anchor Press, London.

Post, F. (1971). The diagnostic process. In: Kay, D.W.K., and Walk, A. (eds.) *Recent Advances in Psychogeriatrics*, British Journal of Psychiatry Special Publication No. 6, Headley Bros.

Rai, G.S., Bielawska, C., Murphy, P.G., and Wright, G. (1986). Hazards for elderly people admitted for respite ("Holiday admissions") and social care ("social admissions"). *Br. Med. J.*, **292**, 240.

Robinson, G.W. (1956). The toxic delirious reactions of old age. In: Kaplan, O.J. (ed.) *Mental Disorders in Later Life*, Stanford University Press, Stanford, California.

Roth, M. (1955). Natural history of mental disorder in old age. *J. Ment. Sci.*, **101**, 281–96.

Roth, M. (1959). Some diagnostic and aetiological aspects of confusional states in the elderly. *Gerontol. Clin.*, **1**, 83–95.

Royal College of Physicians (1982). Organic mental impairment in the elderly implications for research, education and the provision of services: Report of the Royal College of Physicians Committee on Geriatrics.

Seymour, D.G., Henshire, P.J., Cape, R.D.T., and Campbell, A.J. (1980). Acute confusional states in the elderly: the role of dehydration/volume depletion, physical illness and age. *Age Ageing*, **9**, 137–46.

Simon, A., and Cahan, R.B. (1962). The acute brain syndrome in geriatric patients. *Psychiatr. Res. Rep.*, **16**, 8–21.

Simpson, C.J. (1984). Doctors and nurses use of the word confused. *Br. J. Psychiatry*, **145**, 441–3.

Smith, B.A. (1986). What is "Confusion translocation syndrome?" *Am. J. Nurs.*, **11**, 1280–1.

Storand, T. (1986). Psychological aspects of ageing. In: Rossman, I.J.D. (ed.) *Clinical Geriatrics*, third edition, Lippincott, Philadelphia.

Swift, C.J. (1982). Hypnotic drugs. In: Isaacs, B. (ed.) *Recent Advances in Geriatrics*, Vol. II, Churchill Livingstone, Edinburgh.

Thomas, D.J., Zilkha, E., Redmond, S., Du Boulay, G.H., Marshall, J., Russel, R.W., and Symon, L. (1979). An intravenous 133 Xenon clearance technique for measuring cerebral blood flow. *J. Neurol. Sci.*, **40**, 53–63.

Tomlinson, B.E. (1977). Morphological changes and dementia in old age. In: Smith, W.L., and Kingsbourne, M. (eds.) *Ageing and Dementia*, Spectrum Publications, New York.

Vardon, V.M., and Blessed, G. (1986). Confusion ratings and abbreviated mental performance: a comparison. *Age Ageing*, **15**, 139–44.

Wattis, J., and Arie, T. (1984). Further developments in psychogeriatrics in Britain. *Br. Med. J.*, **289**, 77.

Weed, L.L. (1971). *Medical Records and Medical Education and Patient Care*, Yearbook Medical Publishers, Chicago.

Wolanin, M.O., and Philips, L.R.F. (1981). *Confusion: Prevention and Care*, C.V. Mosby, St Louis.

Woods, R.T., and Holden, U.P. (1982). Reality orientation. In: Isaacs, B. (ed.) *Recent Advances in Geriatric Medicine*, Vol. II, Churchill Livingstone, Edinburgh.

The Clinical Neurology of Old Age
Edited by R. Tallis
© 1989 John Wiley & Sons Ltd

Chapter 31

The Neuropathic Bladder

Gerald Tobin

Consultant Physician in Geriatric Medicine, Manor Park Hospital, Bristol, UK

The term neuropathic bladder disorder refers to dysfunction of the lower urinary tract resulting from disease of, or injury to, its neural control.

In the following review, particular emphasis will be placed on the causes and management of the uninhibited neuropathic bladder, as this is the neuropathic bladder disorder most likely to be encountered by those involved in the care of the elderly.

INNERVATION OF THE BLADDER

In addition to its sensory supply, the lower urinary tract is innervated by efferents from the parasympathetic, sympathetic and somatic nervous system.

Efferent Parasympathetic Supply

This arises in the intermediolateral region of the second to fourth sacral segments of the spinal cord. The neurotransmitter released by both preganglionic and postganglionic fibres is acetylcholine. The parasympathetic neurones, which are responsible for detrusor contraction, are evenly distributed to all parts of the bladder except the superficial trigone, which has a sparse cholinergic supply. They also supply the entire length of the urethra in the female and that part of the urethra proximal to the entrance of the ejaculatory ducts in the male (Gosling and Dixon, 1975).

Efferent Sympathetic Supply

The sympathetic nerve supply to the lower urinary tract has its origins in the intermediolateral grey columns of the tenth thoracic to the second lumbar segments of the spinal cord. The superficial trigone has a plentiful supply of alpha adrenergic receptors. The remainder of the detrusor has a sparse supply of beta adrenergic receptors which mediate relaxation. Gosling et al. (1977) have shown that the proximal urethra in the male has a rich sympathetic supply with mainly alpha adrenergic receptors. They have suggested that their function is to prevent reflux ejaculation. In the female, they found only a sparse sympathetic supply to the proximal urethra. This finding was surprising as pharmacological and clinical studies have indicated that there are alpha adrenergic receptor sites in this region in the female. The explanation may lie in the fact that postganglionic sympathetic nerves have been shown to synapse with postganglionic parasympathetic nerves. Thus sympathetic effects may be mediated via an effect on parasympathetic ganglionic transmission.

There is debate concerning the innervation of the striated muscle fibres of the urethra (the rhabdosphincter). Some investigators (Vadusek and Keith-Light, 1983) claim that the dominant innervation is somatic from the pudendal nerve. Koyanagi (1980) believes that there is a dominant alpha adrenergic supply.

The importance of the sympathetic nerve supply for normal micturition is unknown. What is known is that agents that can stimulate or block alpha adrenergic receptors in the human urethra can produce significant changes in intra-urethral pressure. The relaxing effect produced by stimulation of the beta receptors is minimal (Norlen *et al.*, 1978).

Efferent Somatic Supply

The peri-urethral striated muscle fibres of the pelvic floor are supplied by somatic fibres originating in the anterior horn of the second to fourth sacral segments. These travel via the pudendal nerve.

Afferent Nerve Supply

Afferent fibres from the bladder travel with the sympathetic, parasympathetic and somatic fibres. Afferents from the detrusor respond to an increase in bladder wall tension, resulting either from bladder distension or contraction. Because individual receptors have different thresholds, the afferent system can signal pressure status over a wide range of pressures by recruiting more receptors (Fletcher and Bradley, 1978). Afferents from the mucosa respond to touch, pain or temperature.

Within the bladder, nerves pursue a tortuous course. This enables them to accommodate to stretch during bladder filling.

Distinct neuromuscular junctions do not occur in the bladder. Each efferent terminal branch has multiple varicosities resulting from the presence of collections of vesicles containing the neurotransmitter. Vesicles of cholinergic fibres are agranular, while those of the postganglionic sympathetic fibres, which contain noradrenaline, have a central, electron dense core. There is a third type of vesicle which is large and dense cored whose neurotransmitter is unknown.

THE NEURAL CONTROL OF LOWER URINARY TRACT FUNCTION

Although afferents from the bladder synapse on inter-neurones involved in a variety of spinal reflexes, the critical neural circuit involved in normal micturition relays through the brain stem. The brain stem detrusor nucleus is believed to be localized in the nucleus locus coeruleus in the pons. Three efferent pathways descend from the brain stem. The principal descending pathway is in the lateral reticulospinal tract and produces excitation in the preganglionic parasympathetic nerves to the detrusor, along with inhibition of the neurones supplying the smooth and striated muscles of the urethral sphincter (Fletcher and Bradley, 1978).

Lesions above the detrusor nucleus in the brain stem do not affect the characteristic features of a normal detrusor contraction. However, lesions above the sacral cord and below the detrusor nucleus cause a loss of coordination between the detrusor and the sphincter with consequent poor emptying. Normally the peri-urethral striated muscle relaxes at the same time as the detrusor contracts. In this situation it may contract and relax intermittently (clonic sphincter) or may remain contracted (tonic sphincter) (Diokno *et al.*, 1974).

There is no longer believed to be a coordinating centre for the control of micturition in the sacral cord.

Different areas of the brain are involved in the control of micturition. Andrew and Nathan (1964) showed that the area responsible for the cortical control of micturition lies in the anteromedial part of the frontal lobe. The area involved includes the superior frontal gyrus, the anterior cingulate gyrus and the genu of the corpus callosum. This is generally believed to be an inhibitory area. However, Mundy (1984) has argued that it may be a facilitatory area because when Andrew and Nathan's patients had the causative lesion treated surgically, many regained continence. If this were an inhibitory area, surgery would not be expected to have this result. He thus suggests that these lesions resulted in pathological stimulation of a facilitatory area. The basal ganglia have an inhibitory effect on the detrusor centre in the brain stem. Various other areas including the cerebellum, the septal region and the hypothalmus, are known to have an inhibitory or facilitatory effect on the bladder.

THE UNSTABLE BLADDER

The maintenance of urinary continence requires that the pressure in the urethra be greater than that in the bladder except during voluntary micturition. During normal filling there is only a small rise in intravesical pressure. The response of the detrusor to stretch is known as its 'tone'. Tang and Ruch (1955) have shown that this is due to the inherent physical properties of the bladder muscle and is not directly affected by its nerve supply. The nervous system controls the micturition reflex, not bladder tone. The latter, however, is affected by its degree of stretch. Over-stretching leads to hypotonia and lack of stretch leads to hypertonia. As the degree of stretch allowed is determined by the micturition reflex, the nervous system indirectly influences the bladder tone.

Normally there are no bladder contractions during filling. The ability to prevent the bladder contracting, until emptying is convenient, is vital to the maintenance of continence. The bladder is said to be unstable if there is a pressure rise of greater than 15 cm of water during filling cystometry or on the provocative testing of coughing or passive pressure changes. 'The unstable bladder' is thus a urodynamic diagnosis. These involuntary bladder contractions are real and are not just artefacts due to the unphysiological filling of cystometry (Ramsden *et al.*, 1977). As a result of such contractions, patients may experience urinary frequency, nocturia, urgency or urge incontinence. They may also have stress incontinence if contractions are precipitated by rises in intra-abdominal pressure.

The bladder may become unstable as a result of damage to its neural control, either in the cerebrum or in the suprasacral spinal cord. Where bladder instability results from neurological damage, the term detrusor hyperreflexia is used (Bates *et al.*, 1976). Bladder instability may also occur secondary to outflow obstruction (Anderson, 1976; Jones and Schoenberg, 1985). Many young people have unstable bladders in the absence of any other detectable pathology. This idiopathic unstable bladder is generally believed to be a psychosomatic disorder (Cardozo and Stanton, 1980a; Frewen, 1984). There are also many elderly people with unstable bladders in the absence of detectable neurological disease or significant outflow obstruction. It is unknown whether or not these have a psychosomatic disorder or if, as seems more likely, their bladder disorder is secondary to age-related neurone fallout (Cardozo and Stanton, 1980a; Castleden *et al.*, 1985).

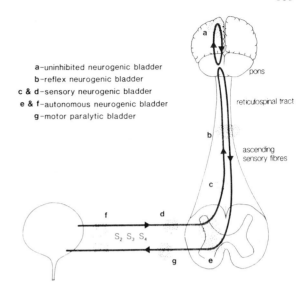

a–uninhibited neurogenic bladder
b–reflex neurogenic bladder
c & d–sensory neurogenic bladder
e & f–autonomous neurogenic bladder
g–motor paralytic bladder

Figure 31.1. Neuropathic bladder disorders.

CLASSIFICATION

The various ways of classifying neuropathic bladder disorders have been reviewed by Wein (1981). The most useful system for general use divides neuropathic bladder disorders as described below (see also Figure 31.1).

The Uninhibited Neuropathic Bladder

This results from damage to the higher centres in the brain or from incomplete spinal cord lesions. It is characterized by unstable bladder contractions. Sensation is generally normal and there is usually no significant residual urine.

Reflex Neurogenic Bladder

This results from complete suprasacral interruption of the fibres to and from the brain stem detrusor nucleus. The patient usually has an unstable bladder with failure of the external sphincter to relax (detrusor sphincter dyssynergia). This may lead to an elevated residual urine. Sensation is usually absent.

Autonomous Neuropathic Bladder

This results from either total destruction of the second to fourth sacral segments of the spinal cord or extensive injury to the motor and sensory innervation of the bladder. There is absent sensation and the patient is unable to initiate voluntary micturition. The residual urine volume depends on the patient's ability to increase intravesical pressure and on the resistance of the sphincter mechanism.

Sensory Neurogenic Bladder

This occurs when either the sensory fibres from the bladder to the spinal cord or the sensory afferent tracts to the brain stem are damaged. Desire to void is lost and unless voiding is initiated out of habit, the bladder becomes over-distended and decompensates.

Motor Paralytic Bladder

This occurs when the motor innervation of the bladder is damaged. The patient cannot initiate voluntary micturition and overflow incontinence results.

Many patients do not fit neatly into this classification system because of mixed or incomplete lesions (Wein, 1981). The clinical presentation may also be altered by secondary changes such as infection, over-distension or reinnervation.

DISEASES CAUSING NEUROPATHIC BLADDER DYSFUNCTION IN THE ELDERLY

There is no neurological disease which affects the bladder alone and it is rare for a neurological disease to present with isolated urinary symptoms. Among the more common disorders causing neuropathic bladder dysfunction in the elderly are cerebrovascular disease, Parkinson's disease and chronic brain failure.

Cerebrovascular Disease

Although incontinence is common in the early stages of a cerebrovascular accident, it is usually transient. Thirty per cent of survivors, however, will be incontinent at 3 months. In the vast majority this is due to an uninhibited neuropathic bladder (Borrie *et al.*, 1986). Lesions in both hemispheres may cause an uninhibited neuropathic bladder (Khan *et al.*, 1981). It is as yet unknown whether or not incontinence is more common with dominant than non-dominant hemisphere lesions. In addition to causing the uninhibited neuropathic bladder, a cerebrovascular accident may lead to incontinence because of impaired mobility, communication problems or confusion. Some patients may have had unstable bladders prior to the cerebrovascular accident and may have coped well with their urgency until the sudden impairment of mobility precipitated incontinence.

Parkinson's Disease

As the basal ganglia have an inhibitory effect on the micturition reflex, Parkinson's disease is usually associated with an uninhibited neuropathic bladder (Anderson and Bradley, 1976; Pavlakis *et al.*, 1983; Fitzmaurice *et al.*, 1985). These patients have been reported to suffer also from sphincter bradykinesia (Pavlakis *et al.*, 1983). However, this finding has been disputed (Fitzmaurice *et al.*, 1985). Incontinence may also be aggravated by impaired mobility and confusion.

Chronic Brain Failure

Both multi-infarct dementia and senile dementia of the Alzheimer's type may lead to the uninhibited neuropathic bladder. Incontinence may be aggravated by difficulty in finding the toilet. Some patients may have lost awareness of the need to micturate in the appropriate setting.

There are many other diseases capable of causing neuropathic bladder disorders. The uninhibited neuropathic bladder may result from multiple sclerosis or intracerebral neoplasms. The reflex neuropathic bladder and the autonomous neuropathic bladder may be caused by multiple sclerosis, traumatic spinal cord damage and tumours. The sensory neuropathic bladder may be a complication of diabetes mellitus, tabes dorsalis or pernicious anaemia. A motor paralytic bladder may result from surgical damage, pelvic fracture, poliomyelitis or herpes zoster.

URODYNAMIC STUDIES

There are many potential hazards in attempting to diagnose a patient's incontinence on purely clinical grounds. This is because the same symptom, or combination of symptoms, can be produced by very different pathophysiological processes. Thus the symptom or sign of stress incontinence may result from genuine stress incontinence or from unstable bladder contractions. Patients with urge incontinence may have stable or unstable bladders. A poor urinary flow may result from outflow obstruction, an underactive detrusor or the frequent passage of small volumes of urine due to severe instability. Thus the clinical diagnosis is frequently incorrect (Powell *et al.*, 1981; Friis *et al.*, 1982). Although the use of algorithms (Hilton and Stanton, 1981; Eastwood and Warrell, 1984) can improve the accuracy of clinical diagnosis and reduce the need for urodynamic studies, these studies are necessary if a definitive diagnosis is required. They are not, however, without risk (Sabanathan *et al.*, 1985) and involve some patient discomfort. In the elderly in particular, their use should be restricted to those cases where the result is likely to affect management (Farrar *et al.*, 1984; Resnick and Yalla, 1985; Abrams *et al.*, 1983).

MANAGEMENT OF THE NEUROPATHIC BLADDER

There are two main considerations in the management of the neuropathic bladder: the preservation of renal function, and the maintenance of continence. Renal failure may result from a combination of infection, calculosis and amyloidosis. If the neurological damage leads to incomplete bladder emptying, residual urine may become infected. In the presence of ureteric reflux or upper tract dilatation, this may lead to renal infection. In addition, stasis and infection may predispose the patient to calculus formation.

DRUG TREATMENT OF THE NEUROPATHIC BLADDER

The Unstable Bladder

Many different drugs have been used in the treatment of the unstable bladder. They include anticholinergics, smooth muscle relaxants, prostaglandin inhibitors and calcium antagonists. Despite the vast literature on the use of these drugs, their clinical efficacy in the management of the unstable bladder of neuropathic origin remains in doubt. There have been few double-blind placebo-controlled trials containing an adequate number of patients. In addition, in most of the trials, the majority of the patients have had an idiopathic unstable bladder. The relevance of these trials, containing mainly patients believed to have a psychosomatic disorder, to the management of neuropathic bladder disorders is questionable.

Recent trials (Ritch *et al.*, 1977; Walter *et al.*, 1982; Robinson and Brocklehurst, 1983; Meyhoff *et al.*, 1983) have shown emepronium bromide, an anticholinergic, to be ineffective when given orally, probably because it is so poorly absorbed. Flavoxate, a smooth muscle relaxant with anticholinergic effects, has also been shown to be ineffective (Robinson and Brocklehurst, 1983; Meyhoff *et al.*, 1983; Cardozo and Stanton, 1979; Briggs *et al.*, 1980).

Despite a wealth of experimental evidence (Kohler and Morales, 1968; Tulloch and Creed, 1979; Gregory *et al.*, 1974) showing that the anticholinergic propantheline has an effect on the unstable bladder, there is a paucity of clinical studies on its use. Blavias *et al.* (1980) used oral propantheline on 26 patients, increasing the dose until it was effective or until side-effects developed. Seventeen required either intermittent or permanent catheterization.

Despite initial favourable results (Farrar and Osborne, 1976), bromocriptine has been shown to be ineffective in the management of the unstable bladder (Cardozo and Stanton, 1980b; Delaere *et al.*, 1978; Abrams and Dunn, 1979).

Imipramine is also widely used in the management of the unstable bladder. Three possible modes of action are postulated: a central action, as a muscarinic blocker and as a sympathomimetic agent. Cardozo and Stanton (1979) and Diokno *et al.* (1972) found it to be ineffective when given parenterally. More recently, Castleden *et al.* (1985) reported favourable results using oral imipramine. However, they combined its use with bladder drill, thus making it difficult to assess whether the benefit resulted from the drug or the voiding regimen. In a later study (Castleden *et al.*, 1986), in which both study and control patients had habit retraining, they found no significant difference in outcome between those receiving imipramine and those receiving placebo.

Dicyclomine and oxybutynin, which like flavoxate are direct smooth muscle relaxants with anticholinergic effects, have been reported to be of use by a number of authors (Moisey *et al.*, 1980; Diokno and Lapides, 1972; Awad *et al.*, 1977; Fischer *et al.*, 1978; Holmes *et al.*, 1985; Gajewski and Awad, 1986). However, none of these trials was sufficiently well designed or analysed to establish the clinical value of these drugs in patients with neuropathic bladder instability. Most studies on terodiline, a drug with combined anticholinergic and calcium antagonistic properties, have excluded patients with neurological disease. Initial favourable reports (Rud *et al.*, 1980; Ekman *et al.*, 1980) are difficult to interpret as the results were not subjected to statistical analysis. More recent studies (McFarlane and Tolley, 1984; Sole and Arkel, 1984; Gerstenberg *et al.*, 1986), while reporting a good symptomatic response, have shown either no significant objective improvement or a significant, but small objective improvement. The prostaglandin synthetase inhibitors indomethacin and flurbiprofen (Cardozo *et al.*, 1980; Cardozo and Stanton, 1980b) appear to be effective, but their use has been attended by an unacceptable level of side-effects.

Although the efficacy of these drugs and others, such as ephedrine (Castleden *et al.*, 1982), baclofen (Taylor and Bates, 1979) and flunarizine (Palmer *et al.*, 1981), in the management of detrusor hyperreflexia remains open to question, their ability to cause side-effects does not. Their overall impact on the management of the unstable bladder of neuropathic origin has so far been unimpressive.

The Underactive Detrusor

For over 40 years the cholinergic agent bethanechol chloride has been the most widely used drug in the treatment of impaired bladder contractility. However, recent clinical studies (Wein *et al.*, 1980; Barratt, 1981) have called its clinical usefulness into question. Finkbeiner (1985) has recently reviewed

the literature on its use. He concluded that although pharmacologically active both in vitro and in vivo, it has not been shown to be effective in promoting bladder emptying, regardless of dose, route of administration or disease state.

An alternative therapy is the use of intravesical prostaglandins (Bultitude *et al.*, 1976). This mode of therapy remains experimental at present.

SURGERY

Various operations are used in the management of the unstable bladder. They all involve surgical interruption of the micturition reflex. Reports on the use of selective sacral neurectomy (Torrens and Griffith, 1974; Clarke *et al.*, 1979; Diokno *et al.*, 1977) and bladder transection (Mundy, 1982; Janknegt *et al.*, 1979; Parsons *et al.*, 1984) have involved small numbers of patients most of whom have had idiopathic bladder instability. Although the majority of patients have been reported to have improved symptomatically, in most the bladder has remained unstable.

More encouraging results have been obtained using the less traumatic procedure of subtrigonal phenol injections. This involves injecting phenol at a point halfway between the ureteric orifice and the urethra on each side at cystoscopy. Phenol is injected to a depth of 2–3 cm and destroys the pelvic plexuses where they lie on the anterolateral vaginal wall. Ewing *et al.* (1982) used this technique on 30 patients, 23 of whom had neuropathic bladder instability. In ten, the bladder became stable within one week of the procedure and the volume at which eighteen of the remainder had their first unstable contraction increased. Five, however, developed chronic retention. Encouraging results have also been obtained by others (Blackford *et al.*, 1984).

VOIDING REGIMENS

Regular toileting, in which the patient is taken to the toilet at fixed intervals and instructed to micturate, has long been used by nurses, particularly in geriatric wards in the management of incontinent patients. If the patient empties her bladder prior to the onset of the unstable contraction, continence is maintained. The regimen may be unsuccessful if the patient has unstable contractions at low volumes of bladder filling or has stress induced unstable contractions. Despite its widespread use and the amount of nursing time involved, there have been few studies on the efficacy of toileting alone. Those that have been done (Sogbein and Awad, 1982; Hardy *et al.*, 1982) indicate that the procedure is worthwhile.

Bladder drill, in which the patient is taught to regain control of her own bladder, is very effective in the management of the idiopathic unstable bladder (Frewen, 1982; Jarvis and Milla, 1980; Jarvis, 1982). However, as a psychological treatment, it would not be expected to be of benefit in those whose instability results from neurological disease.

MANAGEMENT OF THE NON-CONTRACTILE DETRUSOR

Some patients with a non-contractile detrusor may achieve satisfactory emptying by abdominal straining and/or manual compression of the bladder. Even if they fail to do so, the presence of a large residual urine is not, of itself, an indication for treatment, providing there is no infection. Where treatment is required, because of the presence of infection or incontinence, management can be difficult because the balance between continence and effective voiding may be very difficult to achieve. There are various approaches to the management of the non-contractile detrusor:

1. Decrease outflow resistance. If the sphincter function is preserved, the relative outflow resistance that is present may be reduced by urethral dilatation, alpha sympathetic blockade, internal urethrotomy or prostatic resection.
2. Increase contractility. The use of drugs for this purpose had already been discussed.
3. Catheterization. If sphincter function is preserved, clean intermittent self-catheterization may be successful in both sexes. The use of this procedure requires that the patient be sensible, well motivated and have the necessary manual dexterity. If intermittent catheterization is impractical, permanent catheterization can be used.

DETRUSOR SPHINCTER DYSSYNERGIA

There are a number of different approaches to management including antispastic drugs (Florante *et al.*, 1980) and sphincterotomy. A third option is to use anticholinergic agents to convert the hyperreflexive bladder to a non-contractile bladder and to manage this using intermittent self-catheterization.

PERMANENT CATHETERIZATION

This is usually seen as the last resort in the management of incontinence. In some patients, the use of a catheter may lead to a large improvement in their quality of life. In others catheterization may cause more problems than it solves. Bypassing of urine occurs in 40% of continuing care geriatric patients with a catheter in situ (Kennedy, 1983). This can be reduced by using a smaller catheter with the minimum amount of fluid necessary in the balloon. Anticholinergic agents may also help. Infection is an almost invariable accompaniment of long-term indwelling catheters. Neither urinary antiseptics, nor bladder washouts are effective in preventing infection (Brocklehurst and Brocklehurst, 1978). Antibiotics are only indicated if there is evidence of systemic infection (Ferrie *et al.*, 1979). Other problems encountered include catheter encrustation with struvite (Hukins *et al.*, 1983), urethral abscess, calculi and removal of the catheter by confused patients. Silastic catheters, which minimize encrustation by virtue of their smooth surface, are usually recommended for long-term catheterization. However, in geriatric practice there is little difference in the time in situ between Silastic and latex Foley catheters (Brocklehurst and Brocklehurst, 1978).

PROTECTIVE GARMENTS

For many incontinent elderly patients, the use of protective garments is the mainstay of management. Their use is well reviewed in the recent books by Mandelstan (1986) and Norton (1986).

REFERENCES

Abrams, P.H., and Dunn, M. (1979). A double blind trial of bromocriptine in the treatment of idiopathic bladder instability. *Br. J. Urol.*, **51**, 24–7.

Abrams, P., Feneley, R., and Torrens, M. (1983). The clinical contribution of urodynamics. In: Abrams, P., Feneley, R., and Torrens, M. (eds.) *Urodynamics*, Springer Verlag, Berlin, pp. 118–74.

Anderson, J.T. (1976). Detrusor hyperreflexia in benign infravesical obstruction. A cystometric study. *J. Urol.* **115**, 532–48.

Anderson, J.T., and Bradley, W.E. (1976). Cystometric, sphincter and electromyelographic abnormalities in Parkinson's disease. *J. Urol.*, **116**, 75–7.

Andrew, J., and Nathan, P.W. (1964). Lesions of the anterior frontal lobes and disturbances of micturition and defaecation. *Brain*, **87**, 234–6.

Awad, S.A., Blyniak, S., Downie, J.W., and Bruce, A.W. (1977). The treatment of the uninhibited bladder with dicyclomine. *J. Urol.*, **117**, 161–3.

Barrett, D.M. (1981). The effect of oral bethanechol chloride on voiding in female patients with excessive residual urine: a randomized double blind study. *J. Urol.*, **126**, 640–2.

Bates, P., Bradley, W.E., Glen, E., Melchior, H., Rowan, D., Sterling, A., and Hald, T. (1976). First report in the standardisation of terminology of lower urinary tract function. *Br. J. Urol.*, **48**, 39–42.

Blackford, H.N., Murray, K., Stephenson, T.P., and Mundy, A.R. (1984). Results of transvesical infiltration of the pelvic plexuses with phenol in 116 patients. *Br. J. Urol.*, **56**, 647–9.

Blavias, J.G., Labib, K.B., Michalik, S.J., and Zayed, A.A.H. (1980). Cystometric response to propantheline in detrusor hyperreflexia; therapeutic implications. *J. Urol.*, **124**, 259–63.

Borrie, M.J., Campbell, A.J., Cardoc-Davies, T.H. *et al.* (1986). Urinary incontinence after stroke: A prospective study. *Age Ageing*, **16**, 177–82.

Briggs, R.S., Castleden, C.M., and Asher, M.J. (1980). The effect of Flavoxate on uninhibited detrusor contractions and urinary incontinence in the elderly. *J. Urol.*, **123**, 665–71.

Brocklehurst, J.C., and Brocklehurst, S. (1978). The management of indwelling catheters. *Br. J. Urol.*, **50**, 102–5.

Bultitude, M.I., Hills, N.H., Shuttleworth, K.E.D. (1976). Clinical and experimental studies on the action of prostaglandins and their synthesis inhibitors on detrusor muscle in vitro and in vivo. *Br. J. Urol.*, **48**, 631–7.

Cardozo, L.D., and Stanton, S.L. (1979). An objective comparison of the effects of parenterally administered drugs in patients suffering from detrusor instability. *J. Urol.*, **122**, 58–9.

Cardozo, L.D., and Stanton, S.L. (1980a). Genuine stress incontinence and detrusor instability—a review of 200 cases. *Br. J. Obstet. Gynaecol.*, **87**, 184–90.

Cardozo, L.D., and Stanton, S.L. (1980b). A comparison between bromocriptine and indomethacin in the treatment of detrusor instability. *J. Urol.*, **123**, 399–401.

Cardozo, L.D., Stanton, S.L., Robinson, H., and Hole, D. (1980). Evaluation of flurbiprofen in detrusor instability. *Br. Med. J.*, **280**, 281–2.

Castleden, C.M., Duffin, H.M., and Gulati, R.S. (1986). Double-blind study of imipramine and placebo for incontinence due to bladder instability. *Age Ageing*, **15**, 299–303.

Castleden, C.M., Duffin, H.M., Briggs, R.S., and Ogden, B.M. (1982). Clinical and urodynamic effects of Ephedrine in elderly incontinent patients. *J. Urol.*, **128**, 1250–1.

Castleden, C.M., Duffin, H.M., Asher, M.J., and Yeomawson, C.W. (1985). Factors influencing outcome in elderly patients with urinary incontinence and detrusor instability. *Age Ageing*, **14**, 303–7.

Clarke, S.J., Forster, D.M.C., and Thomas, D.G. (1979). Selective sacral neurectomy in the management of urinary incontinence due to detrusor instability. *Br. J. Urol.*, **51**, 510–14.

Delaere, P.J., Debruyne, F.M.J., and Moonen, W.A. (1978). Has bromocriptine a place in the treatment of the unstable bladder? *J. Urol.*, **50**, 169–71.

Diokno, A.C., Koff, S.A., and Bender, L.F. (1974). Periurethral striated muscle activity in neurogenic bladder dysfunction. *J. Urol.*, **112**, 743–9.

Diokno, A.C., and Lapides, J. (1972). Oxybutynin. A new drug with analgesic and anticholinergic properties. *J. Urol.*, **108**, 307–9.

Diokno, A.C., Vinson, R.K., and McGillicuddy, J. (1977). Treatment of the severe uninhibited neurogenic bladder by selective sacral rhizotomy. *J. Urol.*, **118**, 299–301.

Diokno, A.C., Hyndmen, C.W., Hardy, D.A., and Lapides, J. (1972). Comparison of activity of imipramine (Tofranil) and propantheline (Probanthine) on detrusor contraction. *J. Urol.*, **107**, 42–3.

Eastwood, H.D.H., and Warrell, R. (1984). Urinary incontinence in the elderly female: prediction in diagnosis and outcome of management. *Age Ageing*, **13**, 230–4.

Ekman, G., Anderson, K.E., Rud, T., and Ulmsten, U. (1980). A double-blind cross-over study of the effects of terodiline in women with unstable bladder. *Acta Pharmacol. Toxicol.* **46** (Suppl. 1), 39–43.

Ewing, R., Bultitude, M.I., and Shuttleworth, K.E.D. (1982). Subtrigonal phenol injection for urge incontinence secondary to detrusor instability in females. *Br. J. Urol.*, **54**, 689–92.

Farrar, D.J. (1984). Urodynamics in the elderly. In: Mundy, A.R., Stephenson, T.P., and Wein, A.J. (eds.) *Urodynamic Principles, Practices and Applications*, Churchill Livingstone, Edinburgh, pp. 249–55.

Farrar, D.J., and Osborne, J.L. (1976). The use of bromocriptine in the unstable bladder. *Br. J. Urol.*, **48**, 235–8.

Ferrie, B.G., Glen, E.S., and Hunter, B. (1979). Long term urethral catheter drainage. *Br. Med. J.*, **279**, 1046–7.

Finkbeiner, A.E. (1985). Is bethanechol chloride clinically

effective in promoting bladder emptying? A literature review. *J. Urol.*, **134**, 443–4.

Fischer, C.P., Diokno, A.C., and Lapides, J. (1978). The anticholinergic effects of dicyclomine hydrochloride in uninhibited neurogenic bladder dysfunction. *J. Urol.*, **120**, 328–9.

Fitzmaurice, H., Fowler, C.J., Rickards, D. *et al.* (1985). Micturition disturbance in Parkinson's Disease. *Br. J. Urol.*, **57**, 652–6.

Fletcher, T.F., and Bradley, W.E. (1978). Neuroanatomy of the bladder-urethra. *J. Urol.*, **119**, 153–61.

Florante, J., Leyson, J., Boston, F. *et al.* (1980). Baclofen in the treatment of detrusor sphincter dyssynergia in spinal cord injury patients. *J. Urol.*, **124**, 82–4.

Frewen, W.K. (1982). A reassessment of bladder training in detrusor dysfunction in the female. *Br. J. Urol.*, **54**, 372–3.

Frewen, W.K. (1984). The significance of the psychosomatic factor in urge incontinence. *Br. J. Urol.*, **56**, 331.

Friis, E., Hjortrup, A., Runge Nielsen, J.E., Sanders, S., and Walter, S. (1982). A prospective blind study of the value of urodynamic evaluation in urinary incontinence and genital prolapse. *J. Urol.*, **128**, 764–5.

Gajewski, J.B., and Awad, S.A. (1986). Oxybutynin versus propantheline in patients with multiple sclerosis and detrusor hyperreflexia. *J. Urol.*, **135**, 966–9.

Gerstenberg, T.C., Klarskov, P., Ramirez, D., and Hald, T. (1986). Terodiline in the treatment of women with urgency and motor urge incontinence. *Br. J. Urol.*, **58**, 129–33.

Gosling, J.A., and Dixon, J.S. (1975). The structure and innervation of smooth muscle in the wall of the bladder neck and proximal urethra. *Br. J. Urol.*, **47**, 549–58.

Gosling, J.A., Dixon, J.S., and Lendon, R.G. (1977). The autonomic innervation of the human male and female bladder neck and proximal urethra. *J. Urol.*, **118**, 302–5.

Gregory, J.G., Wein, A.J., and Schoenberg, W. (1974). A comparison of the action of Tofranil and Probanthine on the urinary bladder. *Invest. Urol.*, **12**(3), 233–5.

Hardy, V.M., Capuano, E.F., and Worsam, B.D. (1982). The effect of care programmes on the dependency status of elderly residents in and extended care setting. *J. Adv. Nurs.*, **7**, 295–306.

Hilton, P., and Stanton, S.L. (1981). Algorithmic method for assessing urinary incontinence in elderly women. *Br. Med. J.*, **282**, 940–2.

Holmes, D.M., Mortz, F.J., and Stanton, S.L. (1985). Oxybutynin versus Propantheline in the treatment of detrusor instability in the female: a patient regulated variable dose trial. In: *Proceedings 15th Annual Meeting International Continence Society*, Gwynne Printers, Sussex, pp. 63–4.

Hukins, D.W.L., Hickey, D.S., and Kennedy, A.P. (1983). Catheter encrustation by struvite. *Br. J. Urol.*, **55**, 304–5.

Janknegt, R.A., Moonen, W.A., and Schreinemachers, L.M.H. (1979). Transection of the bladder as a method of treatment in adult enuresis nocturna. *Br. J. Urol.*, **51**, 275–7.

Jarvis, G.J. (1982). Bladder drill for the treatment of enuresis in adults. *Br. J. Urol.*, **54**, 118–19.

Jarvis, G.J., and Millar, D.R. (1980). Controlled trial of bladder drill for detrusor instability. *Br. Med. J.*, **281**, 1322–3.

Jones, K.W., and Schoenberg, H.W. (1985). Comparison of the incidence of bladder hyperreflexia in patients with benign prostatic hypertrophy and age matched female controls. *J. Urol.*, **133**, 425–6.

Kennedy, A. (1983). Incontinence advice 1. Long term catheterisation. *Nursing Times*, April 27th, 41–5.

Khan, Z., Hertann, J., Young, W.C., Melman, A., and Eiter, E. (1981). Predictive correlation of urodynamic dysfunction and brain injury after cerebrovascular accident. *J. Urol.*, **126**, 86–8.

Kohler, F.P., and Morales, P.A. (1968). Cystometric evaluation of Flavoxate Hydrochloride in normal and neurogenic bladders. *J. Urol.*, **100**, 729–30.

Koyanagi, T. (1980). The external urethral sphincter revisited. Studies on the sphincteric mechanism located distally in the urethra. *J. Urol.*, **124**, 400–5.

McFarlane, J.R., and Tolley, D.A. (1984). The effect of Terodiline on patients with detrusor instability. *Scand. J. Urol. Nephrol.* **87**, (Suppl.) 51–4.

Mandeltan, D. (1986). *Incontinence and Its Management*, second edition, Croom Helm, London.

Meyhoff, H.H., Gerstenberg, T.C., and Nordling, J. (1983). Placebo—the drug of choice in female motor urge incontinence. *Br. J. Urol.*, **55**, 34–7.

Moisey, C.U., Stephenson, T.P., and Brendler, C.B. (1980). The urodynamic and subjective results of treatment of detrusor instability with oxybutynin chloride. *Br. J. Urol.*, **52**, 472–5.

Mundy, A.R. (1982). The surgical treatment of urge incontinence of urine. *J. Urol.*, **128**, 481–3.

Mundy, A.R. (1984). Clinical physiology of the bladder, urethra and pelvic floor. In: Mundy, A.R., Stephenson, T.P., and Wein, A.J. (eds.) *Urodynamics Principles, Practice and Applications*, Churchill Livingstone, Edinburgh, pp. 14–25.

Norlen, L., Sundin, T., and Waagstein, F. (1978). Beta-adrenoceptor stimulation of the human urinary bladder in vivo. *Acta Pharmacol. Toxicol.*, **43**, 26–30.

Norton, C. (1986). *Nursing for Continence*, Beaconsfield Publishers, Beaconsfield, pp. 219–46.

Palmer, J.H., Worth, P.H.L., and Exton-Smith, A.N. (1981). Flunarizine; a once daily therapy for urinary incontinence. *Lancet*, **ii**, 279–81.

Parsons, S.K.F., Machin, D.G., Woolfenden, K.A., Walmsley, B., Abercrombie, G.F., and Vinnicombe, J. (1984). Endoscopic bladder transaction. *Br. J. Urol.*, **56**, 625–8.

Pavlakis, A.J., Siroky, M.B., Goldstein, I., and Krane, R.J. (1983). Neurourological findings in Parkinson's disease. *J. Urol.*, **129**, 80–3.

Powell, P.H., Shepard, A.M., Lewis, P., and Feneley, R.C.L. (1981). The accuracy of clinical diagnosis assessed urodynamically. In: Zinner, N.R., and Sterling, A.M. (eds.) *Female Incontinence*, Alan R. Liss, New York, pp. 201–3.

Ramsden, P.D., Smith, J.C., Pierce, J.M., and Ardran, G.M. (1977). The unstable bladder, fact or artefact? *Br. J. Urol.*, **49**, 633–9.

Resnick, N.M., and Yalla, S.W. (1985). Management of urinary incontinence in the elderly. *N. Engl. J. Med.*, **313**, 800–4.

Ritch, A.E.S., Castleden, C.M., George, C.F., and Hall, M.R.P. (1977). A second look at emepronium bromide in urinary incontinence. *Lancet*, **i**, 504–6.

Robinson, J.M., and Brocklehurst, J.C. (1983). Emepronium bromide and flavoxate hydrochloride in the treatment of urinary incontinence associated with detrusor instability in elderly women. *Br. J. Urol.*, **55**, 371–6.

Rud, T., Anderson, K.E., Boye, N., and Ulmsten, U. (1980). Terodiline inhibition of human bladder contraction. Effects in vitro and in women with unstable bladder. *Acta Pharmacol. Toxicol.*, **46** (Suppl. 1), 31–8.

Sabanathan, K., Duffin, H.M., and Castleden, C.M. (1985). Urinary tract infection after cystometry. *Age Ageing*, **14**, 291–5.

Sogbein, S.K., and Awad, S.A. (1982). Behavioural treatment of urinary incontinence in geriatric patients. *Can. Med. Assoc. J.*, **127**, 863–4.

Sole, G.M., and Arkell, D.G. (1984). A symptomatic and cystometric comparison of Terodiline with emepronium on the treatment of women with frequency, urgency and incontinence. *Scand. J. Urol. Nephrol.*, Suppl. 87, 35–59.

Tang, P.C., and Ruch, T.C. (1955). Non-neurogenic basis of bladder tonus. *Am. J. Physiol.*, **181**, 249–57.

Taylor, M.C., and Bates, C.P. (1979). A double blind cross over trial of baclofen—a new treatment for the unstable bladder syndrome. *Br. J. Urol.*, **51**, 504–5.

Torrens, M.J., and Griffith, H.B. (1974). The control of the uninhibited bladder by selective sacral neurectomy. *Br. J. Urol.*, **46**, 639–44.

Tulloch, S., and Creed, K.E. (1979). Comparison between propantheline and imipramine on bladder and salivary gland function. *Br. J. Urol.*, **51**, 359–62.

Vadusek, D.B., and Keith-Light, J. (1983). The motor nerve supply of the external urethral sphincter muscles. *Neurourol. Urodynam.* **2**, 193–200.

Walter, S., Hansen, J., Hansen, L., Malgaard, E., Meyhoff, A.H., and Nordling, J.A. (1982). Urinary incontinence in old age. A controlled clinical trial of emepronium bromide. *Br. J. Urol.*, **54**, 249–51.

Wein, A.J. (1981). Classification of neurogenic voiding dysfunction. *J. Urol.*, **125**, 605–9.

Wein, A.J., Molloy, T.R., Shafer, F., and Raezer, D.M. (1980). The effects of bethanechol chloride on urodynamic parameters in normal women and in women with significant residual urine volumes. *J. Urol.*, **124**, 397–9.

SECTION FOUR

Neurological Rehabilitation

Chapter 32

The Assessment of the Neurologically Disabled Elderly Patient

Keith Andrews

Director, Medical and Research Services, Royal Hospital and Home, Putney, London, UK

INTRODUCTION

The assessment of the neurologically disabled patient is not synonymous with examination of the nervous system, which is described in Chapter 5. Conventional neurological examination is important in making the diagnosis whereas the assessment is intended to determine the effect of clinical features will have on the patient's life. The assessment of the neurologically disabled person does not therefore stop at the examination of the nervous system but includes the investigation of the mental, physical, social, environmental and psychological features of the individual.

One approach to 'assessment' is to examine it in the light of the concepts used in defining *disablement*.

Impairment is the damage to an organ or part of the body. In a stroke this would be hemiplegia, sensory loss or homonymous hemianopia. The clinical examination is the prime method of assessing impairment.

Disability is the functional effect of the impairment on the patient, e.g. whether he can dress, make a cup of tea or climb stairs. This is more likely to be accurately assessed in the occupational therapy department or by the nursing staff than as a result of clinical examination. It is less easy to quantify, though more relevant to the patient, than impairment. Since many factors determine the disability, or more accurately the ability, of individual patients it

is not surprising that there is no direct correlation between *impairment* and *disability*. For instance several studies (Jefferys *et al.*, 1969; Stern *et al.*, 1971; Anderson *et al.*, 1974; Andrews *et al.*, 1981) of stroke patients have shown that there was no direct correlation between motor function and the ability to carry out activities of daily living. Whereas the impairment is reasonably specific for a given disorder, the same disability may be produced by a variety of impairments—and similar impairments do not necessarily produce identical disabilities.

Handicap is the effect that the impairment and/or the disability has on the patient's life. It is even more difficult to measure than impairment or disability but it is by far the most important aspect of disablement. It is also the least likely feature to be detected on the clinical examination. Two patients with identical impairment and disability may function entirely differently at home depending on personality, expectations, the attitude of their family and the social environment. This can be seen from the study by Andrews and Stewart (1979) who assessed elderly stroke patients attending a day hospital and measured the ability to carry out specific activities of daily living. The patients were then visited at home to assess the activities which he or she was actually carrying out. About half of the patients were carrying out significantly more activities in the supervised environment of the rehabilitation day hospital than at home. Much of the discrepancy was due to the family's unwillingness to allow the patient to carry out the activities at home—or a lack of knowledge of how far the patient could be allowed to be independent.

Since multiple pathology is common in the elderly the neurological features cannot be considered in isolation when assessing the elderly disabled person. Several authors (Wilson *et al.*, 1962; Green, 1973; Williamson *et al.*, 1964) have found that elderly patients have on average four to seven different problems. Andrews *et al.* (1985), looking at the prevalence of thirteen specified conditions on admission of elderly people to a geriatric unit, found that 19% of males and 12% of females had five or more concurrent problems. Whereas 9% of those under 80 years of age had more than five problems this rose to 18% for those 80 years and over. The commonest problems were balance disturbances (64%), arthritis of the lower limbs (35%), symptomatic heart disease (30%), confusion (25%), chronic chest disease (22%) and stroke (22%). The high prevalence of heart and lung disease is important when considering the additional energy required to cope with neurological dysfunction. For example, whereas the energy required for walking by healthy young individuals is 3.2–3.5 J m^{-1} kg^{-1} body weight (McDonald, 1961; Corcoran and Brengelmann, 1970; Waters *et al.*, 1976), hemiplegic patients expend 4.5–6.3 J m^{-1} kg^{-1} body weight (Bard, 1963; Corcoran *et al.*, 1970). Cardiorespiratory disease or anaemia will, therefore, have a complicating role and must be taken into account in assessing the neurological patient.

When assessing the ability of an elderly patient it is important to come to some conclusion about the *needs* of the patient and, equally importantly, the family. New *et al.* (1969) have demonstrated the difficulty of planning goals when patient, relatives and staff have different expectations. Difficulties arise not only when the patient has lower expectations than his real potential but also when the expectations are unrealistically high. Similar problems arise when the family have differing expectations in relation to reality than the patient or the professional staff. This fits in with the view of Knight and Warren (1978) that 'need' is as important a concept as 'handicap'.

MEASUREMENT

One of the problems of assessing disability is that there are no universally accepted measurement systems. Although several authorities have recommended standardization of tests this is often an excuse to develop yet another 'scale' or 'score'. Moreover, measurements are usually designed for hospital assessment and are not always appropriate for non-institutionalized people (Haber, 1973).

Unlike biochemical tests, measurement of disability requires the cooperation of the patient. Several workers (Jayson, 1974; Nichols, 1975; Hewer, 1974; Huskisson, 1976) have emphasized the role that motivation, intelligence, emotional state and mood play not only in recovery but also in the assessment process.

Several criteria are important in the assessment of disability in the elderly. It is important to be satisfied that:

1. The patient has heard the question. About half of the population 75 years and over have problems with hearing (Herbst and Humphery, 1980; Robinson and Sutton, 1979; Glorig and Roberts, 1970). It is, therefore, important to sit in front of the hard of hearing patient in a good light where the patient can gain visual clues. Many elderly people have hearing aids but do not wear them. It is always worthwhile making sure that the hearing aid is switched on, that the batteries are in working order and that the ear piece is clear of wax. Such simple procedures are rarely carried out.

2. The patient understands the question. Many elderly patients do not always grasp the meaning of what is being said. This is not always due to a cognitive impairment and may arise out of a semantic misunderstanding. Occasionally this may be because the elderly person has some difficulty in grasping the concept of a new idea.

3. The patient is well enough to respond. The patient with pain, for instance, has difficulty in concentrating on long involved questioning. Similarly, the depressed patient may not be in the mood to respond to instructions.

4. The environment is suitable. Testing should take place in an area where the patient is not being

distracted by embarrassment or noise. In addition the patient should be warm since cold increases muscle tone and makes it difficult to respond to the examination.

5. The assessment is simple and does not fatigue the patient. This is important since abnormal responses may be obtained if the patient is tired or bored. Care must be taken to assess patients within their tolerance.

6. The tests are comprehensive but objective (Smith, 1976) and readily accepted in other centres (Hewer, 1974). For the assessment of the individual patient in the clinical setting this is not always essential but it is of value to use tests which have been validated.

7. The tests have good inter- and intra-observer agreement (Garraway *et al.*, 1976; Sheikh *et al.*, 1980; Suchett-Kaye *et al.*, 1971; Nichols, 1975). In other words, the assessment should give the same result when repeated either by the same person or by someone else. This is always difficult since we are dealing with people who fluctuate in their ability to respond or to assess.

8. The assessment is valid, i.e. it must indicate a true disability (Nichols, 1975) and must be meaningful to the patient.

9. Changes in the scores reflect the significance of the changes in the patient. Capildeo and Rose (1979) have pointed out that in several scoring systems there is a disproportionate value given to certain clinical features. One example they quote (Mathew *et al.*, 1972) results in a score of 20 for an unconscious patient which rises to 57 when he regains consciousness; but the score rises by only two points (from 64 to 66) when the patient changes from being bedfast to being able to walk.

MOTOR FUNCTION

Deficits of motor power are some of the most obvious, though not necessarily the most important, signs of neurological damage. There are several problems associated with their measurement. First of all testing is usually subjective. The assessor compares muscle strength by asking the patient to pull against resistance provided by the examiner. This has several disadvantages. It assumes that the examiner

can judge what the strength of the muscle should be for the age, sex, and build of the patient. It also assumes that muscle power is fixed. It may, however, be influenced by tone which in turn changes with the position of the patient. Indeed therapists use positioning to inhibit the development of abnormal tonal patterns. Since muscle power is complicated by spasticity, ataxia, mass motion and motor deficits (Friedland, 1975; Dinken, 1947; Hewer, 1974), assessment of motor function cannot be meaningfully tested by simply moving one section of a limb against resistance. The traditional technique of testing hand function in stroke by asking the patient to grip the fingers of the examiner, for example, simply encourages reflex patterns of movement. A more meaningful test of hand function would be the ability to extend and abduct the fingers. Hewer (1974) has suggested that the assessment of skilled movement patterns which characterize normal motor function is much more useful than testing individual muscle groups. Moreover, the relevance of handgrip in the elderly is limited by arthritis, parkinsonism and confusional states (Milne *et al.*, 1972).

Most methods of testing power are subjective. The early measurement systems varied from simple four-point scales for the whole limb (Tennett and Harman, 1949) to complex thirteen-point scales (Dinken, 1947) ranging from no to normal power with the upper extremity having 20 movements (giving a maximum score of 240 and the lower limb fifteen movements (maximum score 180). Simple testing of movement around the joint has the advantage that it is quick to perform and can easily be understood by elderly people (Carroll, 1965). However, the traditionally accepted MRC six-point muscle testing score has been shown (John, 1984) to be no better than an analogue scale in the assessment of motor deficits. Nevertheless, these techniques have been used to describe the severity of neurological damage in stroke research studies (Sheikh *et al.*, 1980; Andrews *et al.*, 1981).

Several other difficulties arise in motor assessment. For instance, there is wide variation between different observers measuring the same parameters. Garraway *et al.* (1976) showed that there were statistically significant differences between four consultant geriatricians measuring motor function in elderly stroke patients. They also found that there was a tiring effect from repeated testing. Another obvious problem is that change in the score depends on the sensitivity of the testing system, and this includes the number of grades in the score (Andrews *et al.*, 1981). In longitudinal observation, change is more likely to be recorded when there are more grades in the scoring system.

Recently Carr *et al.* (1985) have tried to develop a scale which is brief, easily administered, has a high degree of inter-rater reliability, provides objective results without the use of expensive equipment, produces a change in score only if the patient's performance has changed and measures relevant everyday motor activities. They included a range of activities from moving from the supine position to side lying, to sitting over the side of the bed, balanced sitting, standing, walking, upper arm function, hand movements, advanced hand activities and general tonus. The difficulty here, as with many of the overall scales, is that each item is given the same weighting (all are scored on a 0 to 6 scale); consequently, two patients with the same score do not necessarily have the same dysfunction. Indeed there may be improvement in one parameter and deterioration in another but no change in the total scores.

These criticisms are not specific to this scoring system since they are a common problem when trying to get a meaningful total score from a number of independent heterogeneous variables.

MOBILITY

There is natural progression from the measurement of motor power to the assessment of mobility. Capildeo and Rose (1979) have suggested that the term 'leg function' should be used rather than 'walking function' since the latter depends on the social needs of the patient. It might equally be argued that it is more appropriate to measure the walking needs of the patient rather than isolated leg function. Wright (1979) has pointed out in his description of the 'stammering gait' that many patients with quite severe problems in initiating gait and walking can often move the limbs quite normally whilst sitting or lying. It is therefore essential

to assess mobility by observing the patient walking. This is not as obvious as it sounds since few doctors actually watch their patients walk. Thus medical records of elderly patients may record that the central nervous system, including motor power in the legs, is 'normal' whilst the patient remains immobile or falls.

It is possible to provide very accurate measurements of gait patterns using assessment of the vertical force exerted on the ground (Skorecki, 1966; Jacob *et al.*, 1972), by measuring hip and knee angles in the sagittal plane (Grieve, 1968; Mitchelson, 1979; Herschler and Milner, 1980) or recording the position of the feet (Shore, 1980; Nyak and Gabell, 1983; Jackson, 1981) when walking. The difficulty with all of these measurements is that they require sophisticated equipment which is rarely available outside research centres. These techniques, however, have given us indications as to the important parameters to observe. For instance Guimaraes and Isaacs (1980) have shown that one of the most important gait characteristics of elderly people who fall is the great variability in consecutive step lengths.

A different concept of mobility can be assessed using an overall grading systems such as the following:

1. fully mobile,
2. activities limited but can get away from neighbourhood,
3. activities limited to the immediate neighbourhood,
4. activities limited to the home or one floor in the home,
5. activities limited to one room,
6. chairfast,
7. bedbound.

This categorization says more about the social limitations rather than the actual problems with walking. Much will depend on whether the patient wants to go further than the neighbourhood and will often depend as much on the weather or the availability of family rather than a true physical limitation. At the other end of the scale the difference between being bedbound and chairfast depends on the availability of someone strong enough to help the patient to get out of bed. When discussing mobility outside the home the ability to walk not only on the level but up ramps, on and off kerbs and on stairs should also be taken into account (Adler *et al.*, 1977).

FUNCTIONAL ASSESSMENT

Functional recovery of the patient can occur in spite of relatively poor neurological recovery. Feigenson *et al.* (1979) have suggested that a functional profile is the most important measurement for longitudinal and multidisciplinary studies.

Most of the assessments of general function have looked at specific activities of daily living. There are several problems with this approach: the selected features are obtained by intuitive consensus (Jette, 1980); the measurements are subjective (Mitchelson, 1979); and they are influenced by a multiplicity of intangibles including the personality of the patient, his motivation, the degree of support and encouragement he receives from the family and the personality of the therapist (Auld, 1979).

One of the major difficulties with measurements based on activities of daily living is to obtain a meaningful score. Part of this lies in the problem of defining the individual categories. For instance terms such as 'needs minimum assistance', is 'partially dependent for help' or 'is independent but requires slight modification' are too imprecise for scientific research. On the other hand attempts to be too specific may result in difficulty in placing a patient in any grade. The five-point scale of Baker *et al.* (1968) has the category 'moderate disability' for patients able to care for personal needs and unable to work and 'moderately severe disability' for those requiring help for personal needs and requiring frequent medical care. There is, however, no category for those in the 'moderately disabled' group who can work because of the nature of their occupation and in the 'moderately severe' group for those who do not need medical attention. A grading system which will cover every eventuality must be impossible to develop.

Many research workers have developed scales which will cover different aspects of complex disability. For instance the widely used gradings of Adams and McComb (1953) include intellect as well as use of the limbs and mobility. Even more complex

systems have been used. Moskowitz and McCann (1957) developed the PULSES physical profile where:

'P' represents physical conditions including cardiovascular, pulmonary, gastrointestinal, urological and endocrine disorders,

'U' represents upper extremity functions,

'L' represents the lower extremities function,

'S' represents sensory components relating to speech, vision and hearing,

'E' represents excretory function,

'S' represents mental and emotional status.

Sokolow *et al.* (1962) included cardiopulmonary, neuromuscular, special senses, psychiatric and environmental scores which were multiplied to provide an overall score. The problem is that the more complex the system becomes the lower its specificity. At the other extreme, measurement of disability by recording the patient's dependency on others or on institutional care (Hoberman and Springer, 1958; Shafer *et al.*, 1974) depends as much on social situations as the physical disability. It is, however, a more accurate measurement of the patient's real function.

For research purposes it is preferable to have a score which can be analysed statistically. The obvious variables are the activities of daily living but there are difficulties in knowing which ones to select and what weighting to give to each item. This is relevant when considering the various needs of different individuals and age groups. It is obvious that it is irrelevant to include occupational levels in measurement systems for the elderly whereas they would be very important in systems for the younger disabled.

Ottenbacher (1980), on examining 35 occupational therapy evaluation forms, found that the level of measurement most frequently employed was descriptive, there being a tendency to collect data at a higher or more sophisticated level of measurement in those areas which were most commonly assessed. This collection of a large amount of information of functional activities has been assessed by Jette (1980) who found that, of 36 activities measured, 60% of the total variance was accounted for by mobility, kitchen chores, personal care, home chores and transferring.

TABLE 32.1 THE MODIFIED BARTHEL ADL INDEX

Activity	Independent	Needs help	Unable
Feeding	10	5	0
Chair/bed transfer	15	5–10[a]	0
Personal toilet	5	0	0
Toilet	10	5	0
Bathing	5	0	0
Dressing	10	5	0
Walking on level	5	0	0
Stairs	10	5	0
Bowel control	10	5	0
Bladder control	10	5	0

[a] 10=minimum verbal/physical help, 5=maximal help, but can sit independently.

There have been many attempts to develop a numerical score for functional activities. There are, however, problems. For instance Adler *et al.* (1977) took four activities (feeding, toileting, self-care and dressing) along with perception and awareness of safety and subdivided each into five classifications, e.g. for feeding 'managing without supervision', 'managing with supervision', 'requires constant attention', 'needs to be fed or tube fed'. This system gives the same emphasis to feeding as to dressing. It also implies that the change from being tube fed to being spoonfed is quantitatively as large as the changes from feeding with supervision to feeding independently.

To overcome this problem there have been attempts to provide loading to different activities. One of the most commonly used of these is the Barthel Index (Mahoney and Barthel, 1965) (Table 32.1). Donaldson *et al.* (1973) criticized the Barthel Index on the grounds that it was an insufficiently sensitive measure of self care; whilst Wylie (1964) suggested that the scores 0–100 are not true points, that deterioration can occur beyond these limits and that changes in the same number of points do not reflect precisely the same change in disability. Wade *et al.* (1984) have also pointed out that there is a lack of sensitivity, especially at the upper level of ability, which arises from the pass–fail nature of the scoring. A score of 100 does not imply normality but simply

independence in the activities measured. To this might be added that the grades are artificial since they give the same score to a patient requiring help with feeding as to a patient requiring help with climbing stairs. One further difficulty is that the same score does not necessarily mean the same type of disability for either cross-sectional or longitudinal studies.

In spite of these difficulties Gresham *et al.* (1980) compared several activities of daily living (ADL) scoring systems and found that the Barthel Index had the advantage of completeness, sensitivity to change, amenability to statistical manipulation and greater familiarity due to its widespread use. Granger and Greer (1976) also found it to be effective primarily because of its simplicity and high inter-observer reliability.

Dinken (1947) took a different approach by subdividing each activity into a number of grades according to its importance. Dressing, for example, was given eight grades, toileting seven, and hand activities fifteen. On the other hand, Harris (1971) grouped activities into major and minor activities and gave a different score to each group.

A different approach has been described by the Staff of the Benjamin Rose Hospital (1959) and further validated (Katz *et al.*, 1963; Kelman and Willner, 1962). Instead of giving a numerical score to the disability they classified by a grading system, which allowed some flexibility, based on the recovery pattern, as follows:

A: Independent in feeding, continence, transferring, toileting, dressing and bathing.
B: Independent in all but one of these activities.
C: Independent in all but bathing and one other activity.
D: Independent in all but bathing, dressing and one additional activity.
E: Independent in all but bathing, dressing, toileting and one additional activity.
F: Independent in all but bathing, dressing, toileting, transferring and one additional activity.
G: Dependent in all six functions.
Other: Dependent in at least two functions but not classifiable as C, D, E or F.

The advantage of this system is that the grades are

specific and follow the natural recovery of most disabling conditions. It, however, lacks sensitivity since there are only two points (independent/dependent) for each activity.

The measurement systems described are more applicable to research studies than to daily clinical practice where each activity can be assessed independently from the others without the need to develop an overall score. Nevertheless it is important for the rehabilitation team to keep some record of the patient's progress and this does require some simple measurement system. One of the difficulties is deciding on the relevance of the measurements. Andrews and Stewart (1979) showed that what the patient can do in the rehabilitation setting is not necessarily what he does do in the home environment. One approach to overcoming this is the Goal Attainment Score (GAS) (Kiresuk and Sherman, 1968; Garwick, 1974; Clark and Caudrey, 1983). In the GAS system the main problems requiring management are identified and goals mutually determined by the patient, chief carer and staff. It is important that the goals are relevant and achievable. The success of rehabilitation is then measured by the extent to which the goals are achieved. The assessment of the patient therefore takes into account the individual needs of the patient without depending on artificially set measurement systems. In effect there is a different measurement system for each patient.

Trieschmann (1974) has pointed out that one of the key factors in whether an individual will cope is the number of rewards that are available and the level of motivation needs to be assessed in the early stages of the rehabilitation programme. In an attempt to assess this at an early stage Becker *et al.* (1974) set up a list of 30 items of activity which were discussed with the patient and the family separately. Where there were differences of opinion between the expected goals of the patient, relatives and staff, compromise goals were negotiated and agreed on. They concluded that this method of assessment helped to identify early conflicts of interest, improved the planning of individual treatments whilst encouraging staff–relative interaction. It is obviously more difficult to obtain a neat score from this type of assessment but the result is much more directly related to the patient's needs.

SOCIAL ASSESSMENT

This is one of the most difficult assessments to make. Measurement systems at best can only be vague and, although essential for research purposes, are of little value in the day to day management of individual patients.

It is essential to recognize the differences between the 'wants' and the 'cans'. Many patients want to go home and unrealistically think that they will cope. This is particularly common with left hemiplegic patients (denial of illness) though it is not uncommon in others. Such patients find it difficult to appreciate that it is one thing to cope in a protective hospital environment with plenty of space to move around with a frame, no obstructions to trip over, furniture of the right height and staff to provide stimulation and support; while it is quite another to return to live at home in unsatisfactory conditions without the stimulation of the supportive environment. Some indication of the likelihood of the patient coping at home can be obtained from observing him or her in an Independence Assessment Flat where he or she is expected to cope with daily activities without help or supervision. The environment is still artificial and does not necessarily give a true reflection of how the patient will manage at home. It may, however, bring problems to light which otherwise would have been missed. The assessment of the patient's capability is more appropriately made on a home visit. Since this can last only a short time a true evaluation of the situation may not be obtained even then. For instance the patient may be tired or made apprehensive by the journey home and may not perform well. On the other hand, the patient may be so determined to prove that he will cope that he appears to do better than he actually manages when he is discharged home. To some extent this can be overcome by more prolonged home assessments, either by leaving the patient at home all day (returning in the evening) or on a 24–48 hour trial discharge basis. Follow-up by intensive home support teams and domiciliary physiotherapy services may provide a better assessment than was possible in the protective environment of the hospital.

For those involved in research there are a number of scales and scoring systems which measure various aspects of social functioning. Some measure the amount of social support. For instance the Role Activity Scales (Havinghurst and Albrecht, 1953) examine ten levels of activity in thirteen social roles of the elderly whereas the Mutual Support Index (Kerchoff, 1965) estimates the level of family support by producing a scale of four categories of family.

1. The extended family (a highly supportive family group living near to each other).
2. The modified extended family (family living near to each other but low levels of support).
3. The nucleated family (a highly supportive family but living some distance away).
4. The individuated family (a family living away with little mutual support).

These use objective tests taking account of actual physical relationships. Others are more subjective, assessing satisfaction with family relationship (Smilkstein, 1978) or recording the amount of time spent on specific activities such as watching television, reading and visiting (Graney and Graney, 1973).

Linn *et al.* (1969) attempted to measure social dysfunctioning, taking into account self esteem, personality, reaction with others and attitudes to life. Although not primarily designed for the elderly, it is nevertheless easily adapted for their use. It must also be recognized that most of the items are subjective and depend on the response from the client. Other scales (Platt *et al.*, 1980) have been designed specifically to obtain information about social functioning from the most involved relative.

A number of other scales has been developed to measure life satisfaction (Havinghurst *et al.*, 1961), attitudes (Oberleder, 1961; Cavan *et al.*, 1949), contentment (Bloom and Blenkner, 1970) and morale (Lawton, 1970). In practice these are rarely used though they may be valuable for research projects.

CONCLUSION

The assessment of the neurologically disabled elderly patient is not fundamentally different from the assessment of those whose disability arises from damage in other systems. Most measurement systems are usually more applicable to the research field than to the clinical situation. That is not to say that measurement is not required in the day to day management of patients but there is less need to develop overall grades and numerical scores.

The main reason for having a scoring system in clinical practice is to observe the rate of recovery and the response to therapy. It it therefore important to decide at an early stage which activities are relevant and what will be regarded as the successful outcome. New activities will be added and others dropped from the assessment as the condition changes. This provides a continuous modification of both the goals and the measurement systems.

Since the level of ability required to provide a reasonable quality of life will depend on so many different factors including the personality, mental state and the level of family support these must be of prime concern in the assessment. Although scoring systems satisfy the scientific need of the assessor they must not be allowed to distract from the less easily measured handicap. Counting pieces of a jig-saw puzzle tells us nothing about the final picture. What matters is how the pieces fit together. That is the true art of assessment.

REFERENCES

Adams, G.F., and McComb, S.G. (1953). Assessment and prognosis in hemiplegia. *Lancet*, **ii**, 266–9.

Adler, M., Hamaty, D., Brown, C.C., and Potts, H. (1977). Medical audit of stroke rehabilitation: a critique of medical care review. *J. Chronic Dis.*, **30**, 461–71.

Anderson, T.P., Bourestom, N., Greenberg, F.R., Hilyard, V.G. (1974). Predictive factors in stroke rehabilitation. *Arch. Phys. Med. Rehabil.*, **55**, 545–53.

Andrews, K., Harding, M.A., and Goldstone, D. (1985). The social implications of multiple pathology. *Gerontologia*, **31**, 325–31.

Andrews, K., and Stewart, J. (1979). Stroke recovery—He can but does he? *Rheumatol. Rehabil.*, **18**, 43–8.

Andrews, K., Brocklehurst, J.C., Richards, B., and Laycock, F.B. (1981). The rate of recovery from stroke—and its measurement. *Int. Rehabil. Med.*, **3**, 155–61.

Auld, M. (1979). Problems of evaluating remedial therapy. In: Kenedi, R.M., Paul, J.P., and Hughes, J. (eds.) *Disability—Proceedings of a Seminar on Rehabilitation of the Disabled*, Macmillan Press, London.

Baker, R.N., Schwartz, W.S., and Ramseyer, J.C. (1968). Prognosis among survivors of ischaemic stroke. *Neurology*, **18**, 933–41.

Bard, B. (1963). Energy expenditure of hemiplegic

subjects during walking. *Arch. Phys. Med. Rehabil.*, **44**, 368–70.

Becker, M.C., Abrams, K.S., and Onder, J. (1974). Goal setting: A joint patient staff method. *Arch. Phys. Med. Rehabil.*, **55**, 87–9.

Bloom, M., and Blenkner, M. (1970). Assessing functioning of older persons living in the community. *Gerontologist*, **10**, 331–7.

Capildeo, R., and Rose, F.C. (1979). The assessment of neurological disability. In: Greenhaulgh, R.M., and Rose, F.C. (eds.) *Progress In Stroke Research I*, Pitman Medical, Tunbridge Wells.

Carr, J.H., Shepherd, R.B., Nordholm, L., and Lynne, D. (1985). Investigation of a new motor assessment scale for stroke patients. *Phys. Ther.*, **65**, 175–9.

Carroll, D. (1965). A quantitative test of upper extremity function. *J. Chronic Dis.*, **18**, 479–91.

Cavan, R.S., Burges, E.W., Havinghurst, R.J., and Goldhamer, H. (1949). *Personal Adjustment in Old Age*, Sci. Res. Associates, Chicago.

Clark, M.S., and Caudrey, D.J. (1983). Evaluation of rehabilitation services: the use of goal attainment scaling. *Int. Rehabil. Med.*, **5**, 41–5.

Corcoran, P.J., and Brengelmann, G.L. (1970). Oxygen uptake in normal and handicapped subjects in relation to speed of walking beside velocity controlled cart. *Arch. Phys. Med. Rehabil.*, **51**, 78–87.

Corcoran, P.J., Jebsen, R.H., Brengelmann, G.L., and Simons, B.C. (1970). Effects of plastic and metal leg braces on speed and energy cost of hemiparetic ambulation. *Arch. Phys. Med. Rehabil.*, **51**, 69–77.

Dinken, H. (1947). The evaluation of disability and treatment in hemiplegia. *Arch. Phys. Med. Rehabil.*, **28**, 263–72.

Donaldson, S.W., Wagner, C.C., and Gresham, G.H.E (1973). Unified evaluation ADL form. *Arch. Phys. Med. Rehabil.*, **54**, 175–9.

Feigenson, J., Polkow, L., Meikle, R., and Furguson, W. (1979). Burke stroke time orientated profile: an overview of patient function. *Arch. Phys. Med. Rehabil.*, **60**, 580–11.

Friedland, F. (1975). Physical therapy. In: Licht, S. (ed.) *Stroke and its Rehabilitation*, Waverley Press, Baltimore.

Garraway, W.M., Akhtar, A.J., Gore, S.M., Prescott, R.J., and Smith, R.G. (1976). Observer variation in the clinical assessment of stroke. *Age Ageing*, **5**, 233–40.

Garwick, G. (1974). Recent findings on the use of goal-setting in human service agencies: the implementation, flexibility and validity of goal attainment scaling. *Goal Attain. Rev.*, **1**, 1–4.

Glorig, A., and Roberts, J. (1970). Hearing levels of adults by age and sex: United States 1960–1962. *Vital and Health Statistics*, 1965, Series 11, No. 11.

Graney, M.J., and Graney E.E. (1973). Scaling and adjustment in older people. *Int. J. Ageing Hum. Develop.*, **4**, 351–9.

Granger, C.V., and Greer, D.S. (1976). Functional status measurement and medical rehabilitation outcome. *Arch. Phys. Med. Rehabil.*, **57**, 103–9.

Green, M.F. (1973). Geriatric Medicine. *Br. J. Hosp. Med.*, December, 672–3.

Gresham, G.E., Phillips, T.F., and Labi, M.L.C. (1980). ADL status in stroke: relative merits of three standard indexes. *Arch. Phys. Med. Rehabil.*, **61**, 355–8.

Grieve, D.W. (1968). Gait patterns and the speed of walking. *Bioed Eng.*, **3**, 119–22.

Guimaraes, R.M., and Isaacs, B. (1980). Characteristics of the gait in old people who fall. *Int. Rehabil. Med.*, **2**, 177–80.

Haber, L.D. (1973). Disabling effects of chronic disease and improvement. II Functional capacity limitations. *J. Chronic Dis.*, **26**, 127–51.

Harris, A.I. (1971). *Handicapped and Impaired in Great Britain*, HMSO, London.

Havinghurst, R.J., and Albrecht, R. (1953). *Older People*, Longmans, Green and Company, New York.

Havinghurst, R.J., Newgarten, B.L., and Tobin, S.S. (1961). The measurement of life satisfaction. *J. Gerontol.*, **16**, 134–43.

Herbst, K.G., and Humphery, C. (1980). Hearing impairment and mental state in the elderly living at home. *Br. Med. J.*, **281**, 903–5.

Herschler, C., and Milner, M. (1980). Angle-angle diagrams in assessment of locomotion. *Am. J. Phys. Med.*, **59**, 109–24.

Hewer, R.L. (1974). Quantification in stroke. *Proc. Roy. Soc. Med.*, **67**, 404–6.

Hoberman, M., and Springer, C.F. (1958). Rehabilitation of the 'permanently and totally disabled' patient. *Arch. Phys. Med. Rehabil.*, **39**, 235–40.

Huskisson, E.C. (1976). Measurement in rehabilitation. *Rheumatol. Rehabil.*, **15**, 132.

Jackson, K.M. (1981). Monitoring the position of the feet during human locomotion. *J. Biochem. Eng.*, **15**, 297.

Jacob, N.A., Skorecki, J., and Charnley, J. (1972). Analysis of the vertical component of force in normal and pathological gait. *J. Biomech.*, **5**, 11–34.

Jayson, M.I.V. (1974). Quantification of disability. *Proc. Roy. Soc. Med.*, **67**, 400–1.

Jefferys, M., Millard, J.B., Hyman, M., and Warren, M.D. (1969). A set of tests for measuring motor impairment in prevalence studies. *J. Chronic Dis.*, **22**, 303–19.

Jette, A.M. (1980). Functional capacity evaluations empirical approach. *Arch. Phys. Med. Rehabil.*, **61**, 85–9.

John, J. (1984). Grading of muscle power: comparison of MRC and analogue scales by physiotherapists. *Int. J. Rehabil. Res.*, **7**, 173–81.

Katz, S., Ford, A.B., and Moskowitz, R.W. (1963). Studies of illness in the aged: Index of ADL. *J.A.M.A.*, **185**, 914–19.

Kelman, H.R., and Willner, A. (1962). Problems of measurement and evaluation. *Arch. Phys. Med. Rehabil.*, **43**, 172–81.

Kerchoff, A.C. (1965). Nuclear and extended family relationships: a normative and behavioural analysis. In: Shanas, E., and Streb, G. (eds.) *Social Structure and the Family: Generational Relations*, Prentice-Hall.

Kiresuk, T., and Sherman, R. (1968). Goal attainment scaling: a general method of evaluating comprehensive mental health programmes. *Comm. Ment. Health J.*, **4**, 443–53.

Knight, R., and Warren, M.D. (1978). Physically disabled people living at home: a study of number and needs. *Report on Health and Social Services 13*, HMSO, London.

Lawton, M.P. (1970). Assessment, integration and environments for older people. *Gerontologist*, **10**, 38–46.

Linn, M.W., Sculthorpe, W.B., Evje, M., Slater, P.H., and Goodman, S.P. (1969). A social dysfunction rating scale. *J. Psychiatr. Res.*, **6**, 299–306.

McDonald, I. (1961). Statistical studies of recorded energy expenditure in man. Part II: expenditure on walking related to weight, sex, age, height, speed and gradient. *Nutr. Abstr. Rev.*, **59**, 121–3.

Mahoney, F.I., and Barthel, D.W. (1965). Functional evaluation: the Barthel Index. *Maryland Med J.*, **14**, 61–5.

Mathew, N.T., Meyer, J.S., Rivera, V.M. *et al.* (1972). Double blind evaluation of glycerol therapy in acute cerebral infarction. *Lancet*, **ii**, 127–9.

Milne, J.S., Maule, M.M., Cormack, S., and Williamson, J. (1972). The design and testing of a questionnaire and examination to assess physical and mental health in older people using a staff nurse as an observer. *J. Chronic Dis.*, **25**, 385–405.

Mitchelson, D.L. (1979). Bioengineering in motor function assessment and therapy. In: Greenhalgh, R.M., and Rose, F.C. (eds.) *Progress in Stroke Research I*, Pitman Medical, Tunbridge Wells.

Moskowitz, E., and McCann, C.B. (1957). Classification of disability in the chronically ill and aging. *J. Chronic Dis.*, **5**, 342–6.

New, P.K., Ruscio, A.T., and George, L.A. (1969). Towards an understanding of the rehabilitation system. *Rehab. Lit.*, **30**, 130–9.

Nichols, P.J.R. (1975). Some psychological aspects of rehabilitation and their implications for research. *Proc. Roy. Soc. Med.*, **68**, 537–44.

Nyak, U.S.L., and Gabell, A. (1983). Foot placement analysis in the elderly: practical considerations. *J. Biomed. Engin.*, **5**, 69.

Oberleder, M. (1961). An attitude scale to determine adjustment in institutions for the aged. *J. Chronic Dis.*, **15**, 915–23.

Ottenbacher, K. (1980). Cerebrovascular accidents: some

characteristics of occupational therapy evaluation forms. *Am. J. Occup. Ther.*, **34**, 268–70.

Platt, S., Weyman, A., Hirsch, S., and Hewett, S. (1980). The social behavior assessment schedule (SBAS): rationale, contents, scoring and reliability of a new interview schedule. *Soc. Psychiatry*, **15**, 43–55.

Robinson, D.W., and Sutton, G.J. (1979). Age effect in hearing—a comparative analysis of published threshold data. *Audiology*, **18**, 320–34.

Shafer, S.Q., Brunn, B., Brown, R., and Richter, R.W. (1974). Stroke: early portends of functional recovery in black patients. *Arch. Phys. Med. Rehabil.*, **55**, 264–8.

Sheikh, K., Smith, D.S., Meade, T.W., Brennan, P.J., and Ide, L. (1980). Assessment of motor function in studies of chronic disability. *Rheumatol. Rehabil.*, **19**, 83–90.

Shore, M. (1980). Footprint analysis in gait documentation. *Phys. Ther.*, **60**, 1163.

Skorecki, J. (1966). The design and construction of a new apparatus for measuring the vertical forces exerted in walking: a gait machine. *J. Strain Analysis*, **1**, 429.

Smilkstein, G. (1978). The family APGR: a proposal for a family function test and its use by physicians. *J. Fam. Pract.*, **6**, 1231–9.

Smith, D.S. (1976). The Northwick Park Hospital Stroke Rehabilitation Study. *Rheumatol. Rehabil.*, **15**, 163–6.

Sokolow, J., Silson, J.E., Taylor, E.J., Anderson, M.A., and Rusk, H.A. (1962). A new approach to the objective evaluation of physical disability. *J. Chronic Dis.*, **15**, 105–12.

Staff of the Benjamin Rose Hospital (1959). Multidisciplinary studies of illness in aged persons. II A new classification of functional status in activities of daily living. *J. Chronic Dis.*, **9**, 55–62.

Stern, P.H., McDowell, F., Miller, J.M., and Robinson, M. (1971). Factors influencing rehabilitation. *Stroke*, **2**, 213–15.

Suchett-Kay, A.I., Sarkov, U., Elkan, G., and Waring, M. (1971). Physical, mental and social assessment of elderly patients suffering from cerebrovascular accident, with special reference to rehabilitation. *Gerontol. Clin.*, **1**, 192–206.

Tennett, E.C., and Harman, J.W. (1949). A study of factors affecting the prognosis of C.V.A. *Am. J. Med. Sci.*, **218**, 361–8.

Trieschmann, T.B. (1974). Coping with disability: a sliding scale of goals. *Arch. Phys. Med. Rehabil.*, **55**, 556–60.

Wade, D.T., Skilbeck, C.E., Hewer, R.L., and Wood, V.A. (1984). Therapy after stroke: amount, determinants and effects. *Int. Rehabil. Med.*, **6**, 105–10.

Waters, R.L., Perry, J., Antonelli, D., and Hislop, H. (1976). Energy costs of walking of amputees: influence of the level of amputation. *J. Bone Joint Surg.*, **58A**, 42–6.

Williamson, J., Stokoe, I.H., Gray, S., Fisher, M., and

Smith, A. (1964). Old people at home: Their unreported needs. *Lancet*, **i,** 1117–20.

Wilson, L.A., Lawson, I.R., and Brass, W. (1962). Multiple disorders in the elderly—a clinical and statistical study. *Lancet*, **ii,** 841–3.

Wright, W.B. (1979). Stammering gait. *Age Ageing*, **8,** 8–12.

Wylie, C.M. (1964). A measure of disability. *Arch. Environ. Health*, **8,** 834–9.

The Clinical Neurology of Old Age
Edited by R. Tallis
© 1989 John Wiley & Sons Ltd

Chapter 33

The Role of Remedial Therapists

Peter Chin

Consultant Physician, Department of Geriatric Medicine, Cumberland Infirmary, Carlisle, UK

INTRODUCTION

Until dramatic advances are made in the immediate reversal or limitation of brain damage following vascular, demyelinating and other degenerative insults, the main burden of rehabilitating the afflicted lies in the hands of remedial therapists. Even when skilled use of drugs improves prognosis and functional performance (as in Parkinson's disease), the part played by therapists remains substantial. Clinicians, whose main preoccupation is with diagnosis and the role of pharmaceutical agents, ought to take a greater interest in the work of these professionals who make such a remarkable contribution to the welfare of their patients.

Much remedial therapy is empirical, and estimates of its efficacy are heavily reliant on anecdotal accounts. There is also a considerable placebo effect derived from the use of impressive electronic gadgetry and other physical devices. There is much to be gained from collaboration between clinicians and therapists in separating folk remedies (on which much time and energy is dissipated) from effective practice demonstrated by controlled trials (Tallis, 1984).

This account of the role of remedial therapists is not intended to be comprehensive, but will focus on aspects relevant to the rehabilitation of the elderly neurological patient.

COMMON GROUND

The Elderly Disabled

Most therapists involved with neurologically damaged patients recognize that, although the technical expertise that each has to offer may be different from that offered by the others, there are certain aspects of the rehabilitation of elderly people which are common to all. These include the special effects of disease in the context of old age, with particular reference to physical, psychological and environmental aspects of the patient.

First, the aims and objectives of the overall regimen have to be tailored to the response capability of the elderly person, and realistic goals have to be set that take account of overall prognosis and concurrent pathology. Isaacs (1984) put it succinctly when he stated that rehabilitation should aim at restoring lost function, and the person to his or her former role, with maximal use of the remaining function. Sometimes this means that the sufferer has to be helped to adapt and accept an altered role. With individually prescribed targets, rehabilitation failure should be rare.

The presence of multiple pathology not only makes it difficult to estimate how much of a patient's disability is due to neurological damage, but also interferes frustratingly with the assessment of the outcome even when standardized techniques are applied under controlled conditions. This makes the evaluation of physical techniques in the rehabilitation of elderly patients particularly difficult. It also invites a proliferation of different empirical approaches, so that neurological disability is a happy hunting ground for practitioners of alternative medicine.

Definitions and Evaluation

Some of the controversy surrounding the measurement of success of remedial therapy may arise out of confusion over definitions. Three words, which are now widely used in the terminology of rehabilitation, encapsulate the effect of physical or neurological insult in a patient. These are impairment, disability and handicap.

Impairment refers to the pathological damage and its manifestations, such as paralysis, imbalance, disordered speech, cognition, or perception or superadded features, such as abnormal movements and spasticity.

Disability is the reduction in functional ability, consequent upon the neurological damage, such as the inability to walk, talk or move freely.

Handicap is the disadvantaged or restricted life style imposed by disability.

Remedial therapy is unlikely to have a substantial influence on impairment, though contrary claims are made. The best hope for containing the burden of neurological impairment, as in strokes, lies in prevention. Remedial therapy can, however, make a major impact on disability and handicap. In evaluating the effectiveness of interventions, therapists need to be clear about where they are targeting their efforts—impairment, disability or handicap—and make measurements accordingly. The switch from maximum therapeutic effort in the direction of restoring ability to optimizing function with aids and gadgetry has to be achieved without harming expectations too drastically. It also therefore means that therapists may have to change tack, abandoning special treatment regimens, and this may complicate evaluation of these methods of treatment; cynics would call it 'fudging'.

Where Therapists Work

The best places to observe various remedial therapy techniques and the individualized approaches of enthusiasts are probably centres of excellence or the home base of particular proponents of techniques. These special settings have an important role in teaching and research, where staff are highly trained and in abundance—for example the Wolfson Centre or the Bobath Clinic.

The concentration of specialist therapists in disease-specific wards in hospitals (such as stroke units) remains a matter for debate (Hewer, 1972; Garaway, 1982). However, regional centres for rehabilitation of head injury and spinal injuries are well established. In practice they cater for very few elderly patients, and usually only for the acute phase of treatment.

For most physicians dealing with the majority of elderly neurologically damaged patients, the practical delivery of care by therapists is severely constrained, not least by the lack of therapists trained in specialized techniques. Such therapists as are available face other constraints—most importantly limitation of time, the sheer numbers of patients to be treated, and the pressures of inpatient bed space. In some instances, there is a conflict between those who need to ensure a high turnover of beds to make room for the acutely ill, and therapists who are required to expedite patient discharge when rehabilitation may be incomplete and the place of discharge not ideal for further rehabilitation. These apparently mundane issues can have a demoralizing effect on all carrying out practical rehabilitation. Some patients may achieve remarkable independence in activities of daily living in wards but make no use at all of their skills when they go home. This may be due to 'learned dependency', when the dependent role is more gratifying, but more often misguided carers become over-protective and undo much that has been gained through treatment (Andrews, 1979).

Despite these problems, some therapists manage to motivate not only the patients, but also nurses, relatives and even physicians, all of whose expectations of recovery may be discouragingly low. The role of friend, comforter and counsellor is one of the most important aspects of the work of a remedial therapist treating neurological patients.

Collaboration

The last two decades have seen not only the emergence of specific therapeutic programmes propounded by individual therapists, but also a mood of assertive professionalism. In Britain, various re-organizations of the National Health Service have encouraged the professions allied to medicine to be managerially as well as professionally independent. Nowadays, remedial therapists no longer work under the direct supervision and guidance of consultants in rehabilitation medicine. Sadly, in some places, this has had a disruptive influence, but it is encouraging to note from Gloag's (1985) account of rehabilitation services, that there is much evidence of cooperation. The close and successful interdisciplinary collaboration between therapists, nurses, doctors and social workers fostered in the departments of geriatric medicine (which care for the bulk of stroke and parkinsonian patients) is the hallmark of British geriatrics, emulated in many parts of the world.

Formal and informal case conferences are useful not only to review the patients' progress but also to identify potential barriers to progress. This will ensure that different groups do not vie with each other to 'kick patients through the goals', instead of letting patients kick their own goals. Moreover, the case conference acts as a focal point for teaching and for inspiration and sustenance of the exhausted and discouraged. The danger is that the conference becomes an end in itself and a means of postponing decisions and avoiding responsibility.

The concept of a generic therapist versed in most aspects of remedial treatment for specific diseases has been advocated by, for example, Hopkins (1975). Feldman (1961) has demonstrated that nurses trained in a functionally orientated approach improved stroke patients' levels of function to the same degree as a rehabilitation ward staffed by professional therapists in all respects except gait. Whether this idea, which has some merit, will catch on or succumb to the politicking of the respective professional bodies only time will tell. In neurological conditions which make a heavy demand on a numerically large and diverse multidisciplinary team this approach to management should at least be evaluated.

PHYSIOTHERAPY

In the last 25 years, some remarkable changes have taken place in physiotherapy for the neurological patient. Until the late 1960s, the prevailing methods of restoration of function relied heavily on a pragmatic approach. For example, in stroke rehabili-

TABLE 33.1   ROLE OF PHYSIOTHERAPY

1. Manual techniques
   a. Passive movements and massage
   b. Active and resistive exercises
   c. Facilitation and inhibition (for stroke patients particularly)
2. Use of physical agents, e.g. heat, ice, ultrasound and electricity.
3. Orthotic advice
4. Education and counselling—relatives and other carers

tation, therapists concentrated on making full use of the normal side, and training it to compensate for the loss of function in the hemiplegic limbs. Lately, the emphasis has shifted to the hemiplegic limbs in an attempt to overcome disability by improving control of them. The pursuit of symmetry in gait and posture has shaped much of current physiotherapy in stroke rehabilitation. Techniques evolved with such aspirations are collectively known as 'facilitation and inhibition movement therapies'. Aside from the preoccupation of physiotherapy with these relatively new techniques, various functions of physiotherapists are given in Table 33.1.

Passive Movements and Massage

When limbs are paralysed, passive movements ensure that major joints are put through the functional range of movements to prevent, for example, the frozen shoulder syndrome and contractures. These movements are usually applied in the early phase of neurological damage, but they also have a major role in the late stages of such conditions as motor neurone disease, Parkinson's disease, and when spasticity supervenes in multiple sclerosis and stroke.

In stroke patients the use of asymmetrical pulley exercises, in which the normal limb is used to pull the hemiplegic arm and shoulder through its paces, is outmoded. The vigour with which some patients pursued this exercise occasionally damaged the capsule and pericapsular muscles and tendons, producing more pain than the frozen shoulder syndrome which it was intended to prevent.

Some patients have the unshakeable belief that hemiplegic limbs may be restored through massaging the offending part. Though massage is unlikely to restore power or control, it has a soothing effect on any painful area, and also increases proprioception in limbs which are bereft of position sense. Passive positioning of the patient to avoid exaggeration of abnormal reflexes and increased spasticity in stroke is an important early rehabilitation manoeuvre. Breathing exercises are important in patients with motor neurone disease, Parkinson's disease and the acute phase of stroke.

Active and Resistive Exercises

Active exercises require the participation of patients, either individually or in a group. Conventional regimens incorporating the Swedish exercises were initially designed for the treatment of injury. The particular exercises used are based on the principle of progressive strengthening of muscles through isotonic and isometric contractions. These exercises are performed against graded resistance, provided by weights and springs, or by the therapist. Sometimes they are combined with circuit training and gymnastic exercises which may not be applicable to the elderly patient. On the other hand, group exercises aimed at putting joints through full ranges of movement, are widely practised, often to the accompaniment of music. Such group therapy sessions are particularly valuable in stroke and Parkinson's disease, helping to maintain current levels of performance.

In stroke rehabilitation, the 'traditional' functionally orientated approach used early passive movements to ensure maintenance of range of joint movement, and then active and resistive exercises to re-establish sitting, standing, and walking as soon as possible. If there was no rapid return of control or power in the hemiplegic limbs, physiotherapists concentrated on training the normal side, particularly in right-sided hemiplegics, whose normal left side did not have the dexterity of the right-sided limbs in the pre-morbid stage. The instability of the hemiplegic knee would be controlled with braces and the flail hemiplegic upper limb supported by a sling.

This approach enabled the patient to regain independence, subordinating elegance of gait to the exigencies of daily living. In this unsightly gait pattern the hemiplegic arm was held adducted tightly across the body, with the knee joint in hyperextension in the stance phase. Ambulation was achieved by circumduction of the hemiplegic leg. Usually a below knee caliper would be prescribed to control equino-varus deformity at the ankle joint (Chin, 1980). Patients trained in this way had often to rely on either a tripod or quadropod for stabilization (Perry, 1969; Chin, 1982). The exaggeration of the abnormal reflex activity resulted in a tight flexor synergy in the upper limb, making dressing difficult and hygiene of the hemiplegic palm almost impossible to maintain. In later stages braces and calipers seldom controlled an increasing equino-varus deformity, and the heel of the hemiplegic foot usually rose out of the shoe. Painful callosities of the forefoot were not uncommon.

Facilitation and Inhibition Techniques
(used mainly for stroke patients and following head injury) (Chin *et al.*, 1982; see also appendix to this chapter)

In the late 1950s, physiotherapists working with cerebral palsied children saw that their approach in the management of these patients could be applied to adults with cerebrovascular accidents. These techniques were based upon a resurgence of interest in the neurophysiological studies of Jackson (1882), Sherrington (1906), Magnus and De Kleijn (1912) and Simons (1923) as well as the observations made by Twitchell (1951) on the recovery pattern of motor deficit in stroke patients.

The four main schools of facilitation techniques are: (a) Rood (1954), (b) Knott (1967), (c) Brunnstrom (1970), and (d) Bobath (1978). Followers of particular schools highlight the differences, but examination of the general principles underlying most of the facilitation shows more similarities than differences in the basic concept and practice (Flanagan, 1976).

Knott (1967) expanded and consolidated the early work of Fay (1948) and Kabat (1952), and called her approach 'proprioceptive neuromuscular facilitation' (PNF), which had a wide following in the USA, and in this country, until recently, when the Bobath techniques overtook it in popularity. Mobility is augmented by proprioceptive stimulation through stroking or brushing the skin, as well as using various flavours to stimulate movement of facial, tongue and oropharyngeal musculature. Movement patterns commence after stability has been achieved in a particular position, progressing to mobility from various functional postures. In this country, PNF is now usually used in conjunction with Bobath techniques.

Brunnstrom (1970), unlike Bobath or Knott, developed her technique through direct observation of adult hemiplegics, and has a wide following in the USA. The claim that the facilitation techniques can produce restoration of function through the reversal of neurological impairment has not been objectively substantiated by hard evidence. However, the reduction in spasticity in hemiplegic limbs, which follows careful positioning and manipulation of key joints, is unequivocal. It defies current neurophysiological explanation. Brodal (1973), a neuroanatomist gave a vivid personal account of the effect of facilitation techniques following his own stroke.

Whether these relatively recent techniques are more effective in overcoming disability when compared with the traditional functional approach, or even reverse neurological impairment as is sometimes claimed, is still hotly debated. At present enthusiasm, seemingly impervious to the discipline of controlled trials, is sweeping many physiotherapists and occupational therapists along the tide of facilitation techniques. The consensus among therapists is that the Bobath method prepares hemiplegics better for walking, and patients achieve a symmetrical gait more quickly at the expense of more physiotherapy time spent in individual instruction. Unfortunately, symmetry of gait is difficult to maintain and by about 6 months or a year, increasing spasticity may require the patient to use a stick—or to undergo a further course of Bobath therapy.

The paucity of controlled trials evaluating efficacy of individual techniques is a reflection of the great difficulties faced by therapists involved in designing and organizing trials (Smith *et al.*, 1981). Trials investigating the influence of specific exercise regimens will need to take into account other factors such as concurrent illness, patient motivation, variations in the expertise of therapists in interpreting and executing exercise programmes, as well as other aspects of patient/therapist interaction. Stratification to produce groups with comparable neurological impairment results in small unrepresentative numbers when single departments attempt to recruit patients. Small trials with unselected patients generate more questions than answers. Clearly a multicentre effort is indicated—but this too has problems.

In the application of facilitation techniques physiotherapists tend to exhibit loyalty to a particular theoretical school, with rival supporters contesting the opinions of others. In a review, Chin (1982) concluded that there was as yet no convincing evidence of the superiority of facilitation techniques over that of the traditional functional approach in the restoration of function in the hemiplegic patients. As already indicated, the similarities between all these facilitation techniques may be more important than the differences. Studies designed to distinguish intermethod effectiveness may not yield significant differentiating results, however elegant the design of these trials. Wescott (1967), in a study of traditional exercise regimens, observed that the movement patterns described, for example by Clayton (1924), were not too dissimilar to those proposed in some of the facilitation techniques.

For the therapists, the essence of successful rehabilitation, whatever techniques are used, is to know when to diligently intervene to maximize recovery, when to discreetly withdraw, accepting fixed disability and optimizing function with aids. Perhaps an eclectic approach to the use of the various exercise regimens would be the most expedient, until there is clear guidance from controlled trials. In fact, nowadays, this is what most therapists working in hospitals practise (Johnstone, 1976).

Conductive Education

Just after the Second World War, Andreas Peto in Budapest developed an approach to the management of physical disability, now referred to as conductive education. It involves teaching children and adults with various types of motor disability how to regain control of disordered movement. It is based on the concept of 'plasticity of the brain', and the re-awakening or re-establishing of new patterns of movement in undamaged areas (Devor, 1982; Gazzaniga, 1982). The aim is to achieve performance of activities as near to normality as possible without the use of aids. The early work concentrated on children; recently the same approach has been used in adults and the elderly with Parkinson's disease, multiple sclerosis and other neurological diseases. Patients are treated in groups, stratified by diagnosis, and led by trained 'conductors'. The general principles are:

a. Verbal regulation, by which a patient is made to vocalize an action which is taking place. The patient repeats the command for the action, and then performs it over and over again, until it becomes automatic.
b. Rhythmic intention. This refers to the way in which a smooth fluent execution of a movement pattern takes place. Before the full sequence of movement can be executed, the patient is taught to break the whole sequence into small achievable portions. These are then strung together again—'concatenated'—and reinforced by mentally stating the intention, and then carrying out the movement.

At the same time, patients are taught the best way to overcome difficulties in activities of daily living, such as writing, dressing, grooming and toilet training, by the same 'conductors'—an example of 'generic' therapists at work.

Anecdotal accounts of success of this approach have encouraged the Parkinson's Disease Society in this country to support a research fellowship in the investigation of the applicability of the technique and its possible introduction to Britain (Nanton, 1984).

Use of Physical Agents

Although most physiotherapy for neurological disease consists of the application of techniques described above, the public and physicians are more aware of the way physiotherapists use physical agents and gadgetry. Where pain is the major problem (as in the hemiplegic shoulder, or muscle spasms as in multiple sclerosis), heat in the form of an infra-red lamp or diapulse using interrupted short wave may be used to soothe away the discomfort (Licht, 1969). Ultrasound is preferred for the pain due to tendonitis (Coakley, 1978; Munting, 1978). Ice packs and immersion of the limbs in ice have been used to control spasticity. Release from marked spasticity lasts for about 30–45 minutes and therapists use this period of relaxation to put joints through their full range of movements. Some physiotherapists have learnt to use Chinese acupuncture for chronic pain, such as that due to post-herpetic neuralgia; others use transcutaneous nerve stimulators.

In patients with persistent and recalcitrant oedema (such as may occur in a hemiplegic limb) physiotherapists may either manually massage it or use an electric vibrator or a Flowtron. The last encases the limb in a plastic bag and applies intermittent graduated pressure by means of an electrically driven air pump. Low frequency faradic current is sometimes used to stimulate tendon movement within their sheaths. Pulsed current is occasionally used to maintain muscle tone in patients with Bell's palsy or other peripheral nerve damage. In the past electrical stimulation has also been used for persistent flaccidity. Interferential current stimulation is a method for enhancing pelvic muscle activity in neurogenic incontinence. Physiotherapists have experimented with functional electrical stimulation (FET) for correction of 'drop foot' (Liberson, 1979; Condie and Treithuysen, 1979). This is occasionally used for gait training in hemiplegia. Feedback in the form of videotape recordings may also be employed in walking training (Chin, 1982).

Education and Counselling

Much of the work of a trained physiotherapist involves personal contact with patients. As interest in time consuming facilitation techniques grows, physiotherapists will find it increasingly difficult to cope with the vast number of elderly stroke patients. It seemed, sensible, therefore, that in the early 1970s physiotherapy departments should begin to recruit 'aides', who did not have formal training in basic sciences or physiotherapy, but received in-service instruction in specific exercise programmes. These 'physiotherapy helpers', seconded to departments of geriatric medicine and working under supervision, reinforced formal sessions of physiotherapists, as much of rehabilitation in motor disability is repetitious. Teaching these 'helpers' is a major commitment. Physiotherapists also have to instruct relatives, friends and other volunteers to continue rehabilitation when the patient is discharged home, as well as helping the patient to adapt to fixed disability.

It is incumbent on physiotherapists to continue research into specific physiotherapy techniques, to ascertain which is the most effective, both in terms of time and manpower. Brocklehurst *et al.* (1978) noted that in hemiplegia physiotherapy is sometimes continued long after improvement has ceased and most of it is given to severely damaged individuals with little prospect of recovery. One way forward is collaborative research and evaluation in the context of a multidisciplinary research forum, such as the Society for Research in Rehabilitation inaugurated in 1978.

An emphasis on scientific evaluation of physiotherapy should not detract from the art of its practice. For when all the excitement of diagnosis and medical treatment has subsided, the patient has to face anxieties and doubts and the struggle to overcome disability. The kindly therapist, with a warm reassuring disposition, can do much to restore self-respect and hope, to encourage maximum effort, or help the patient to come to terms with a reduced role in life.

OCCUPATIONAL THERAPY (see Table 33.2)

Gone are the days when occupational therapists (OTs) were regarded as domestic science teachers misplaced in hospitals, or as the purveyors of diversional activities for the mentally ill and physically disabled, venturing occasionally into vocational training with a fretsaw and discarded industrial machinery. In 1982, The British Association of

TABLE 33.2   ROLE OF OCCUPATIONAL THERAPISTS

1. Assessment
   a. Motor, sensory and perceptual problems
   b. The degree of disability and handicap
2. Training
   a. In techniques of self-care and social interaction
   b. Collaboration with other remedial therapists
   c. Use of microelectronic technology
3. Provision of aids and resettlement
   a. Provision of aids and tools for living—including electronic environmental control systems
   b. Liaison with community services initiating structural alteration to homes, and other environmental changes
4. Education of family and health professionals
5. Diversional therapy
   a. Purposeful diversional activity incorporating remedial exercises
   b. Recreation

Occupational Therapists defined their role as 'the treatment of physical and psychiatric conditions through specific activities in order to help people reach their maximum level of function and independence in all aspects of daily life'. Bumphrey (1984), in an overview of the work of occupational therapists in a health district, reported that it was the fastest growing group within the National Health Service (7.9% increase from 1980 to 1984) in spite of which there still is a marked shortfall necessitating the appointment of OT aides. The ratio of qualified OTs to OT aides is 1:1.19. Bayliss *et al.* (1983) reviewed the referral profile, and found just over half the work concerned psychiatric patients. Among physical disorders, those affecting the central nervous system were the most important (39%).

In contrast to the physician's emphasis on loss of function as a pointer to the nature and site of the lesion, the OT is concerned to assess the patient's residual capabilities. Their primary function in hospitals, among elderly patients with neurological problems, is to help them to regain independence in activities of daily living (ADL), such as feeding, grooming, toileting, cooking and other household tasks. They are pre-eminent in contriving aids and adaptations for patients struggling to overcome the tyranny of established neurological disability. They are increasingly involved in using microcomputers to help the disabled (Ediss and Grove, 1983).

Assessment and Training

In the past, OTs were involved comparatively late in the treatment of neurological disease. It was only when fixed disability had supervened that the OT was called in to deal with adaptations of the patient to the neurological deficit and of the environment to the patient. In the major neurological diseases of old age, such as stroke and Parkinson's disease, OTs are now involved much earlier. They pay particular attention to residual functional ability, assessing ADL performance, to gauging progress, and to evaluating the effectiveness of various types of treatment. Testing for perceptual disorders has been improved, avoiding the use of demeaning children's toys, and refining it with the help of microcomputers (Johnson and Garvie, 1985). OTs are particularly interested in proprioceptive and motor disorders of the upper limb, and work closely with physiotherapists, using the same 'therapeutic approach' to the patient. They no longer concentrate on training the normal side to compensate for failure in ADL or teach unilateral skills.

In keeping with the Bobath approach they have altered their traditional games and other diversional activities, as well as their methods of teaching ADL. In following this approach for stroke rehabilitation, OTs also avoid introducing aids too early and have redesigned the way patients use traditional OT pursuits, such as printing, writing, sanding and remedial games. (Details of these are well documented in Eggers, 1983.)

As they are involved much earlier in neurological disease, occupational therapists now assist in the assessment of cognitive and speech disorders, working in close collaboration with speech therapists, augmenting the training programme, as well as enhancing communication skills. They use behavioural modification techniques, as well as other psychological approaches to the patients. In some geriatric, as well as psychogeriatric, wards they are the catalyst in organizing and sustaining sessions in reality orientation and reminiscence for the management of patients with chronic confusional states. In psychiatric hospitals they are the prime movers in arranging art, music and group therapy, helping depressed elderly patients to re-engage in social activities.

Aids and Adaptations

The occupational therapist is best known as the adviser and provider of aids. A whole industry has grown around the provision of tools for living for the disabled and keeping abreast of the availability, as well as the ingenuity of designs of these aids, has been a major problem for OTs. Some of them now work exclusively in centres demonstrating the use of aids for disabled patients, run under the aegis of the Disabled Living Foundation. The OT has to be familiar with aids for use in motor disability, and also for other problems in symptom control, such as incontinence, hearing and visual impairment, as well as orthotic devices. There is also a burgeoning array of electronic gadgetry and microelectronic environmental control systems for which a few elderly patients will need training and advice. It is not difficult to see why the College of Occupational Therapy has an active 'interest group' in computing.

Assessment and selection of wheelchairs for the disabled is one of the main activities of the OT. Knowing when to begin training the neurologically disabled patient to be wheelchair independent requires considerable judgement and skill. In hemiplegics, for example, the physician, anxious that the patient should make some kind of progress, may urge the early provision of a wheelchair. But using the normal arm for propulsion and leg for control can exaggerate abnormal reflex activity and undo what the physiotherapists are attempting with their facilitation techniques. In contrast, for paraplegics the sooner mobility in a wheelchair is advised the better for their morale. The OT must also take account of the patient's home circumstances and the need of carers to manoeuvre the chair.

When resettling patients and, for example, advising on internal house adaptations and ways of facilitating access, hospital based OTs will need to work in cooperation with colleagues in the community and to know how best to manipulate local

TABLE 33.3 ROLE OF SPEECH THERAPY

1. Assessment of speech and language disorders
2. Organizing treatment programmes
   a. Carrying out treatment
   b. Organizing volunteers and other helpers
   c. Advising on communication aids
3. Education and counselling

authority machinery to their patient's advantage. In Britain, the cost of adaptations is charged to local authorities and sometimes stifling bureaucracy delays authorization. The OT can act as the patient's advocate urging housing committees and architects to design special housing with the neurologically disabled in mind and to ensure that access to public buildings is readily available to the wheelchair user.

In the new age of microelectronics, it is possible that much of the disability resulting from neurological disease, even in old age, may be minimized by the introduction of cheap and efficient gadgetry, thus mitigating the demoralizing effect of restricted life styles.

SPEECH THERAPY (Table 33.3)

For a long time speech therapists concentrated on the education of children with language problems. Lately the growing stroke population, with its confusing varieties of aphasias, has attracted greater involvement of speech therapists. The Quirk report on Speech Therapy in (1972) highlighted the need for an expansion of speech therapy services. Since then, there has been an encouraging increase in the numbers of studies concerning the use of speech therapy in stroke and other neurological conditions. There has also been an interest in language disorders, and communication problems in old age (Edwards, 1982).

Apart from dealing with aphasias, speech therapists are playing an increasingly effective role in the management of dysarthrias associated with cerebellar disorders, parkinsonism, motor neurone disease and stroke and other diseases affecting articulation. The proliferation of electronic communication aids

for those with severe dysarthria calls for careful appraisal by therapists.

There is much debate concerning the effectiveness of speech therapy in the restoration of language loss (Sarno, 1976; David *et al.*, 1979; Lincoln *et al.*, 1984) but this should not detract from the important role of speech therapists in the overall rehabilitation of the patient with aphasia. Central to this is restoring the ability to communicate in spite of language difficulties, using non-verbal channels.

Assessment

Loss of language is one of the most devastating aspects of neurological damage. Of the protean manifestations of stroke illness, speech loss causes the greatest anxiety in relatives in the aftercare of these patients. Attitudes are now somewhat less pessimistic, in response to the contributions of enthusiasts. This has been accompanied by a wider interest among physicians. Hopkins (1975) outlined the current position of speech therapy in stroke rehabilitation perceptively. Geschwind's reclassification of dysphasias, provides a useful framework for further study (Geschwind, 1971).

In the past, the testing of speech and language loss was a tedious and time consuming exercise. The more recent methods for assessment are less lengthy and now await validation as tools for evaluating treatment programmes, as well as use in the day-to-day assessment of patients (Schuell, 1965; Porch, 1972).

Another aspect of assessment, becoming increasingly important as the surviving number of aphasic patients increases, is the question of testamentary capacity. A number of patients will not have made wills prior to their stroke. Speech impairments may post major legal problems. It may be difficult for the non-specialist medical practitioner to ascertain whether the aphasic patient is in fact capable of making a will. The contribution of a speech therapist may be crucial (Udell *et al.*, 1980).

Treatment Programmes

Common experience shows that most spontaneous recovery from dysphasia occurs in the first few weeks following a stroke. Some patients recover completely while others make little or no recovery. Coulton (1969), Geschwind (1971), Kertesz and McCabe (1977), Brust *et al.* (1976), Demeurisse *et al.* (1980) have contributed most helpfully in the delineation of recovery patterns following stroke aphasia. In the light of these observations the timing of speech therapy needs to be considered carefully in any controlled trial. Occasionally, progress may occur in fits and starts, making assessment of the effect of therapy even more difficult. Nonetheless, speech therapists have evolved specific strategies in helping patients with this problem. For a detailed account, the reader is referred to Darley (1972) and Sarno and Levita (1979). There is considerable overlap between the various strategies adopted.

1. The traditional approach. This method relies on getting the patient to speak in whatever way he or she wishes. Much use is made of nursery rhymes and repetition of words. There is, however, no clear evidence that the words used in the context of treatment are subsequently utilized in other contexts.

2. Programmed instruction—Sarno and Sands (1970). The basic premise of this approach is that the acquisition of language is an educational process. The patient is taught language all over again, using learning techniques, such as repetition and association of pictures with words rather than actual letters.

3. Group therapy—Darley (1972). Mixed groups of dysphasic patients are allowed to interact freely under the guidance of the therapists. Use is made of role play and charades.

4. Melodic intonation—Albert *et al.* (1973). This is a one-to-one relationship between the therapist and the patient, in which the patient is made to repeat phrases and words in unison with the therapist. These are intoned with an emphasis on certain parts of the phrase to achieve association of ideas.

Other methods of helping the patient to regain speech include visual communication therapy, in which the patient is taught to recognize words on flash cards and to associate them with action. In others, the main emphasis is on the recognition of symbols, such as the 'Bliss' symbols. Other therapists prefer to combine encouraging the re-acquisition of language with the use of non-verbal methods of communication, such as 'Amerind', which is a simple sign system using internationally accepted gestures. For example, hunger is depicted by pointing to the upper abdomen and accompanied by a clockwise rubbing action.

The efficacy of these methods remains controversial. Sarno and Sands (1970), in a controlled trial of 31 severely disabled patients, compared those who were given programmed therapy with those receiving non-programmed therapy and a third group given no treatment. They showed that there were small gains in the areas of functional communication in the patients receiving programmed therapy and non-programmed therapy. There was no significant improvement in any of the three groups in important areas such as imitation, writing, auditory comprehension, and expressive speech.

Lincoln *et al.* (1984) studied aphasic stroke patients randomly, allocating them either to a speech therapy group receiving two 1 hour speech therapy sessions per week, or to a non-treatment group. Although some improvement in communication was seen in both groups, there was no significant difference in language recovery between those receiving speech therapy and the controls. They concluded that the treatment regimen, which is representative of clinical practice in Britain, is ineffective for most aphasic stroke patients. This has at least narrowed the current gap of ignorance; nevertheless further elucidation of the role of specific treatment programmes is much needed.

In view of the scale of aphasia as a problem among the stroke population, and the shortage of trained speech therapists, attempts have been made to recruit and train volunteers to help aphasic patients. The work of Griffith (1975) is now well publicized and has been taken up by other speech therapists. Volunteers are carefully trained by speech therapists and help patients with communication difficulties (Editorial, 1975). They also act as friends, and help with social activities (Meikle *et al.*, 1979). David *et al.*

(1979) compared the effect of speech therapy delivered by professionally trained therapists and volunteers and demonstrated that the stimulation provided with either form of intervention had an effect over and above that of spontaneous recovery. On the whole, volunteers achieve as good results as speech therapists.

Much of what has been said so far refers to the management of patients with aphasia. Speech therapists are also involved in the treatment of patients with other impairments, in particular dysarthria, where the results have been encouraging. Robertson and Thompson (1984) reported on the efficacy and long-term effects of intensive speech therapy in patients with Parkinson's disease. The benefit of speech therapy involvement has also been demonstrated by Scott *et al.* (1983). Although the dysarthria in Parkinson's patients improves with speech therapy, the degree of dysphonia is more sensitive to levodopa. In patients with motor neurone disease, although specific speech therapy may not improve articulation, speech therapists can advise on the use of alternative communication aids, such as the microcomputer system. With recent advances in microelectronics, handheld or table top communicators have found their way into the homes of these patients.

Education and Counselling

Perhaps the best use to be made of our scarce speech therapists is for them to act as advisers and counsellors to families, patients and other therapists involved in the management of patients with aphasia. There should be an intermittent review of actual treatment given to individual patients as well as a validation of the techniques used. To this end therapists ought to retain a small case load of identified slow recoverers.

CLINICAL PSYCHOLOGY

Clinical psychology is the discipline in which knowledge of human behaviour is applied to diseased populations (Liberman, 1972; Larner and Leemming, 1984). The work of clinical psychologists is perceptively summarized by Watts (1985), who pointed out that it is a relatively new health profession in Britain, having grown up largely since the inception of the National Health Service in 1948. The uneven distribution of qualified clinical psychologists means that not many physicians dealing with the elderly will have come into close contact, or worked with, psychologists regularly. It is therefore worth mentioning that the training of clinical psychologists currently takes 5 years, with a basic honours degree in psychology followed by a 2–3 year postgraduate course, in a university or polytechnic or as part of in-service training, leading to a diploma in clinical psychology from the British Psychological Society.

This background places clinical psychologists in the enviable position of being trained not only in the observation of human behaviour, but also theories of learning, as well as the scientific method and statistical analysis of experimental work. Watts (1985) indicated that clinical psychology is probably better than most health service professions in submitting its procedures to scientific scrutiny. Nevertheless, a substantial number of reports on the efficacy of psychological interventions are anecdotal (Holden and Woods, 1982). This may be inevitable as behavioural treatments have to be tailored to individual circumstances.

In the early years, clinical psychologists were mainly involved with patients in psychiatric institutions and their chief role was in assessment and testing of higher mental function. Lately, the greater opportunities for study, as well as direct involvement, have brought a number of psychologists into the arena of behaviour problems in old age (Larner and Leemming, 1984; Leng, 1982; Holden and Woods, 1982; Church, 1986). The main areas of involvement relevant to neurological diseases are:

1. Psychological testing of cognitive function and personality.
2. Behavioural assessment and therapy.
   a. Identifying 'barriers' to recovery.
   b. Disruptive problem behaviours.
   c. Specialist schemes, reminiscence therapy, reality orientation, behavioural psychotherapy.
3. Teaching and counselling.

Cognitive Assessment

Physicians dealing with the neurologically damaged call on clinical psychologists most frequently to seek help in testing cognition or intellect. Larner and Leeming (1984) instance the case of a stroke patient who wished to take an Open University degree course following his stroke. Superficially, this seemed over-ambitious, but psychological testing showed that the patient had a reasonable chance of success. Community physicians may refer a patient to a clinical psychologist to determine the presence or absence of a dementing process or of mental retardation, before the nowadays rare recourse to compulsory removal to hospital under Section 47 of the National Assistance Act.

Psychological Treatments

Recently, psychologists have developed treatment schedules, which are dependent on manipulation of 'cognitive processes'. Depression is characterized by negative thoughts about current experience, self-image and the future. Cognitive therapy for depression is directed at refocusing the patient's attention away from gloomy preoccupations, patients are taught to look at the more positive aspects and to re-engage in activities of daily living, so that each event is seen as a successful achievement. It is claimed that this approach is just as effective as antidepressant medication (Williams, 1984).

Behavioural Assessment and Treatments

The involvement of psychologists in 'behaviour therapy' has produced ingenious and engaging schemes for dealing with elderly patients, who shout incessantly, swear, nip, bite and spit 'intolerably' (Birchmore and Clague, 1983). Occasionally, they quell the disordered behaviour successfully, but sadly, not for long; and sometimes it returns with a vengeance.

The most commonly used form of behavioural treatment is directed at reducing abnormal anxiety reactions, such as phobias using carefully controlled exposure to whatever arouses the phobia. The exposure is graduated and in a 'de-sensitization' process patients are helped to overcome their phobias. Simple phobias appear to respond best to this form of management, but more complex problems, such as agoraphobia, respond less well (Richman, 1979; Salter and Salter, 1975). Obsessive compulsive disorders are also amenable to de-sensitization (O'Brien, 1978). The other commonly used behaviour modifying device is the application of rewards, with reinforcements for desirable behaviour and the withdrawal of 'privileges' when unwanted behaviour is manifested. Variations on the same theme, such as earning 'tokens' for good behaviour, are used to enhance activity and the atmosphere in long stay institutions. The objective is to mitigate the effect of institutionalization. Occasionally, such treatment is counterproductive, provoking tension and feelings of oppression in patients which generates even more disruptive behaviour.

Another approach is based on the premise that relative sensory deprivation leads to confusion and apathy (Cameron, 1941; Corso, 1967). Stimulation programmes, including occupational therapy and recreational activities, produce positive and purposive behaviour in elderly patients with dementia (Pappas *et al.*, 1958; Cosin *et al.*, 1958; Bower, 1967). Improved cognitive function was reported by Loew and Silverstone (1971).

Due to a lack of well-trained psychologists to oversee the behaviour altering programmes through to conclusion, many well-intentioned schemes fall by the wayside. This leads to disillusionment in patients and others involved in the treatment with clinical psychologists. If psychologists believe that behaviour and cognitive treatment programmes are effective, their validity needs to be tested under controlled conditions (Leng, 1985). Physicians have a responsibility to ensure that programmes initiated are pursued with sustained vigour, and not run by 'remote control'; otherwise beneficial treatments may be lost to patients by default.

Other behaviour modifying methods, such as stimulus control for the treatment of insomnia (Puder *et al.*, 1983) and biofeedback in the treatment of stroke patients (Leng, 1982) and incontinence (Ehrman, 1983) have yet to be validated.

Reminiscence

Butler (1963) studied the use that elderly people made of 'reminiscence'. Since then others have found and argued that reminiscence may be a useful approach to the psychological treatment of the elderly (Pincus, 1976; Merriam, 1980). It is a common experience of all age groups, that when friends meet after an interval apart, reminiscing is the major activity, often helped along by a 'wee dram'. Both of these can have mood elevating effects.

Reminiscence can be carried out in a number of ways. It can either be unstructured, where a group sits together and talks about a subject with staff prompting. The usual topics are the major wars, Christmas, and significant events such as weddings and anniversaries. The sessions can also be structured and the topics pre-selected, the discussion being supported by slides, photographs and video tapes. Age Concern (UK) has produced a package for reminiscence therapy. These sessions also have a group leader, who may be a psychologist, a trained nurse, an occupational therapist or a social worker. Apart from their undoubted warm after-glow, the effectiveness of these seminars in altering behaviour or cognitive function is still a matter for investigation.

Reality Orientation

Reality orientation (RO) has in the last decade captured the imagination of health professionals dealing with the elderly confused. Folsom originated this psychological approach in geriatric wards of the Veterans Administration Hospital (VA) in Topeka, Kansas in 1958. He developed and refined it when he moved to the VA Hospital in Tuscaloosa, Alabama (Folsom, 1967, 1968). By the 1980s over 20 000 workers from all over the USA had been trained in RO. It had also been enthusiastically received in this country, and Brooks *et al.* (1975) published the first encouraging controlled trial. Since then, Degun (1976), Green (1979), Hanley (1981, 1984) and Holden and Woods (1982) have been the main proponents of RO for the elderly confused. Patients treated in this way fall into different diagnostic categories, although the main target population is those with dementia.

Methodology

The American Psychiatric Association's booklet on the subject described RO as a technique to rehabilitate elderly and brain damaged patients, with a moderate to severe degree of disorientation. The RO package consists essentially of two main components: (a) informal 24 hour RO, and (b) formal classroom RO.

a. Informal 24 hour RO. This requires staff to give patients as much information as possible about activities in the ward. For example, at lunchtime patients would be greeted with the comment that lunch was being served, the contents of the meal would be described and the setting in which lunch was to be taken would be clearly signposted. Staff constantly remind patients of who they are, what time of the day it is, and what is happening to them. The surroundings are modified to provide clearly identifiable markings of ward amenities. Information bulletins posted in large print for easy reading are designed to attract and explain topics simply and concisely.

b. Formal classroom RO. Small groups of patients, usually about two to five, meet daily with a carer in a special room equipped with materials for social engagement, such as familiar adult games. Teaching aids encourage the relearning or reinforcing of vocabulary. The room also contains orientating devices, such as clocks, calendars, maps and newspapers. Groups may be led didactically or allowed to interact informally. The degree of complexity of teaching and interaction is dependent on the severity of confusion.

As RO has developed over the years, variations on the same theme have emerged, but the common aim is to reduce confusion and to enable the patient to realize the meaningfulness of time, place and related activity. It is also designed to restore some measure of independent living, within the context of the institution or other current living conditions. Details of the methods are available in comprehensive accounts by Cornbleth and Cornbleth (1977, 1979), and Holden and Woods (1982).

Evaluation

Early proponents of RO in uncontrolled trials were impressed by the changes in the life style of patients (Salter and Salter, 1975). There were gains in social ability, and cooperativeness. These have been followed in the last few years by controlled trials, measuring the effectiveness of RO in cognitive function, as well as behaviour (Brooks *et al.*, 1975; Burton and Spall, 1982). A report by Holden and Sinebruchow (1978), using RO in a group of patients with mixed diagnoses (depression, dementia, stroke and Parkinson's disease), was not able to demonstrate cognitive improvement.

Holden and Woods (1982) have carefully reviewed the literature on controlled trials and categorized them into two main groups.

1. Those which demonstrate that improvements occur in cognitive functions, using memory and recall tests (Barnes, 1974; Harris and Ivory, 1976; Citrin and Dixon, 1977; Woods, 1979; and Hanley *et al.*, 1981).
2. Those which show an improvement in behaviour, but little or no improvement in cognitive function (Brooks *et al.*, 1975; Holden and Sinebruchow, 1978).

Burton's critique (1981) of the studies of RO highlighted several problems. The use of RO in different patient groups makes it difficult to compare the studies across samples. The memory tests employed also differed, as did the setting in which RO was used.

Despite the shortcomings of these controlled trials there is substantial evidence that 24 hour RO and classroom RO have some positive effect in orientation (Reeve and Ivison, 1985). There is conflicting evidence of behavioural changes mediated by RO. Those behavioural changes that have been noted are those approved within the discipline of the institution. There is little evidence to show that these changes in behaviour have any effect in regulating or organizing new forms of behaviour related to social integration and self-care.

Conclusions

Reality orientation, as a philosophical approach to the care of the confused institutionalized elderly patients, has many converts in different parts of the English speaking world. Like so many 'movements', its wide acceptance is taken as a token of success. Whether its effects are attributable to the techniques themselves, or to the whole ambience created by the use of the technique, remains uncertain. Nonetheless, RO appears to have improved the outlook and atmosphere of some of the institutions in which it has been applied. It appears to encourage a positive outlook and stimulates greater contact with patients, as all levels of staff participate in 'therapy'. It does not appear to require an injection 'of Utopian levels of resources', which makes it attractive to managers. Another asset of RO is that it can be used in conjunction with reminiscence therapy and is used in different contexts—such as the day hospital—or indeed in ordinary households, where the vast majority of patients with dementia live. One drawback is that, once the enthusiasm of the staff has been fired, it seems to have limited momentum, and needs the sustaining influence of a charismatic psychologist, a committed psychiatrist or an interested physician, like so many other cognitive and behavioural treatment regimens.

CREATIVE ARTS AS THERAPY

The use of art and music as adjuncts to the main therapeutic thrust has had a fluctuating popularity in psychiatric hospitals in this country. Occupational therapists use art, not only as a diversion from boredom, but also in remedial training of the hemiplegic upper limb, and to motivate depressed patients.

Creative arts are used more widely in the treatment of mental illness, and are better established in the USA. The American Psychiatric Association organized a national conference on Creative Art Therapies in Washington in 1980. It is noteworthy that in the USA, professionals in the various fields have developed a corpus of knowledge, and instituted training programmes and accreditation procedures for aspiring practitioners. There is an American Art Therapy Association, Dance Therapy Association, a National Association for Music Therapy and Society for Group Psychotherapy and Psychodrama. There is a British Association for Art

Therapy, and a British Society for Music Therapy, whose offices are in London; the latter runs courses for interested individuals.

Gibson (1982) postulated that creative art therapies tap emotional rather than cognitive responses and therefore deal more directly with primary mental processes than do the verbal ones. Zwerling (1979) considers that creative arts therapies evoke responses at the level at which psychotherapists seek to engage their patients, only more directly and more immediately than the traditional verbal therapies. As verbal response is not required to a great extent these creative art therapies are useful across ethnic language barriers and in diverse neurological deficits.

Art

Art has been used mainly for diversional work in neurological disability. In mental illness, psychologists and psychiatrists have found that it facilitates the uncovering of unconscious feelings and out of this has emerged the use of art for interpreting the inner emotions of patients (Willmuth and Broedy, 1979). Erikson (1979) sounds a warning against too much reliance on the diagnostic aspect of art. She observed that the releasing effect of pent-up feelings through art may be sacrificed to an inordinate preoccupation with it as a means of diagnosis. Gombrich (1977) has explored the psychological processes behind the imageries of pictures. More on this subject is available from British Association of Art Therapy, 13c Northwind Road, London N6 5TL.

Dance

Dance is part of the cultural expression of many ethnic groups. In primitive societies it operated as a means of releasing collective emotions, and as a prelude to battle. It forms part of the ritual surrounding the dispensing of traditional medicine in Africa and South-East Asia. As part of the healing process and in the maintenance of wellbeing, practitioners of traditional Chinese medicine advocate a system of callisthenics with movement patterns, not unlike those of western ballet, though it is performed in silence. The American Dance Therapy Associ-ation has more than 1000 members, over 250 of whom are accredited therapists. The essence of dance therapy is to give vent to self expression with a deliberate avoidance of a set pattern of steps. This means that patients with all forms of disability can participate. Dance enhanced by rhythmic music and verbal imagery is used to provoke motor responsiveness, all of which is alleged to culminate in a kind of emotional catharsis. Some dance therapists profess expertise in the interpretation of the mental state through observation of posture and the repertoire of movement patterns.

Choreographers have also contributed to the investigation of abnormal movement patterns in neurological disease, through their notation of abnormal postures, with symbolic representation of these on paper—the Benesche notations.

Apart from lifting mood and altering behaviour, dance is a form of exercise, and Powell (1974) has demonstrated that regular exercise programmes in the elderly improve cognition and behaviour. Tea dances organized for the elderly may therefore do more than merely encourage physical contact and social interaction.

Music (Alvin, 1966)

Piped or performed music is widely used to keep institutionalized patients amused and entertained, and most hospitals have volunteers operating a radio station broadcasting record requests or relaxing music (Cook, 1972).

The participation by the elderly in group sing-song sessions lifts mood as well as encouraging social interaction, and can be very enjoyable, both for patients and staff (Bright, 1981). Unfortunately, this is sometimes portrayed by the media as demeaning—we are shown elderly demented patients, swaying bemusedly in concert, with ragdolls clutched tightly or waved rhythmically. Physiotherapists, however, use music for group work in the form of movement to music; and some patients, who would not participate in simple verbally instructed exercises, are seen to move rhythmically with the music, and participate more readily in these exercise sessions (Kennard, 1983).

In the USA, music as therapy is practised more extensively. It has been used as adjunctive treatment for autism, schizophrenia and behavioural disturbance in adolescent and geriatric patients. Van de Wall, a professional harpist, organized the first formal sessions of 'music therapy' in psychiatric hospitals in the USA. He demonstrated that music altered muscle tension, produced generalized relaxation, raised the threshold to sensory stimuli, and had other physiological effects on the cardiovascular and respiratory system. Kaplan cites anecdotal accounts of its effectiveness in improving self-image and behaviour. In group psychotherapy sessions, patients' verbal interactions were increased when background music with a smooth and unchanging rhythm was played.

There are about 3000 members (2000 of them registered therapists) in the National Association for Music Therapy, which certifies some as music therapists (Gibson, 1982). The successful application of creative art therapy seems to be heavily dependent on the charisma and enthusiasm of individuals. The address of the British Society for Music Therapy is: Guildhall School of Music and Drama, Barbican, London EC2Y 8DT (Tel: 01-368-8879).

APPENDIX:

FACILITATION TECHNIQUES

Facilitation therapy techniques are based on the premise that alterations of posture and sensory stimuli can modify primitive synergistic reflex patterns which emerge after vascular or traumatic damage to the brain. Rigidly organized stereotyped reflexes are seen by some as having an adverse effect on restoration of normal function. Control of motor function could be effected by identifying the stroke patient's abnormal reflex pattern and then altering this reflex pattern by positioning and specific exercise regimens. In general, facilitation techniques are practised with close contact between therapists and patient. Bobath maintains that the tactile cues given to the patient, and an active change of position of various joints by the therapist, allows her to treat some patients in total silence, so that her technique can be applied to patients with aphasia. The proper

application of the facilitation techniques consumes a great deal of the therapist's time and physical energy (Flanagan, 1967).

The Bobath Method (1978)

This facilitation technique claims a theoretical basis in the neurophysiological observation of Sherrington (1906), and Magnus and De Kleijn (1912). Bobath first worked with cerebral palsied children and has translated some of the therapeutic principles assumed in treating this group of patients to the adult hemiplegic. The basic premise is that it is sensory information arising out of movement (not the actual movement pattern) which is imprinted during maturation of the nervous system, overriding primitive reflex activity. Thus, skilled movement takes place under the modulating influence of proprioception, touch and equilibrium, righting and other protective reactions. Brain damage disrupts these controls as well as unmasking abnormal primitive reflex synergies. Suppression of spasticity and pathological reflex activity brought about by cutaneous and joint proprioceptive stimulation and through adjustment of posture is the prelude to relearning of controlled movements. The therapist alters her handling of the patient according to the observed response to these stimuli.

After spasticity and unwanted patterns of movement have been overcome, the patient is taught how to rebuild control of movement by repetition of simple exercises, chaining successful control of each fragment until fluent execution is achieved. The watchword of Bobath devotees is a 'bilateral' approach. This calls for a concentration on the hemiplegic limbs, and retraining them to function as near as possible to normal. In the majority of stroke patients, this is not an achievable goal, and the relentless pursuit of symmetry of movement leads some practitioners to condemn the use of tripods, quadropods or other aids held in one arm for walking purposes. Fortunately, this purist approach is not commonly practised and a compromise is often accepted. In the elderly, at an early stage, they are given pulpit-type walking aids, which at least favours a semblance of 'symmetry'; later they may graduate to a cane (Chin, 1982).

The Brunnstrom Approach

(Perry, 1967; Brunnstrom, 1970)

Signe Brunnstrom in the USA developed facilitation techniques based on her experience and observations of adult stroke patients referring also to the studies of Magnus and De Kleijn (1912), Simons (1923) and Twitchell (1951), who described the motor recovery patterns of hemiplegics. She accepted that in the natural history of strokes spasticity was a necessary stage through which the patient passed.

The programme of exercises she teaches her patients is based on the principle of eliciting abnormal reflex patterns and then attempting to break these reflex synergies down through posture and sensory stimulation such as stretching and tapping. She claims that once these synergies are voluntarily 'captured', conditioning of the synergy for functional use is attempted. Interestingly, whilst the aim is to take the patient through various phases of recovery, Brunnstrom accepts that there are stroke patients who plateau at a certain level, and in these patients the use of aids, such as short leg braces, is encouraged. She also accepts that if the tight extensor synergy seen in the hemiplegic lower limb cannot be re-educated then gait training should go ahead with the acceptance of this and trick movements, such as circumduction, could be used to overcome difficulties in stepping. In this there is much resemblance to the pragmatic approach of the traditional exercise regimens propounded prior to the upsurge of interest in facilitation techniques, though the underlying principles differ sharply from Bobath's precepts.

Proprioceptive Neuromuscular Facilitation (PNF) (Kabat, 1952; Knott, 1967)

Kabat in the mid-1940s proposed a new set of facilitation exercises. These were based on the concept that early motor behaviour is dominated by reflex activity, and that mature motor behaviour is modulated by postural reflex mechanisms. He described a pattern of diagonal and oscillatory movements between extremes of flexion and extension, pronation and supination, designed to re-establish interaction of agonist and antagonist muscles. One such movement pattern begins with the right arm being placed in pronation on the greater trochanter of the left hip and moves in a diagonal direction to end up in the fully abducted and extended supinated position above the head on the right side. Kabat's observations are based on phylogenetic patterns of development emerging from primitive amphibians through to the mammalian patterns of movement.

Knott consolidated and refined the exercise regimens, calling them 'proprioceptive neuromuscular facilitation exercises', proprioceptors being the receptors which respond to pressure and stretch and situated in muscle spindles and Golgi tendon organs. They are responsible for setting muscle tone and also for those subtle alterations necessary to ensure correct posture and positioning of joints. In response to activation of these proprioceptors, purposeful movements may be carried out involving control of several muscle groups, so that synergists contract at the same time as antagonists relax.

In proprioceptive neuromuscular facilitation exercises, muscle movements are facilitated by the bombardment of anterior horn cells by impulses arising from pressure and stretch receptors. The therapists, therefore, assist the patient's initial movements, and then, as the muscle power and control return, add on resistive measures to train better control by the muscle groups. Clearly PNF exercises will not be applicable when there is total paralysis. Because the patient has to respond to verbal commands, it is difficult to use PNF exercises in patients with disordered comprehension, unlike those used by Bobath.

Rood's technique includes sensory stimulation, which is applied more widely throughout the body, and consists of skin brushing and stroking to enhance the receptivity of proprioceptors. She advocated the use of cold or ice to effect muscle function. Her movement patterns commence with stabilization of joint posture, progressing to control other joint positions (Rood, 1954).

These various techniques are now widely practised in the treatment of adult hemiplegics. Whilst there are purists and unswerving devotees of a particular technique, the consensus among physiotherapists is that no single technique is applicable to all stroke patients. Physiotherapists tend to use the most appropriate facilitation technique, attempting to match the exercise regimen with a response capability, as well as the neurological impairment seen in the stroke patients (Johnstone, 1976).

REFERENCES

Albert, M., Sparks, R., and Helm, M. (1973). Melodic intonation therapy for aphasia. *Arch. Neurol.*, **29**, 130–1.

Alvin, J. (1966). *Music Therapy*. J. Baker, London.

Andrews, K. (1979). Stroke recovery: he can but does he? *Rheum. Rehab.*, **18**, 43–5.

Barnes, J.A. (1974). Effects of reality orientation classroom on memory loss, confusion and disorientation in geriatric patients. *Gerontologist*, **14**, 138–42.

Bayliss, D.E., Goble, R.E.A., King, D.J., and Mendez, M.A. (1983). Present trends in occupational therapy practice. *Br. J. Occup. Ther.*, **46**, 216–19.

Birchmore, T., and Clague, S. (1983). A behavioural approach to reduce shouting. *Nursing Times*, **79**(16), 37–9.

Bobath, B. (1978). *Adult Hemiplegia Evaluation and Treatment*, second edition, Heinemann, London.

Bower, H.N. (1967). Sensory stimulation and the treatment of senile dementia. *Med. J. Aust.*, **1**, 1113–19.

Bright, R. (1981). *Music in Geriatric Care*, Belwyn Mills, London.

Brocklehurst, J.C., Andrews, K., Richards, B., and Laycock, P.J. (1978). How much physical therapy for patients with stroke? *Br. Med. J.*, **1**, 1307–10.

Brodal, A. (1973). Self observations and neuro-anatomical considerations after a stroke. *Brain*, **96**, 675–94.

Brooks, P., Degun, G., and Mather, M. (1975). Reality orientation, a therapy for psychogeriatric patients: A controlled study. *Br. J. Psychiatry*, **127**, 42–5.

Brunnstrom, S. (1970). *Movement Therapy in Hemiplegia*, Harper and Row, New York.

Brust, J.C.M., Shafer, S.Q., Richter, R.W., and Bruun, B. (1976). Aphasia in acute stroke. *Stroke*, **7**, 167–74.

Bumphrey, E.E. (1984). The role of occupational therapy. *Health Trends*, **16**, 80–90.

Burton, M., and Spall, R. (1981). Contributions of the behavioural approach to nursing the elderly. *Nursing Times*, **77**(6), 247–8.

Butler, R.M. (1980). The life review—an interpretation of reminiscence in the aged. *Psychiatry*, **163**, 26, 65–76.

Cameron, D.E. (1941). Studies in senile nocturnal delirium. *Psychiatric Quarterly*, **15**, 47–53.

Chin, P.L., Rosie, A., Irving, M., and Smith, R. (1980). *Final Report on Hemiplegic Gait Studies*, Regional Research Committee, Northern Regional Health Authority, Newcastle-upon-Tyne, UK.

Chin, P.L., Rosie, A., Irving, M., and Smith, R. (1982).

Studies in hemiplegic gait. In: Rose, F.C. (ed.) *Advances in Stroke Therapy*, Raven Press, New York.

Chin, P.L. (1982). Physical techniques in stroke rehabilitation. *J. Roy. Coll. Phys. Lond.*, **16**(3), 165–9.

Church, M. (1986). Issues in psychological therapy with elderly people. In: Hanley, I., and Gilhooly, M. (eds) *Psychological Therapies for the Elderly*, Croom Helm, London.

Citrin, R.S, and Dixon, D.N. (1977). Reality orientation: A milieu therapy used in an institution for the aged. *Gerontologist*, **17**, 39–43.

Clayton, E.B. (1924). *Physiotherapy in General Practice*, W. Wood, New York.

Coakley, W.T. (1978). Biophysical effects of ultrasound at therapeutic intensities. *Physiotherapy*, **64**(6), 166–79.

Condie, D.M., and Threithuysen, C.V. (1979). Use of functional electrical stimulation for gait training. In: Keendie, R.M. (ed.) *Disability*, Macmillan, London.

Cook, J.D. (1972). The therapeutic use of music—A literature review. *Nursing Forum*, **20**(3), 253–66.

Cornbleth, R., and Cornbleth, C. (1977). Reality orientation for the elderly. Journal Supplement Abstract Services of the American Psychological Association, MS 1539.

Cornbleth, R., and Cornbleth, C. (1979). Evaluation of the effectiveness of reality orientation classes in a nursing home unit. *J. Am. Geriatr. Soc.*, **27**, 522–4.

Corso, J.F. (1967). *The Experimental Psychology of Sensory Behaviour*, Holt, Rinehart and Winston, New York.

Cosin, L.Z., Mort, M., Post Fm Westropp, C., and Williams, M. (1958). Experimental treatment of persistent senile confusion. *Int. J. Soc. Psychiatry*, **4**, 24–42.

Coulton, G. (1969). Spontaneous recovery from aphasia. *J. Speech Hearing Dis. Res.*, **12**, 825–32.

Darley, F.C. (1972). The efficacy of language rehabilitation in aphasia. *J. Speech Hearing Dis. Res.*, **37**, 3–21.

David, R.M., Enderby, P., and Bainton, D. (1979). Progress report on an evaluation of speech therapy for aphasia. *Br. J. Dis. Comm.*, **14**, 85–8.

Degun, G. (1976). Reality orientation: A multidisciplinary therapeutic approach. *Nursing Times*, **72**, 117–20.

Demeurisse, G., Demol, O., Derouk, M., de Beuckelaer, R., Coekaerts, M.-J., and Capon, A. (1980). Quantitative study of the rate of recovery from aphasia due to ischaemic stroke. *Stroke*, **11**, 455–8.

Devor, M. (1982). Plasticity in the adult nervous system. In: Illis, L.S., Sedgwick, E.M., and Glanville, H.J. (eds) *Rehabilitation of the Neurological Patient*, Blackwell Scientific Publications, Oxford.

Ediss, P.B., and Grove, E. (1983). Microcomputers in occupational therapy departments of hospitals and day centres. *Br. J. Occup. Ther.*, **46**, 222–6.

Editorial (1975). Experts and amateurs in stroke therapy. *Lancet*, **ii**, 859.

Edwards, M. (1982). Communication changes in elderly people. *Br. J. Dis. Comm.*, Monograph no. 3, College of

Speech Therapists, Harold Poster House, Letchmere Road, London NW2 5BU.

Eggers, O. (1983). *Occupational Therapy in the Treatment of Adult Hemiplegia*, W. Heinemann, London.

Ehrman, J.G. (1983). Use of biofeedback to treat incontinence. *J. Am. Geriatr. Soc.*, **31**, 182–4.

Erikson, J. (1979). The arts and healing. *Am. J. Art Ther.*, **183**, 75–80.

Fay, T. (1948). The neurological aspects of therapy in cerebral palsy. *Arch. Phys. Med.*, **29**, 327–31.

Feldman, D.J., Lee, P.R., Unterecker, J., Lloyd, K., Rusk, H.A., and Toole, A. (1961). A comparison of functionally orientated medical care and formal rehabilitation in management of patients with hemiplegia due to cerebrovascular disease. *J. Chronic Dis.*, **15**, 297–82.

Flanagan, E.M. (1967). Methods for facilitation and inhibition of motor activity. *Am. J. Phys. Med.*, **46**, 1006–23.

Folsom, J.C. (1967). Intensive hospital therapy of geriatric patients. *Current Psychiatric Therapies*, **7**, 209–15.

Folsom, J.C. (1968). Reality orientation for the elderly mental patient. *J. Geriatr. Psychiatry*, **1**, 291–307.

Garraway, W.M. (1982). Stroke unit or medical units in the management of acute stroke. Lessons from a controlled trial. In: Rose, F.C. (ed.) *Advances in Stroke Therapy*, Raven Press, New York.

Gazzaniga, M.S. (1974). Determinants of cerebral recovery. In: Stein, D.G. (ed.) *Plasticity and Recovery of Function in the Central Nervous System*, Academic Press, New York.

Geschwind, N. (1971). Aphasia. *N. Engl. J. Med.*, **284**, 654–6.

Gibson, R.W. (1982). The creative arts therapies. In: Masserman, J.H. (ed.) *Current Psychiatric Therapies*, Grune and Stratton, Washington, DC, pp. 185–8.

Gloag, D. (1985). Needs and opportunities in rehabilitation—rehabilitation of the elderly. Settings and services. *Br. Med. J.*, **290**, 455–7.

Gombrich, H.E. (1977). *Art and Illusion—Study in the Psychology of Pictorial Representation*, Phaidon, London.

Green, E.J.G., Nicol, R., and Jamieson, H. (1979). Reality orientation with psychogeriatric patients. *Behav. Res. Ther.*, **17**, 615–17.

Griffith, V.E. (1975). Volunteer scheme for dysphasia and allied problems in stroke patients. *Br. Med. J.*, **3**, 633–5.

Griffith, V.E. (1980). Observations on patients dysphasic after stroke. *Br. Med. J.*, **281**, 1608–9.

Hanley, I.G., McGuire, R.J., and Boyd, W.D. (1981). Reality orientation and dementia: a controlled trial of two approaches. *Br. J. Psychiatry*, **138**, 10–14.

Hanley, E.G. (1984). Theoretical and practical considerations in reality orientation therapy with the elderly. In: *Psychological Approaches to the Care of the Elderly*, Croom Helm, London.

Harris, C.S., and Ivory, P.B.C.B. (1976). An outcome evaluation of reality orientation therapy with geriatric patients in a state mental hospital. *Gerontologist*, **16**, 496–503.

Hewer, R.L. (1972). Stroke units. *Br. Med. J.*, **1**, 52.

Holden, U.P., and Sinebruchow, A. (1978). Reality orientation therapy: A study investigating the value of the therapy in the rehabilitation of elderly people. *Age Ageing*, **7**, 83–90.

Holden, U.P. (1976). A flexible technique for rehabilitating the confused. *Geriatr. Med.*, **9**(7), 49–60.

Holden, U.P., and Woods, R.T. (1982). *Reality Orientation—Psychological Approaches to the Confused Elderly*, Churchill Livingstone, Edinburgh, London.

Hopkins, A. (1975). The need for speech therapy for dysphasia following stroke. *Health Trends*, **7**, 58–60.

Isaacs, B. (1984). Rehabilitation for the elderly. *Int. Rehabil. Med.*, **6**, v–vi.

Jackson, J.H. (1882). On some implications of dissolution of the nervous system. *Medical Press Circular*, **2**, 411–18.

Johnson, R., and Garvie, C. (1985). The BBC microcomputer for therapy of intellectual impairment following acquired brain damage. *Occup. Ther.*, **2**, 46–8.

Johnstone, M. (1976). *The Stroke Patient: Principles of Rehabilitation*, Churchill Livingstone, Edinburgh.

Kabat, H. (1952). Studies on neuromuscular dysfunction. XV The role of central facilitation in restoration of motor function in paralysis. *Arch. Phys. Med.*, **33**, 521–3.

Kaplan, E.I. (1985). Hospitalisation and milieu therapy, music therapy. In: *Comprehensive Textbook of Psychiatry*, Vol. 32, pp. 2388–9.

Kennard, D. (1983). A touch of music for physiotherapists. *Physiotherapy*, **69**(4), 114–16.

Kertesz, A., and McCabe, P. (1977). Recovery patterns and prognosis in aphasia. *Brain*, **100**, 1–18.

Knott, M. (1967). Introduction to and philosophy of neuromuscular facilitation. *Physiotherapy*, **53**, 2–5.

Larner, S.L., and Leemming, J.T. (1984). The work of a clinical psychologist in cases of the elderly. *Age Ageing*, **13**, 29–33.

Leng, N. (1982). Behavioural treatment of the elderly. *Age Ageing*, **11**, 235–43.

Liberman, R.P. (1972). *Guide to Behavioural Analysis and Therapy*, Pergamon Press, Oxford.

Liberson, W.T. (1979). Electrical aids in hemiplegia. In: Licht, S. (ed.) *Stroke and Its Rehabilitation*, New Haven, Connecticut.

Licht, S. (1969). *Therapeutic Heat and Cold*, E. Licht, New Haven, Connecticut.

Lincoln, N.B., McQuirk, E., Mulley, G.P., Lendrem, W., Jones, A.C., and Mitchell, J.R. (1984). Effectiveness of speech therapy for aphasic stroke patients. A randomised controlled trial. *Lancet*, **i**, 1197–200.

Loew, C.A., and Silverstone, B.M. (1971). A programme of intensified stimulation and response facilitation for the senile aged. *Gerontologist*, **11**, 341–7.

Magnus, R., and De Kleijn, A.S. (1912). A Bliangigkeit des Tonus der Extremitatien musketn. Von der Kopfstellung. *Pflugers Arch.*, **145**, 455–8.

Meikle, M., Wechsler, E., Tupper, A., Beneson, M., Butler, J., Mulhall, D., and Stern, G. (1979). Comparative trial of volunteer and professional treatments of dysphasia after stroke. *Br. Med. J.*, **ii**, 87–9.

Merriam, S. (1980). The concept and function of reminiscence—a review of the research. *Gerontologist*, **20**, 605–9.

Munting, E. (1978). Ultrasonic therapy for painful shoulders. *Physiotherapy*, **64**(6), 180–1.

Nanton, V. (1984). Conductive education and Parkinson's disease or, "Why I went to Hungary". Birmingham Conductive Education Project, University of Birmingham.

O'Brien, J.G. (1978). The behavioural treatment of a thirty year smallpox obsession and hand washing compulsion. *J. Behav. Ther. Exp. Psychol.*, **9**, 365–8.

Pappas, W., Curtis, W.P., and Baker, J. (1958). A controlled study of an intensive treatment programme for hospital geriatric patients. *J. Am. Geriatr. Soc.*, **6**, 17–25.

Perry, C.E. (1967). Principles and techniques of the Brunnstrom approach, treatment of hemiplegia. *Am. J. Phys. Med.*, **46**, 789–812.

Perry, J. (1969). The mechanics of walking in hemiplegia. *Clin. Orthop.*, **63**, 23–31.

Pincus, A. (1976). Reminiscence in ageing and its implications for social work practice. *Social Work*, **15**, 47–53.

Porch, B.E. (1972). *Porch Index of Communications Ability*, Consulting Psychology Press, Palo Alto.

Powell, R.R. (1974). Psychological effects of exercise therapy upon institutionalized geriatric mental patients. *Gerontologist*, **14**, 157–61.

Puder, R., Lacks, P., Bertleson, A.D, and Storandt, M. (1983). Short-term stimulus control treatment of insomnia in older adults. *Behaviour Therapy*, **14**, 424–9.

Quirk, R. (1972). Department of Education and Science. *Report of the Committee on Speech Therapy Services Appointed by the Secretaries of State for Education and Science*, HMSO, London.

Reeve, W., and Ivison, D. (1985). Use of environmental manipulation and classroom, and modified informal Reality Orientation with institutionalized confused elderly patients. *Age Ageing*, **14**, 119–21.

Richman, L. (1969). Sensory training for geriatric patients. *Am. J. Occup. Ther.*, **23**, 254–7.

Robertson, S.J., and Thompson, F. (1984). Speech therapy in Parkinson's disease. A study of the efficacy and long term effects on intensive treatment. *Br. J. Dis. Comm.*, **19**, 213–24.

Rood, M.S. (1954). Neurophysiological reactions as a basis for physical therapy. *Phys. Ther. Rev.*, **34**, 444.

Salter, C.L., and Salter, C.A. (1975). Effects of an individualized activity programme on elderly patients. *Gerontologist*, **15**, 404–6.

Sarno, M.T. (1976). The status of research in recovery from aphasia. In: Leburn, Y., and Hoops, R. (ed.) *Recovery in Aphasics Neurolinguistics*, Swets and Zeitlinger, Amsterdam.

Sarno, M.T., and Sands, E.C. (1970). An objective method for evaluation of speech therapy in aphasia. *Arch. Phys. Med. Rehabil.*, **51**, 44–54.

Sarno, M.T., and Levita, E. (1979). Recovery in treated aphasia in the first year post-stroke. *Stroke*, **10**, 663–70.

Schuell, H.S. (1965). *The Minnesota Test for Differential Diagnosis of Aphasia*, University of Minneapolis.

Scott, S., Caird, F., and Williams, B.O. (1983). Speech therapy for Parkinson's disease. *J. Neurol. Neurosurg. Psychiatry*, **46**, 140–4.

Sherrington, C.S. (1906). *The Integrative Action of the Nervous System*, second edition, 1947, Yale University Press, New Haven.

Simons, A. (1923). Z. Kopfhalting and Muskeltonus. *Neurology*, **80**, 499–549.

Smith, D.S., Gordenberg, E., Ashburn, A., Kinsella, E., Sheikh, K., Breunan, P.J., Meade, T.W., Zutsh, D.W., Perry, J.D., and Reeback, J.S. (1981). Remedial therapy after stroke: a randomised controlled trial. *Br. Med. J.*, **282**, 517–20.

Tallis, R. (1984). Neurological rehabilitation: the next thirty years. *Physiotherapy*, **70**(5), 196–9.

Twitchell, T.E. (1951). The restoration of motor function in hemiplegia in man. *Brain*, **74**, 443–54.

Udell, R., Sullivan, R.A., and Schlanger, P.H. (1980). Legal competency of aphasic patients; role of speech language pathologists. *Arch. Phys. Med. Rehabil.*, **61**, 374–5.

Watts, F.N. (1985). Clinical psychology. *Health Trends*, **17**, 28–30.

Westcott, E.J. (1967). Traditional exercises regimens for hemiplegic patients. *Am. J. Phys. Med.*, **46**, 1012–23.

Williams, J.M.G. (1984). Cognitive behaviour therapy for depression: problems and perspectives. *Br. J. Psychiatry*, **145**, 254–62.

Willmuth, M.E., and Broedy, D.L. (1979). The verbal diagnostic and art therapy combine, an extended evaluation procedure with family groups. *Art Psychotherapy*, **6**(1), 11–18.

Woods, R.T. (1979). Reality orientation and staff attention. A controlled study. *Br. J. Psychiatry*, **134**, 502–7.

Zwerling, I. (1979). The creative arts therapies as "real therapies". *Hosp. Community Psychiatry*, **30**, 12–21.

The Clinical Neurology of Old Age
Edited by R. Tallis
© 1989 John Wiley & Sons Ltd

Chapter 34

Aids for the Neurologically Disabled

Ted Cantrell

Senior Lecturer in Rehabilitation

Susan Farr

Senior Occupational Therapist, Aid and Equipment Centre, Rehabilitation Unit, Southampton General Hospital, Southampton, UK

The major issue in relation to equipment for the disabled is whether we can find good ways of matching up the huge variety of gadgets and devices with the finance and needs of the people who need them. The range of answers to disabilities and the number of suppliers is so massive that it would take volumes to describe them. This chapter will not, therefore, describe individual aids for the handicapped but rather will concentrate on information systems and how to match equipment with people in need.

SOURCES OF EQUIPMENT AND INFORMATION

Disabled elderly persons may find out about or obtain special equipment from six sources, all of which may present difficulties.

Self-bought in Shops

The wide selection may be bewildering to a disabled person who has poor mobility, lacks information about best buys or has inadequate funds—in other words for most severely disabled people, particularly pensioners. The most lavishly advertised goods can be the most expensive buys and the worst designed.

Occupational Therapy Guided

A far better approach is to make sure that a professionally trained occupational therapist (OT)

does a proper assessment of all the person's needs, and the home, and advises on the best equipment. Such a person may also be able to help to find some sources of funds. Many old people in need have no knowledge of OTs and may not be referred by their GP. Moreover, they may be willing to put up with diminishing independence. In many areas the OTs are so busy that the waiting list for assessment may be many months; in addition, funds are often extremely short.

DSC (ALAC) Provided

Most GPs are aware that they are able to prescribe equipment from a relatively local Disablement Services Centre (DSC), the new name for the Artificial Limb and Appliance Centre (ALAC). If the request is approved, the provision of equipment (e.g. wheelchairs) is free. Nevertheless, assessment could involve a journey of many miles (50–100 in some parts of the UK). The DSC staff may also find it impossible to know enough about the design of the home to approve sensible and practical answers, unless they do a home visit.

Book-guided Buys

Excellent reference books give a choice of alternatives that are available if funds are forthcoming. (A list is included at the end of this chapter.) This may allow intelligent relatives to see what is available, and where to get it. The trouble is that such books may present a range of alternatives (such as the various hand-rails in the *Which* guide). The problem for the untrained family is then to know exactly which is best for their house and their elderly dependent's particular disability. The precise matching of ergonomic design with the specific abilities of the person in need is a very skilled task, much better done by an OT than by a lay person relying on pictures or drawings.

Phone-advice Centres

There are several important telephone answering services in Britain (e.g. DIAL (Disabled Information and Advice Line), DLF (Disabled Living Foundation), DLCs (Disabled Living Centres), Help for Health). These are usually open 8 hours/day with responding staff, and some with 24 hour answerphone recorders. They provide an essential contact point for the anxious but confused disabled person. Public libraries may offer access to an extensive (paper or computer) database, and information about a far greater range of alternatives than almost any professional. They may, however, for this very reason confuse the lay person who does not have the benefit of professional advice.

Self-designed

Very rarely there are relatives who design ingenious hoists, lifts and gadgets for their own family and some fascinating inventions have resulted from this. The real danger lies in the amateur with good ideas but no concept of safety, so that serious electrical, mechanical or other catastrophes may result from faulty equipment.

THE DISABILITY ENQUIRY NETWORK (DEN)

It is clear that the pathway from an elderly disabled person with special disability needs to a carefully matched and funded answer is not straightforward. Many elderly people, especially those with dwindling intellectual powers and diminishing confidence, may feel unable to ask for help. Far too often they sit at home increasingly unable to do things, depressed by the frustration of being unable to cope,

and withdrawn from a society that often does not care about the elderly or the disabled. They may regard GPs or hospital doctors as too busy for anything but acute medical needs and yet not know who else they can turn to. The problems of such patients will not be answered unless they are regularly visited by someone prepared to field every sort of question, however 'irrelevant' it may seem, and to ask questions themselves.

If queries do reach the GPs there is no guarantee that they will find an answer, because the range of possible solutions is sufficient to fill the database of a very large computer (such as at the Disabled Living Foundation) and is far greater than any one person can carry in his head. Excellent books exist but they need to be regularly updated, and are not free.

We suggest that there should be a disability enquiry network (DEN) (Figure 34.1) of information suppliers that may be able to offer several types of answer to the disability/equipment needs of the most isolated and reticent disabled people in the community.

The diagram (Figure 34.1) shows some of the common systems used with the advantages and disadvantages of each (talking to relatives or neighbours, local doctors and social services). New systems that can improve the speed or quality of information-gathering are as follows:

1. A regular visitor to the house (e.g. health visitor) may pick up a person's needs informally and quickly.
2. Reports back to the local GP alert the practitioner.
3. Direct enquiries to a local information centre (e.g. Help for Health) may find an immediate suggested answer.
4. GP teams may get help via the local Citizens' Advice Bureau or local library, or may ring an information centre.
5. Direct suggestions can be made to the local community OT and speed up the process of home assessment and equipment advice.

THE ANALYSIS OF PROBLEMS PRESENTED

It is possible to consider the myriad of problems of the elderly at two levels: firstly the lay phase that will

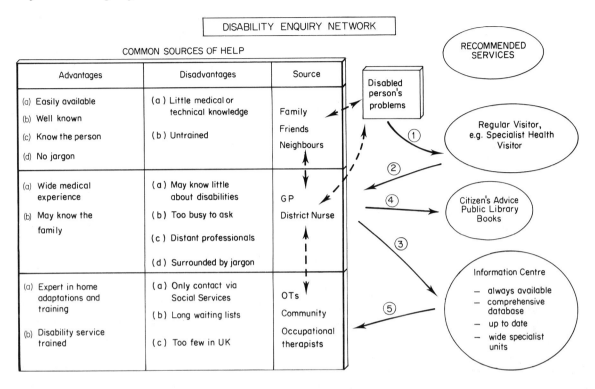

Figure 34.1

be the tentative remark of the family or the patient; and secondly some of the medico-social explanations that must be sorted out before answers are looked for (Table 34.1).

The most important step is to think through (or rehearse) the essential daily activities in order to identify those which are difficult or impossible. The list should also encompass unfulfilled ambitions so that it can extend to a range of interests, hobbies and dreams. It is possible that people lack motivation for the mundane functions of life until they are helped to extend themselves into the risky or 'impossible' areas. Breaking new ground may bring back excitement and the will to succeed. Digging, one may uncover an enthusiasm for needlework, knitting, birdwatching, sea fishing, academic work, reading, mountain watching or creative arts. A determined

effort to make these possible can be a great stimulus to live. An elderly person with neurological disease still needs to be helped to develop any submerged enthusiasm, even if it is a penchant for talking about the First World War. There are some classic examples of retired people who have set up museums, started evening classes or achieved amazing results in life because they have been fired with enthusiasm. Sadly, many people enter retirement with no preparation and no concrete plans and they have simply given up because their joints creak, their memories are poor, their strength is low.

Full assessment of a disabled person (of any age) may therefore generate a long list of things which he or she is prevented from doing. As an adaptation of the Weed system (1969) of problem orientated records we suggest a more positive rehabilitation version.

TABLE 34.1   ANALYSIS OF PROBLEMS PRESENTED

Presentation	Some explanations	
Cannot Walk	Spastic legs Poor balance Painful feet Painful arthritis	Uneven floor coverings Too cold Cannot see to walk Frightened to move
Poor speech	Profoundly depressed Dysarthria Dyspraxia Dysphasia Dysphonia	No teeth, mouth ulcers Dementia Drugs inappropriate Drinking alcohol Deaf
Poor hygiene	Depressed No motivation Bereaved Relatives do not care Battered/neglected Inadequate finance	Physically unable to wash Cannot afford hot water Outside WC Incontinent Malnourished
Incontinent	Painful knees, Confusional state Outside WC Too much tea	Drugs or alcohol Neurogenic bladder Cannot dress/undress Depressed
Bored	Isolated from neighbours Family never visit No hobbies Cannot use arms	No ideas to follow Uninspired No helpers
Unmotivated	Retired No interests Housebound	Too unwell for original interests

PAOMR—Problem and Asset Oriented Medical Records

In this scheme a simple matrix of statements can be compiled from a full assessment (Cantrell and Dawson, 1983) whereby a person's positive and negative attributes can be derived, and compared with those of the main relative or companion (or outside helpers). The end result of a PAOMR matrix could be something like that shown below:

Name: A.P. Erson (aged 70)

Diagnoses: OA knees
CVA—left hemiplegia
Bronchitis and effort dyspnoea

	Problems	*Assets*
Patient	Slurred speech Reduced left-sided function Breathless on exertion Night pain, poor sleep Slow on stairs Limited walking	Nearly ADL independent Sense of humour Music Birdwatching
Wife	Hypertension Chronic back pain Blackouts Has fallen × 3 Isolation	Enthusiastic home-maker Needlework/tapestry Daughter lives near

The problem list provides a more complete picture of practical needs than will be found in a bald statement of medical diagnoses. An item on the list may imply a need for special training (physiotherapy, occupational therapy or speech therapy training) and possibly specific aids:

Problem	Equipment
e.g. slow on stairs	stair rail portable step aid
e.g. reduced left-sided function	feeding aids dressing aids
Asset	
e.g. birdwatching	portable tripod seat binocular support thermal protection clothing rough ground transport

In order that this exercise can succeed, three things are needed. Firstly, there must be a key worker who is prepared to spend time with Mr Erson and think through the possible dreams he and his wife have for the future, however idiosyncratic or unrealistic, in order to find out what may make them tick. Secondly, there needs to be a proper assessment unit with appropriate professional support. Thirdly, there needs to be access to a local DEN (disability enquiry network) or a detailed and comprehensive resource centre, for advice on facilities, equipment, finance, supplies, so that any answers can be looked at in detail. For the example given, this may include contacts with local ornithological groups, special groups for the disabled, or those who can offer voluntary assistance or drivers, and advice on rough ground transport, special clothing and binoculars.

Clearly these approaches become more difficult for a disabled elderly person with mental impairment, perception defects, poor vision, lack of concentration or deteriorating general health. The difference is only quantitative, since even the person confined to bed may have needs for special equipment to keep him hygienic and also be helped to follow his wishes. Sometimes this may be simply a matter of providing old familiar pictures and furniture round the room. These may be augmented by visual aids linking the patient with relatives, special telephone equipment, radio or taped music. Modern information technology based communication methods may be especially relevant here.

FINANCING

Money is sometimes in short supply, but the following sources should always be considered, though success sometimes needs persistent enquiry.

Local Authority Social Services Department

Legally, provision is made for home equipment, as described in the Chronically Sick and Disabled Persons Act 1970—Section 2: 'practical assistance in the home' and 'assistance in arranging for the carrying out of any works of adaptation in the home or provision of any additional facilities designed to secure greater safety, comfort or convenience'. The local authority should provide these services for a disabled person 'if they are satisfied they are necessary in order to meet the person's needs and that it is necessary for it to provide them'. The 1986 Disabled Persons Act obliges social services departments to carry out an assessment of need if requested to do so by the disabled person. They also have a duty to inform them of the services available. It does not, however, oblige them to provide any new services.

This is open to a variety of interpretations and so the services vary considerably from county to county. Most areas have an aids loan service; some make provision for all disabled people; some only for those with long-term problems but excluding those who need items on a temporary basis at pre- or post-surgery; some provide only the more expensive items, expecting clients to purchase small items, e.g. under £10 in cost; and some only those items which are specially made for disabled people (an armchair, though needed for an arthritic, may be excluded). Most local authorities employ their own occupational therapists to advise and assess people in their own homes. Sometimes this work is carried out for them by the health authority. They will accept a referral for assessment from the client, relatives or other social services or health care staff. However, they will usually accept specific requests for equipment only from other occupational therapists or trained staff such as physiotherapists and district nurses.

Local Health Authorities

Most health authorities provide a medical or home nursing equipment loan service. This includes items like hospital beds, cot sides, pressure reducing mattresses and urinals. The supply of incontinence pants, pads and bed pads is usually included in this service.

The service and range of equipment varies considerably between health authorities. Requests for equipment can be made by district nurses, health visitors and family doctors; sometimes occupational therapists and physiotherapists are required especially for assessing items such as walking aids.

Occasionally the local authority and health authority combine their community loan services, and have centralized ordering and delivery, and provide access and training to all health care staff. A very successful scheme of this type has been running for some years in the Salisbury Health District.

District health authorities appliance departments, whilst normally concerned with the provision of body worn appliances, e.g. braces, surgical footwear and orthoses, can also usually supply, on loan, special equipment requested by a hospital consultant. This can include items like standing frames, special walking aids or vacuum moulded body supports. There is, however, again, considerable variation between districts.

District health authorities can also set aside monies for special categories of equipment (e.g. communication aids), or consider individual requests. These are purely local decisions.

Regional Health Authorities

Regional health authorities are normally involved only in the provision of one type of equipment: environmental controls. The procedure for applying is laid down in the DHSS booklet 'Arrangements for the Provision of Environmental Control and Communication Equipment through the DHSS'.

There are two makes of system available, and the regional health authorities provide the control and switch units. Equipment to be used with the system is either loaned by the social services department (e.g.

page turner) or purchased by the user. The procedure for these items involves application to a special office at the regional health authority, the appointment of a medical assessor, and then (if approved) the free provision of the equipment to the home. Many requests are refused since referrals may be better answered by personal visitors (e.g. home helps) than by impersonal switching gear.

DHSS Regional Services: Disablement Services Centres or Artificial Limb and Appliance Centres (ALAC)

This service is being reorganized following the McColl report; by 1991 the regional centres will become part of their regional health authority. This will mean that each region will be able to make its own decisions about the makes of equipment that it supplies, depending on its budget. They provide, on loan, wheelchairs and their accessories, e.g. pressure reducing cushions and bicycles and tricycles. A complete list is given in the 'Handbook of Wheelchairs' Bicycles and Tricycles'—MHM 408 available from the DHSS Store, No. 2 Site, Manchester Road, Heywood, Lancs. This book is currently being updated and some models listed are no longer available. A self propelling wheelchair, a pushchair, or accessories can be requested from the local DSC on form AOF 5G, signed by a doctor.

DSCs supply only indoor electric powered chairs, or one type of attendant controlled electric powered outdoor wheelchair. These are not listed in the handbook or on the form as DSCs will want to carry out their own assessment. DSCs normally supply wheelchairs that are listed in the handbook; however, it does state that 'the majority of wheelchairs shown in manufacturers' catalogues can be supplied to meet proven clinical needs where in the Department's view, these can be met only by the supply of such wheelchairs. DSCs have their own medical and technical officers who can carry out assessments at DSC or in the client's own home.

Doctor's Prescription

The DHSS Drug Tariff book gives a list of items that can be prescribed. This includes such items as condom drainage incontinence appliances and surgical stockings.

DHSS—Social Security

Mobility allowance is a tax-free cash payment for anyone who is unable or virtually unable to walk out of doors and likely to be in this condition for at least one year. The patient has to be at least 5 years old or under 65 years old when the first claim is made. If he is in receipt of the allowance when he reaches 65 years, it can continue until he is 75 years old. It is a usual source of funding particularly for powered wheelchairs.

Manpower Services Commission (MSC)

MSC will provide equipment on loan to enable someone to remain in or take up employment. Their Disablement Advisory Service (DAS) or the Disablement Resettlement Officer (DRO) can give advice on the type of item they would consider.

Voluntary Organizations

Red Cross: almost all areas of the country have an equipment loan service run by the Red Cross. Sometimes the equipment is bought with Red Cross money; sometimes the social services department or the health authority give the Red Cross money to buy equipment. Many depots prefer their equipment to be for short-term loan, e.g. a wheelchair for 2 weeks' holiday, and would expect a long-term user to apply to the relevant statutory authority.

Many other voluntary organizations will provide equipment on loan to their members or help to raise money to buy equipment for individuals or special units.

BUYING EQUIPMENT

There are many companies which manufacture and/ or sell special aids and equipment for disabled people. Some produce a wide range of items and some only one or two. Many of them advertise in therapy or nursing magazines or those magazines produced by voluntary organizations like RADAR

(Royal Association for Disability and Rehabilitation), and the Multiple Sclerosis Society. However, few advertise in the national or local press, with the notable exception of the stairlift and electric wheelchair companies. Most companies offer a mail order service and have either local representatives or agents who can demonstrate the equipment to the individual at home. Most will consider 'sale or return' so that the item can be tried out. There are few retail shops specializing in aids but the number is increasing.

The quality of advice offered depends on the training of the staff. Chemists often stock small items like feeder cups and incontinence garments and some have introduced a wide range of aids into their larger stores. Many ordinary stores keep items which, whilst not specially made for disabled people, are of help to some of them, e.g. high seat chairs, jar openers. The large mail order companies now also include a few items in their catalogues. However, they do not have as much information as is contained in the literature from the specialist companies.

SOURCES OF INFORMATION AND ADVICE
(full list at the end of the chapter)

Information on aids and equipment is more readily available than advice for individuals. The Research Institute for Consumer Affairs (RICA) produced a comprehensive book *Aids for People with Disabilities; a Review of Information Services* which lists most sources of information. *Occupational therapists (OTs)* with their training in assessing and advising on problems associated with activities of daily living, are perhaps the most readily available source of advice as well as information.

Hospital OTs will see in- and outpatients and will require a consultant's or doctor's referral. They will often carry out pre-discharge home visits for inpatients to check on conditions at home.

Social services OTs can visit people in their own homes. They will usually accept a referral from anyone (via social services area offices). The availability of these services depends on local factors, such as the number of therapists and the demand on the services. Other health care professionals can usually give some advice or can refer someone to the local OT service.

Disabled Living Centres or Aid and Equipment Centres provide information and advice on aids and equipment, and have a permanent display of such equipment for visitors to try. They are open to the general public and act as a resource and exhibition centre for therapists, health care and social services staff and others who may work with disabled people. All visitors need to make an appointment and disabled visitors do not usually need a referral. There are twenty centres in Britain plus one travelling centre. They all employ suitably qualified staff, usually OTs or physiotherapists. Most centres do not sell or loan equipment but can put the person in contact with the correct source of supply. A complete list of centres can be obtained from the Disabled Living Centres Council (DLCC) Secretary, Trent Region Aids Information and Demonstration Service, 76 Clarendon Park Road, Leicester LE2 3AD.

The Disabled Living Foundation (DLF) is recommended as having the most comprehensive information on aids, equipment and related matters, in Britain. It can be contacted by letter or telephone. It produces sets of information sheets in sixteen categories, e.g. 'chairs', 'personal toilet', 'household equipment'. These list and briefly describe aids, give addresses of manufacturers, often a price, and notes on supply and publications. They are updated throughout the year and once a year each sheet is completely renewed. They can be obtained on subscription and most health authorities and social services departments subscribe. The lists are usually kept by the occupational therapy department, but many hospital libraries have a set. Individual lists can be bought separately and the DLF prepare some special lists for particular conditions or subjects e.g. 'Aids for People who have had Strokes' and 'Notes on Equipment Designed to Reduce Pressure'. The DLF also have specialist advisers in, for example, incontinence and clothing.

Equipment for the Disabled is a series of books produced by staff at Mary Marlborough Lodge, Oxford for the DHSS. There are thirteen titles, e.g. 'Communication', 'Outdoor Transport', 'Hoists and Lifts'. They are less comprehensive than the DLF lists but the equipment has been assessed in use and they have fuller notes on use and are illustrated with some idea of costs. They are updated periodically.

Six *Communication Aids Centres* have been established in Britain. They can provide advice and information on communication equipment and can assess individuals referred by a consultant and speech therapist. They require that funding be obtained to pay for the equipment they may recommend.

The Royal National Institute for the Blind (RNIB) has a central resource centre in London, and local centres and officers who can advise on aids for the visually handicapped.

The Royal National Institute for the Deaf (RNID) has an advice and information service at its London headquarters.

Social services departments often have specialist officers for the visually handicapped and hearing impaired.

REMAP (Rehabilitation Engineering Movement Advisory Panels) are voluntary groups consisting of qualified engineers, skilled craftsmen, therapists and other health care staff who consider unusual daily living problems referred to them. They design and make one-off aids when commercially produced aids are not suitable.

Voluntary organizations, usually for specific conditions, often produce guidance leaflets and can answer individual queries. They often have regular magazines or newsletters which can include information on new aids and equipment.

Local information services vary greatly throughout the country. There are two nationwide networks that can offer information on equipment or provide contacts with local therapy services. These are: Citizens' Advice Bureaux; and DIAL (Disabled Information and Advice Line) which is run by disabled people. Local libraries often have books on various disabilities, which may include sections on aids, and information on local services. Many local radio stations have information and 'phone-in' programmes on topics to do with disability, and these can reach a large number of people.

National radio has specialist programmes, e.g. 'In Touch', which can supply relevant information, and fact sheets. Specialist television programmes like 'Link' and 'See Hear' give a great deal of valuable information. Some programmes provide written information and are assisted in this by Broadcasting Support Services.

Details of suppliers vary so much with each health district and social services area that it would not be helpful to describe suppliers in more detail. Any person needing advice on suppliers should either contact one of the national bodies (addresses at the end of the chapter) or research the local facilities in their own district.

WHO SHOULD ASSESS PEOPLE FOR SPECIAL EQUIPMENT?

Supposing we are concerned about a very heavy old lady who has had a stroke, can barely move herself without help, wants to live at home, but only has a rather small arthritic husband at home. Quite a few important decisions need to be made which have a bearing on her plans including the provision of some kind of hoisting or 'bulk handling' equipment.

The couple themselves may have clear, perhaps fixed, ideas about what they regard as the ideal life for them, and they are entitled to be involved in the decision. Their understandable preference for their familiar surroundings should be taken seriously and, indeed, should have priority. They may, however, be totally out of touch with the practical details of daily nursing needs, the medical prognosis, the availability of special hoists and the practicality of using any hoist in their house full of Victorian furniture. The medical staff may also have relevant information about the prognosis and the presence of mental impairment interfering with rational decision making.

An occupational therapist is also essential to the decision and is the closest in skills to the ideal person to make an equipment plan. Her training and experience make her well informed about the wide range of hoists available, their relative safety for a large patient, the problems of home ergonomics (floor surfaces, under-bed access, turning circles, activating controls, release mechanisms and safety maintenance). She also will know enough about the medical conditions to plan for the likely future.

A home visit will be essential to make sure that the equipment being considered will get to the parts of the house other systems do not reach, whether there is storage when it is not in use, and that the spouse can control it. It is also essential to look at other features of house design to check the common items essential to the daily routine (access, WC, washing, cooking, feeding, leisure).

Thus the apparently simple question as to who should assess is really not so simple, since there are many components (family, medical prognosis, functional capacity and equipment) which need to be taken account of for a fully informed, rational decision. This is especially true where expensive items of equipment, such as stairlifts, are being considered. All this takes time, but where finance is short (as for most elderly and disabled people) this is the only approach. A case conference between the experts and the family is usually essential.

Training in the use of special items (e.g. bath aids) is of great importance, and several surveys have shown that people do not use equipment properly at home unless they have been fully trained to use it, and visited in their own homes. Since elderly people may have memory problems, instructions may need to be repeated and written down.

REHABILITATION UNITS

Many hospitals do have a centre where several professions can get together to offer a combined approach to disabled people. The importance of a rehabilitation unit is that the combination of professionals in assessment and training may achieve quicker results than in a general ward, special hostel, rest home or own home, so that the final placement will be after a careful evaluation of all the possibilities. The decision must take into account all aspects of the assessment. Financial constraints and lack of resources often reduce options greatly, but a team discussion involving the family is an ideal to aim for.

ACKNOWLEDGEMENTS

We are particularly grateful to Bob Gann and Marilyn Jamieson in the Help for Health office for all their guidance on information resources.

REFERENCES

Cantrell, E.G., and Dawson, J. (1985). Young disabled in the community. In: Barbenel, J., Forbes, C.D., and Lowe, G.D.O. (eds.) *Pressure Sores*, Macmillan Press.

Weed, L. (1969). *Medical Records, Medical Education and Patient Care*, Case Western Reserve University.

BOOK GUIDE

Directory of Aids for Disabled and Elderly People (1986). Anne Darnborough and Derek Kinrade. Woodhead-Faulkner, Cambridge.

Disabled Living Foundations Information Service Sheets. 16 catalogues providing a comprehensive list of equipment. Essential for those who need a complete list for reference, regularly updated.

Equipment for the Disabled. A series of 13 carefully researched books which are very useful for showing the range and cost of equipment available, and well illustrated (from Mary Marlborough Lodge, Dept 405, Nuffield Orthopaedic Centre, Headington, Oxford).

The New Source Book for the Disabled (1983). Edited by Glorya Hale. Published by Heinemann. A practical, well-illustrated book dealing with many aspects of daily living, work and leisure including many suggestions of aids and equipment.

Directory for Disabled People (1985). Compiled by A. Darnborough and D. Kinrade. Published by Woodhead-Faulkner (renewed every 2–3 years). Has a chapter on 'Aids—their provision and availability' plus many useful addresses throughout the book.

Signpost (1984). Where to go for advice, information and help. RICA (Research Institute for Consumer Affairs). As the name implies, it directs you to further detailed help. Has a chapter on 'Aids to make life easier'.

Compass (1984). The direction finder for disabled people. DIG (Disabled Income Group). Has a chapter on 'Aids, Equipment and Services' and detailed advice on finance and welfare benefits.

Physical Handicap (1981). A guide for the staff of social services departments and voluntary agencies. L. Bell and A. Klemz. Published by Woodhead and Faulkner. Gives advice and examples of basic daily living problems and solutions.

Disabled—An Illustrated Manual of Help and Self Help (1981). P. Nichols, R. Haworth and J. Hopkins. Published by David and Charles. A practical and well-illustrated book dealing with many aspects of daily living and leisure.

Coping with Disability (1984). Peggy Jay. Published by Disabled Living Foundation. A practical, illustrated book on aspects of daily living, problems and solutions.

Motoring and Mobility for Disabled People. A. Darnborough and D. Kinrade. Published by RADAR. Practical advice and information on all aspects of mobility plus useful addresses including suppliers of special equipment.

Choosing the Best Wheelchair Cushion for Your Needs, Your Chair and your Lifestyle (1983). P. Jay. Published by RADAR. A useful guide to the large range of cushions available and what factors to consider when choosing one.

In Touch Handbook. Aids and services for blind and partially sighted people. Published by BBC Publications. A practical and very useful guide; also available on tape or in braille.

Incontinence (1977). D. Mandelstam. Published by Heinemann. A practical book on aids to help maintain continence and manage incontinence.

Disabled Living Foundation have a large selection of books dealing with specific areas of practical problems and solutions, e.g. *Kitchen Sense for Disabled and Elderly People, Footwear for Problem Feet, Dressing for Disabled People.* It is well worth sending for their complete book list.

Help Yourselves (1985). A handbook for hemiplegics and their families. P. Jay. Fourth edition 1985. Published by Ian Henry Pub. A practical book that covers many of the everyday problems arising from hemiplegia.

Aid for People Who Have Had a Stroke. DLF Information Service. Notes and advice on some of the commonest problems following a stroke and their solutions.

Parkinson's Disease Day-to-Day. Parkinson's Disease Society. Contains a section on 'aids for the home'.

Living with Parkinson's Disease. Parkinson's Disease Society. Contains a chapter on 'aids to daily living'.

Learning to live with MS. R. Davie, R. Povey, and G. Whitley. MS Society 1981. Has a short section with suggestions for some practical problems and addresses of where to obtain further help.

MS Society's Information Sheets. 'Motoring' February 1984, 'Sports and Hobbies' August 1983, 'Government and Local Authority Help' April 1985. Very useful information sheets on specific topics.

So, You're Paralysed (1978). Bernadette Fallon. Spinal Injuries Association. Advice for the recently spinal injured on specific problems and concerns, e.g. spasticity, pressure and continence. This is directed mainly at young people, but easy to read.

With a Little Help. Series of eight. Philippa Harpin. Published by Muscular Dystrophy Group of Great Britain. An excellent series of booklets with many practical suggestions of use to many people with neuromuscular problems not just muscular dystrophy. Very well illustrated.

Upper Limb Disability—A Guide to Aids. *Lower Limb Disability*—A Guide to Aids. Motor Neurone Disease Association 1985. Short but helpful guides to aids that might help those with MND, plus useful addresses.

Your Rights for Pensioners. Age Concern. Annually rewritten. A very clearly written guide for retired people with problems. Age Concern also produce detailed factsheets (25) and information handbooks on diverse topics.

Disability Rights Handbook. Annual guide to financial benefits, home adaptations, equipment, etc. Disability Alliance, 10 Denmark Street, London WC2.

ADDRESS LIST

Broadcasting Support Services, Room 17, 252 Western Avenue, London, W3 6XJ. Tel. 01-992-5522.

DHSS Store, No. 2 Site, Manchester Road, Heywood, Lancs., OL10 2PZ.

DIAL (UK), 117 High Street, Clay Cross, Derbyshire, S45 9D2. Tel. 026-864498.

Disablement Advisory Service—consult Disablement Resettlement Officer and local Jobcentre.

Disablement Income Group (DIG), Attlee House, Toynbee Hall, 28 Commercial Street, London, EC1 6LR. Tel. 01-790-2424.

Disabled Living Foundation, 380–384 Harrow Road, London, W9 2HU. Tel. 01-289-6111.

DLCC Disabled Living Centres Council, Secretary, Trent Region Aids, Information and Demonstration Service, 76 Clarendon Park Road, Leicester, LE2 3AD.

Equipment for the Disabled, Mary Marlborough Lodge, Department 405, Nuffield Orthopaedic Centre, Headington, Oxford, OX3 7LD.

Help for Health (Wessex Information Centre), Southampton General Hospital, Tremona Road, Shirley, Southampton, SO9 4XY. Tel. 0703-777222, Ext. 3753.

Motor Neurone Disease Association, 61 Derngate, Northampton, NN1 1UE. Tel. 0604-22269/250505.

Multiple Sclerosis Society, 25 Effie Road, Fulham, London, SW6 1EE. Tel. 01-381-6267.

Muscular Dystrophy Group of Great Britain, Nattrass House, 35 Macauley Road, London, W4 0QP. Tel. 01-720-8055.

Northern Ireland Information Service for Disabled People, 2 Annadale Avenue, Belfast, BT7 3JH. Tel. 0232-640011.

Parkinson's Disease Society, 36 Portland Place, London, W1N 3DG. Tel. 01-323-1174.

RADAR (Royal Association for Disability and Rehabilitation), 25 Mortimer Street, London, W1N 8AB. Tel. 01-637-5400.

REMAP—As for RADAR.

RICA (Research Institute for Consumer Affairs), 14 Buckingham Street, London, WC2N 6DS.

RNIB (Royal National Institute for the Blind), 224 Great Portland Street, London, W1N 6AA. Tel. 01-388-1266.

RNID (Royal National Institute for the Deaf), 105 Gower Street, London, WC1E 6AH. Tel. 01-387-8033.

Scottish Council on Disability, Information Department, 5 Shandwick Place, Edinburgh, EH2 4RG. Tel. 031-229-8632.

Spinal Injuries Association, Yeomans House, 76 St James Lane, London N10. Tel. 01-444-2121.

Wales Council for the Disabled, Caerbragdy Industrial Estate, Bedwas Road, Caerphilly, Mid Glamorgan, CF8 3SL. Tel. 0222-887325.

The Clinical Neurology of Old Age
Edited by R. Tallis
© 1989 John Wiley & Sons Ltd

Chapter 35

Social Services for the Neurologically Disabled

Ruth Eley

Principal Social Worker and Head of Department, Social Work Department, Royal Liverpool Hospital, Liverpool, UK

INTRODUCTION

The origins of the present day health and social services are varied. The current structure did not emerge as a coherent entity, but grew piecemeal and often in an uncoordinated way. Some services exist as a result of the gradual dismantling of the Poor Law and the final abolition of workhouses in 1948, others followed the greater involvement of the state in providing for its citizens, and yet others were created or adapted as a response to changing population trends or economic constraints. This has resulted in a complex system of social welfare affecting the elderly no less than any other group of people. Indeed, the elderly have fared worse in many ways, as a financially dependent group in society, some of whom will inevitably develop severe problems of ill-health and disability. Services for the neurologically disabled elderly usually come under the umbrella of services for elderly, rather than disabled people, and are therefore not always adapted for particular disability needs.

One aspect of provision for elderly people is the number of different agencies and professionals involved. These include the public, voluntary and private sectors. There is inevitably some overlap and duplication. Day care may be provided in day centres run by local authorities or voluntary agencies such as Age Concern, or in day hospitals run by local health authorities. Although theoretically they may all serve different functions, from the patient's point

of view the activities and pattern of the day may be very similar. An Appendix summarizing the range of resources available appears at the end of this chapter. Your local social services department can provide you with details of provision in your area.

In 1971, local authority services, previously divided into three separate departments of welfare, children, and mental health, were reorganized into single generic social services departments. These new departments, run by directors of social services, assumed responsibility for all resources previously provided under the old structure. For old people this meant domiciliary services such as the home help service, day care service, and residential homes. The new structure also introduced the concept of generic (or non-specialist) social workers, so that one social worker would work with the family as a whole and tackle all its problems, rather than having a child care officer and a welfare officer involved in the same family.

Since its foundation in 1948, the National Health Service has also had its fair share of reorganization, in 1974 and again in 1983. As the largest consumers of the National Health Service, elderly people are inevitably affected by any change in emphasis or direction. Although geriatric services have been developed extensively over the last 10 years, most elderly people never reach a geriatric unit and are directly affected by any reduction in general medical or surgical beds, or diversion of resources into high technology areas, e.g. cardiac transplantation.

I shall look at the provision of services in three sections: state benefits, domiciliary and day care services, and residential services.

STATE BENEFITS

Although provision had been made for elderly people over 70 outside the Poor Law by the 1908 Old Age Pension Act, the National Insurance system introduced in 1946, based on the Beveridge Report (1942), provided retirement pensions for all elderly people. Although this system was confidently expected to reduce poverty amongst old people, significant numbers had to apply to the National Assistance Board (created in 1948) for extra, means-tested, financial support. Peter Townsend's study in Bethnal Green in 1957 found that one-third of the respondents had a personal income below the National Assistance Board's subsistence minimum (Townsend, 1957). In 1966, the National Assistance Board was merged with the Ministry of Pensions and National Insurance to become the Ministry of Social Security, which set up the Supplementary Benefit Commission. Originally conceived as a safety net for a small number of people, supplementary benefit is now a significant provider of pensioners' resources. Hunt (1976) found that 13.3% of elderly married couples on their own and 39.5% of elderly non-married persons living alone were receiving supplementary benefit. In 1977, 58% of the three million people receiving supplementary benefit were pensioners. An estimated 35% of elderly people are eligible for the benefit but do not claim.

Apart from an additional weekly income, claimants of supplementary benefit can receive financial help towards extra heating, laundry, diet (paid as weekly additions), travelling expenses for attending hospital, and essential items of clothing and furniture. For those people in private residential care, application can be made to the Department of Health and Social Security for payment to be made through supplementary benefit, of board and lodging fees. To be eligible for supplementary benefit, claimants have to have less than £3000 in savings and an income less than the statutory minimum laid down by government—currently £51.45 for a cou-

ple and £33.40 for a single person plus weekly rates for disabled and elderly people. Help with housing costs can be met by housing benefit, which replaced the rent and rate rebates and is paid by the local authority housing department. The benefit is means tested but it is possible to receive housing benefit on an income quite a bit higher than that required to obtain supplementary benefit.

A benefit of major importance to elderly disabled people is attendance allowance. This is paid to people who need help with bodily functions or supervision to prevent harm to self or others. It is paid at a lower rate for day *or* night time, currently £22.00, or the full rate for day *and* night time, currently £32.95 (July 1988). It is tax free.

In 1966 the National Insurance Act introduced a graduated pension scheme, the aim of which was to enable people to receive a pension related to their earnings rather than a basic minimum. This scheme was discontinued in 1978 when a new state earnings related pension scheme was introduced. This is now under threat following the reviews of social security and pensions undertaken in the spring of 1985. It has also been decided to remove pensions from their statutory link to rises in prices or earnings, a measure introduced in 1975.

One of the greatest preoccupations of policy makers over the past 40 years has been the amount that the younger working population can afford—or tolerate—to pay in contributions to provide for retired people. The 1949 Royal Commission on Population was most concerned about the increasing levels of consumption by old people and a corresponding reduction in their productivity (Phillipson, 1982). The expected increases in population of the old has produced a similar sense of foreboding amongst cabinet ministers of the present—'affordability' has become one of the main criteria for assessing what the state should provide in the way of pensions, and the elderly are constantly portrayed as a burden which the working population cannot afford.

Beveridge based his proposals on the expectation of full employment. With several million people unemployed, and a growing elderly population, it is not surprising that a Conservative government should question the concept of the state taking prime responsibility for the financial wellbeing of its citizens. Norman Fowler, the cabinet minister who carried out the review of social security in 1985, has emphasized the need for a partnership between the state and informal support from families and friends. Private pension schemes are actively encouraged so that individuals take responsibility for their own financial security. The Fowler review also proposed changes to the supplementary benefit system, which would abolish weekly additions and special payments and replace it by a Social Fund. This Fund would be of a fixed amount, which could run out halfway through the year, so payments would be rationed and could not be based on individual need.*

Elderly people are discriminated against by the benefits system. Mobility allowance, for example, is not payable to people whose onset of disability occurred after the age of 65. Even where it did occur below this age, the allowance is only payable up to the age of 75. Similarly, the board and lodging payments in private and voluntary homes vary according to age, rather than degree of disability. The maximum payment for an elderly person in a nursing home is £185 per week, whereas a physically handicapped person can claim up to £230 per week. The only exception is when it can be proven that disability began before pensionable age. The majority of disabled people are elderly and both these measures are therefore particularly unjust. They reinforce the view that disability is a normal part of ageing, that it is therefore less tragic and there is less need for compensation.

The system also discriminates against women. Invalid care allowance is paid to people who give up work to care for a dependent person, who must be in receipt of attendance allowance. Despite the fact that most carers are women, invalid care allowance was not payable to women who are married or living with a man, until a recent ruling by the European Court that this condition was illegal under the European Economic Community regulations governing equal opportunities. Private pension schemes also discriminate against women, who are more likely to be part-time workers, or to lose contributions while having children or looking after elderly or disabled relatives.

* See *Note added in proof* at end of chapter.

DOMICILIARY SERVICES AND DAY CARE SERVICES

The Home Help Service

The home help service is probably the most widely known and widely used resource for old people. Hunt (1976) found that 15.8% of those aged 75–84 and 27.3% of those aged 85 and over received home help. Like other services, it has had to adapt its provision to meet the needs of a frailer and older population. Although the traditional role of help with housework and shopping is still very important, the home help of the 1980s is more likely to be providing a personal care service—help with washing and dressing, preparing meals, general supervision—which may overlap with or be very close to the care provided by the district nursing service. Many local authorities now offer a 7 day service, with help available morning, afternoon and evening for its most vulnerable clients. Some authorities also provide services on the home help model but which vary slightly to meet the needs of particular groups of people. The most common is an intensive, guaranteed service for elderly people being discharged from hospital, in recognition of the fact that this is a very vulnerable time for older people who may be profoundly affected by illness and may, therefore, need a longer period to recover fully. For stroke patients, discharge from hospital may be to a totally new situation brought about by the illness, e.g., having to sleep downstairs because of inability to manage stairs, using a commode because the outside toilet is now inaccessible, being unable to light the coal fire without help, being dysphasic and unable to communicate needs to shopkeepers, all of which may make it essential for the patient to have help, where previously they had been totally independent.

One criticism of the home help service is that it has not been very responsive to the needs of carers. In the face of a growing population of frail elderly people it has seen as its priority for those people who live alone and have no family close at hand to provide help. Understandable though it is, this approach has meant that many families have struggled to continue to support their elderly relatives without help from the statutory services. There is now, however, a growing recognition of the needs of carers, aided by groups such as the National Association of Carers and the National Council for Single Carers and their Dependants.

There is strong evidence that men are more likely to receive home help than women, and that male carers receive help more often than women carers. Hunt (1970) found that of the men receiving home help, 98.1% were able to go out compared with 67.8% of the women, and that only 8% of the women had no difficulty with any of the personal tasks involving mobility compared with 29.1% of men. A study carried out in the research section of the psychogeriatric unit in South Manchester University Hospital (Charlesworth et al., 1984) found that male carers were considerably more likely than women in the sample to be receiving home help service, and that at each level of dependency of the elderly persons being cared for, more male than female carers received the service. From 1971 to 1979 the percentage of married women in work or seeking work has risen from 46% to 58% in the 25–44 age group and from 53% to 61% in 45–59 age group (Department of Employment, 1980). Given this shift in employment patterns, the home help service must review the way the service is allocated to ensure that women carers have equal access to its benefits.

Meals on Wheels

A second service which is used extensively by old people is the meals service. The extent of the provision varies considerably from authority to authority, sometimes being organized and delivered by voluntary organizations such as the WRVS (Women's Royal Voluntary Service), sometimes run entirely by the local authority. Meals are not only provided in people's own homes, but for the more active and mobile elderly, meals are served at luncheon clubs, often meeting in local church halls and community centres and run by voluntary organizations such as Age Concern and, again, the WRVS. Local authorities were given the power to provide a meals service under the 1962 Amendment to the 1948 National Assistance Act, and one of the intentions of this Amendment was not only to meet the nutritional needs of those old or disabled people at risk, but also to provide a means of monitoring

recipients so that difficulties can be picked up early. It is true that having a meal delivered ensures that people have a personal contact with an outsider as well as receiving a hot meal, but the time available per client to a driver is so limited that it is questionable whether this secondary role of monitoring can be adequately carried out, other than checking that the client is alive. The effectiveness of a meals service also depends on ensuring access to bed- or chair-fast clients, and the old person being able to eat the meal unaided. Unless these issues are considered properly, a meals service may not be able to meet the needs of the most vulnerable clients.

Many local authorities are now paying particular attention to the needs, previously overlooked, of black old people and providing additional services for them. A service which is staffed by white people is probably geared towards meeting the needs of white people and is less likely to be seen as relevant by the black population, even though individual officers and care staff are not intentionally racist in their delivery of the service. Some local authorities provide Moslem meals and others, such as Liverpool, offer a special home help service, employing black staff aimed at the black population. The success of such a scheme in reaching the black community can be measured by the fact that prior to its introduction, Liverpool Social Services Department had fifteen black old people in receipt of home help, while now the new service looks after 46 such people (Liverpool Social Services Department, internal paper).

Day Care

Day care services meet a variety of needs and are provided in a range of settings. Day centres provide social facilities for people who are lonely and isolated, including those who can no longer get out of doors unaided. A hot meal and the opportunity for social activities are normally included. Day centres are increasingly providing personal care for more dependent people in the form of bathing, toileting, chiropody, laundry facilities and hairdressing. An old person attending a day centre 5 days a week can receive far more care and attention than is available from the home help service, yet is still enabled to remain in their own home. It can also provide a valuable breathing space for carers, although the availability of transport may be inappropriate for carers who go out to work. The day is a short one, people normally arriving at the centre at about 9.30–10.00 a.m., and leaving again from 3.30 p.m. onwards. Considerable time may also be spent on the bus or ambulance, and arrival times are not always reliable. There is a need for day care services to extend their hours to include early evenings and weekends, so that the needs of working families can be catered for without them having to give up their job or the old person having to go into residential care.

Day hospitals are provided by health authorities. Normally they are for people who require rehabilitation and medical treatment and do not aim to provide merely a social function. They normally have occupational and physiotherapy services and can usually call upon the services of a chiropodist, dentist, speech therapist and other specialists when required, as well as full medical diagnostic and treatment facilities.

Nursing Services

The community nursing service provides a vital resource of particular benefit to elderly people. As well as carrying out basic nursing duties such as giving injections and changing dressings, community nurses also assist immobile people to get up, washed and dressed in the morning and back to bed in the afternoon or evening. They may also assist with bathing. Incontinence aids and advice are provided and some health authorities also offer a laundry service for incontinent patients. Home nursing aids, such as commodes, rubber rings, back rests etc., are provided through the community nursing services. Some health authorities provide a night sitting service for patients to enable carers to get adequate rest. Although aimed primarily at terminally ill people, the service may also be provided for elderly people who require care and supervision at night.

Community psychiatric nurses provide a specialized service to elderly mentally infirm people. They

can supervise medication and offer advice to carers (both professionals and informal carers) on the management and care of mentally infirm people.

Voluntary Agencies

Voluntary agencies also provide domiciliary services for elderly people. The largest and most active is Age Concern, a national charity which through its local branches provides day care services, good neighbour schemes, which offer befriending and shopping services, and advice and information services. They also act as a pressure group on behalf of old people.

Some voluntary agencies are organized around particular disabilities or diseases, e.g., Parkinson's Disease Society, Multiple Sclerosis Society, Chest, Heart and Stroke Association, Alzheimer's Disease Society. They often have local groups which may provide social events, voluntary visiting schemes, news letters and advice and information services. Such voluntary associations are often major providers of funds for research into their particular disability, and may employ staff as counsellors or welfare officers. Many hospitals organize social clubs for stroke victims. Such stroke clubs may be the gateway to a restored social life for people who would otherwise find it extremely difficult to overcome their embarrassment about their unusual gait or speech difficulties. In a stroke club, such disabilities are accepted and the individual can gain confidence without constant fear of ridicule or avoidance. The danger is that people never move on to participate in other social activities, and the stroke club becomes their only social outlet. Even so, such a situation must be better than being afraid to go out at all and remaining totally isolated.

RESIDENTIAL CARE

General Comments

Residential care for old people is provided from three sources: the local authority, voluntary organizations and the private sector. During the last decade there has been a shift in emphasis away from long-term hospital care towards care in the community, which has inevitably put greater strain not only on domiciliary services and informal carers, but also on residential resources. At the same time, there has been active encouragement by the government to the private sector to expand, and following the changes in the supplementary benefit system, private homes are now accessible to people with low incomes as well as those who are well off. In theory, therefore, the expansion of the private sector has widened the choice for old people requiring residential care. In practice, however, the choice will depend on the local distribution of homes, the level of charges compared with the maximum benefits payable by the Department of Health and Social Security, and the extent of local authority provision.

Local Authority

Part III of the 1948 National Assistance Act laid a duty on local authorities to provide residential accommodation for those in need of care and attention—hence the term 'Part III accommodation'. Application procedures vary but usually include an assessment by a social worker. Applicants normally go on a waiting list with some rating to indicate priority. Allocation systems vary from authority to authority; decisions may be made by a panel of various professional staff, or by individual social workers or headquarters staff. Some authorities include a geriatric or psychogeriatric assessment in their application procedures, in recognition of the fact that a significant number of elderly people referred for residential care have been found to have medical problems that can be treated or alleviated (Brocklehurst *et al.*, 1978).

The population in old people's homes has changed significantly over the last 10 to 15 years, with a much higher degree of mental and/or physical frailty. The improvement in domiciliary services, health care and housing provision has enabled old people to remain at home for much longer; admission to residential care is now more likely to occur because of the need for help or supervision with personal care, rather than loneliness or social isolation. Unfortunately, there has been little corresponding change in staffing ratios or training opportunities, so that residential staff find themselves providing a high level of personal care, including nursing care, to the

majority of residents, many of whom would have been cared for on a long stay hospital ward a decade ago. The emphasis on care in the community and the run down of long stay hospitals has resulted in residential homes being squeezed between the diminishing long stay resources and the domiciliary services struggling to keep pace with an increasing very elderly population. Understaffing means that staff usually have little opportunity to do anything more than ensuring that basic needs of food, warmth, shelter and hygiene are met. A home of 55 residents may only have three care staff on duty in an afternoon and evening, and two or even one during the night. The main functional criterion for admission is independent mobility, including a walking aid or wheelchair. With such low staffing ratios, those who require help with mobility from another person are usually regarded as needing nursing care and more appropriately cared for in a nursing home or hospital.

One issue which has prompted much debate within health and social services recently is whether people suffering from dementia should be cared for in the same or separate facilities as the mentally alert. It is very distressing to be disturbed in the middle of the night by someone who is looking for their mother, or trying to get into bed with you, or who urinates on the floor, or who simply cannot remember where their own room is. Some local authorities, for example Newcastle, do provide separate residential facilities for elderly mentally infirm people. Admission procedures for such a home would normally include a psychogeriatric assessment, to ensure that all possible treatable or avoidable causes of the disturbed behaviour have been excluded. Unfortunately, all too often such behaviour is accepted as a normal and inevitable part of ageing, and is not taken seriously. Although separate facilities may be desirable from the point of view of the mentally alert residents, some consideration has to be given to the desirability of depriving confused people of normal conversation and behaviour. Demented people do copy each other and pick up each other's bad behaviour; from their point of view it would seem preferable to provide them with as normal an environment as possible.

Much debate has also taken place on the design of

residential homes, many of which are adapted buildings or were built in the 1960s and early 1970s before the importance of single room accommodation or the need for mobility standards were evident or accepted. A study by Dianne Willcocks and colleagues of the consumer view of residential care (Willcocks *et al.*, 1982) commissioned by the Department of Health and Social Security, came up with the suggestion of the residential flatlet, larger than the normal bedroom and with its own toilet and shower unit en suite, which would ensure greater privacy and provide more personal space than is currently available in most residential homes. Unfortunately, the economic constraints of the 1980s mean that few local authorities are in a position to make large capital investments into what is an already expensive resource. Furthermore, at a time when the private sector is flourishing, it is tempting for local authorities to allow private home owners to spend money and provide additional resources.

Charges for residential care vary from authority to authority, but there is a minimum charge laid down by central government which is currently (July 1988) £32.95 per week. All income is included in the assessment and any capital over £1200 including property, is taken into account when determining the weekly charge to the resident, up to a maximum set by the social services committee. Each resident receives a statutory amount per week as a personal allowance, currently £8.25 per week.

Voluntary Organizations

These are non-profit making organizations which provide residential (and other) resources for specific groups of people, often on the basis of religious or cultural affiliation. All the main church denominations provide residential homes, as do other bodies such as the British Legion, Freemasons, trade related benevolent associations and trade unions. Methods of application vary considerably. This may be to the matron of the home, the local branch, or to the head office of the organization, and usually includes an assessment by a social worker, although some people may apply directly or through another representative such as their local priest or vicar. Local authorities are empowered under the 1948 National Assist-

ance Act to supplement the contributions of residents in voluntary homes to meet the charges. Since the change in regulations which enable the Department of Health and Social Security to meet costs under the supplementary benefit system, however, some local authorities have discontinued this practice except for residents who do not qualify for supplementary benefit.

The Private Sector

There have always been those who have provided accommodation and care for other people in exchange for a fee and in order to make a living. It is in the last decade, however, that the private residential sector has mushroomed. Demographic changes, restrictions on local authority spending and allowances to individual residents being made available through the supplementary benefits system, have produced a lucrative market. Large multinational companies, as well as those running small businesses, are investing in private residential care. Unfortunately, the money making aspects of the business have sometimes taken over from the responsibility for providing good standards of care.

The highlighting of cases of abuse, coupled with the huge amounts of public money being spent in the private sector, resulted in the reform of the legislation governing private and voluntary homes, not just for the elderly but also for physically and mentally handicapped and mentally ill people. The 1984 Residential Homes Act laid down regulations governing the registration and inspection of all private and voluntary residential care homes, and the Department of Health and Social Security set up a working party, under the auspices of the Centre for Policy on Ageing, to produce a code of practice. The report, 'Home Life: a Code of Practice for Residential Care' (1984), is an extremely comprehensive document covering all aspects of care. All local authorities are required to draw up their own criteria for registration, based on the code. Unfortunately the code is a voluntary one, although 'commended' by the Secretary of State for Social Services, and only ten recommendations which apply to the elderly, out of a total of 218, are legal requirements. It is yet to be seen how seriously local authorities take the code of practice, and how enforceable it will be in law. There are large cost implications for local authorities if they are to employ registration officers to carry out properly the inspection requirements of the code. It is unfortunate, to say the least, that 'Home Life' does not apply to homes run by local authorities, who may lay themselves open to charges of double standards by expecting of the private sector high standards which they cannot afford to implement in their own establishments.

Private residential homes tend to be adapted buildings rather than purpose-built establishments, and are often smaller than local authority homes. Facilities vary considerably from establishment to establishment. The Department of Health and Social Security will pay up to a maximum of £130 per week for a resident in a private home, and up to £155 per week for very dependent elderly people who are eligible for the higher rate of attendance allowance (July 1988). Many homes charge far more than this, and choice for people dependent on supplementary benefit may therefore be limited. Private nursing homes, catering for very dependent elderly people, have to be registered with the local health authority. The limit for Department of Health and Social Security payments is £185 per week, but most nursing homes charge at least £225. It is a condition of registration that qualified nursing staff have to be on duty 24 hours a day.

Making the Right Decision

The need for residential care may seem obvious to medical staff and other professionals involved in the care of a neurologically disabled patient who has not made sufficient progress to return home. Moving into a home is a very difficult decision, however, and patients may prefer to run the risks of being alone at home in familiar surroundings, than give up their privacy for the safety and security of residential care. Living in an old people's home means spending a lot of your time with other people, with little choice over meals or mealtimes, limited privacy for entertaining visitors and restricted personal space. This may be unacceptable to someone who has been used to spending most of their time alone and deciding for

themselves what to have for a meal and what time to eat it. Such a crucial decision as giving up your home needs careful thought, and it is essential that people are given sufficient time and access to information to enable them to make a realistic decision, even though the professional staff may be impatient for a speedy outcome. The social worker can explain to the patient the available options and help them to choose the outcome which is right for them.

With such a wide range of services spread among so many different agencies, it is essential that there is good communication and liaison. It is pointless for an occupational therapist to carry out a home visit with the patient and establish the need for a daily home help service, if no-one informs the home help organizer of the patient's discharge home. The Continuing Care Project (1975, 1979) has highlighted the severe problems which can arise if proper liaison does not take place. Ward staff should ensure that they involve the social worker in the planning of a patient's rehabilitation, so that aims are realistic as far as home circumstances are concerned. It is the role of the social worker to liaise with the appropriate services, and interested relatives and friends, to ensure that the right service gets to the right person at the right time, in order to achieve a minimum risk discharge.

As people's needs change, and their dependency increases, there is an expectation that people will move to where more appropriate care is available. Tenants in sheltered housing who need help with personal care are expected to move on to a residential home, while residents in rest homes who become immobile must usually move on to a nursing home or continuing care bed. Medical resources are organized in a similar way, with patients progressing through acute, rehabilitation and continuing care beds as appropriate. People also move the other way along the care continuum; those who improve gradually after transfer to a continuing care bed will be expected to move out of hospital to a residential home. Generally speaking, the organization of services is such that people have to move to care, rather than care moving to people (Eley and Middleton, 1983). The provision of a more flexible system of domiciliary care, so that frail elderly people have a real choice about whether to remain at home or go into institutional care, would be expensive, and would require a radical rethink of the whole spectrum of health and social services.

REFERENCES

Beveridge Report (1942). *Social Insurance and Allied Services*, HMSO, London.

Brocklehurst, J., Carty, H.W., Leeming, J.T., and Robinson, J.M. (1978). Medical screening of old people accepted for residential care. *Lancet*, **ii**, 141–2.

Charlesworth, A., Wilkin, D., and Duria, A. (1984). *Carers and Services: a comparison of men and women caring for dependent elderly people*, Manchester, Equal Opportunities Commission.

Continuing Care Project (1975, 1979). *Going Home* and *Organising Aftercare*, Continuing Care Project, Centre for Policy on Ageing, London.

Department of Employment (1980). *Background Paper to the Green Paper on the Taxation of Husband and Wife*, Department of Employment, London.

Eley, R., and Middleton, L. (1983). Square pegs, round holes? The appropriateness of providing care for old people in residential settings. *Health Trends*, **15**, August, pp. 68–9.

Home Life: a Code of Practice for residential care (1984). Centre of Policy on Ageing, London.

Hunt A. (1970). *The Home Help Service in England and Wales*, HMSO, London.

Hunt, A. (1976). *The Elderly at Home*, O.P.C.S. Social Survey Division, HMSO, London.

Phillipson, C. (1982). *Capitalism & the Construction of Old Age*, Macmillan, London.

Royal Commission on Population (1949). *Report*, HMSO, London.

Townsend, P. (1957). *The Family Life of Old People*, Routledge & Kegan Paul, London.

Willcocks, D., Peace, S., and Kellaher, L. (1982). *The Residential Life of Old People; a Study in 100 local authority homes*; Polytechnic of North London Department of Applied Social Studies—Survey Research Unit Reports No. 12 (Vol. I) and No. 13 (Vol. II).

Note added in proof: The proposals referred to on pp. 524–5 became law in April 1988. Supplementary benefit has been replaced by Income Support, weekly additions abolished, and the Social Fund introduced. Housing Benefit has also been revised, so that all claimants now have to pay at least 20% of their rates. These measures have had a significant impact on the financial circumstances of elderly people.

APPENDIX

Resource	Provided for	Provided by	Referral via
A. Domiciliary services			
1. Home help	People requiring help with personal care, housework and shopping	Social services department	Social worker or direct to home help organizer
2. Meals on wheels	People unable to prepare a meal for themselves, usually living alone, usually housebound	Social services department or voluntary organization	Social worker
3. Bath attendant	People unable to bath themselves	Health Authority	District nurse
4. Laundry service	Incontinent people	Health authority	District nurse
5. Home nursing aids	People being nursed at home	Health authority, voluntary organizations like Red Cross	District nurse
6. Aids to daily living, adaptations to home	People requiring aids or adaptations to achieve maximum independence	Social services department	Occupational therapist
7. Sheltered housing	People requiring alarm system, oversight by a warden (NB not a personal care service)	Local authority housing department, housing associations, some private schemes	Housing department, housing advice centre or social worker
8. District nurse	People requiring nursing at home or in residential care	Health authority	Refer direct
9. Community psychiatric nurse	Mentally ill people needing nursing support, carers needing advice regarding management	Health authority	Refer direct
10. Health visitor	People at home needing advice about diet, general health care	Health authority	Refer direct
11. Chiropody	People in any setting needing foot care	Health authority (some private practitioners)	Refer direct
12. Social worker	People requiring practical help and support, and counselling	Local authority social services department; some voluntary organizations	Refer direct to hospital social work department, or local services office

APPENDIX (*continued*)

Resource	Provided for	Provided by	Referral via
13. Occupational therapist (OT)	People needing rehabilitation advice or treatment	Health authority, local authority social services department	Refer direct to hospital OT department or local social services office
B. Day care services			
14. Day centre	Those requiring social stimulation or personal care	Social services department or voluntary organization	Refer direct
15. Geriatric day hospital	Physically ill or frail people requiring rehabilitation or medical treatment	Health authority	Consultant geriatrician
16. Psychogeriatric day hospital	Mentally ill or infirm people requiring rehabilitation or maintenance	Health authority	Consultant psychogeriatrician
17. Luncheon club	People able to make their own way to a centre, benefiting from company and having a meal provided	Voluntary organizations	Refer direct or via social worker
C. Residential Services			
18. Residential care	People requiring help or supervision with personal care, usually independently mobile (including with walking aid or wheelchair)	Social services department, voluntary organizations, private owners	Social worker
19. Nursing home	People requiring nursing care, usually immobile or needing help to walk from another person	Some voluntary organizations, but mostly privately owned	Social worker
20. Continuing hospital care	People requiring nursing care, usually immobile or needing help to walk from another person	Health authority, geriatric or psychogeriatric units	Consultant geriatrician or psychogeriatrician

The Clinical Neurology of Old Age
Edited by R. Tallis
© 1989 John Wiley & Sons Ltd

Chapter 36

Counselling the Neurologically Disabled

Anne Gibson

*formerly Principal Social Worker, Royal Liverpool Hospital, Liverpool; now,
Methodist Minister and Tutor, Wesley College, Henbury Road, Westbury-on-Trym, Bristol, UK*

INTRODUCTION

Unless you have experienced it, it is impossible to understand the awful feelings of aloneness when suddenly faced with the care of a sick and disabled person you love. The ups and downs are innumerable, the sudden freezing when walking, the awful loss of temper on both sides, the tears of sheer despair because he cannot express himself and constantly says 'Yes' when he means 'No'. The shouting and calling the minute I go out of sight. The swings of mood, obsession with times of meals, the minor falls. All this and more. The strain on my patience and his has been almost unendurable and yet, it is still wonderful to have him home because I am so fortunate in being backed by a wonderful team who have always got time to listen and reassure (Wicke, 1978).

This quote from the wife of a 71 year old man when he came home from hospital after suffering a stroke, reminds us of the personal and family strains inherent in coping with disability and of the need of patient and carer for support and advice. We must be aware of the needs of both, for disability disrupts not only the life of the patient, but also the family. It is a family matter and requires adjustments in family life (Holbrook, 1981). The family whose member has had a stroke or been diagnosed as having multiple sclerosis is facing an unknown, bewildering situation.

It needs help in charting a course through unfamiliar waters. This includes practical information and advice, guidance and support. The staff involved can help most effectively through team work, with a good understanding of each other's roles and good communication in the team as well as with the patient and his family.

EXPLAINING NEUROLOGICAL DISABILITY TO THE PATIENT AND HIS FAMILY

In the case of stroke patients admitted to hospital in the acute phase, few relatives may in fact have seen the consultant physician prior to discharge. They will probably have been interviewed by a junior doctor and it is unlikely that aspects of rehabilitation will have been discussed (Murray *et al.*, 1982). Communication with the doctor is of primary importance to the patient and his family and it is therefore unfortunate if there is inadequate medical information about the diagnosis, treatment, rehabilitation and likely course of the patient's condition. There should be the opportunity for an interview with the consultant. Time needs to be set aside for this and wherever possible a private room; it is hard to communicate sensitively in a ward corridor!

Before seeing the patient and his family, the doctor should gather any information, perhaps from the nursing staff, about how they have reacted so far and what information if any, they have acquired already.

They may have some idea of the implications of their situation, or none at all. The doctor's approach will vary accordingly; if in doubt, it is better to let them state at the outset what they know, or to assume that they have not picked up any information.

The time when the diagnosis is made (soon after, say, a stroke) is one of shock and high anxiety. This limits the ability of the patient and family to absorb what is said to them. Sometimes, if they do not ask questions, they receive little information. It is important to recognize that they may be too shocked or uncertain to know what to ask or to have prepared specific queries. This does not mean to say that they will not have anxieties and not be wanting information. The doctor, therefore, needs to volunteer it and to know at the outset what general areas the interview should cover. This will, however, need to be modified in the light of the response of the patient and family. During the interview, it is important to check how much they are taking in and how they are reacting. Rather than overwhelm or shock them with too much information at once, it is better to recognize the need for repeated explanations and opportunities to return for more later. The important thing is to establish, at the outset, a relationship based on sensitive, honest communication and ease of access to staff for further advice. This will do much to reassure the patient and his family and help them to face the situation.

It is likely that staff from a number of disciplines will be treating the patient who is neurologically disabled. This should be acknowledged by all those involved, so that there is as much understanding of each other's contribution as possible. Multidisciplinary discussion ensures all are planning and working along the same lines, information is shared and team work enhanced; otherwise the patient and his family become confused about who is doing what, they may receive conflicting advice or some responsibilities may go by default.

Nursing staff, the physiotherapist or social worker may have more day to day contact with the patient and his family than the doctor. His responsibility for communication is therefore better shared with other staff. The doctor may also lack the essential counselling skills and the time necessary to allow the patient and his family to ask questions and express their feelings. If another member of staff is included in the doctor's interview, she or he can give this opportunity, staying on after the doctor leaves or arranging a further meeting. The doctor's words may have been misinterpreted, some things not taken in at all, and clarification may be necessary. If the opportunity is given to reflect on what has been said and to voice fears and anxieties, tension is often relieved and help can be focused appropriately.

ADJUSTING TO NEUROLOGICAL DISABILITY

The impact on the patient and his family of a condition such as stroke will obviously differ in some respects from a chronic disease such as multiple sclerosis, with its remissions and relapses. After a stroke, a patient may be plunged from being fit and able to complete dependence; from this, depending on the condition and its management, he will emerge to make some kind of recovery. However, with chronically deteriorating conditions the sufferer may start at a level of independence and it may be some time before any substantial level of disability appears. The patient and his family have to live with great uncertainty about the future and the course the disease will take. Each relapse or new deterioration may produce shock and fresh anxieties.

Whilst there are differences, there are also common features in the problems of adjustment presented by the varied causes of neurological disability. Once people become ill, they are generally exempted temporarily from social responsibility and not expected to take care of themselves. The sick role, particularly in a general hospital ward, is a passive one; things are done to and for you. However, once a patient is pronounced 'disabled' instead of 'ill' he is expected to behave in a totally different manner. Rehabilitation staff expect him to accept his disability and start learning how to live with it; to be motivated to do better and be actively involved in his rehabilitation. We ask the patient to accept his condition and yet, at the same time, to fight it. Patients who are depressed, or who are denying their disability—such as the stroke patient who is expecting that one day he will awake to find himself back to normal—will find it hard to adjust to this rehabilitation role.

Staff need to be aware of the patient's state of mind and make sure that he has received adequate explanations and consistent messages about what is required of him in treatment and rehabilitation. Two way communication is vital; the giving of information and advice is important; but so too is the need to listen. Counselling has been defined as a process whereby a person can express his thoughts and feelings in such a way as to clarify his situation, come to terms with some new experience, see the difficulty more objectively and so face it with less tension and anxiety (British Association of Counselling, 1979). Listening is the principal therapy. If we do not listen we are simply isolating the patient with his problems. When people face loss of bodily function, independence or a healthy identity, there is a grief reaction, just as in bereavement. This is characterized by shock, denial, mourning for the loss, and depression, hopefully followed by some degree of acceptance or adjustment (Ross, 1970; Parkes, 1975). The stages of adjustment to disability can be seen in these terms and a similar model has for example been suggested for stroke families (Holbrook, 1982). (See Table 36.1.)

Not all patients and their families will experience these reactions and they are unlikely to be distinct, separated phases. However, they are part of a commonly observed pattern. Adjustment, if achieved, can take a long time. In order to help patients adjust and cooperate with rehabilitation treatment, it is necessary to understand their reactions. It has been pointed out that the second stage may coincide with discharge from hospital and the third with discharge from active treatment (Holbrook, 1982). For the patient who remains disabled these can both be crisis points, particularly if he has not adjusted to his disability. Discharge may convey that 'nothing more can be done'; unfortunately this is sometimes said to the patient and he may well feel let down, abandoned by those who have treated him, or angry and depressed.

It is important that the patient is offered the opportunity to talk through what has happened to him—to voice his shock, grief and fears for the future. He may do this with a friend or family member or

TABLE 36.1   REACTION OF STROKE FAMILIES

First stage:	*Crisis*
	Shock
	Confusion
	High anxiety
Second stage:	*Treatment stage*
	High expectation of recovery
	Denial that disability is permanent
	Periods of grieving
	Fears for future—job
	mobility
	lifestyle
	about coping
Third stage:	*Realization of disability*
	Anger
	Feelings of rejection
	Despair
	Frustration
	Depression
Final stage:	*Adjustment*

From Holbrook (1982) with permission.

with any of the staff involved with him; alternatively he may not wish, or be able, to express his thoughts and feelings. One member of the staff team should, however, be able to encourage him to do so. The family are often too emotionally involved to help in this way and may not be fully aware of the adjustments required. The initial reaction to depressed people is to try to cheer them up. Whilst this may have its place, the patient should be allowed to air his grief and sorrow to someone who can sit and listen without constantly telling him to pull himself together. Often it is only in talking it through that he begins to adjust to the reality of the situation facing him and if his feelings are accepted as a natural reaction, it will help him to adapt and engage in rehabilitation.

Anger and frustration at what has happened to him may be violent and may be directed at staff. Nurses in particular, may be a target of anger, as well as visiting family and friends. This should not be taken as a personal attack when it has originally little or nothing to do with the people it is directed at. Returning the anger will only feed the patient's hostility. Relatives or staff may then avoid him, by shortened visits or ward rounds, which only makes his situation worse. Instead staff and family should be encouraged to listen, in the knowledge that the relief in expressing himself will help towards better adaptation. Through gaining awareness of causes for the patient's anger, it becomes possible to open up communication.

The social worker, by virtue of training and concern for the patient's return to the community, has a particular responsibility for counselling and for understanding the family dimension. She needs to be aware of the social, emotional and financial impact of the patient's disability as this will be important in helping the patient and other staff to plan future care and treatment. In addition, the social worker has a continuing responsibility to follow up the patient in the community and to ensure that any statutory help required is provided. This involves arranging specific services such as home help and monitoring the effectiveness of arrangements made prior to discharge in relation to the needs of the patient and his family.

ASSESSMENT AND PLANNING

With patients admitted to hospital, the social worker can do an initial assessment of their home circumstances at an early stage. Rehabilitation has to be directed towards the patient's needs in the community, so information is required about the type of accommodation the patient lives in and about those living with him. The family's ability to cope with disability is often difficult to predict and is not necessarily related to the degree of disability. The quality and history of family relationships prior to the illness may be a significant factor in determining the type and degree of dependence carers will tolerate. The frequency of contact with other family members and friends is also important in establishing the type of support a patient will have in the community. Neighbourly help can mean anything from help in an emergency to practical assistance on a daily basis. The domiciliary services which are available or appropriate are another important factor.

Even when patients are mentally impaired, it is important that they are involved in planning for their future as far as is possible. In addition, it is

necessary to see relatives or significant others in the patient's life. As stated previously, it is important, in any case, to involve them at an early stage. The level of anxiety in an acute admission or phase of illness is usually high. Some relatives are frightened to get involved because they fear that they will not cope, or because of uncertainties about the future. Therefore, whilst the social worker may be gathering information at this stage, it is important to allow relatives to give expression to their anxieties. Also, it will help the family to know at the outset the kind of support network which would be available to them should they require it in the future.

Some families may require no services or follow-up after discharge. It can, however, be reassuring for them to have a reference point, someone they know they can contact in the event of a crisis, or if they need advice. The social worker is in a good position to fulfil this role, arranging further services which may be required, providing guidance or fielding enquiries to other members of the team or other agencies.

Planning for the future may involve helping the family to come to a decision about whether the patient can be cared for at home, or perhaps helping the patient who lives alone to decide whether he is going to return to the community or consider residential care. The alternatives should be discussed as openly as possible, planning with the patient and his family. Indeed, underlying the social worker's approach is a concern to involve them in such a way that some of the sense of meaning and purpose, disrupted by illness and disability, begins to return. This means sorting out practical problems in a way which marshalls their practical and emotional resources, maintaining their self respect by working with rather than for them and, above all, listening with sensitivity.

It is important that there is adequate preparation for discharge from hospital. All too often, discharge comes as a surprise to the family with only a few days' notice; indeed they may only hear about it from the patient. This is bad practice as both patient and family need to gear themselves emotionally for discharge. Also, there may be practical chores to do such as moving furniture at home, or purchasing a new bed. Trial weekends or pre-discharge visits home can be very valuable, giving a chance to iron out problems at an early stage, with the help of the hospital team. Unfortunately, however, it seems that these are by no means a standard procedure (Murray *et al.*, 1982).

Many families do have a feeling of aloneness when faced with the discharge and for the patient there may well be a crisis of confidence, even though the return home may have been eagerly awaited. It is important that the family is aware of the patient's capabilities and the assistance they can give in order to help them attain their full potential. People can perform tasks of daily living within the structured environment of a hospital which they cannot, or do not, do at home. This is possibly because relatives find it easier or quicker to do tasks themselves, resulting in a lack of motivation in the patient, or because relatives have not been sufficiently involved in the rehabilitation process to understand its objectives (Andrews and Stewart, 1979).

Within the community the patient and his family are likely to face many changes in life style. There may be a need for role adjustments within the family. For example, the husband may have to take over domestic duties because of his wife's disability; or a partner may suddenly have to manage all the family's financial affairs. These adjustments may come easily, or alternatively they may not be readily accepted. The patient who has to take a more passive, dependent role may feel useless and unwanted; the carer may feel burdened and anxious. Practical advice and guidance can help here and again the chance to talk through their situation with someone outside the family.

Awareness of being at risk is felt most by those living alone. They may feel unsupported and frightened to pursue their former daily routine. This can be exacerbated after a stay in hospital with a great deal of attention from staff and other patients, leading to a sense of loss and decline in morale on going home. By helping the patient to describe his fears and reasons for insecurity it may be possible to improve the situation by domiciliary or voluntary services.

There is also likely to be a change in the pattern of the patient's social contacts and activities. These are commonly more restricted—even where physical disability is not severe. A lack of confidence, a feeling of not being back to 'normal', memory or minor speech difficulties may mean that those who could physically take up their previous social activities are reluctant to do so. Also, the patient may suffer from excess fatigue and the time and effort required to get ready to go out may deter him. There may be transport problems, difficulty in finding usable toilets and embarrassment at having to rely on others. If his attempts to socialize lead to disappointment and an unchanged, or increased, sense of stigmatization, he may be tempted to give up. For all these reasons there is a tendency on the part of the patient to withdraw from social contact. At the same time there is also a tendency for family and friends to withdraw, to stop visiting or making social arrangements. One study reported that 55% of stroke patients sampled reported less contact with friends and relatives than before; only 14% reported more contact (Chester Royal Infirmary, 1981). This is a commonly reported reaction to people with disability and illness in general. Obviously in part, this is a response to the patient's withdrawal. However, it also reflects a more general unease in coping with disability, a discomfiture in the face of physical symptoms, an uncertainty about what to do and say. The patient and his family may need these social contacts more than ever; any difficulties they face are likely to cause added strain if accompanied by loss of support from their social network.

Neurological disease societies such as the Alzheimer's Disease Society, the Parkinson's Disease Society and locally run stroke clubs can play a vital role in this situation. Sometimes they act as pressure groups for the improvement of services, but they also serve to lessen the isolation of the patient and his carer. Meetings where they can get together with others in similar situations, share experiences and exchange ideas, are a valuable support. They can also provide an opportunity for the patient to test himself out socially in a safe environment where his difficulties are accepted and understood.

THE IMPACT ON CARERS

It is a common misconception that the modern family no longer cares for its elderly dependants. The evidence in fact documents the central role played by families in caring for the elderly. Whilst the absolute number of elderly people in residential care has grown over the past 20 years, the proportion admitted to residential care has not. Only a tiny minority are in residential or hospital care, and the proportion has not increased significantly since the turn of the century (Parker, 1985).

One study found more people now caring for an elderly or disabled relative than were responsible for the day to day care of children under 16 years (Briggs, 1981). At the most conservative estimate there are 1.5 million people who act as principal carers to adults and children with disabilities severe enough to warrant support in daily living tasks (Parker, 1985). An elderly person may be cared for by someone in the same household or be receiving a substantial amount of help from a relative who visits frequently. A study of elderly stroke patients found that two-thirds of carers were of the same generation as the patient and in a majority of cases this was a spouse and therefore also elderly. One-third were of a younger generation and normally a daughter or daughter-in-law (Murray et al., 1982). There is often inadequate preparation of the family for the role they are to take on and little help or support once active treatment or rehabilitation is completed. Most family members are unprepared for the major changes in their life style. Services too have tended to be geared to the needs of the patient rather than helping those looking after them. The trend in government policy itself has been towards greater emphasis on care in the community, but has not always reflected a recognition of the burdens or costs of care for individuals or families.

Hopefully, there is beginning to be an increased awareness among professionals involved in this field of the impact on carers and the problems they face. A growing number of voluntary and self-help organizations have helped to highlight carers' needs, as well as provide them with information and advice about sources of help.

However, there is often a tendency to take informal carers for granted, a feeling that it is their 'duty' to provide care. This can lead to a defensive, even aggressive attitude on the part of staff when families voice anxieties or uncertainty about caring. This is counterproductive. It is important to remember that most families provide excellent support and they will be encouraged in their task if they can air their anxieties, knowing there is someone they can turn to if difficulties arise and that they are not expected to 'go it alone'. If there is a refusal to take the patient home or continue to provide care, it is likely to be because relationships were poor prior to the illness, or that there are major practical problems in providing care at home. Another reason may be that the family has been let down by the lack of provision of help promised in the past; once their trust has gone, it may be difficult to restore it.

Caring for a dependent person consists in the main of a daily round of domestic and physical activities. The housework, dressing, feeding, toileting and extra laundry take up much of the time and effort. The physical demands associated with heavy lifting and disturbed nights may be considerable. Carers may face the strain of being on duty 24 hours a day, having an ear cocked even if they are watching television. The carer looking after an elderly relative along with a husband and children can face conflicting demands and recriminations and stress within the family.

Often carers neglect their own health. Many are anxious that their own health may break down and worry about the implication of this for the relative. As a result, they may delay seeking medical advice or treatment on their own account. Sainsbury and Grad de Alarcon (1971) found that three-fifths of families caring for elderly relatives reported a decline in the physical wellbeing of the principal care-giver. The health of carers may be directly affected by providing the care, whether it be through back pain associated with lifting the non-ambulant, or depression and anxiety associated with the strains of caring over a long period of time.

The emotional and psychological demands of caring may be considerable. To care for a parent who has now become totally dependent on you, or a spouse who needs help with toileting and eating obviously affects the whole relationship. Accepting the dependence involved can be difficult to both carer and patient. Feelings about being a burden can lead to guilt but also resentment and the carer may resent the restrictions imposed on his or her life. The expression of anger in this situation is a natural reaction but it may be difficult to deal with. It may increase feelings of guilt, the patient feeling he should be more grateful and the carer feeling she should be more accepting. It may be hard for them to help each other in this context and the chance to 'let off steam' to someone outside the family can help them to understand each other. To prevent or alleviate the build up of this kind of stress can be an important feature of the social worker's role.

There may be psychological or personality changes in the patient or behavioural problems associated with mental deterioration. The family need to be made aware of the effect of these so they are prepared, for example, for the emotional lability of the stroke patient. Mental infirmity is commonly regarded as one of the most difficult problems faced by care-givers. The patient suffering from senile dementia may present excessive demands for help and attention or may have to be watched constantly because of the danger of unwittingly harming himself. Problems in communicating may cause a great deal of frustration; indeed it may be no longer possible to relate to the patient in a meaningful way.

One of the most common problems faced by carers is that of isolation; a restricted life with little leisure time. Restrictions on freedom can range from being unable to go to the shops or have a lie in, to being unable to go on holiday. The provision of alternative care for the patient on a regular planned basis can do much to relieve the physical and emotional burden on the carer.

Financial considerations are of importance to the patient and his carer. All studies of long-term sickness and poverty have found a correlation between the two. Disability creates extra needs and entails extra expense, e.g. for heating, nutrition, laundry and transport. In addition, there may be a direct cost to the carer of being unable to take up paid work. The carer may in fact have to resign from employment; if she continues she may frequently lose work time or forgo training or promotion opportunities. Nine of the fifteen carers in Nissel and Bonnerjea's pilot study who were not in paid employment had given up their jobs because of their dependent relative and most would have liked to take up paid work again (Nissel and Bonnerjea,

1982). See also Equal Opportunities Commission (1980).

Family income may therefore drop, just at a time when expenses increase, making it hard to finance basic needs, let alone anything to provide a fuller existence. It is essential that families know what statutory allowances are available, how to claim them and appeal if at first unsuccessful. The social worker should ensure this information is provided, along with advice about the range of support services available in the area.

The provision of practical help can enable carers to continue with their work in spite of great difficulties. However, even when the social worker can offer little on a practical level, the commitment to keep in touch and enable patient and carer to share their concerns and problems, can sustain them. Also, if there is a relationship of trust with the social worker, painful decisions, for example about admission to residential care, are likely to be easier for patient and carer to resolve.

The family is the most important resource available to the patient and those treating him. Treatment, rehabilitation and the way professional staff communicate with them, should reflect this. The help we offer should be geared to their needs as well as those of the patient to enable them to continue in their task of caring.

REFERENCES

Andrews, K., and Stewart, J. (1979). Stroke recovery: he can but does he? *Rheumatol. Rehabil.*, **18**, 43–8.

Briggs, A. (1981). *Who Care?—Report of a door to door survey of people caring for dependent relatives*, The Association of Carers.

British Association of Counselling (1979). Counselling. Definition of terms in use with expansion and rationale. (Reissued 1985.)

Chester Royal Infirmary (1981). Unpublished Study: Social Work Department.

Equal Opportunities Commission (1980). *The Experience of Caring for Elderly and Handicapped Dependants*, Equal Opportunities Commission, Manchester.

Holbrook, M. (1981). Stroke is a family matter. *Community Care*, 21.5.81, pp. 12–13.

Holbrook, M. (1982). Stroke: social and emotional outcome. *J. Roy. Coll. Phys. Lond.*, **16**(2), 100–4.

Murray, S.K., Garraway, W.M., Akhtar, A.J., and Prescott, R.J. (1982). Communications between home and hospital in the management of acute stroke in the elderly: results from a controlled trial. *Health Bulletin*, **40,** 214–19.

Nissel, M., and Bonnerjea, L. (1982). *Family care of the Handicapped Elderly: Who Pays?*, Policy Studies Institute, London.

Parker, G. (1985). *With due Care and Attention: a review of research on informal care*, Family Policy Studies Centre.

Parkes, C.M. (1975). *Bereavement: Studies of Grief in Adult Life*, Penguin, Harmondsworth.

Ross, E.K. (1970). *On Death and Dying*, Tavistock Publications, London.

Sainsbury, P., and Grad de Alarcon, J. (1971). The psychiatrist and the geriatric patient. *J. Geriatr. Psychiatry*, **4**(1), 23–41.

Wicke, M. (1978). Time to go home. *New Age*, Summer, pp. 20–1.

SECTION FIVE

Epilogue

Chapter 37

Research Trends in Neurological Diseases that Affect the Elderly

Donald Calne

Professor and Head of Division of Neurology,

H. Teravainen and J. Tsui

Division of Neurology, University of British Columbia, Health Sciences Centre Hospital, Vancouver, British Columbia, Canada

Over the last few decades, there has been a rapid increase in both the absolute and the relative number of persons over 60 years of age and the neurological problems of the elderly are consequently receiving increasing attention. While efforts are being made to advance knowledge and improve treatment over a wide range of diseases that afflict the nervous system in the elderly, the major focus is on degenerative disorders of unknown aetiology, and the commonest of these are senile dementia of Alzheimer's type (SDAT) and Parkinson's disease (PD). In this chapter we shall confine our attention to these disorders since they also constitute an area in which substantial developments have occurred over recent years.

SENILE DEMENTIA OF ALZHEIMER'S TYPE

The importance of this disease can hardly be exaggerated, not only because of the increasing number of affected persons, but also because of the major impact of the loss of the most valuable assets of human behaviour. Many aspects of dementias have been discussed at length in several recent articles and reviews (Brun, 1982; Cummings and Benson, 1983;

Terry and Katzman, 1983; Gaitz and Samorajski, 1985) and we shall limit our discussion to problems related to SDAT that we consider either controversial or of major significance.

Dementia (Table 37.1) in the elderly often occurs as one manifestation of more generalized neurological disorders (Table 37.2). Alzheimer's disease and SDAT are the most common forms of dementia and consist of at least 50% of all dementias after the age of 30 years. The second major group (40%) comprises patients with multiple brain infarcts; the remaining secondary dementias account for some 10% of cases (Sulkava *et al.*, 1985).

Diagnosis of SDAT has to be made by clinical assessment and exclusion of secondary forms of dementia (Table 37.3). Computed tomography (CT) may show diffuse cerebral atrophy but as this may occur in elderly subjects without dementia, its main value is for ruling out dementias secondary to other CNS diseases such as multiple infarcts, or tumour. Even the most sophisticated measurements of cerebral atrophy or densitometric analysis utilizing CT are unable to establish SDAT in the majority of patients (Wilson *et al.*, 1982; Yerby *et al.*, 1985). Similarly, other objective measures, such as EEG,

TABLE 37.1   CLINICAL CRITERIA FOR DEMENTIA

1. Loss of intellect sufficient to impair social or occupational function
2. Memory impairment
3. At least one of the following:
   impaired abstraction
   impaired judgement
   aphasia
   agnosia
   constructional difficulties
   personality change
4. Alert state of consciousness

Modified DSMIII, Mayeux and Stern (1983).

TABLE 37.2   DISEASE ACCOMPANIED BY DEMENTIA

Primary degenerative
  Cortical dementias
    Alzheimer's disease
    Pick's disease
  Extrapyramidal
    Huntington's disease
    Multiple system atrophies
    Parkinson's disease
    Spinocerebellar degenerations
    Progressive supranuclear palsy
    Wilson's disease
    Hallervorden–Spatz disease
Vascular
  Multi-infarct degeneration
Infectious
  General paresis
  Slow virus infections
Toxic and metabolic
  Alcoholism
  B12 deficiency
  Drug intoxications
  Hypothyroidism
  Heavy metal poisoning
Miscellaneous
  Anoxic
  Hydrocephalic
  Neoplastic
  Traumatic

evoked potential studies, haematology, blood chemistry and examination of cerebrospinal fluid are normal in most cases.

What, then, are the clinical characteristics of the disease that are required to establish a diagnosis? Patients experience a slow and gradual decline in intellectual functions, with insidious onset. Impairment of memory is usually the first symptom and some patients may be depressed. Decline in specific cognitive functions (aphasia, agnosia), changes in personality and loss of insight occur as the disease progresses. Patients later lose their ability to read and write and are sometimes completely helpless long before death.

The neurological examination is normal in early stages of SDAT but extrapyramidal signs, similar to those seen in Parkinson's disease (rigidity, poverty of movement, postural changes, tremor), may emerge later (Molsa *et al.*, 1984; Chui *et al.*, 1985) and primitive reflexes (such as suck, grasp and pout) are usually present in advanced cases. Early in the disease we are thus faced with one of the most difficult tasks in clinical neurology, that of proving minimal abnormality of intellectual function. Global neuropsychological evaluation (Reisberg *et al.*, 1982) may have to be repeated, if initial findings are marginal, to demonstrate progression.

Pathology

The extent of neuronal loss in SDAT is controversial. Current estimates of drop out range from 11 to 80%,

the observations depending upon the severity of the disease, the type of neurone counted, and the area studied. Does the loss of neurones correlate with dementia? The count is usually performed over a specified area of the brain and yields a neuronal index relative to other tissue components such as glial cells, dendrites and axons. The integrity of connections (synapses, dendrites and axons) between neurones is likely to be important for mental function and the relative loss of these tissue components would actually increase the index of neuronal cell bodies expressed as the neurone/extraneuronal tissue ratio. Characterized in this way, the neuronal density in monkey is clearly higher than in man (Sholl, 1956; Cragg, 1967). These analyses are manifestly difficult to interpret.

The shape of the neurones may be altered in SDAT and the number of dendritic spines may

TABLE 37.3   CRITERIA FOR CLINICAL DIAGNOSIS OF ALZHEIMER'S DISEASE

Probable
    Dementia established by clinical evaluation and verified by neuropsychological examination
    Deficits in at least two cognitive areas
    Progressive worsening of memory and other cognitive functions over a period of months
    Alert state of consciousness
    Absence of systemic disorders that could account for progressive deterioration
    Diagnosis is supported by
        progressive deterioration of specific cognitive functions such as language (aphasia), motor skills (apraxia), and perception (agnosia);
        impaired activities in daily living and altered behaviour;
        positive family history particularly if confirmed neuropathologically;
        normal cerebrospinal fluid, normal or non-specific changes in EEG, normal drug screen and analysis of heavy metals, normal blood chemistry and cell count, normal serum thyroxine and B12 levels, negative tests for syphilis;
        normal clinical general and neurological examination;
        CT evidence of cerebral atrophy
Definite
    Clinical criteria for probable Alzheimer's disease fulfilled
    Histopathological evidence obtained from a biopsy or autopsy

Modified from McKhann *et al.* (1984)

decrease (Mehraein *et al.*, 1975; Scheibel and Scheibel, 1975). Further research in this field is desirable. Previously much attention has been focused on the presence of neurofibrillary tangles, neuritic (senile) plaques and accumulation of lipofuscin in SDAT. This work has not yet contributed significantly to understanding the pathogenesis of SDAT and it is possible that some of these changes are simply an indication of one category of neuronal degeneration. Qualitatively similar but quantitatively different changes have been observed in the brains of both demented and non-demented persons suffering from a wide variety of neurological diseases (Steele *et al.*, 1964; Corsellis *et al.*, 1973; Boller *et al.*, 1980; Chen, 1981; Uhl *et al.*, 1982; Ulrich, 1985; Wisniewski *et al.*, 1985). The number of neurofibrillary tangles and neuritic plaques found in SDAT significantly exceeds that observed in other conditions including normal ageing. Similarities and differences between SDAT neuropathology and that of normal ageing have recently been compared (Kokmen, 1984; Berg, 1985); from such considerations the pattern of SDAT appears to be distinct from premature ageing.

Normally, the number of the neurones in the nucleus basalis does not seem to decrease between the ages of 25 and 87 years (Chui *et al.*, 1984), yet there is a substantial depletion in SDAT (see below).

The cerebral cortex receives cholinergic innervation from the basal forebrain and the loss of nerve cells in this region has recently received much attention (Whitehouse *et al.*, 1982; McGeer *et al.*, 1984; Perry *et al.*, 1985; Rogers *et al.*, 1985; Saper *et al.*, 1985). Depletion of neurones in the basal forebrain does not appear to be the only reason for cognitive decline: patients with Parkinson's disease and Huntington's disease can be demented with or without significant neuronal losses in the nucleus basalis (Clark *et al.*, 1983; Tagliavini *et al.*, 1984; Heilig *et al.*, 1985).

In SDAT, the primary motor, somatosensory and visual cortical areas are better preserved than the association areas (frontal, temporal and parietal cortex) and hippocampus (cf. Mountjoy *et al.*, 1983; Terry and Katzman, 1983). The vulnerable regions are especially well developed in human subjects, compared with phylogenetically lower species.

Whereas significant cell loss occurs in the nucleus basalis of Meynert, amygdala and locus coeruleus (Herzog and Kemper, 1980; Mann *et al.*, 1982; Arendt *et al.*, 1985; Rogers *et al.*, 1985), other subcortical structures are relatively intact.

Recent biochemical observations have raised the possibility that SDAT may be a generalized systemic disease, not limited to the brain. Various biochemical changes have been reported in non-neuronal tissues (Diamond *et al.*, 1983; Krause, 1983; Zubenko *et al.*, 1984; Peterson *et al.*, 1985; Skias *et al.*, 1985). The importance of these observations is not currently understood. They may reflect a systemic disorder but may alternatively be secondary to diminished ability of the nervous system to maintain homeostasis.

Biochemistry

A significant decrease of markers for cholinergic neurotransmission (acetylcholine and choline acetyltransferase) is well documented (cf. Gottfries *et al.*, 1983; McGeer *et al.*, 1984; DeKosky *et al.*, 1985; Perry *et al.*, 1985) and has been claimed to correlate with cognitive impairment (Francis *et al.*, 1985). There are no cholinergic cells in the cerebral cortex, though there are numerous muscarinic receptors for acetylcholine, which appear to be normal in SDAT (Lang and Henke, 1983).

Anticholinergic drugs impair memory and cognition in patients with parkinsonism, whether they are demented or not (Syndulko *et al.*, 1981; Sadeh *et al.*, 1982; Koller, 1984). In normal subjects these drugs can induce transient deficits resembling SDAT (Fuld, 1984; Brinkman and Brain, 1984). Furthermore, it is possible to ameliorate these effects with cholinomimetics (e.g. Harbaugh *et al.*, 1984; Muramoto *et al.*, 1984). Similarly, models of SDAT in experimental animals benefit from cholinomimetics (Flood *et al.*, 1983). Significant decreases in other neurotransmitters have been reported but they do not seem to correlate with the severity of the cognitive impairment (Francis *et al.*, 1985).

Cerebral cortical glucose metabolism is decreased (Foster *et al.*, 1984; Cutler *et al.*, 1985) but there is no cogent evidence that this is a primary defect.

Epidemiology

SDAT is two to three times commoner in women compared with men (Roth, 1978; Sulkava *et al.*, 1985). There is no satisfactory explanation for this distribution (Weitkamp *et al.*, 1983; Crapper McLachlan and Lewis, 1985).

There is a familial predisposition to SDAT (Chui *et al.*, 1985) but the quantitative estimates of clustering show considerable variation (Larsson *et al.*, 1983; Heston *et al.*, 1981; Heyman *et al.*, 1983) so genetic studies are desirable.

There is an increased incidence of Down's syndrome in families with SDAT (Heyman *et al.*, 1983, 1984) as well as histology resembling SDAT in patients with Down's syndrome (Wisniewski *et al.*, 1985).

Epidemiological observations indicate that women (but not men) with SDAT have a higher prevalence of previous thyroid disease, compared with a control population (Heyman *et al.*, 1984). A history of head injury is also more frequent in SDAT, but there have been no differences observed between the patients and controls in toxic environmental exposure, dietary habits, smoking, alcohol intake or animal contacts (Heyman *et al.*, 1984).

Subclinical infection is a possible aetiology, but SDAT is not transmissible, and its epidemiology does not suggest infection (Goudsmit *et al.*, 1980).

Primary dementia may comprise a group of diseases. Rossor *et al.* (1984) have reported that there are multiple neurochemical abnormalities in cases with early onset (Alzheimer's disease) whereas a substantial cholinergic abnormality confined to temporal lobe and hippocampus was present in the brains of patients with late onset (SDAT). The loss of neurones in both nucleus basalis (Candy *et al.*, 1983; Tagliavini and Pilleri, 1983) and locus coeruleus (Bondareff *et al.*, 1982) is more marked in patients with early onset. Bird *et al.* (1983) reported that language disorder was prominent in the early onset cases which showed severe decreases in both cortical and hippocampal choline acetyltransferase (ChAT), whereas the late onset cases had more severe impairment in recent memory and low ChAT values confined to the hippocampus. Division into four distinct clinical subgroups has been recently suggested (Mayeux *et al.*, 1985):

1. Benign with little or no progression.
2. Myoclonic with severe intellectual decline.
3. Extrapyramidal with severe intellectual and functional decline.
4. Typical.

This grouping may be clinically useful, but as yet no inferences on aetiology can be drawn. It may prove relevant that familial cases of primary dementia tend to start at a relatively young age (Chui *et al.*, 1985).

PARKINSON'S DISEASE (PD)

Little was known about the pathogenesis of Parkinson's disease before the discovery of dopamine deficiency in the substantia nigra. Subsequently, the therapeutic effects of L-dopa (Birkmayer and Hornykiewicz, 1962) have been extensively investigated. The introduction of bromocriptine (Calne *et al.*, 1974) led to another wave of research into developing new dopamine agonists and subdividing dopamine receptors. The toxic effects of manganese (Mena *et al.*, 1967) and 6-hydroxydopamine (Cohen and Heikkila, 1974) generated theories about the pathogenetic mechanisms of the illness, and the concept of nigral damage by free radicals emerged (Cohen and Heikkila, 1974; Donaldson *et al.*, 1980). More recently, parkinsonism induced by methylphenyl-tetrahydropyridine (MPTP) (Langston and Ballard, 1985) shed more light on toxic mechanisms of producing the syndrome. Another approach to therapy has involved studies with monoamine oxidase inhibitors aiming at decreased rate of destruction of dopamine, and more recently trials with antioxidants are under preparation with an attempt to slow down the disease process.

Research in Aetiology and Pathogenesis

The relationship between PD and normal ageing is intriguing (Calne *et al.*, 1983). In both there is reduction of enzymatic activity (tyrosine hydroxylase and dopa decarboxylase) concerned with dopamine metabolism (McGeer and McGeer, 1976; McGeer *et al.*, 1977) and loss of nerve cells in the locus coeruleus (Brody, 1976) and the substantia nigra (McGeer *et al.*, 1977). Deterioration of parkinsonian deficits in patients in the seventh decade has been reported to occur more rapidly than in the fourth decade (DeJong and Burns, 1967). Since the individual's DNA is generally regarded as an important determinant of ageing, the low concordance of PD in identical twins (Ward *et al.*, 1983) can be construed as evidence against an aetiological hypothesis of premature or exaggerated ageing. Incidentally, this finding also militates against any genetic factor playing a major role in the cause of PD.

Toxic agents that produce irreversible parkinsonian syndromes include carbon monoxide (Ringel and Klawans, 1972), manganese (Mena *et al.*, 1967), and MPTP (Langston and Ballard, 1985). Positron emission tomography (PET) with 6-fluorodopa has demonstrated impairment of the nigrostriatal pathway in subjects exposed to MPTP who are clinically normal (Calne *et al.*, 1985).

Viral infection has been proposed as the cause of PD ever since the outbreak of encephalitis lethargica and its aftermath of parkinsonism. However, extrapyramidal syndromes following other viral infections, though reported (Duvoisin and Yahr, 1965; Hoehn, 1971), are rare. Herpes simplex virus (HSV) had long been suspected (Levaditi, 1929), but antibody studies had failed to demonstrate any significant increase in neutralizing antibodies in PD (Andrews and Carmichael, 1930; Gay and Holden, 1931) compared with control groups. Other immunological techniques (complement fixation and immunofluorescence) were claimed to show increased humoral HSV antibody in PD (Marttila *et al.*, 1977; Marttila and Rine, 1978), but another group has reported contradictory results, a tendency for HSV antibodies to be lower in PD (Elizan *et al.*, 1979). While direct evidence of the presence of HSV DNA sequences in parkinsonian brains has not been found (Wetmur *et al.*, 1979), indirect evidence links the virus to cerebral monoamine metabolism in mice (Lycke *et al.*, 1970; Lycke and Roos, 1972).

Initial epidemiological studies have suggested a higher prevalence of the disease among whites compared with blacks (Kessler, 1972; Paddison and Griffith, 1974; Reef, 1977). However, more recently, this difference has not been confirmed (Schoenberg *et al.*, 1985). PD is less common in Japan (Kondo, 1984) and China (Li *et al.*, 1985), the prevalence being some 0.57 per 1000, in these countries, compared with 1 per 1000 in Europe, North America, and Australia (Kurland *et al.*, 1973).

Parkinsonism is particularly common in Guam, where it has a special propensity to be linked with dementia. This focus is likely to reflect an environmental risk factor, since the high prevalence has been falling dramatically in recent years (Gajdusek, 1977). The nature of this risk factor has yet to be established.

One current hypothesis is that PD derives from subclinical damage to the nigrostriatal pathway, followed by age-related depletion of the compromised zona compacta of the substantia nigra, so that ultimately symptoms appear and progressively increase with the passage of time (Calne and Langston, 1983). Clinically normal subjects exposed to MPTP constitute a unique population to follow in order to confirm or refute this concept.

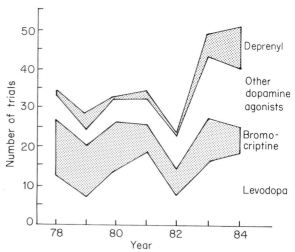

Figure 37.1. Number of trials each year for various antiparkinsonian agents.

Therapy

Anticholinergic agents have been used in the treatment of Parkinson's disease since the late nineteenth century (reviewed by Aquilonius, 1979) and had remained the only effective treatment until the 1960s. Following the advent of levodopa (L-dopa), anticholinergic agents became adjuvant therapy and studies with these drugs have become scanty. Although much newer, amantadine occupies a similar position to anticholinergic agents in the therapy of Parkinson's disease.

Over the last 7 years, the therapeutic agents most frequently studied have been levodopa, various dopamine agonists, and deprenyl. The trend is shown in Figure 37.1, which illustrates the number of trials each year for levodopa remaining in the range of 10–20, and dopamine agonists running at about 20–25. Bromocriptine represents consistently half of the studies with dopamine agonists. A notable feature is that the number of trials with deprenyl has increased substantially over the past 2 years.

Levodopa still remains the most important drug in the treatment of Parkinson's disease. Its therapeutic effects have been proven, but its long-term appli-

cation is problematic because of fluctuations in response, increasing dyskinesia, and psychiatric difficulties. It is not clear whether the increasing prevalence of these problems is due to the inexorable advance of PD, or the cumulative dosage of levodopa. Recent studies have been directed towards the arguments for *early* (Markham and Diamond, 1981) or *late* (Fahn and Bressman, 1984) administration. Combination with peripheral inhibitors of dopa decarboxylase has also been studied extensively (Barbeau and Roy, 1976).

Bromocriptine is still the most commonly used dopamine agonist despite the development of congeners such as mesulergine, pergolide, and lysuride. As in the case of levodopa, there are unresolved questions on whether bromocriptine should be used early or late; there is also controversy over whether the dosage should be high or low (above or below 25 mg daily). Our view is that levodopa and bromocriptine can usefully be employed together, in low doses, early in the disease. As symptoms increase, the dose of both drugs needs to be raised, to levels determined by the balance between efficacy and adverse reactions.

Deprenyl, a monoamine oxidase (MAO) B inhibitor, was introduced in the late 1960s (Knoll *et al.*, 1968), and its therapeutic effect in PD was soon established (Birkmayer *et al.*, 1975). Initially considered as palliative therapy in combination with levodopa, this drug has received more attention recently because it has been claimed that progress of the underlying pathology may be slowed (Birkmayer and Riederer, 1984). This possibility has been argued on theoretical grounds because MAO enhances the production of toxic free radicals. A multicentre trial in North America is now in preparation with the object of studying deprenyl prospectively. To pursue the free radical hypothesis of neuronal damage, it would be logical to investigate other antioxidants, such as vitamin E.

Research in Other Areas

Research into the pathophysiology of parkinsonism has been undertaken over many years. Various techniques are available to measure the individual deficits such as tremor, rigidity, and bradykinesia (Teravainen and Calne, 1979).

The role of surgery in PD had declined considerably (Siegfried, 1979); this is exemplified by the dramatic fall in the number of publications on surgical treatment over the period 1958 to 1978.

Studies on CSF (Kartzinel *et al.*, 1976; Lakke *et al.*, 1972) and neuroendocrine (prolactin) changes in PD have been pursued over the last two decades, but interest in these approaches has been waning, and is likely to be replaced by PET studies with various agents thought to provide more direct information on the integrity of the nigrostriatal pathway and dopamine receptors (Martin *et al.*, 1985).

SUMMARY

Chronic diseases of the elderly comprise the major challenge to health economists and those concerned by the inexorably deteriorating quality of life of the population as a whole. The elderly are suffering proportionately more than any other section of the community. Degenerative disease of the nervous system constitutes a substantial component of this problem and the only reasonable approach to a solution is research to elucidate the cause and hence develop rational strategies to prevent or at least alleviate the pathology. In this review we have

discussed research trends in two of the more important quantitative and qualitative disorders of the elderly nervous system, dementia and parkinsonism.

REFERENCES

Andrews, C.H., and Carmichael, E.A. (1930). A note on the presence of antibodies to herpes virus in postencephalitic and other human sera. *Lancet*, **i**, 857–8.

Aquilonius, S.M. (1979). Cholinergic mechanisms in the CNS related to Parkinson's disease. In: Rinne, U.K., Klinger, M., and Stamm, G. (eds.) *Parkinson's Disease: Current Progress, Problems and Management*, Elsevier, North-Holland, pp. 17–27.

Arendt, T., Bigl, V., Ennstedt, A., and Arendt, A. (1985). Neuronal loss in different parts of the nucleus basalis is related to neuritic plaque formation in cortical target areas in Alzheimer's disease. *Neuroscience*, **14**, 1–14.

Barbeau, A., and Roy, M. (1976). Six-year results of treatment with levodopa plus benzerazide in Parkinson's disease. *Neurology*, **267**, 399–404.

Berg, L. (1985). Does Alzheimer's disease represent an exaggeration of normal aging. *Arch. Neurol.*, **42**, 737–43.

Bird, T.B., Strahanan, B.S., Sumi, S.M., and Raskind, M. (1983). Alzheimer's disease: choline acetyltransferase activity in brain tissue from clinical and pathological subgroups. *Ann. Neurol.*, **14**, 284–93.

Birkmayer, W., and Hornykiewicz, O. (1962). Der L-dioxyphenylalanin (= L-Dopa)-Effekt beim Parkinson Syndrom des Menschen: Zur Pathogenese und Behandlung der Parkinson-Akinese. *Arch. Psych. Zeit. Neurol.*, **203**, 560–74.

Birkmayer, W., and Riederer, P. (1984). Deprenyl prolongs the therapeutic efficacy of combined L-dopa in Parkinson's disease. In: Hassler, R.G., and Christ, J.F. (eds.) *Advances in Neurology*, Vol. 40, Raven Press, New York, pp. 475–81.

Birkmayer, W., Riederer, P., Youdim, M.B.H., and Lihauer, W. (1975). Responsibility of extrastriatal areas for the appearance of psychotic symptoms: clinical and biochemical human post-mortem findings. *J. Neurol. Transm.*, **36**, 303.

Boller, F., Mizutani, T., Roessman, V., and Gambetti, P. (1980). Parkinson disease, dementia and Alzheimer disease: clinicopathological correlations. *Ann. Neurol.*, **7**, 329–35.

Bondareff, W., Mountjoy, C.Q., and Roth, M. (1982). Loss of neurons of origin of the adrenergic projection to cerebral cortex (nucleus locus ceruleus) in senile dementia. *Neurology*, **32**, 164–8.

Brinkman, S.D., and Brain, P. (1984). Classification of dementia patients by a WAIS profile related to central cholinergic deficiencies. *J. Clin. Neuropsychol.*, **6**, 393–400.

Brody, H. (1976). An examination of cerebral cortex and

brainstem aging. In: Terry, R.D., and Gershon, S. (eds.) *Neurobiology of Aging*, Raven Press, New York, pp. 177–81.

Brun, A. (1982). Alzheimer's disease and its clinical implications. In: Platt, D. (ed.) *Geriatric*, Vol. 1, Springer, Berlin, pp. 342–40.

Calne, D.B., Duvoisin, R.C., and McGeer, E. (1983). Speculations on the etiology of Parkinson disease. In: Hassler, R.G., and Christ, J.F. (eds.) *Advances in Neurology*, Vol. 40, Raven Press, New York, pp. 353–60.

Calne, D.B., and Langston, J.W. (1983). Aetiology of Parkinson's disease. *Lancet*, **ii**, 1457–9.

Calne, D.B., Teychenne, P.F., Claveria, L.E., Eastman, R., Greenacre, J.K., and Petrie, A. (1974). Bromocriptine in Parkinsonism. *Br. Med. J.*, **iv**, 442–4.

Calne, D.B., Langston, J.W., Martin, W.R.W., Stoessl, A.J., Ruth, T.J., Adam, M.J., Pate, B.D., and Schulzer, M. (1985). Positron emission tomography after MPTP: observations relating to the cause of Parkinson's disease. *Nature*, **317**, 246–8.

Candy, J.M., Perry, R.H., Perry, E.K., Irvin, D., Blessed, G., Fairbairn, A.F., and Tomlinson, B.E. (1983). Pathological changes in the nucleus Meynert in Alzheimer's and Parkinson's diseases. *J. Neurol. Sci.*, **59**, 277–89.

Chen, L. (1981). Neurofibrillary change on Guam. *Arch. Neurol.*, **38**, 16–18.

Chui, H.C., Bondareff, W., Zarov, C., and Slager, U. (1984). Stability of neuronal number in the human nucleus basalis of Meynert with age. *Neurobiol. Aging*, **5**, 83–8.

Chui, H.C., Teng, E.L., Henderson, V.W., and Moy, A.C. (1985). Clinical subtypes of dementia of the Alzheimer type. *Neurology*, **35**, 1544–50.

Clark, A.W., Parhad, I.M., Folstein, S.E., Whitehouse, P.J., Hedreen, J.C., Price, D.L., and Chase, T.N. (1983). The nucleus basalis in Huntington's disease. *Neurology*, **33**, 1262–7.

Cohen, G., and Heikkila, R.E. (1974). The generation of hydrogen peroxide, superoxide radical, and hydroxyl radical by 6-hydroxydopamine, dialuric acid, and related cytotoxic agents. *J. Biol. Chem.*, **249**, 2447–52.

Corsellis, J.A.N., Bruton, C.J., and Freeman-Browne, D. (1973). The aftermath of boxing. *Psychol. Med.*, **3**, 270–303.

Cragg, B.G. (1967). The density of synapses and neurones in the motor and visual areas of the cerebral cortex. *J. Anat.*, **101**, 639–45.

Crapper McLachlan, D.R., and Lewis, P.N. (1984). Alzheimer's disease: errors in gene expression. *Can. J. Neurol. Sci.*, **12**, 1–5.

Cummings, J.L., and Benson, D.F. (eds.) (1983). *Dementia: A Clinical Approach*, Butterworth, Sevenoaks.

Cutler, N.R., Haxby, J.V., Duara, R., Grady, C.L., Kay, A.D., Kessler, R.M., Sundaram, M., and Rapoport, S.I. (1985). Clinical history, brain metabolism, and neuropsychological function in Alzheimer's disease. *Ann. Neurol.*, **18**, 298–309.

DeJong, J.D., and Burns, B.D. (1967). Parkinson's disease—a random process. *Can. Med. Assoc. J.*, **97**, 49–56.

DeKosky, S.T., Scheff, S.W., and Markesbery, W.R. (1985). Laminar organization of cholinergic circuits in human frontal cortex in Alzheimer's disease and aging. *Neurology*, **35**, 1425–31.

Diamond, J.M., Matsuyama, S.S., Meier, K., and Jarvik, J.F. (1983). Elevation of erythrocyte countertransport rates in Alzheimer's dementia. *N. Engl. J. Med.*, **309**, 1061–2.

Donaldson, J., LaBella, F.A., and Gesser, D. (1980). Enhanced autoxidation of dopamine as a possible basis of manganese neurotoxicity. *Neurotoxicology*, **2**, 53–64.

Duvoisin, R.C., and Yahr, M.D. (1965). Encephalitis and Parkinsonism. *Arch. Neurol.*, **12**, 227–39.

Elizan, T.S., Madden, D.L., Herrman, K.L., Gardner, J., Schwartz, J., Smith, H., Sever, J.L., and Yahr, M.D. (1979). Viral antibodies in serum and cerebrospinal fluid of parkinsonian patients and controls. *Arch. Neurol.*, **36**, 529–34.

Fahn, S., and Bressman, B. (1984). Should levodopa therapy for parkinsonism be started early or late? Evidence against early treatment. *Can. J. Neurol. Sci.*, **11**, 200–5.

Flood, J.F., Smith, G.E., and Cherkin, A. (1983). Memory retention: potentiation of cholinergic drug combinations in mice. *Neurobiol. Aging*, **4**, 37–43.

Foster, N.L., Chase, T.N., Mansi, L., Broos, R., Fedio, P., Patronas, N.J., and Di Chiro, G. (1984). Cortical abnormalities in Alzheimer's disease. *Ann. Neurol.*, **16**, 649–54.

Francis, P.T., Palmer, A.M., Sims, N.R., Bowen, D.M., Davison, A.N., Esiri, M.M., Neary, D., Snowden, J.S., and Wilcock, G.K. (1985). Neurochemical studies of early onset Alzheimer's disease. *N. Engl. J. Med.*, **313**, 7–11.

Fuld, P.A. (1984). Test profile of cholinergic dysfunction and of Alzheimer-type dementia. *J. Clin. Neuropsychol.*, **6**, 380–92.

Gaitz, C.M., and Samorajski, T. (eds.) (1985). *Aging 2000: Our Health Care Destiny*, Vol. I, Biomedical Issues, Springer, Berlin.

Gajdusek, D.C. (1977). Unconventional viruses and the origin and disappearance of Kuru. *Science*, **197**, 943–60.

Gay, F.P., and Holden, M. (1931). Loss of viricidal property in serums from patients with herpes and encephalitis. *J.A.M.A.*, **96**, 2028–9.

Gottfries, C.G., Adolfsson, R., Aquilonius, S.M., Carlsson, A., Eckernas, S.A., Nordberg, A., Oreland, I., Svennerholm, L., Wiberg, A., and Winblad, B. (1983). Biochemical changes in dementia disorders of Alzheimer type (AD/SDAT). *Neurobiol. Aging*, **4**, 261–71.

Goudsmit, J., Morrow, C.H., Asher, D.M., Yanagihard, R.T., Master, C.L., Gibbs, C.J. Jr, and Gajdusek, D.C.

(1980). Evidence for and against the transmissibility of Alzheimer disease. *Neurology*, **30**, 945–50.

Harbaugh, R.E., Roberts, D.W., Combs, D.W., Saunders, R.L., and Reeder, T.M. (1984). Preliminary report: intracranial cholinergic drug infusion in patients with Alzheimer's disease. *Neurosurgery*, **15**, 514–18.

Heilig, C.W., Knopman, D.S., Mastri, A.R., and Frey, W., II (1985). Dementia without Alzheimer pathology. *Neurology*, **35**, 762–5.

Herzog, A.G., and Kemper, T.L. (1980). Amygdaloid changes in aging and dementia. *Arch. Neurol.*, **37**, 625–9.

Heston, L.L., Mastri, A.R., Anderson, V.E., and White, J. (1981). Dementia of the Alzheimer type: clinical genetics, natural history and associated conditions. *Arch. Gen. Psychiatry*, **38**, 1085–90.

Heyman, A., Wilkinson, W.E., Hurwitz, B.J., Schmechel, D., Sigmon, A.H., Weinberg, T., Helms, M.J., and Swift, M. (1983). Alzheimer's disease: genetic aspects and associated clinical disorders. *Ann. Neurol.*, **14**, 507–15.

Heyman, A., Wilkinson, W.E., Stafford, J.A., Helms, M.J., Sigmon, A.H., and Weinberg, T. (1984). Alzheimer's disease: a study of epidemiological aspects. *Ann. Neurol.*, **15**, 335–41.

Hoehn, M.M. (1971). The epidemiology of parkinsonism. In: de Ajuriahuera, J., and Gauther, G. (eds.) *Monoamines Noyaux Gris Centraux et Syndrome de Parkinson*, Georg et Cie SA, Geneva, pp. 281–300.

Kartzinel, R., Perlow, M.D., Carter, A.C., Chase, T.N., Calne, D.B., and Shoulson, I. (1976). Metabolic studies with bromocriptine in patients with idiopathic Parkinsonism and Huntington's chorea. *Trans. Am. Neurol. Assoc.*, **101**, 53–6.

Kessler, I.I. (1972). Epidemiologic studies of Parkinson's disease II. A hospital based survey. *Am. J. Epidemiol.* **95**, 308–18.

Knoll, J., Vizi, E.S., and Somogyi, G. (1968). Phenylisopropyl-methylpropinylamine (E250), a monoamine oxidase inhibitor antagonizing effects of tyramine. *Arzneim. Forsch.*, **18**, 109–12.

Kokmen, E. (1984). Dementia—Alzheimer type. *Mayo Clin. Proc.*, **59**, 35–42.

Koller, W.C. (1984). Disturbance of recent memory function in Parkinsonian patients on anticholinergic therapy. *Cortex*, **2**, 307–11.

Kondo, K. (1984). Epidemiological clues for the etiology of Parkinson's disease. In: Hassler, R.G., and Christ, J.F. (eds.) *Advances in Neurology*, Vol. 40, Raven Press, New York, pp. 345–51.

Krause, L.J. (1983). Decreased natural killer activity in Alzheimer's disease. *Neurosci. Abstr.*, **9**, 115.

Kurland, L.T., Kurtzke, J.F., Goldberg, I.D., Choi, N.W., and Williams, G. (1973). Parkinsonism. In: Kurland, L.T., Kurtzke, J.F., and Goldberg, I.D. (eds.) *Epidemiology of Neurologic and Sense Organ Disorders*, Harvard University Press, Cambridge, Massachusetts, pp. 41–63.

Lakke, J.P.W.F., Korf, J., Van Praag, H.M., and Schut, T. (1972). Predictive value of the probenecid test for the effect of L-dopa therapy in Parkinson's disease. *Nature*, **236**, 208–9.

Lang, W., and Henke, H. (1983). Cholinergic receptor binding and autoradiography in brains of non-neurological and senile dementia of Alzheimer-type patients. *Brain Res.*, **267**, 271–80.

Langston, J., and Ballard, P.A. (1985). Parkinsonism induced by 1-methyl-4-phenyl-1,2,3,5-tetrahydropyridine: Implications for treatment and the pathophysiology of Parkinson's disease. *Can. J. Neurol. Sci.*, **11**, 160–6.

Larsson, T., Sjogren, T., and Jacobson, G. (1983). Senile dementia: a clinical, sociomedical and genetic study. *Acta Psychiatr. Scand.* **39** (Suppl. 167), 1–25.

Levaditi, C. (1929). Aetiology of epidemic encephalitis, its relation to herpes, epidemic poliomyelitis, and postvaccinal encephalopathy. *Arch. Neurol. Psychiatry*, **22**, 767–803.

Li, S., Schoenberg, B.S., Wong, C., Cheng, X., Rui, D., Bolis, C.L., and Schoenberg, D.G. (1985). A prevalence of Parkinson's disease and other movement disorders in the People's Republic of China. *Arch. Neurol.*, **42**, 655–7.

Lycke, E., Modigh, K., and Roos, B.E. (1970). The monoamine metabolism in viral encephalitides of the mouse. I. Virological and biochemical results. *Brain Res.*, **23**, 235–46.

Lycke, E., and Roos, B.E. (1972). The monoamine metabolism in viral encephalitides of mouse. II. Turnover of monoamines in mice infected with herpes simplex virus. *Brain Res.*, **44**, 603–13.

McGeer, E., and McGeer, P.L. (1976). Neurotransmitter metabolism in the aging brain. In: Terry, R.D., and Gershon, S. (eds.) *Neurobiology of Aging*, Raven Press, New York, pp. 389–403.

McGeer, P.L., McGeer, E.G., and Suzuki, J.S. (1977). Aging and extrapyramidal function. *Arch. Neurol.*, **34**, 33–5.

McGeer, P.L., McGeer, E.G., Suzuki, J., Dolman, C.E., and Nagai, T. (1984). Aging, Alzheimer's disease, and the cholinergic system of the basal forebrain. *Neurology*, **34**, 741–5.

McKhann, G., Drachman, D., Folstein, M., Katzman, R., Price, D., and Stadlan, E.M. (1984). Clinical diagnosis of Alzheimer's disease: Report of the NINCDS-ADRDA Work Group under the auspices of the Department of Health and Human Services Task Force on Alzheimer's disease. *Neurology*, **34**, 939–44.

Mann, D.M., Yates, P.O., and Hawkes, J. (1982). The noradrenergic system in Alzheimer and multi-infarct dementias. *J. Neurol. Neurosurg. Psychiatry*, **45**, 113–19.

Markham, C.H., and Diamond, S.G. (1981). Evidence to support early levodopa therapy in Parkinson's disease. *Neurology*, **31**, 125–31.

Martin, W.R.W., Stoessl, A.J., Adam, M.J., Ammann,

W., Bergstrom, M., Harrop, R., Laihinen, A., Rogers, J.G., Ruth, T.J., Sayre, C.I., Pate, B.D., and Calne, D.B. (1987). Positron emission tomography in Parkinson's disease: Glucose and DOPA metabolism. *Advances in Neurology*, Raven Press, New York, Vol. 45, pp. 95–8.

Marttila, R.J., and Rine, U.K. (1978). Herpes simplex virus antibodies in patients with Parkinson's disease. *J. Neurol. Sci.*, **35**, 375–9.

Marttila, R.J., Arstila, P., Nikoskelainen, J., Halonen, P.E., and Rinne, U.K. (1977). Viral antibodies in the sera from patients with Parkinson's diseases. *Eur. Neurol.*, **15**, 25–33.

Mayeux, R., and Stern, Y. (1983). Intellectual dysfunction and dementia in Parkinson's disease. In: Mayeux, R., and Rosen, W.B. (eds.) *The Dementias*, Raven Press, New York, pp. 211–27.

Mayeux, R., Stern, Y., and Spanton, S. (1985). Heterogeneity in dementia of the Alzheimer type: evidence of subgroups. *Neurology*, **35**, 453–61.

Mehraein, P., Yamada, M., and Tarnowska-Dzidusko, E. (1975). Quantitative study on dendrites and dendritic spines in Alzheimer's disease and senile dementia. In: Kreutzberg, G.W. (ed.) *Physiology and Pathology of Dendrites. Advances in Neurobiology*, Vol. 12, Raven Press, New York, pp. 453–8.

Mena, I., Martin, O., Fuenzalida, S., and Cotzias, G.C. (1967). Chronic manganese poisoning. Clinical picture and manganese turnover. *Neurology*, **17**, 128–36.

Molsa, P.K., Marttila, R.J., and Rinne, U.K. (1984). Extrapyramidal signs in Alzheimer's disease. *Neurology*, **34**, 114–16.

Mountjoy, C.W., Roth, M., Evans, N.J.R., and Evans, H.M. (1983). Cortical neuronal counts in normal elderly controls and demented patients. *Neurobiol. Aging*, **4**, 1–11.

Muramoto, O., Sugishita, M., and Ando, K. (1984). Cholinergic system and constructional praxis: a further study of physostigmine in Alzheimer's disease. *J. Neurol. Neurosurg. Psychiatry*, **47**, 485–91.

Paddison, R.M., and Griffith, R.P. (1974). Occurrence of Parkinson's disease in black patients at Charity Hospital in New Orleans. *Neurology*, **24**, 688–90.

Perry, E., Curtis, M., Dick, D.J., Candy, J.M., Atack, J.R., Bloxham, C.A., Blessed, G., Fairbairn, A., Tomlinson, B.E., and Perry, R.H. (1985). Cholinergic correlates of cognitive impairment in Parkinson's disease: Comparisons with Alzheimer's disease. *J. Neurol. Neurosurg. Psychiatry*, **48**, 413–21.

Peterson, C., Gibson, G.E., and Blass, J.P. (1985). Altered calcium uptake in cultured skin fibroblasts from patients with Alzheimer's disease. *N. Engl. J. Med.*, **312**, 1063–5.

Reef, H.E. (1977). Prevalence of Parkinson's disease in a multiracial community. In: den Hartog Jager, W.A.H., Bruyn, G.W., and Heijstee, A.P.J. (eds.) *11th World Congress of Neurology, International Congress Series*, No. 427, Excerpta Medica, Amsterdam, pp. 125.

Reisberg, B., Ferris, S.H., DeLeon, M.J., and Crook, T. (1982). The global deterioration scale for assessment of primary degenerative dementia. *Am. J. Psychiatry*, **39**, 1136–9.

Ringel, S.P., and Klawans, H.L. Jr (1972). Carbon monoxide-induced parkinsonism. *J. Neurol. Sci.*, **16**, 245–51.

Rogers, J.D., Brogan, D., and Mirra, S.S. (1985). The nucleus basalis of Meynert in neurological disease: A quantitative morphological study. *Ann. Neurol.*, **17**, 163–70.

Rossor, M.N., Iversen, L.L., Reynolds, G.P., Mountjoy, C.Q., and Roth, M. (1984). Neurochemical characteristics of early and late onset types of Alzheimer's disease. *Br. Med. J.*, **288**, 961–4.

Roth, M. (1978). Epidemiological studies. In: Katzman, R., Terry, R.D., and Bick, K.L. (eds.) *Alzheimer's Disease, Senile Dementia and Related Disorders*, Raven Press, New York, pp. 337–9.

Sadeh, M., Braham, J., and Modam, M. (1982). Effects of anticholinergic drugs on memory in Parkinson's disease. *Arch. Neurol.*, **39**, 666–7.

Saper, C.B., German, D.C., and White, III C.L. (1985). Neuronal pathology in the nucleus basalis and associated cell groups in senile dementia of the Alzheimer's type. Possible role in memory loss. *Neurology*, **35**, 1089–95.

Scheibel, M.E., and Scheibel, A.B. (1975). Structural changes in the aging brain. In: Broody, H., Harman, D., and Ordy, J.M. (eds.) *Clinical, Morphological, and Neurochemical Aspects in the Aging Central Nervous System*, Aging Series, Vol. 1, Raven Press, New York, pp. 11–37.

Schoenberg, B.S., Anderson, D.W., and Haerer, A.F. (1985). Prevalence of Parkinson's disease in the biracial population of Copiah County, Mississippi. *Neurology*, **35**, 841–5.

Sholl, D.A. (ed.) (1956). *The Organization of the Cerebral Cortex*, Wiley, New York.

Siegfried, J. (1979). Neurosurgical treatment of Parkinson's disease. Present indications and value. In: Rinne, U.K., Klinger, M., and Stamm, G. (eds.) *Parkinson's Disease: Current Progress, Problems and Management*, Elsevier, North-Holland, pp. 369–76.

Skias, D., Bania, M., Reder, A.T., Luchins, D., and Antel, J.P. (1985). Senile dementia of Alzheimer's type (SDAT): Reduced T8 + -cell-mediated suppressor activity. *Neurology*, **35**, 1635–8.

Steele, J.C., Richardson, J.C., and Olszewski, J. (1964). Progressive supranuclear palsy. *Arch. Neurol.*, **1**, 333–59.

Sulkava, R., Wikstrom, J., Aromaa, A., Raitasalo, R., Lehtinen, V., Lahtela, K., and Palo, J. (1985). Prevalence of severe dementia in Finland. *Neurology*, **35**, 1025–9.

Syndulko, K., Gilden, E.R., Hansch, E.C., Potvin, A.R., Tourtelotte, W.W., and Potvin, J.H. (1981). Decreased verbal memory associated with anticholinergic treatment in Parkinson's disease patients. *Int. J. Neurosci.*, **14**, 61–6.

Tagliavini, F., and Pilleri, G. (1983). Neuronal counts in the basal nucleus of Meynert in Alzheimer disease and simple senile dementia. *Lancet*, **i**, 469–70.

Tagliavini, F., Pilleri, G., Bouras, C., and Constantinidis, J. (1984). The basal nucleus of Meynert in idiopathic Parkinson's disease. *Acta Neurol. Scand.*, **69**, 20–8.

Teravainen, H., and Calne, D.B. (1979). Quantitative assessment of parkinsonian deficits. In: Rinne, U.K., Klinger, M., and Stamm, G. (eds.) *Parkinson's Disease: Current Progress, Problems and Management*, Elsevier, North-Holland, pp. 145–64.

Terry, R.D., and Katzman, R. (1983). Senile dementia of the Alzheimer type. *Ann. Neurol.*, **14**, 497–506.

Uhl, G.R., McKinney, M., Hedreen, J.C., White, III C.L., Coyle, J.T., Whitehouse, P.J., and Price, D.L. (1982). Dementia pugilistica: loss of basal forebrain cholinergic neurons and cortical cholinergic markers. *Ann. Neurol.*, **12**, 99.

Ulrich, J. (1985). Alzheimer changes in nondemented patients younger than sixty-five: possible early stages of Alzheimer's disease and senile dementia of Alzheimer type. *Ann. Neurol.*, **17**, 273–7.

Ward, C.D., Duvoisin, R.C., Ince, S.E., Nutt, J.D., Eldridge, R., and Calne, D.B. (1983). Parkinson's disease in 65 pairs of twins and in a set of quadruplets. *Neurology*, **33**, 815–24.

Weitkamp, L.R., Nee, L., and Keats, B. (1983). Alzheimer disease: evidence for susceptibility ioci on chromosomes 6 and 14. *Am. J. Hum. Genet.*, **35**, 443–53.

Wetmur, J.G., Schwartz, J., and Elizan, T.S. (1979). Nucleic acid homology studies of viral nucleic acid in idiopathic Parkinson's disease. *Arch. Neurol.*, **36**, 529–34.

Whitehouse, P.J., Price, D.L., Strutle, R.G., Clark, A.W., Coyle, J.T., and Delong, M.R. (1982). Alzheimer's disease and senile dementia: loss of neurons in the basal forebrain. *Science*, **215**, 1237–9.

Wilson, R.S., Fox, J.H., Huckman, M.S., Bacon, L.D., and Lobick, J.J. (1982). Computed tomography in dementia. *Neurology*, **32**, 1054–7.

Wisniewski, K.E., Wisniewski, M.H., and Wen, G.Y. (1985). Occurrence of neuropathological changes and dementia of Alzheimer's disease in Down's syndrome. *Ann. Neurol.*, **17**, 278–82.

Yerby, M.S., Sundsten, J.W., Larson, E.B., Wu, S.A., and Sumi, S.M. (1985). A new method for measuring brain atrophy: The effect of aging in its application for diagnosing dementia. *Neurology*, **35**, 1316–20.

Zubenko, G.S., Cohen, B.M., Crowdon, J., and Corkin, S. (1984). Cell membrane abnormality in Alzheimer's disease. *Age*, **2**, 235.

Subject Index

Note: 'vs' denotes differential diagnosis
Abbreviations:

EEG	Electroencephalogram
EMG	Electromyography
GABA	Gamma aminobutyric acid
SDAT	Senile dementia of the Alzheimer type
TIA	Transient ischaemic attack